The Knee

AANA Advanced Arthroscopic Surgical Techniques

AANA Advanced Arthroscopic Surgical Techniques
Series

Series Editors, Richard K. N. Ryu, MD and Jeffrey S. Abrams, MD

The Knee

AANA Advanced Arthroscopic Surgical Techniques

EDITED BY

NICHOLAS A. SGAGLIONE, MD

Professor and Chair, Department of Orthopaedic Surgery
North Shore–Long Island Jewish Health System
Hofstra North Shore–Long Island Jewish School of Medicine
Great Neck, New York

JAMES H. LUBOWITZ, MD

Director, Taos Orthopaedic Institute, Research Foundation, and
Orthopaedic Sportsmedicine Fellowship
Taos, New Mexico

MATTHEW T. PROVENCHER, MD, CDR MC USNR

Chief, Sports Medicine Service, Massachusetts General Hospital
Head Team Physician and Medical Director, New England Patriots
Visiting Professor, Harvard Medical School
Boston, Massachusetts
Professor of Surgery and Orthopaedics
Uniformed Services University of Health Services
Bethesda, Maryland

CRC Press
Taylor & Francis Group
Boca Raton London New York

CRC Press is an imprint of the
Taylor & Francis Group, an **informa** business

First published 2016 by SLACK Incorporated

Published 2024 by CRC Press
2385 NW Executive Center Drive, Suite 320, Boca Raton FL 33431

and by CRC Press
4 Park Square, Milton Park, Abingdon, Oxon, OX14 4RN

CRC Press is an imprint of Taylor & Francis Group, LLC

Library of Congress Cataloging-in-Publication Data
AANA advanced arthroscopic surgical techniques. The Knee / edited by Nicholas A. Sgaglione, James H. Lubowitz, Matthew T. Provencher.
p. ; cm.
Advanced arthroscopic surgical techniques
Knee
Preceded by: AANA advanced arthroscopy. The knee / [edited by] Robert E. Hunter, Nicholas A. Sgaglione. Philadelphia, PA : Saunders/Elsevier, c2010.
Includes bibliographical references and index.
ISBN 9781617119996 (alk. paper)
I. Sgaglione, Nicholas A, editor. II. Lubowitz, James H., editor. III. Provencher, Matthew T., editor. IV. Arthroscopy Association of North America, issuing body. V. AANA advanced arthroscopy. The knee. Preceded by (work): VI. Title: Advanced arthroscopic surgical techniques. VII. Title: Knee.
[DNLM: 1. Arthroscopy--methods. 2. Knee Joint--surgery. WE 870]
RD561
617.5'820597--dc23
2015030718

ISBN: 9781617119996 (hbk)
ISBN: 9781003524755 (ebk)

DOI: 10.1201/9781003524755

Dedication

To my loving and wonderful family, for all your patience and support.

I dedicate this work to my beautiful children, Nicholas, Caroline, Jonathan, and Matthew.

And to Ela, for making me smile again.

I honor the life and celebrate the achievements and rich memory of Dr. Leslie Sgaglione; your balance, unconditional love, and extraordinary existence continue to inspire me every day.

In memory of my close friend and colleague, Benjamin Shaffer, MD; your light shines bright.

Nicholas A. Sgaglione, MD

Thank you to Gina for her inspiration, dedication, patience, and tolerance, and to the Editors, as well as the AANA Past Presidents, for their mentorship.

James H. Lubowitz, MD

To my incredible family for all of your dedication and steadfast support, and my wonderful wife, Melissa, and children, Connor, Brody, Caroline, and Catherine. You inspire me every day. To my dear friend Colonel Warren Kadrmas, whose legacy in the military sports community lives today.

Matthew T. Provencher, MD, CDR MC USNR

CONTENTS

Acknowledgments

We wish to thank all the contributing authors who are responsible for *The Knee: AANA Advanced Arthroscopic Surgical Techniques*. This work is a timely, comprehensive, state-of-the-art publication that progressed from inception to publication in just over 12 months. The topics, practical tabulated pearls, images, and technique videos represent the very best contributions of current expert thought leaders. Many thanks to all of our colleagues for your expertise and efforts in synthesizing and delivering a landmark compilation. Your enduring work and effective collaboration are a testimony to teamwork, timeliness, and excellence.

Nicholas A. Sgaglione, MD
James H. Lubowitz, MD
Matthew T. Provencher, MD, CDR MC USNR

About the Editors

Nicholas A. Sgaglione, MD is Professor and Chairman of the North Shore–Long Island Jewish Medical Center Department of Orthopedic Surgery and at the Hofstra North Shore–Long Island Jewish School of Medicine. He also serves as the Senior Vice President for Orthopaedics for the North Shore–Long Island Jewish Health System and Executive Director of the Orthopaedic Institute. Dr. Sgaglione graduated from the Mount Sinai School of Medicine and completed his residency in orthopaedic surgery at the Hospital for Special Surgery in New York, followed by a fellowship in sports medicine at the Southern California Orthopaedic Institute in Los Angeles, California.

Dr. Sgaglione served as President of the Arthroscopy Association of North America for 2012 to 2013 and also served on its Board of Directors beginning in 2008. He was elected to the American Orthopaedic Association in 2006 and is a trustee of the AANA Education Foundation and Association Member Representative for the Orthopaedic Learning Center in Rosemont, Illinois. He is currently serving on the *Arthroscopy: The Journal of Arthroscopic and Related Surgery* Board of Trustees.

Dr. Sgaglione specializes in sports medicine and has served as the Team Orthopaedist for numerous Long Island High Schools and the US Merchant Marine Academy for the past 24 years and more recently New York's professional Major League Lacrosse team, the New York Lizards. He has also served as an orthopaedic consultant to the US Ski Team and US Professional Golf Association. Dr. Sgaglione has authored more than 75 peer-reviewed published scientific articles. He was a co-editor of *AANA Advanced Arthroscopy: The Knee* and has recently co-edited the Fourth Edition of the textbook *Operative Arthroscopy*.

James H. Lubowitz, MD is founding Director of Taos Orthopaedic Institute and Taos Orthopaedic Institute Orthopaedic Sportsmedicine Fellowship. He is Editor-in-Chief of *Arthroscopy: The Journal of Arthroscopic and Related Surgery* and *Arthroscopy Techniques*. Dr. Lubowitz is founding Director, emeritus, of Taos Orthopaedic Institute Research Foundation and Editor-in-Chief, emeritus, of the *ISAKOS Newsletter*. Dr. Lubowitz is Clinical Associate Professor, University of New Mexico, Department of Orthopaedics and Rehabilitation. Dr. Lubowitz attended the University of Pennsylvania School of Medicine, and served as intern, resident, and Chief Resident at the University of California, Los Angeles, and as Orthopaedic Sportsmedicine Fellow at Thomas Jefferson University.

Dr. Lubowitz has served on committees of the Arthroscopy Association of North America, ISAKOS, American Orthopaedic Society for Sports Medicine, and the ACL Study Group, including both the AANA and AOSSM Education Committees, and is Chairman, emeritus, of the AANA Research Committee. He is designated by AANA as a Master Knee Surgeon at the Orthopaedic Learning Center in Chicago, Illinois. Dr. Lubowitz is a member of the Medical Staff of the US Ski and Snowboard Team.

CDR Matthew T. Provencher, MD, MC USN, a native of Barrington, New Hampshire, attended the US Naval Academy, where he was appointed the Deputy Brigade Commander (Second in Command), graduated with Distinction with a Major in Electrical Engineering, and was designated Secretary of the Navy Distinguished Graduate. He was also a 4-year varsity oarsman and First-Team All-American at Navy, and named Most Valuable Oarsman. He completed his medical education at Dartmouth Medical School where he graduated with honors and was elected to the Alpha Omega Alpha Honor Society.

Dr. Provencher completed his orthopaedic residency at the Naval Medical Center San Diego and his orthopaedic shoulder, knee, and sports surgery fellowship at Rush University. He also served as an Orthopaedic Surgeon at the Naval Medical Center San Diego from 2004 to 2013, and was Director of the Sports Division from 2007 to 2013. In addition to his orthopaedic duties, CDR Provencher performed extensive Humanitarian and Disaster Relief training as the Director for Surgical Services on the USNS Mercy (TAH-19) during Pacific Partnership 2012.

Currently, Dr. Provencher is the Chief of Sports Medicine and Surgery at Massachusetts General Hospital, is Visiting Professor of Surgery and Orthopaedics at Harvard Medical School, and Professor of Surgery and Orthopaedics at the Uniformed Services University of the Health Sciences. As Chief of Sports Surgery at Massachusetts General Hospital, he is the Head Team Physician and Medical Director for the New England Patriots, and is a Past-President of the Society of Military Orthopaedic Surgeons. He was elected into the Herodicus Society, which identifies excellence in Orthopaedic Sports Surgery as well as was nominated to the Board of Directors of the American Orthopaedic Society for Sports Medicine. He serves on numerous national committees and was the Arthroscopy Association of North America 2014 Program Director and is the Assistant Editor-in-Chief of *Arthroscopy: The Journal of Arthroscopic and Related Surgery*. He was recently named one of the Top 20 Shoulder Surgeons in the United States and Top 28 Knee Surgeons in the United States by *Orthopaedics Today*. His research includes more than 150 peer-reviewed publications and 150 chapters, and he has written 5 textbooks. Dr. Provencher resides in Massachusetts with his wife and 4 children.

Contributing Authors

David A. Abrutyn, MD (Chapter 24)
Sports Medicine, Shoulder and Knee Surgery
Summit Medical Group
Bridgewater, New Jersey

Annunziato Amendola, MD (Chapter 22)
Professor
Department of Orthopedic Surgery
Chief
Division of Sports Medicine
Duke University
Durham, North Carolina

Jack Anavian, MD (Chapter 2)
Trauma Fellow
Department of Orthopedic Surgery
Warren Alpert Medical School of
Brown University
Providence, Rhode Island

Jack M. Bert, MD (Chapter 14)
Adjunct Clinical Professor
University of Minnesota School of Medicine
Cartilage Restoration Center of Minnesota
Minnesota Bone & Joint Specialists, Ltd
St. Paul, Minnesota

Timothy M. Bert, MD (Chapter 14)
Hedley Orthopedic Institute
Phoenix, Arizona

Andrew J. Blackman, MD (Chapter 33)
Sports Medicine Fellow
Department of Orthopedic Surgery
Mayo Clinic Sports Medicine Center
Rochester, Minnesota

Trevor Born, MD (Chapter 2)
Sports Medicine Fellow
Department of Orthopedic Surgery
Warren Alpert Medical School of
Brown University
Providence, Rhode Island

Joel Boyd, MD (Chapter 30)
TRIA Orthopaedic Center
Bloomington, Minnesota
University of Minnesota
Minneapolis, Minnesota

Joseph Brunkhorst, DO (Chapter 28)
Department of Orthopaedic Surgery
University of Kentucky School of Medicine
Lexington, Kentucky

William Bugbee, MD (Chapter 18)
Attending Physician
Director
Cartilage Transplantation Program
Division of Orthopaedic Surgery
Scripps Clinic
La Jolla, California

James M. Bullock, MD (Chapter 26)
Department of Orthopaedic Surgery
University of Pittsburgh
Pittsburgh, Pennsylvania

Joseph Carney, MD (Chapter 12)
Department of Orthopaedic Surgery
Naval Medical Center San Diego
San Diego, California

Thomas Carter, MD (Chapter 9)
Emeritus Head of Orthopedic Surgery
Arizona State University
Tempe, Arizona

Brian J. Cole, MD, MBA (Chapters 18, 21)
Professor and Vice-Chairman
Department of Orthopedics
Section Head
Rush Cartilage Restoration Center
Midwest Orthopedics at Rush
Chicago, Illinois

Austin Crow, MD (Chapter 31)
Department of Orthopaedic Surgery
University of Virginia
Charlottesville, Virginia

Umer R. Dasti, MD (Chapter 25)
Instructor of Orthopaedic Surgery
Tufts University School of Medicine
Sports Medicine Fellow
New England Baptist Hospital
Boston, Massachusetts

Julie A. Dodds, MD (Chapter 3)
Associate Clinical Professor
Division of Sports Medicine
Michigan State University
East Lansing, Michigan

Ryan Dunlay, MD (Chapter 30)
TRIA Orthopaedic Center
Bloomington, Minnesota

Neil C. Dunleavy, MD (Chapter 10)
Orthopaedic Sports Medicine and Arthroscopic Surgery
KSF Orthopaedic Center
Houston, Texas

Paul Fadale, MD (Chapter 2)
Professor and Chief of Sports Medicine
Sports Medicine Fellowship Director
Department of Orthopedic Surgery
Warren Alpert Medical School of Brown University
Head Team Physician
Brown University Athletics and Providence Bruins Professional Hockey Team (AHL Affiliate of the Boston Bruins)
Providence, Rhode Island

Gregory C. Fanelli, MD (Chapter 29)
GHS Orthopaedics
Danville, Pennsylvania

Jack Farr, MD (Chapter 19)
Cartilage Restoration Center of Indiana
OrthoIndy Hospital
Greenwood, Indiana
Voluntary Professor of Orthopedic Surgery
Department of Orthopedic Surgery
Indiana University Medical Center
Indianapolis, Indiana

Donald C. Fithian, MD (Chapter 12)
Department of Orthopedics
Southern California Kaiser Permanente
San Diego, California

Freddie H. Fu, MD, DSc (Hon), DPs (Hon) (Chapter 26)
Chairman
Department of Orthopaedic Surgery
University of Pittsburgh School of Medicine
University of Pittsburgh Medical Center
Pittsburgh, Pennsylvania

John P. Fulkerson, MD (Chapter 13)
Orthopedic Associates of Hartford, PC
Clinical Professor of Orthopedic Surgery
University of Connecticut School of Medicine
Farmington, Connecticut

Theodore J. Ganley, MD (Chapter 15)
Director of Sports Medicine
The Children's Hospital of Philadelphia
Associate Professor of Orthopaedic Surgery
The University of Pennsylvania School of Medicine
Philadelphia, Pennsylvania

Brian B. Gilmer, MD (Chapter 4)
Mammoth Orthopedic Institute
Mammoth Lakes, California

Andrew D. Goodwillie, MD (Chapter 7)
North Shore–Long Island Jewish
Department of Orthopaedic Surgery
North Shore–Long Island Jewish
Hofstra School of Medicine
Great Neck, New York

Vipool K. Goradia, MD (Chapter 1)
G2 Orthopedics and Sports Medicine
Richmond, Virginia

Nathan L. Grimm, MD (Chapter 15)
Department of Orthopaedic Surgery
Duke University Hospital
Durham, North Carolina

Jeffrey Halbrecht, MD (Chapter 11)
Private Practice
San Francisco, California

Christopher D. Harner, MD (Chapter 8)
Blue Cross of Western Pennsylvania
Endowed Professor
UPMC Center for Sports Medicine
Department of Orthopaedic Surgery
University of Pittsburgh
Pittsburgh, Pennsylvania

Nathan Jacobson, MD (Chapter 30)
TRIA Orthopaedic Center
Bloomington, Minnesota
Great Plains Orthopaedics
North Platte, Nebraska

Evan W. James, BS (Chapter 32)
Department of BioMedical Engineering
Steadman Philippon Research Institute
Vail, Colorado

Adam M. Johannsen, MD (Chapter 32)
Department of BioMedical Engineering
Steadman Philippon Research Institute
Vail, Colorado

Darren L. Johnson, MD (Chapter 28)
Department of Orthopaedic Surgery
University of Kentucky School of Medicine
Lexington, Kentucky

Ethan Kellum, MD, MS (Chapter 16)
Department of Orthopedic Surgery
New England Baptist Hospital
Boston, Massachusetts

Jason L. Koh, MD (Chapter 10)
NorthShore University HealthSystem
Evanston, Illinois

Peter R. Kurzweil, MD (Chapter 24)
Memorial Orthopaedic Surgical Group
Long Beach, California

Robert F. LaPrade, MD, PhD (Chapter 32)
Complex Knee Surgeon, The Steadman Clinic
Chief Medical Officer, Steadman Philippon Research Institute
Co-Director, Sports Medicine Fellowship Program
Director, International Scholar Program
Adjunct Professor, Orthopaedic Surgery
University of Minnesota
Minneapolis, Minnesota
Affiliate Faculty, College of Veterinary Medicine and Biomedical Sciences
Colorado State University
Vail, Colorado

Bruce A. Levy, MD (Chapter 33)
Professor of Orthopedic Surgery
Department of Orthopedic Surgery
Mayo Clinic Sports Medicine Center
Rochester, Minnesota

Darius Lin, MD (Chapter 16)
Department of Orthopedic Surgery
New England Baptist Hospital
Boston, Massachusetts

Robert Litchfield, MD, FRCSC (Chapter 22)
Associate Professor of Surgery
Western University
London, Ontario, Canada

Jonathan R. Maher, MD (Chapter 25)
Instructor of Orthopaedic Surgery
Tufts University School of Medicine
Sports Medicine Fellow
New England Baptist Hospital
Boston, Massachusetts

Randy Mascarenhas, MD, FRCSC (Chapter 19)
Assistant Professor of Orthopaedic Surgery and Sports Medicine
University of Texas—Houston
Houston, Texas

Taylor Mathis, MD (Chapter 23)
University of Mississippi Medical Center
Jackson, Mississippi

Owen P. McGonigle, MD (Chapter 6)
Instructor of Orthopaedic Surgery
Tufts University School of Medicine
Tufts University Combined Orthopaedic Program
Boston, Massachusetts

Sanjay Menon, MD (Chapter 5)
Suncoast Medical Clinic
Saint Petersburg, Florida

David B. Merkow, BA (Chapters 18, 21)
Sidney Kimmel Medical College
Thomas Jefferson University
Philadelphia, Pennsylvania

Adam V. Metzler, MD (Chapter 28)
Commonwealth Orthopaedic Centers
Edgewood, Kentucky

Ryan Michels, MD (Chapter 17)
Orthopaedic Surgery Resident
Department of Orthopaedic Surgery
North Shore–Long Island Jewish Health System
New Hyde Park, New York

Mark Miller, MD (Chapter 31)
Department of Orthopaedic Surgery
University of Virginia
Charlottesville, Virginia

Kai Mithoefer, MD (Chapter 16)
Department of Orthopedics and Sports Medicine
Harvard Vanguard Medical Associates
Harvard Medical School
Boston, Massachusetts

Kevin R. Myers, MD (Chapter 7)
Orthopaedic Surgery Resident
Department of Orthopaedic Surgery
North Shore–Long Island Jewish Health System
New Hyde Park, New York

Shane J. Nho, MD, MS (Chapter 19)
Assistant Professor
Department of Orthopedic Surgery
Division of Sports Medicine
Rush Medical College of Rush University
Chicago, Illinois

Clayton W. Nuelle, MD (Chapter 34)
Department of Orthopaedic Surgery
University of Missouri
Columbia, Missouri

Benjamin R. Parker, MD (Chapter 13)
University of North Carolina Orthopaedics
Durham, North Carolina

Leon (Lonnie) Paulos, MD (Chapter 5)
Paulos-Toronto Sports Medicine and Orthopedics Clinic
Salt Lake City, Utah

Matthew A. Pifer, MD (Chapter 12)
Orthopaedic Specialists of Wilkes
North Wilkesboro, North Carolina

John D. Polousky, MD (Chapter 15)
Surgical Director of Sports Medicine
The Rocky Mountain Youth Sports Medicine Institute
Centennial, Colorado

John C. Richmond, MD (Chapters 6, 25)
Professor of Orthopaedic Surgery
Tufts University School of Medicine
New England Baptist Hospital
Boston, Massachusetts

V. Franklin Sechriest II, MD (Chapter 18)
Commander
Medical Corps
United States Naval Reserve
Chief of Orthopaedic Surgery
Minneapolis Veteran Affairs
Health Care System
Adjunct Associate Professor
Department of Orthopaedic Surgery
University of Minnesota
Minneapolis, Minnesota

Kevin G. Shea, MD (Chapter 15)
St. Luke's Health System
Boise, Idaho
Department of Orthopedics
University of Utah
Salt Lake City, Utah

Walter Shelton, MD (Chapter 23)
Mississippi Sports Medicine and
Orthopaedic Center
Jackson, Mississippi

Robby Sikka, MD (Chapter 30)
TRIA Orthopaedic Center
Bloomington, Minnesota

Patrick A. Smith, MD (Chapter 27)
Columbia Orthopaedic Group
Head Team Physician
Division Director of Sports Medicine
University of Missouri
Columbia, Missouri

Paul L. Sousa, MD, MBA (Chapter 33)
Orthopedic Resident
Department of Orthopedic Surgery
Mayo Clinic Sports Medicine Center
Rochester, Minnesota

Jeffrey T. Spang, MD (Chapter 13)
Assistant Professor
Department of Orthopaedics
University of North Carolina
Chapel Hill, North Carolina

James P. Stannard, MD (Chapter 34)
Department of Orthopaedic Surgery
University of Missouri
Columbia, Missouri

James Starman, MD (Chapter 31)
Department of Orthopaedic Surgery
University of Virginia
Charlottesville, Virginia

Alexandra Styhl, BA (Chapter 15)
University of Washington School of Medicine
Seattle, Washington

Kentaro P. Suzuki, MD (Chapter 12)
Ventura Orthopedics
Ventura, California

Annemarie K. Tilton, BS (Chapter 21)
Department of Orthopedic Surgery
Rush University Medical Center
Chicago, Illinois

Garth N. Walker, MD (Chapter 26)
Department of Orthopaedic Surgery
University of Pittsburgh
Pittsburgh, Pennsylvania

Amanda L. Weller, MD (Chapter 8)
Orthopaedic Surgeon
Wardell Orthopaedics/
Harbour View Sports Medicine
Suffolk, Virginia

Adam Wilson, MD (Chapter 31)
Department of Orthopaedic Surgery
University of Virginia
Charlottesville, Virginia

Adam B. Yanke, MD (Chapter 21)
Assistant Professor
Department of Orthopedics
Assistant Director
Cartilage Restoration Center
Sports Medicine Division
Rush University Medical Center
Chicago, Illinois

Kenneth R. Zaslav, MD (Chapter 20)
Director of Cartilage Repair Center
Advanced Orthopedic Centers
Clinical Professor of Orthopedic Surgery
Virginia Commonwealth University
Company Physician
Richmond Ballet
Richmond, Virginia

Foreword

In 1918, a Japanese surgeon named Kenji Takagi used a cystoscope to view the inside of a knee, but it was not until 1955 that "true surgery under arthroscopic control" was performed. In the 1950s, Takagi, Watanabe, Takeda, and Ikeuchi were the first "to develop single and multipuncture techniques for performing arthroscopic surgery of the knee."[1]

It was not until the 1970s, however, that arthroscopy of the knee became more widely available in the United Sates, although we were still removing meniscus through an open procedure using Smillie knives when I was a junior orthopedic surgery resident in 1975. By the time I was a chief resident we were struggling to see meniscus in the knee using the arthroscope alone, without the aid of a camera. Shahriaree's textbook, published in 1984, had black and white pictures demonstrating arthroscopy of the knee looking directly through the scope. This was state of the art then and once when watching the head of our department attempting to do a knee arthroscopy, he pulled the scope out of the knee of his patient and said "this is going nowhere!"

I had already spent time with some of the great arthroscopic surgeons of that time: Jack McGinty, Jan Gillquist, Russ Warren, Lars Peterson, Ejnar Erickson, and Per Renstrom. I had watched Lanny Johnson and Bob Jackson move the scope gracefully around the knee and demonstrate what was possible. I knew that arthroscopic surgery was here to stay. That was about 30 years ago, and few orthopedic surgeons had developed the skills necessary to do arthroscopic procedures. The first arthroscopic cameras were becoming more widely available. Arthroscopic anterior cruciate ligament reconstruction and rotator cuff repair were dreams at best.

Fast forward to 2015 and *The Knee: AANA Advanced Arthroscopic Surgical Techniques* by Drs. Sgaglione, Lubowitz, and Provencher, 3 of the most influential and skilled arthroscopic surgeons of the new millennium. This comprehensive textbook brings together experts in the field to produce a definitive update for those wishing to study the cutting edge of arthroscopic surgery in 2015.

The new approaches and level of sophistication presented in this volume far exceed what I learned in the early 1980s, which doesn't seem so long ago… The editors of this current concepts compendium cover some topics not imaginable in 1985—arthroscopic treatment of tibial plateau and eminence fractures, arthroscopic treatment of arthrofibrosis, arthroscopic meniscal repair, and autogenous osteochondral transplantation.

This book is an important resource for those who wish to understand the depths and breadth of arthroscopic knee surgery and related procedures in 2015. We have come a very long way in relatively few years. Thank you, Drs. Sgaglione, Lubowitz, and Provencher, for leading the way in the 21st century and new millennium.

John P. Fulkerson, MD
Orthopedic Associates of Hartford, PC
Clinical Professor of Orthopedic Surgery
University of Connecticut School of Medicine
Farmington, Connecticut

Reference

1. Shahriaree H, ed. *O'Connor's Textbook of Arthroscopic Surgery.* Philadelphia, PA: Lippincott; 1984.

Foreword

Why buy *The Knee: AANA Advanced Arthroscopic Surgical Techniques*? This Foreword is written from the perspective of a fictitious potential purchaser.

Like most orthopedic surgeons, I like to do knee surgery, especially by arthroscopy. So I looked beyond the title.

I looked at the list of authors. It was long and has many recognizable names. The latter is known as the main motivator for a potential purchaser. I should get it for this reason alone. I then looked at the list of topics. The list includes topics of my interest, but more than that the list includes topics I rarely see or do. For that reason alone it gives me a ready reference on synovial chondromatosis or osteotomy, which I have little experience in my residency. I like the list of authors in the patella section that will serve as a ready referral reference for problem patellar cases I do not like to get involved with.

The text has really good illustrations of arthroscopy and radiology. I really liked the summation box of pearls. I will always open the book and read these from time to time. The numerous up-to-date journal reference citations are important to me, especially in the unfolding area of articular cartilage treatment methods. The editors sure got it right by making the contributors conform to the "pertinent" sections.

Will I buy it and not use it? I am pretty experienced in arthroscopy of the knee. I have heard the many authors' presentations at AANA, but I would like to see in more depth what Chris Harner says about meniscus root tears and what Bert and Cole have written about cartilage and arthritis. This is an area of increasing patient requests.

The bonus is the video where the devil is in the details. Probably a must have. I may not read it all, but will use it, even right now on those topics of particular interest to my practice.

Lanny L. Johnson, MD
Clinical Professor
Department of Radiology
College of Human Medicine
Michigan State University
East Lansing, Michigan

Introduction

The *AANA Advanced Arthroscopic Surgical Techniques Series* represents the very best that AANA has to offer the practicing orthopedic surgeon. With premier arthroscopic surgeons taking the lead, each book in the series presents the latest diagnostic, therapeutic, and reconstructive techniques available in arthroscopic surgery today.

Each technique-based chapter is consistently organized with a user-friendly interface allowing for a quick reference or for prolonged study. Bulleted lists of easily accessed, high-yield information, including preoperative planning, patient selection, equipment checklists, step-by-step descriptions of procedures, and essential technical pearls, in addition to indications, contraindications, postoperative protocols, and potential complications, make this an invaluable resource for surgeons who want to improve not only their skill level, but also their mastery of the fundamentals that define arthroscopic surgery. Well-edited videos, accompanied by narration, further serve to support the materials systematically outlined in each chapter for each volume.

Education and innovation continue to be the top priority for AANA and its leadership. As such, all proceeds from this Series will be donated to the AANA Education Foundation, which, among other endeavors, helps support resident education at the Orthopedic Learning Center, The Traveling Fellowship, the Society of Military Orthopedic Surgeons (SOMOS)–AANA collaboration, resident scholarships to the Annual Meeting, as well as numerous research grants and awards. With the purchase of this book, AANA will also provide free electronic access to the text and videos from the same book in their initial series, *AANA Advanced Arthroscopy* (2010).

We believe that this 5-volume series is a "must have" resource for those who rely on their arthroscopic skills and knowledge to improve patient outcomes. Concise, current, and cogent help describe the impact that these textbooks will have on your practice and in your clinical successes. AANA is delighted to have again taken on this critical leadership position in surgeon education, and is proud of the quality and immediacy of these 5 outstanding volumes.

Richard K. N. Ryu, MD
Jeffrey S. Abrams, MD
Series Co-Editors

Section I

General

1

Knee Arthroscopy
Setup, Diagnosis, Portals, and Approaches

Vipool K. Goradia, MD

Anatomy

The knee joint, as other joints, is composed of a synovial lining within the capsule. Superior to the patella, the synovium extends to form the suprapatellar pouch (Figure 1-1).[1] Superior medial and superior lateral portals are sometimes placed within this pouch. A layer of fat separates the pouch from the distal anterior femoral shaft. The pouch extends medially and laterally along the femoral condyles into the medial and lateral gutters. The suprapatellar pouch and gutters are frequent locations for loose bodies.

Articular cartilage covers the tibial plateau as well as anterior, distal, and posterior condyles of the femur, along with the patella. Iatrogenic injury to articular cartilage should be avoided at all times. Forceful insertion and movement of the arthroscopic camera and/or instruments cause most iatrogenic injuries during arthroscopy. Knowledge of anatomy, portal placement, and constant visualization of instruments are also required to avoid iatrogenic injury to articular cartilage and other structures.

The bony anatomy of the knee relevant to arthroscopic knee surgery includes the distal femur, the proximal tibia, and the patella. With the knee at 60 degrees of flexion, the inferior pole of the patella is located above the lateral joint line and is an important guide for anterolateral portal placement (Figure 1-2). Exceptions to using this landmark, however, occur in cases of patellar alta, baja, dysplasia, or congenital absence. These conditions should be identified preoperatively with physical examination and standard radiography.

The femoral trochlea consists of medial and lateral trochlear ridges that arise from the corresponding femoral condyle.[1] The medial femoral condyle is larger than the lateral from proximal to distal and anterior to posterior. The lateral femoral condyle, however, is wider at the level of the femoral notch. Distally, the femur opens into a notch that contains the femoral origins of the anterior cruciate ligament (ACL) and posterior cruciate ligament (PCL). The notch serves as a target for careful, controlled introduction of cannulas and instruments from anterior portals to avoid injury to articular cartilage (Figure 1-3). When using the scalpel for anterior portal placement, the

Sgaglione NA, Lubowitz JH, Provencher MT, eds. *The Knee: AANA Advanced Arthroscopic Surgical Techniques* (pp 3-22).

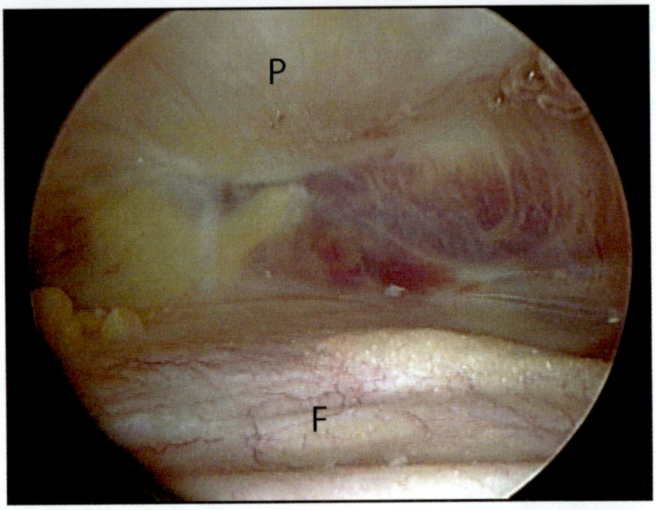

Figure 1-1. Arthroscopic view of suprapatellar pouch as viewed from the high anterolateral portal. The pouch is the space proximal to the patella (P) and superior to fat (F) overlying the distal femur.

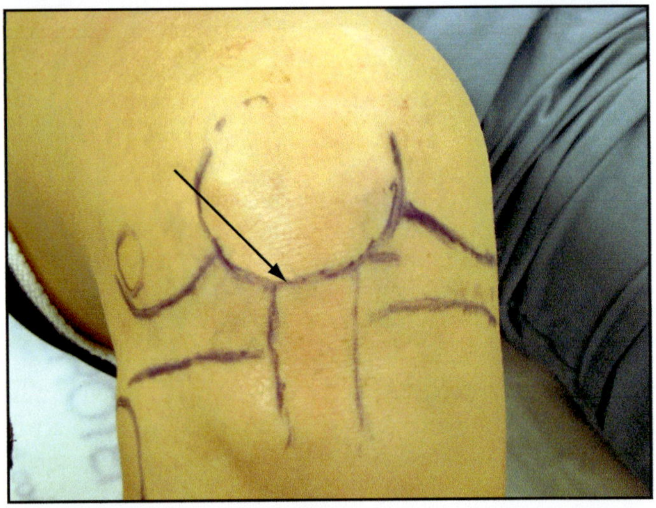

Figure 1-2. Photograph of a right knee with arrow pointing to inferior pole of patella. The high anterolateral portal would be placed just lateral to this point.

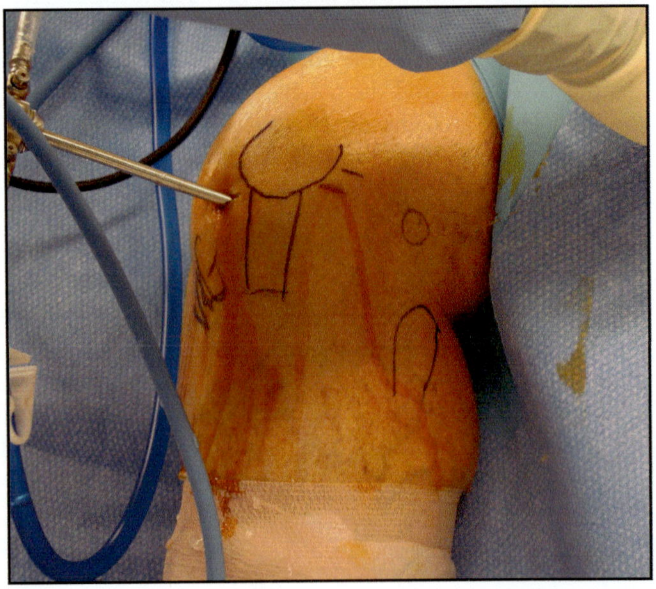

Figure 1-3. The arthroscope in the high anterolateral portal of this right knee is being directed toward the intercondylar notch.

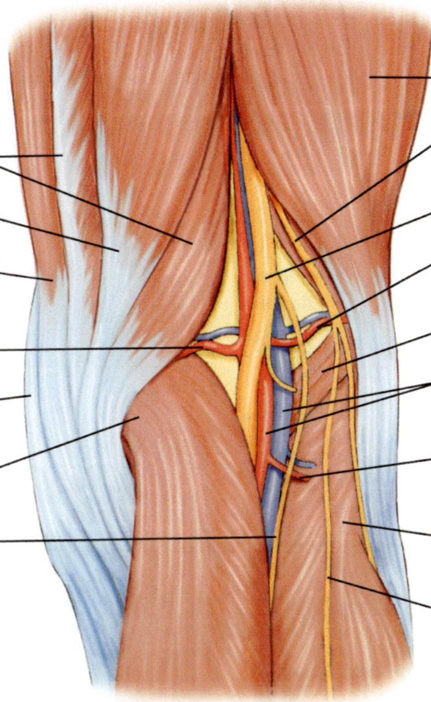

Figure 1-4. Posterior aspect of right knee showing the tibial nerve, popliteal artery, and vein within the popliteal fossa. (This figure was published in *Insall & Scott Surgery of the Knee,* 4th ed, Scott WN, Copyright Elsevier 2006.)

blade should be pointed toward the notch, but blind insertion beyond the skin and capsule should be avoided because this will risk injury to the cruciate ligaments.

The medial tibial plateau is larger than the lateral plateau; the 2 are separated by an intercondylar sulcus or fossa.[1] Adjacent to the fossa is a medial and lateral tibial spine that separates the fossa from the corresponding tibial plateau. The femoral condyles and tibial plateaus are incongruous without the medial and lateral menisci. The fibula, although extra-articular, has direct relevance to arthroscopic knee surgery because it serves as a landmark for portals and surgical approaches. The proximal fibula forms a joint with the proximal posterior surface of the tibia (tibiofibular joint). It also serves as an insertion for the lateral collateral ligament and biceps femoris tendon.

Knowledge of neurovascular anatomy around the knee joint is important for preventing iatrogenic injury during portal placement and surgical approaches.[2] Posteriorly, in the midthigh, the sciatic nerve branches into the tibial (or popliteal) and common peroneal nerves. At the posterior joint line of the knee just posterior to the joint capsule, the tibial nerve passes between the 2 heads of the gastrocnemius muscles, along with the popliteal artery and vein. From medial to lateral, the structures include the nerve, artery, and vein (Figure 1-4).[1] Makridis et al[3] showed that knee flexion increases the distance between the tibial insertion of the PCL and the popliteal neurovascular structures.

The common peroneal nerve passes posterior to the biceps femoris tendon and courses between it and the lateral head of the gastrocnemius toward the fibular head (Figure 1-5).[1,2] It then courses laterally around the fibular neck and into the peroneus longus tendon. In most individuals, the biceps femoris tendon insertion onto the fibular head can be palpated in 90 degrees of knee flexion. Placing incisions, portals, and retractors anterior to this landmark will help avoid injury the common peroneal nerve.

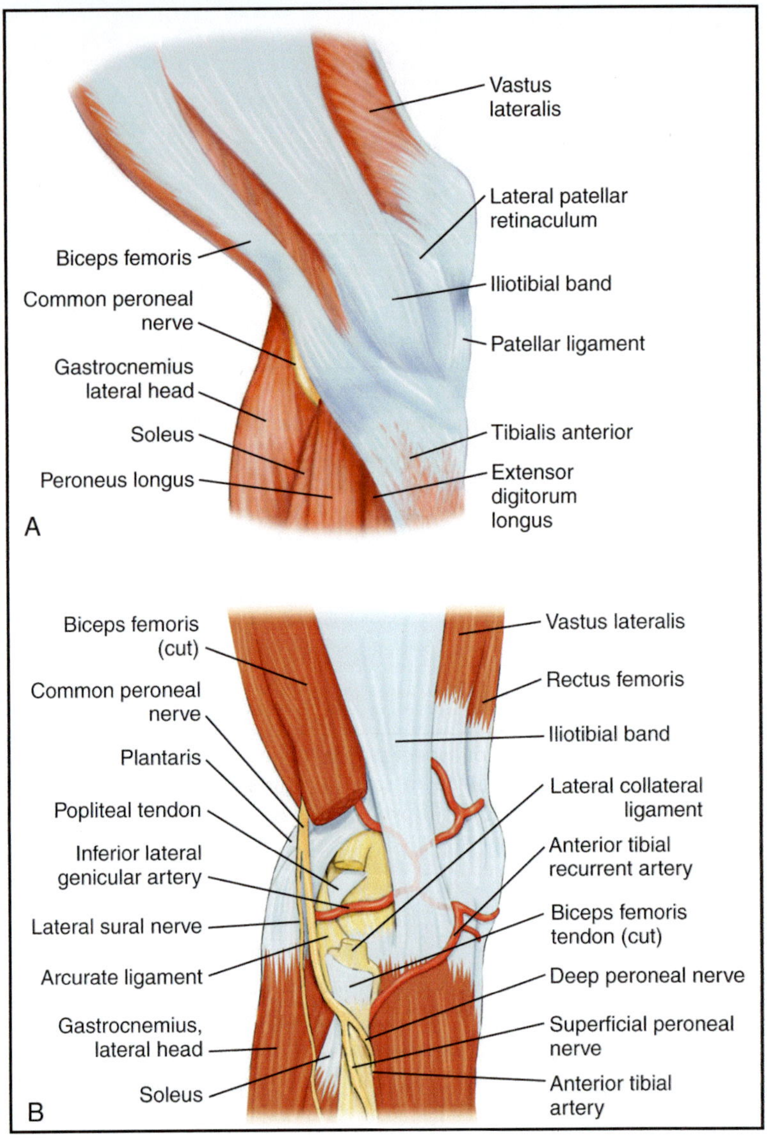

Figure 1-5. Lateral aspect of the right knee. (A) Common peroneal nerve passing posterior to the biceps femoris tendon. (B) The common peroneal nerve passes laterally around the fibular neck. (This figure was published in *Insall & Scott Surgery of the Knee,* 4th ed, Scott WN, Copyright Elsevier 2006.)

On the medial aspect of the knee, the saphenous nerve and its infrapatellar branch are at risk for injury during placement of medial and posteromedial portals, as well as during all medial approaches to the knee. The nerve and its branch have a variable course and number of terminal branches.[1,2] In general, the saphenous nerve passes between the gracilis and sartorius muscles approximately 3 cm posterior to the medial femoral epicondyle. The infrapatellar branch courses beneath the sartorius (ie, posterior to it) and runs along the anteromedial aspect of the knee, where it can terminate medially or laterally to the medial border of the patellar tendon (Figure 1-6).

Pertinent Physical Findings

Each patient undergoing knee arthroscopy should have a complete history, physical examination, and informed consent that are well documented. Anesthetic, medical, and deep venous

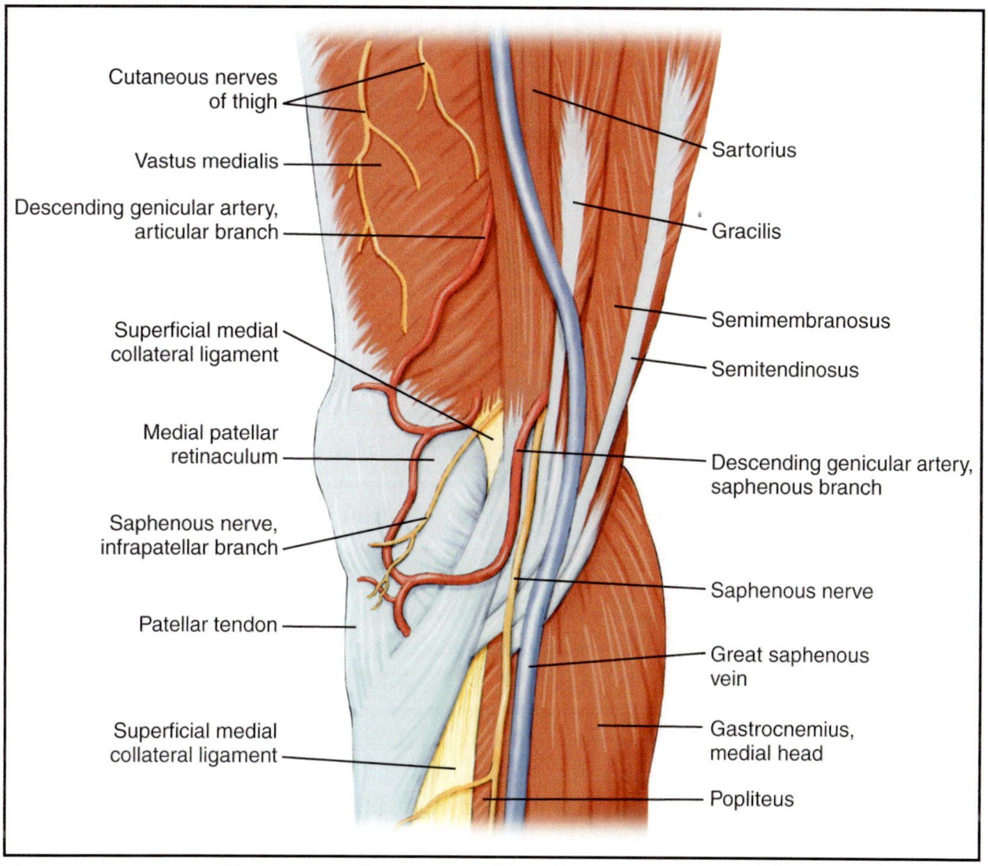

Figure 1-6. Anteromedial superficial structures of right knee showing the saphenous nerve and its infrapatellar branch. (This figure was published in *Insall & Scott Surgery of the Knee,* 4th ed, Scott WN, Copyright Elsevier 2006.)

thrombosis risks should be identified and addressed preoperatively. Details of the history and examination for specific diagnoses will be covered in the appropriate chapters elsewhere in this text. On the day of surgery, the surgeon should speak with the patient prior to him or her receiving sedation. The patient's history should be reviewed and the appropriate knee marked with the surgeon's initials.

Pertinent Imaging

At a minimum, all patients should have preoperative radiography, including a standing posteroanterior view with the knees flexed 45 degrees, a lateral view, and a Merchant or sunrise view. These x-rays can be useful for identifying degenerative joint disease, osteochondral or other injuries, tumors, loose bodies, and patellar pathology, such as patella alta or baja, bipartite, or dysplasia.

The need for magnetic resonance imaging, computed tomography, and other imaging is based on the initial history, examination, x-rays, and response to prior treatment and will be discussed in the appropriate chapters.

Equipment

Gravity inflow, in which multiple bags of fluid are raised to 8 to 10 feet, is a common method for infusing the joint with fluid. Although more popular in the early days of arthroscopy, it continues to be used today by many surgeons. As technology has improved, the fluid pump has gained popularity. It provides the advantage of improved hemostasis and higher pressures.[2] There are a variety of different pumps available, so it is important for the surgeon to have a thorough understanding of the pump that he or she is using. Each pump has different controls for pressure and flow maintenance, and the surgeon cannot assume that a set pressure on one pump is equal to the same pressure on another pump. It is also important to recognize that intra-articular pressures can be increased by simply manipulating the knee in flexion or extension.[4] Muellner et al[5] compared 4 pump systems and concluded that there is a significant difference among pumps in the pressure that was set and the actual measured intra-articular pressure. They also noted that all pumps were accurate at pressures below 60 mm Hg but not above this setting.

Selection of outflow methods also plays an important role in distention of the joint and providing a clear view. The options include suction or gravity outflow through the arthroscope sheath or through a separate outflow cannula. Continuous outflow, whether gravity or suction, will result in greater fluid use; therefore, intermittent outflow controlled by the surgeon or an assistant may be preferable. The author's preferred technique is presented later in this chapter.

Also, shoulder suction can be connected to the shaver or burr and, similar to another type of outflow, can be used continuously or intermittently. Again, it is generally preferable to use suction on an intermittent basis to clear debris; continuous use can make it difficult to maintain joint distention. Although different manufacturers have small variations in shavers and burrs, they are usually available in different sizes and levels of aggressiveness. In general, the smallest, least aggressive instrument that can perform the desired task should be used. However, some smaller shavers and burr tend to become clogged more easily from debris, which can require frequent cleaning. Regardless of which instrument is selected, it is important for the surgeon to be familiar with its characteristics. In particular, the surgeon should know which part of the burr or shaver is the working side and which is the nonworking side. A clear video of the working side should always be maintained in order to reduce risk of iatrogenic injury (Figure 1-7). The instrument must be carefully placed (without force) into the joint, moved with the joint, and removed. Minimal, if any, torque should ever be applied to the shaft, and the surgeon should never shave or burr blindly. The surgeon also should not select the most aggressive burr just because it will perform faster. Slow, steady controlled movements are necessary when using a shaver, but especially a burr.

The selection and proper use of an arthroscopic camera allow the surgeon to examine all areas of the knee joint efficiently. The arthroscope is available in 0, 30, and 70 degrees, although the 0-degree arthroscope is rarely used today because it provides the smallest field of view. As the light cord is rotated, the end of the arthroscope also rotates, resulting in a wide field of view. Most surgeons prefer the 30-degree arthroscope for most procedures. The 70-degree arthroscope should be available if a larger view is needed (looking around a corner), such as in the posterior aspect of the knee. Although it is important to use rotation of the arthroscopic camera to increase the field of view, it is also important to maintain the orientation of the arthroscope with the anatomic position of the joint. For example, with the leg hanging off the end of the bed, the arthroscope power cord and camera should be maintained in a vertical orientation. This orientation should be maintained, even as the arthroscope is moved throughout the joint (Video).

Most systems allow the surgeon to document the arthroscopic findings and treatment with photographs and/or video. Documentation can serve as an important reference for the surgeon, an educational tool for the patient, and support for the charges to an insurance carrier. However, surgeons should discuss giving videos to their patients with their malpractice carrier because some recommend against it for medicolegal reasons.

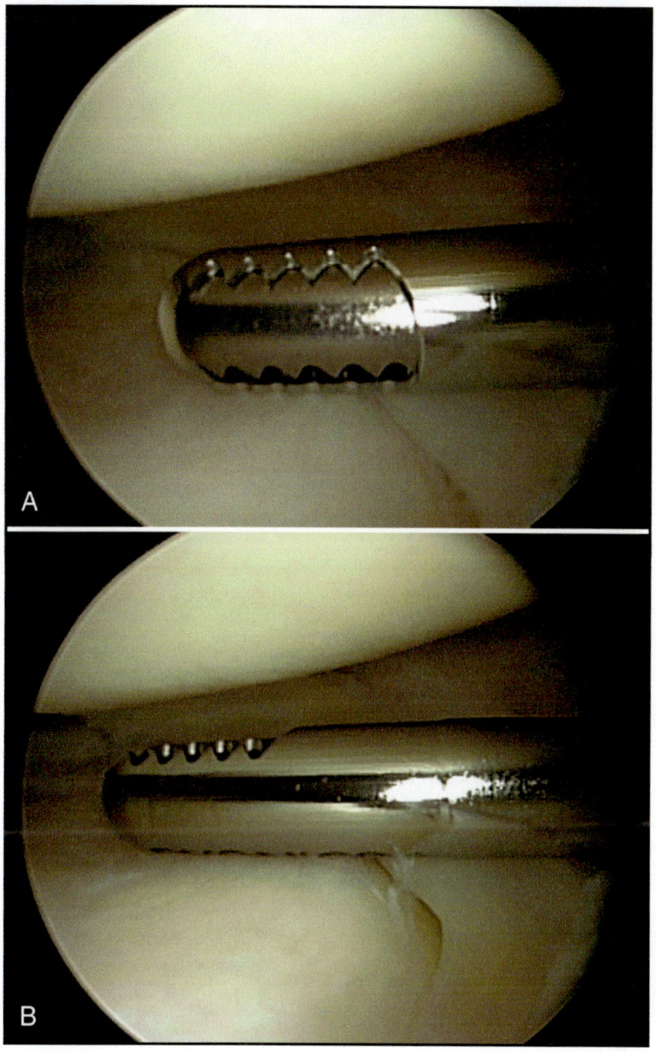

Figure 1-7. The working end of a shaver is kept in view during arthroscopy to reduce the risk of iatrogenic injury. (A) Arthroscopic view of the working end of a shaver. (B) Arthroscopic view of the shaver without view of its working end.

Cannulas are not used as frequently in the knee as in other joints, but they can be useful for posterior portals. Disposable cannulas come in a variety of sizes. You should have several sizes available and should know in advance the minimum cannula diameter required by various instruments that you plan to use. Metal cannulas are useful for posterior portals because shavers can screw into the cannula directly and, with the use of an adapter, the camera can also be exchanged between cannulas.

With repeat use and normal wear, it is common to have to repair or replace cameras and light cords. It is therefore important to have extra cameras and light cords available during surgery. Other basic working instruments needed for knee arthroscopy include a probe, spinal needle, basket punches (narrow, wide, straight, up-biting, up curved, left, right, and back), graspers, cutters, and varying types of shavers, burrs, and cautery. Basket punches are available in various shapes, and their selection largely depends on surgeon preference. More important than the shape, a variety of different angled and curved basket punches should be available so that all areas of the joint can be accessed.

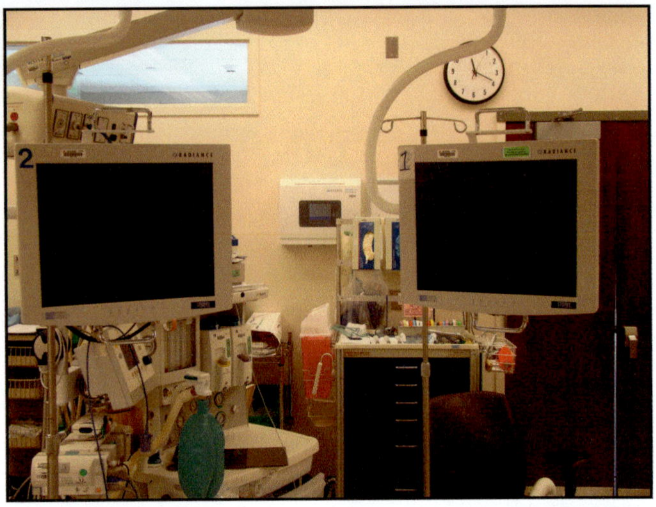

Figure 1-8. The use of 2 liquid crystal display video monitors permits the surgeon and assistant to work and comfortably view the arthroscopic video.

Treatment

Anesthesia Options

Knee arthroscopy can be performed under general, spinal, or local anesthesia. The choice primarily depends on surgeon and patient preference but in some cases may be influenced by the patient's medical history. In a prospective randomized study of 400 patients, Jacobson et al[6] compared 3 anesthesia options and concluded that local anesthesia was technically feasible in 92% of patients undergoing elective knee arthroscopy. However, when comparing patient satisfaction, the local anesthetic group had 90% satisfaction vs 97% for the general anesthesia group. Horlocker and Hebl[7] performed an evidence-based review of published studies comparing various anesthetic methods for knee arthroscopy. They reported that the results of most studies were biased by surgeon and patient expectations as well as by differences in postoperative management. They concluded that a single method of anesthesia could not be recommended for all surgeons performing or patients undergoing knee arthroscopy.

Operating Room Setup

One or more video monitors are required. Traditionally, cathode ray tube monitors have been the standard. New flat screen liquid crystal display monitors are increasingly being used (Figure 1-8), and most manufacturers of arthroscopic video equipment also currently offer high-definition monitors. Although only one monitor is needed, many operating rooms use 2 or more monitors (Figure 1-9). Although there is less benefit of multiple monitors for knee arthroscopy, they can be very useful for shoulder and hip arthroscopy.

The control boxes for the arthroscopic camera, shavers, pump, and other devices can be placed on a mobile tower (see Figure 1-9A) that is easily moved from room to room or can be contained on a boom (see Figure 1-9B). The advantage of the boom is that there are less electrical cords across the floor and that the monitor(s) can be positioned independently of the tower.

Operating Room Team

Most basic arthroscopic knee procedures, such as meniscectomies, chondroplasties, lateral releases, and loose body removals, can be performed by the surgeon with the assistance of a single surgical scrub technician. More advanced procedures, such as ligament reconstructions, meniscal

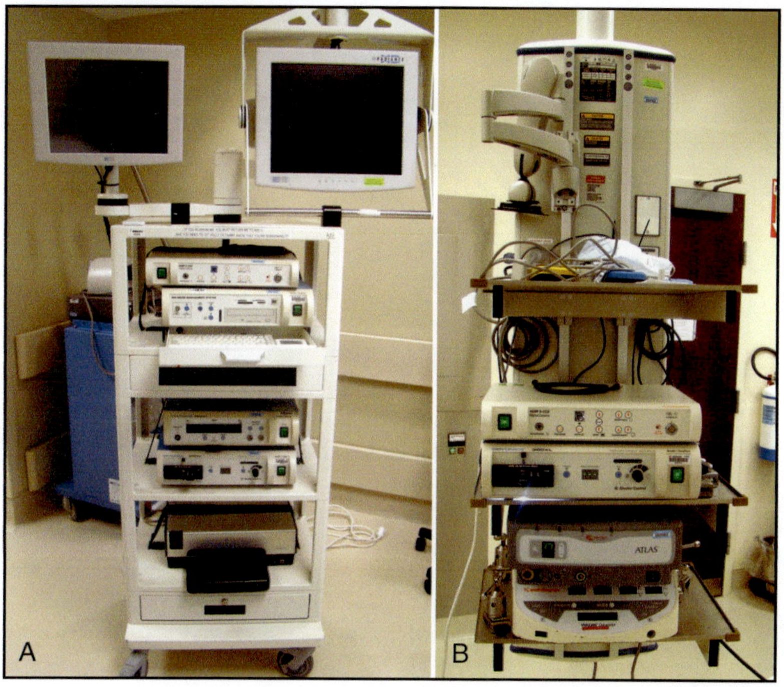

Figure 1-9. (A) Mobile arthroscopic tower that contains 2 monitors. (B) Arthroscopic boom that is connected overhead within the operating room.

repairs, cartilage restoration, and osteotomies, may be easier to perform with a second surgical assistant.

Similarly, all members of the operating room team should be informed well in advance of possible variations in the planned procedure(s) and the instruments required. It is important to discuss required instruments in advance with the surgical team and/or coordinator. Staff in the room must also know where instruments are located in case they are requested during the surgery.

Positioning and Portals

Prior to patient positioning, an initial time-out should be performed by the operating room staff to confirm the correct extremity. Proper patient positioning is extremely important in terms of patient safety and surgical efficiency. A standard operating room bed is needed, with a leg portion that lowers. If fluoroscopy is planned, a radiolucent table may be needed. It is important to make certain that you can obtain the needed fluoroscopic images prior to prepping and draping the patient. It is the surgeon's responsibility to oversee the positioning of the patient. In situations in which you frequently perform surgery at a given center or hospital, you may want to train the staff to position patients for you. Even if you delegate this task, it is still your responsibility to make sure that they are positioned correctly. When training staff, it is important to explain your rationale for patient positioning instructions because they may not readily understand the importance of specific instructions relative to surgical efficiency and patient safety.

The use of leg holders or posts is determined by the preoperative diagnosis, surgical plan, and surgeon preference. A variety of different commercial leg holders are available for the operative and nonoperative leg. When operating on both knees, bilateral leg holders are also available (Figure 1-10A). In most cases, a unilateral leg holder (Figures 1-10B and 1-10C) or lateral post (Figure 1-10D) is used for the operative leg. Leg holders may include padding, and some others require you to apply padding to the leg prior to securing it within the holder. Some holders are designed to hold the leg with a tourniquet (see Figure 1-10B), and others require the tourniquet to

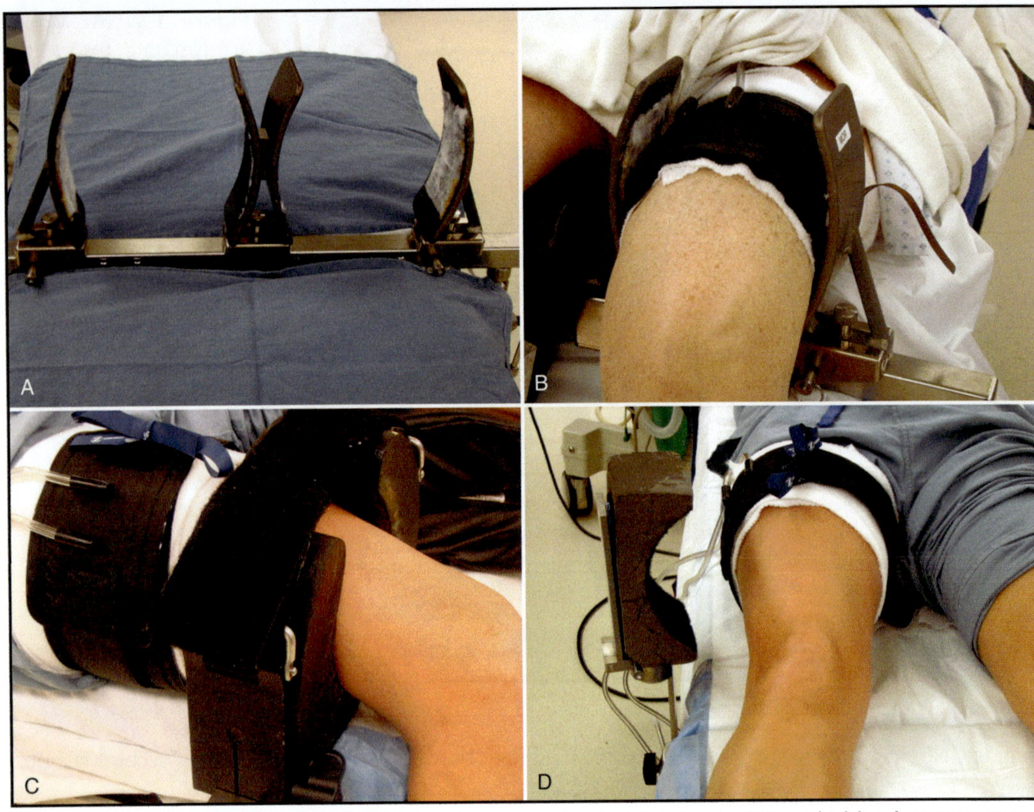

Figure 1-10. Different types of leg holders and an example of a lateral post. (A) Leg holder that can accommodate both legs. (B) Unilateral leg holder with the tourniquet positioned within holder. (C) Unilateral leg holder with the tourniquet outside of the holder. (D) Lateral post.

be outside the holder (see Figure 1-10C). If you prefer a unilateral holder or lateral post, it will be important to determine how to protect the contralateral leg. The use of a leg holder for the nonoperative leg has been shown to increase the risk of compression to the peroneal nerve as it courses around the fibular neck.[2] Nonoperative leg holders can also cause a stretch injury to the femoral nerve if the hip is held extended. If the foot of the bed is left up for a lateral post, then positioning the nonoperative leg does not require anything special. If the foot is dropped, it is often easiest to place a large pad under the nonoperative thigh to keep the hip flexed (Figure 1-11). If there is concern about pressure on the peroneal nerve, additional foam padding can be applied in this region, particularly in thin patients.

Other issues related to the leg holder include the position of the foot of the bed and the use of hip bumps. For lateral post use, the foot of the bed can remain up (see Figure 1-10D) or it can be lowered. The advantage of the lateral post is faster setup and positioning, ability to move the leg freely during surgery, ability to hyperflex the knee, and ease of placing the knee in a figure-4 position. The primary disadvantage is that the leg tends to slide over the post when placing valgus stress on the knee for access to posterior horn of medial meniscus.

This can be prevented, however, by having an assistant place downward pressure on the thigh (Figure 1-12). The major disadvantage associated with a fixed leg holder is the risk of rupturing the medial collateral ligament with excess valgus stress[2]; knee flexion is limited by the lowered portion table and inability to move the leg freely.

The inability to abduct the leg can sometimes pose difficulties in posteromedial portal placement. If this occurs, you can have an assistant carefully abduct the nonoperative leg or the leg holder can be loosened or removed beneath the sterile drapes. Femur fractures have also been

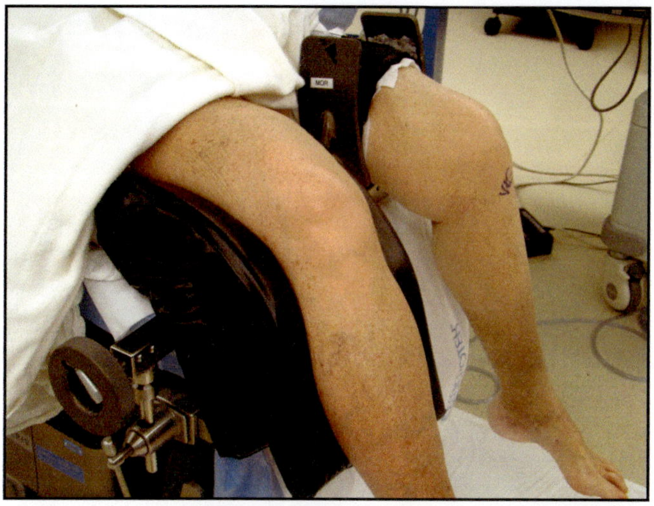

Figure 1-11. The black pad beneath the right nonoperative leg should be placed during knee arthroscopy. The pad protects the nonoperative leg.

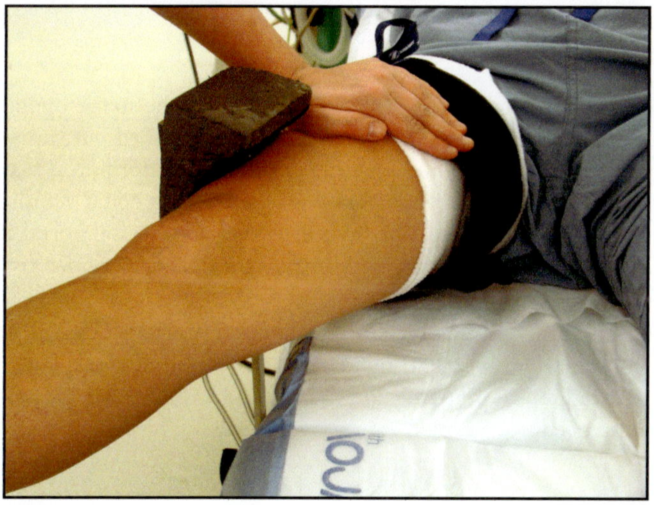

Figure 1-12. Valgus stress can be applied to the knee against a lateral post while an assistant applies downward pressure on the thigh. This prevents the thigh from sliding over the post.

reported with the use of a leg holder, but these are rare.[8] Regardless of choice of leg holder, a small sandbag or other hip bump may be helpful for larger patients who tend to rotate their legs excessively externally when lying supine.

The next consideration is the decision on tourniquet usage. There are conflicting reports in the literature as to the usefulness of tourniquets in improving visualization and potential decreased recovery of muscle strength. Johnson et al,[9] in a randomized prospective evaluation of 109 patients undergoing knee arthroscopy, reported that routine knee arthroscopy could be performed adequately with no tourniquet. Kirkley et al,[10] in a similar evaluation of 120 patients, reported no complications associated with tourniquet use, with a slight trend toward less early postoperative pain and better isokinetic strength at 2 weeks postoperatively in patients in whom a tourniquet was not used. Tourniquets with a wide and/or curved cuff have been shown to decrease the risk of muscle and nerve injury. Rodeo et al[11] recommended that tourniquet time less than 2 hours and pressures less than 350 mm Hg lower the risk of neuropraxia. Several authors have also shown that a tourniquet should not be reinflated during an operative procedure after it is deflated for a period of reperfusion.[12,13]

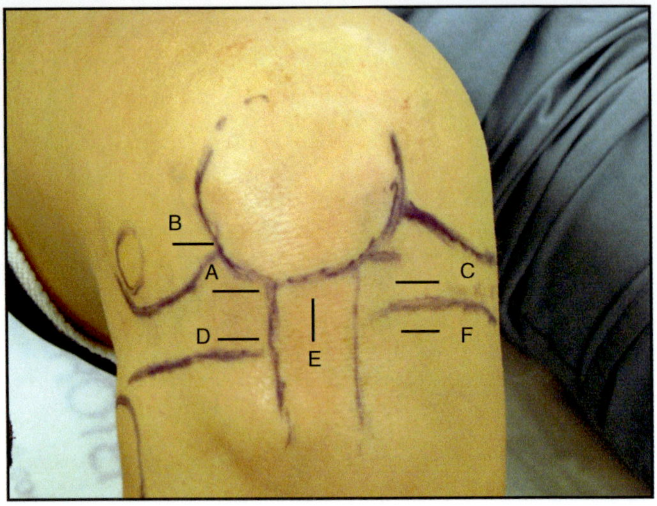

Figure 1-13. Various anterior portals are demonstrated for a right knee: (A) the high anterolateral portal, (B) patellofemoral axillary portal, (C) standard anteromedial portal, (D) accessory low anterolateral portal, (E) transpatellar tendon portal, and (F) accessory low anteromedial portal.

Potential Problems With Setup

If the tourniquet is placed too low on the thigh or if the leg holder is too low, the sterile operative field may be limited during the surgery. If a 2-portal knee arthroscopy is planned but suprapatellar pathology is found and cannot be accessed via anterior portals, then a superior portal may be needed. The limited sterile field superiorly may prevent portal placement and could require repeat prepping and draping. Similarly, it may not be possible to create a posteromedial portal if posterior pathology is identified. Most importantly, the surgeon's initials on the correct operative knee should be visible before and after sterile draping.

Any potential need to convert a routine arthroscopic procedure to an open surgery or to a more involved procedure, such as ACL reconstruction, meniscal repair, or osteochondral transplantation, must be anticipated in advance to avoid repeat prepping and draping. The use of a lateral post may make conversion to more involved procedures simpler.

Portals

Vertical vs horizontal portal incisions are primarily based on surgeon preference. A vertical portal provides greater options for extension in situations in which the pathology cannot be accessed because the initial portal is too high or low.

High Anterolateral Portal

The high anterolateral portal is the most common initial diagnostic portal. It is located above the lateral joint line, adjacent to the patellar tendon's lateral margin.[14] The inferior pole of the patella with the knee in 60 degrees of flexion is a good landmark for the inferior margin of this portal (Figure 1-13, A and Video). It is important, however, to review the preoperative x-rays to make certain that the patient does not have patella alta or baja. The anterolateral portal is useful for examining the medial, lateral, and patellofemoral compartments; visualizing the notch during ACL reconstruction; and treating medial meniscus pathology.[15] In addition to a viewing portal, it can be also used for fluid inflow.

In general, basic knee arthroscopy can be performed with a 2- or 3-portal technique. The 2-portal technique requires inflow through the arthroscopic camera sheath, whereas the 3-portal technique requires a separate superior portal for inflow. Most commonly, this superior portal is placed superolaterally. Stetson and Templin[16] have shown faster return to activities and return of quadriceps strength with the 2-portal technique.

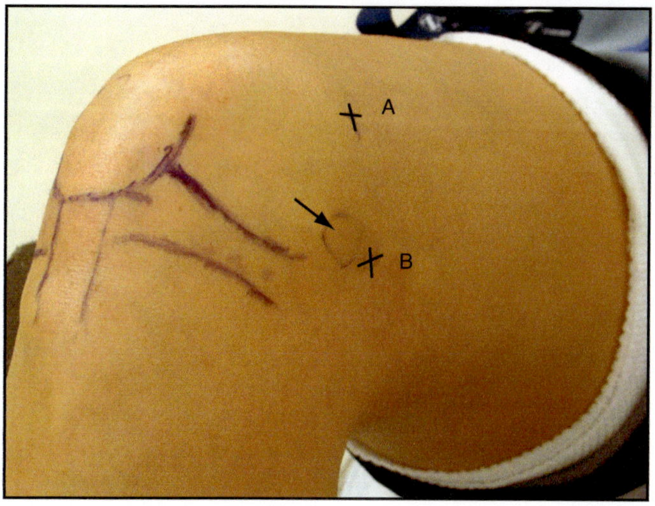

Figure 1-14. Anteromedial view of the right knee demonstrating the (A) superomedial portal, which accesses the (B) suprapatellar space and the posteromedial portal, which is created just proximal and inferior to the medial femoral epicondyle (black arrow).

When pathology is expected in the lateral compartment based on the preoperative diagnosis, Kim and Kim[15] have recommended that the initial portal be placed more laterally and higher (patellofemoral axillary portal) than a standard high anterolateral portal. The patellofemoral axillary portal is at the junction or axilla of the lateral edge of the patella and the anterior edge of the lateral femoral condyle (Figure 1-13, B). The authors stated that this portal allows excellent visualization of the popliteal hiatus, lateral gutter, and lateral compartment.

Anteromedial Portal

A second working portal is created after performing an initial diagnostic examination through the first portal. Most often, the second portal is the anteromedial portal. The exact position of the portal is determined by the pathology (Figure 1-13, C and Video). As with all working portals, a spinal needle is used to determine its precise location. If access to the posterior horn of the medial meniscus is needed, the portal should be just above the anterior horn of the medial meniscus. If lateral compartment access is needed, the portal should be high enough to pass over the tibial spines. Alternatively, if pathology in the posterior horn of the lateral meniscus cannot be accessed through the anteromedial portal, a low anterolateral portal (Figure 1-13, D) can be placed just above the anterior horn of the lateral meniscus.[15]

Accessory and Other Portals

A transpatellar tendon or central portal can be created as an accessory working or viewing portal. The portal must be made vertically in line with the tendon fibers to avoid transecting the tendon. The portal is placed at the inferior pole of the patella (Figure 1-13, E). It can be particularly useful in situations in which the anterolateral portal is too lateral and/or the anteromedial portal is too medial. In these cases, the transpatellar tendon portal can provide excellent visualization and access to the notch. Even when the other portals are placed appropriately, the transpatellar portal can be used as an accessory portal during ACL reconstruction.[14]

Additional anterior accessory portals can be placed at any location necessary for working or viewing. Most commonly, they are used to access a torn meniscus, articular cartilage defect, loose body, or the femoral tunnel placement for ACL or PCL surgery. The landmarks to avoid for accessory anterior portals are the menisci, articular cartilage, and inferior branch of the saphenous nerve. An accessory low anteromedial portal (Figure 1-13, F) is often used for placement of a femoral tunnel during ACL reconstruction.

The superomedial portal is placed 3 to 4 cm superior to the superior pole of the patella (Figure 1-14, A and Video). It should be in line with the medial border of the patella or just posterior to it.

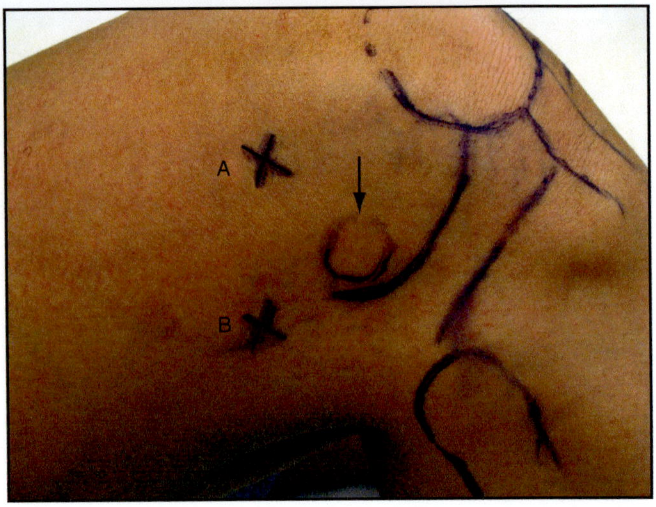

Figure 1-15. Anterolateral view of right knee demonstrating the (A) superolateral portal, which accesses the (B) suprapatellar space and posterolateral portal. The black arrow points to the lateral femoral epicondyle.

The cannula and obturator should aim toward the suprapatellar pouch, just posterior to the patellar articular cartilage. This is an excellent portal for viewing patellofemoral tracking or the lateral retinaculum during release. Because the portal violates the vastus medialis obliquus, it can affect the return of postoperative knee function and quadriceps strength.[16] The superolateral portal is placed 3 to 4 cm superior to the superior pole of the patella and in line with the lateral border of the patella (Figure 1-15, A and Video). It also provides excellent visualization of patellofemoral tracking. Either superior portal can also be used for fluid inflow.

All arthroscopic knee surgeons should be comfortable with access to the posterior compartments of the knee via posteromedial and posterolateral portals (Figures 1-14, B and 1-15, B, respectively, and Video). If unfamiliar with these portals, they should be practiced in the laboratory setting prior to attempting them in the operating room. With the arthroscope in the high anterolateral portal, the camera is advanced into the notch at the interval between the medial femoral condyle and PCL (Figure 1-16A). Next, the arthroscopic sheath is held in place while the camera is replaced with a blunt trocar. The sheath and trocar are then gently advanced into the posteromedial compartment with the knee in 45 to 60 degrees of flexion. It is helpful to have the index finger of the hand holding the sheath positioned along its shaft. As the sheath is advanced, the index fingertip can be positioned so that it abuts the outside of the knee prior to penetrating the posterior capsule with the sheath and trocar. If difficulty is encountered during attempted passage, a limited inferior medial notchplasty can be performed, taking care to avoid injury to the PCL. This notchplasty may be required in cases of osteoarthritic spurs or otherwise stenotic notches.[17] Once in the compartment, the trocar is replaced with the camera and the posteromedial knee is palpated with a gloved finger. This will help in identifying the general area for placement of a spinal needle. The posteromedial portal is approximately 2 cm superior to the medial femoral epicondyle and 1 cm posterior (Figure 1-14, B and Video). With the knee in 90 degrees of flexion, the needle is directed toward the posterior aspect of the intercondylar notch (ie, where the camera is located; Figures 1-16B and 1-16C). The exact position is dependent on the pathology present. Care should be taken to avoid injury to the popliteal neurovascular structures with transverse insertion of the needle posterior to the posterior capsule. A recent cadaver study reported that 90 to 120 degrees of knee flexion are safe for establishing posteromedial portals and 30 degrees is not recommended.[3] Once the correct needle position is attained, a small skin incision is created. A hemostat is then used for blunt separation of soft tissues. This is helpful to prevent injury to the saphenous nerve or its branches. Next, a blunt obturator and cannula are inserted along the same direction as the spinal needle. The entry through the capsule can be directly visualized with the camera. In some cases, the blunt obturator will slide off the capsule in a posterior direction. If the

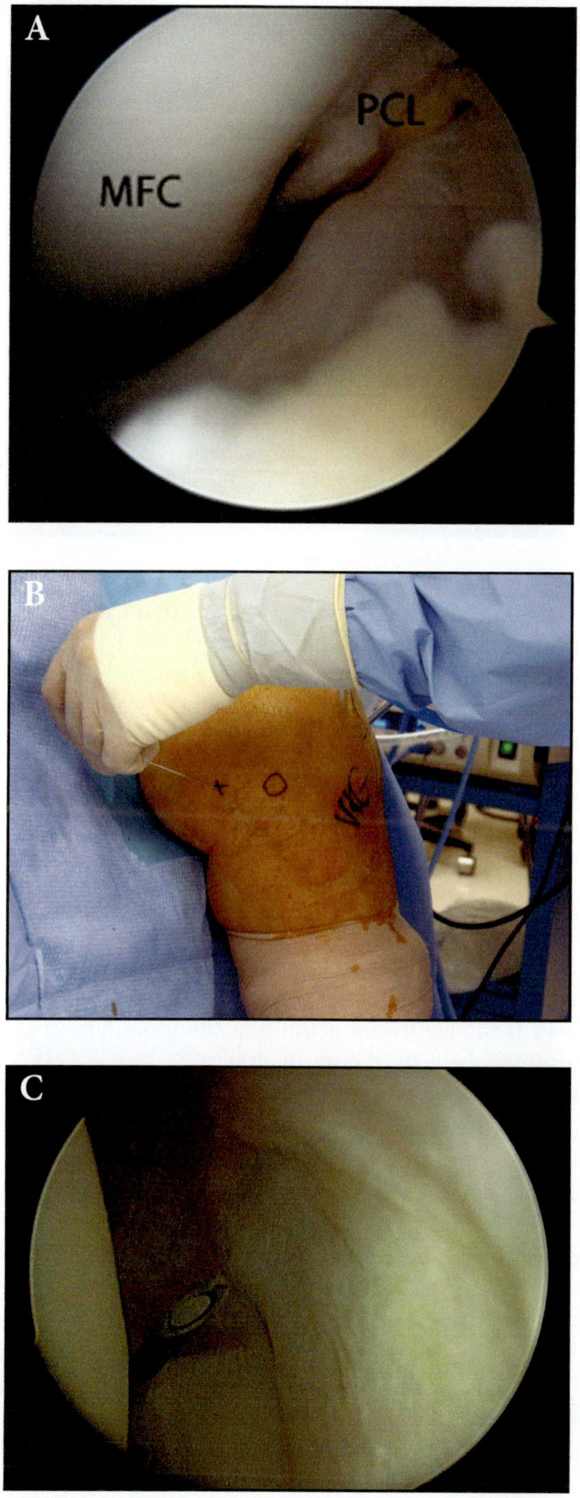

Figure 1-16. Creation of a posteromedial portal in the right knee. (A) Arthroscopic view of the interval between the medial femoral condyle (MFC) and PCL used for passage of arthroscope into the posteromedial compartment of the knee. (B) External view of needle insertion proximal to the medial femoral condyle (circle) for the posteromedial portal. (C) Arthroscopic view of the needle entering the posteromedial compartment.

capsule cannot be penetrated after a few careful attempts, the sharp obturator may be needed. This can be safe if you are confident in the direction required to penetrate the capsule. Once the obturator is against the capsule, it can be more easily pushed through it. The sharp obturator, however, increases the risk of injury to neurovascular structures if directed incorrectly.

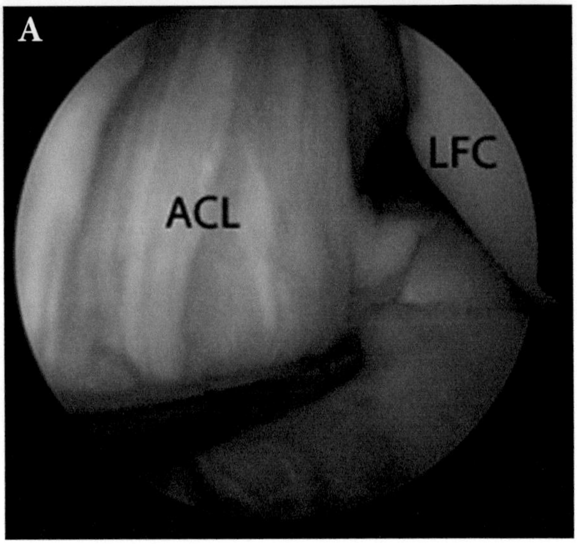

Figure 1-17. Creation of a posterolateral portal. (A) Arthroscopic view of the interval between the lateral femoral condyle and ACL used for passage of the arthroscope into the posterolateral compartment of the knee. *(continued)*

In a similar fashion, a posterolateral portal can be established with the camera in the anteromedial portal. It is advanced through the notch between the ACL and lateral femoral condyle (Figure 1-17A and Video). This can often be done without replacing the camera with a trocar, but do not use excessive force. If the camera does not pass easily, it is safest to use a blunt trocar. A spinal needle is again used posterolaterally 2 cm superior to the lateral femoral epicondyle and anterior to the biceps femoris to avoid injury to the common peroneal nerve (Figures 1-15, B and 1-17B). The needle is directed toward the tip of the camera (Figure 1-17C), a skin incision is created, and the cannula is inserted. For posterolateral portals, 90 degrees of knee flexion is safe but 120 degrees risks injury to common peroneal nerve.[3]

Author's Diagnostic Arthroscopy Technique (Video)

A standard leg holder is used for most arthroscopic procedures, and a lateral post is used for cruciate ligament reconstruction, patellofemoral realignment, and osteochondral autograft transfer procedures requiring extreme knee flexion. If the leg holder is limiting the procedure in any way, the circulating nurse removes it during surgery beneath the sterile drapes.

Prior to examination under anesthesia, the circulating nurse reads the consent and all staff confirm that the correct extremity has the surgeon's initials. A routine knee examination for range of motion and ligament stability is performed. The tourniquet is placed over soft cotton roll approximately one handbreadth above the patella. The extremity is exsanguinated with an Esmarch bandage, and the tourniquet pressure is set to 300 mm Hg for most patients. For children or those with very small legs, the tourniquet pressure may be decreased to 250 mm Hg. For obese patients or those with elevated blood pressure, the tourniquet pressure may be increased to 350 mm Hg.

A large foam pillow is placed beneath the contralateral leg. After sterile prepping and draping, a time-out is performed to again confirm the correct side. Next, a horizontal high anterolateral portal is created. The arthroscopic camera sheath and blunt obturator are then carefully inserted through the capsule. The knee is extended and the sheath is further inserted into the suprapatellar pouch, just lateral to the patella. Care is taken to avoid injury to the femoral or patellar articular cartilage. A fluid pump is used for inflow through the arthroscopic sheath. Suction is also connected to the arthroscopic sheath and controlled by the surgeon. Suction is only used to clear cloudy fluid on an intermittent basis. Routine continuous suction of gravity outflow is not used.

Next, a quick initial diagnostic examination is performed. The sequence of the exam should be a routine that works for the surgeon. The author's preference is first to examine the suprapatellar pouch, lateral gutter, patellofemoral joint, and medial gutter. The knee should be flexed and

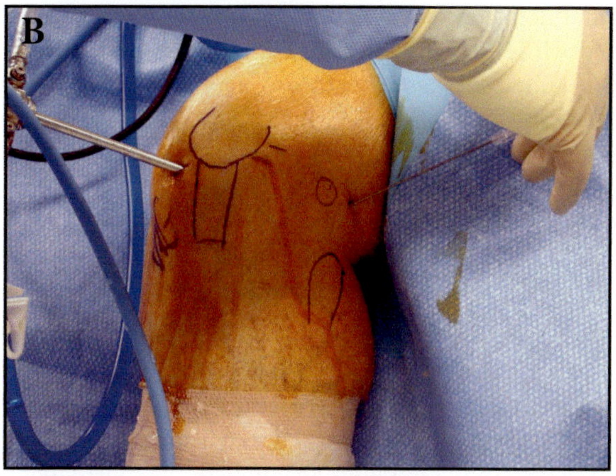

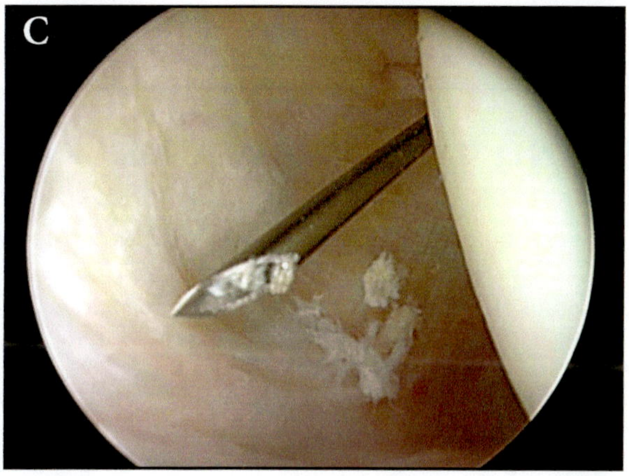

Figure 1-17 (continued). (B) External view of needle insertion for the posterolateral portal. (C) Arthroscopic view of the needle entering the posterolateral compartment.

extended during examination of the patellofemoral joint. The knee is then flexed with gentle valgus stress applied as the camera is moved from the medial gutter into the medial compartment. The camera is then rotated to view the posterior horn, body, and anterior horn of the medial meniscus. The knee is flexed and extended to view the entire articular cartilage of the medial femoral condyle.

The camera is then withdrawn slightly as the notch is entered. In some cases, it may be difficult to visualize the ACL fully because of a thick ligamentum mucosum. In this case, gently pass the camera over the top of the ligamentum and push it slightly so that there is a close view of the medial portion of the lateral femoral condyle. The knee is then gently placed into a figure-4 position and rested on the surgeon's thigh. This provides excellent visualization of the posterior horn of the lateral meniscus. As the knee is slowly extended, the lateral femoral condyle, body of the lateral meniscus, and anterior horn can be examined.

At this stage, an anteromedial working portal is created for most pathology. The superior-inferior position depends on the location of the pathology in the medial vs lateral compartments (see earlier). A spinal needle is inserted prior to creating a horizontal portal incision under direct visualization with the camera.

Next, a probe is inserted through the anteromedial working portal into the medial compartment. Although some have suggested that routine examination of the posterior compartment may be unnecessary,[18] result in increased morbidity, and decrease efficiency of the procedure, the author prefers to examine posteromedially and posterolaterally through the notch in all knee arthroscopies to avoid missing pathology.[19] Usually, this pathology includes a loose body or section of torn meniscus that is flipped posteriorly and not seen from an anterior view of the meniscus. The posteromedial compartment is examined while the arthroscope is still in the high anterolateral portal. If complete visualization is difficult, a 70-degree arthroscope is used, but this is extremely rare.

While the arthroscope is in the anteromedial viewing portal, it is passed into the posterolateral compartment for examination. If any additional pathology is identified from the anteromedial viewing portal, it is addressed at this time with existing portals or new portals as needed.

Postoperative Protocol

At the end of the arthroscopic procedure, the joint is thoroughly irrigated and fluid is suctioned. The portals are each closed with a nylon suture. The joint is injected for postoperative pain control with 30 mL of 0.5% bupivacaine (Marcaine). Dressings are applied, the tourniquet is deflated, and a warm pink foot is confirmed. The postoperative protocol is based on the specific pathology treated and is discussed in the relevant chapters.

Pearls, Pitfalls, and Complications

Pearls

1. Identify and address medical and deep venous thrombosis risks when discussing surgery with the patient in the office.
2. Develop a list of instruments and implants needed for the planned surgery, along with a second list of instruments that may be needed and thus should be available in the room. These lists should be provided to the operating room well in advance of the surgery.
3. Prior to surgery, it is important for the surgeon to notify the operating room about assistants that will be required for the planned procedure(s) and their expected roles. The surgeon should briefly meet with the operating room staff and make certain that everyone is familiar with the planned procedure and that all equipment, instruments, and implants are available.
4. The surgeon must see the patient preoperatively prior to him or her receiving sedation to review and update the history and physical and initial the operative knee.
5. Rather than having a set protocol for always or never using a tourniquet, it may be more important to use a tourniquet judiciously based on the planned procedure, patient-specific risk factors, and bleeding conditions during surgery.
6. Risk of injury to branches of the saphenous nerve may be diminished with horizontal portals, careful dissection during meniscal repair, and hamstring tendon harvest and transillumination of the skin with the arthroscope.
7. The arthroscopic field of view is not improved by changing the orientation of the camera but by rotating the light source. It is important to use the correct instrument for the required task and to examine the joint prior to placement of a working portal because the location of this portal may be affected by the pathology identified.

(continued)

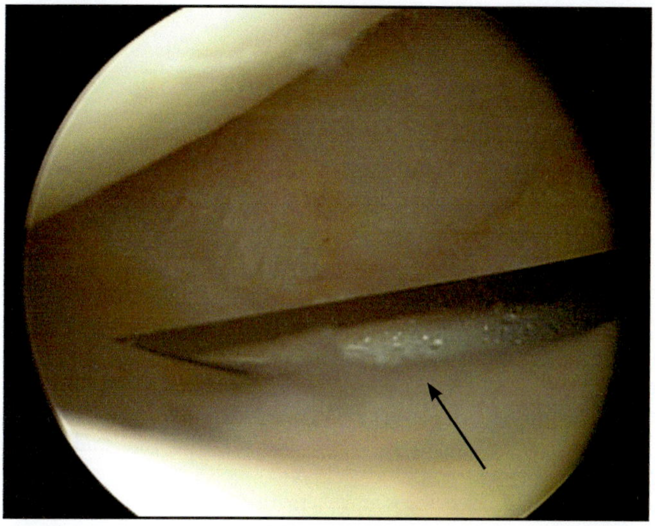

Figure 1-18. Arthroscopic view with the camera in the anterolateral portal showing the scalpel (black arrow) penetrating the joint capsule, creating an anteromedial portal, and making it easier to pass instruments because the capsule has been incised.

8. The #11 blade is inserted completely through the capsule for greater ease in passing instruments in and out of the working portal (Figure 1-18 and Video).
9. While viewing from the anterolateral portal, perform any required work through the anteromedial or other working portals. Once the work is completed, the arthroscope is moved to the anteromedial portal or other viewing portals. This limits movement of the arthroscope back and forth and improves efficiency.

Pitfalls

1. Failure to complete a time-out prior to beginning the surgery may lead to wrong-site surgery.
2. Injury to sensory nerves can result in loss of sensation and painful neuromas.
3. Failure to have the needed instruments during surgery may result in inefficiency, complications, and potentially poor outcomes.
4. If the orientation of the camera is continuously changed, the surgeon will have difficulty triangulating instruments.
5. Trying to use an instrument to perform a task for which it is not designed can result in iatrogenic injury to the joint and/or damage to the instrument.
6. Proceeding immediately to the expected pathology based on the preoperative diagnosis, treating it, forgetting to examine the rest of the joint, and missing unexpected pathology should be avoided.
7. The working end of all instruments should remain in view in order to prevent iatrogenic injury to the joint.
8. The initial quick diagnostic examination may have been limited because of synovitis, thickened ligamentum, or hypertrophic fat pad. Failure to go back, remove obstructions as needed, and perform a thorough examination can result in missed pathology.
9. Do not eliminate moving the camera into another portal just to complete the procedure faster. Complete examination and treatment often require viewing from different portals.

References

1. Clarke HD, Scott WN, Insall JN, et al. Anatomy. In: Scott WN, ed. *Insall & Scott Surgery of the Knee.* Vol 1. 5th ed. Philadelphia, PA: Churchill Livingstone; 2011:2-47.
2. Kim TK, Savino RM, McFarland EG, Cosgarea AJ. Neurovascular complications of knee arthroscopy. *Am J Sports Med.* 2002;30(4):619-629.
3. Makridis KG, Wajsfisz A, Agrawal N, Basdekis G, Djian P. Neurovascular anatomic relationships to arthroscopic posterior and transeptal portals in different knee positions. *Am J Sports Med.* 2013;41(7):1559-1564.
4. Funk DA, Noyes FR, Grood ES, Hoffman SD. Effect of flexion angle on the pressure-volume of the human knee. *Arthroscopy.* 1991;7(1):86-90.
5. Muellner T, Menth-Chiari WA, Reihsner R, Eberhardsteiner J, Engebretsen L. Accuracy of pressure and flow capacities of four arthroscopic fluid management systems. *Arthroscopy.* 2001;17(7):760-764.
6. Jacobson E, Forssblad M, Rosenberg J, Westman L, Weidenhielm L. Can local anesthesia be recommended for routine use in elective knee arthroscopy? A comparison between local, spinal, and general anesthesia. *Arthroscopy.* 2000;16(2):183-190.
7. Horlocker TT, Hebl JR. Anesthesia for outpatient knee arthroscopy: is there an optimal technique? *Reg Anesth Pain Med.* 2003;28(1):58-63.
8. Cautilli R Jr. Introduction to basics of arthroscopy of the knee. *Clin Sports Med.* 1997;16(1):1-16.
9. Johnson DS, Stewart H, Hirst P, Harper NJ. Is tourniquet use necessary for knee arthroscopy? *Arthroscopy.* 2000;16(6):648-651.
10. Kirkley A, Rampersaud R, Griffin S, Amendola A, Litchfield R, Fowler P. Tourniquet versus no tourniquet use in routine knee arthroscopy: a prospective, double-blind, randomized clinical trial. *Arthroscopy.* 2000;16(2):121-126.
11. Rodeo SA, Forster RA, Weiland AJ. Neurological complications due to arthroscopy. *J Bone Joint Surg Am.* 1993;75(6):917-926.
12. Mohler LR, Pedowitz RA, Myers RR, Ohara WM, Lopez MA, Gershuni DH. Intermittent reperfusion fails to prevent post tourniquet neurapraxia. *J Hand Surg Am.* 1999;24(4):687-693.
13. Rorabeck CH, Kennedy JC. Tourniquet-induced nerve ischemia complicating knee ligament surgery. *Am J Sports Med.* 1980;8(2):98-102.
14. Cohen SB, Fu FH. Three-portal technique for anterior cruciate ligament reconstruction: use of a central medial portal. *Arthroscopy.* 2007;23(3):325.e1-325.e5.
15. Kim SJ, Kim HJ. High portal: practical philosophy for positioning portals in knee arthroscopy. *Arthroscopy.* 2001;17(3):333-337.
16. Stetson WB, Templin K. Two-versus three-portal technique for routine knee arthroscopy. *Am J Sports Med.* 2002;30(1):108-111.
17. León HO, Blanco CE, Guthrie TB, Martínez OJ. Intercondylar notch stenosis in degenerative arthritis of the knee. *Arthroscopy.* 2005;21(3):294-302.
18. Lubowitz JH, Rossi MJ, Baker BS, Guttmann D. Arthroscopic visualization of the posterior compartments of the knee. *Arthroscopy.* 2004;20(7):675-680.
19. Amin KB, Cosgarea AJ, Kaeding CC. The value of intercondylar notch visualization of the posteromedial and posterolateral compartments during knee arthroscopy. *Arthroscopy.* 1999;15(8):813-817.

Please see videos on the accompanying website at www.routledge.com/9781617119996

2

Arthroscopic Synovectomy

Jack Anavian, MD; Trevor Born, MD; and Paul Fadale, MD

Introduction

The knee joint has the largest and most extensive synovial membrane compared to any other joint. Thus, pathologic conditions involving the synovium of the knee can be symptomatic and debilitating. Benign and malignant processes can involve the synovial membrane. For most conditions that require surgical treatment, arthroscopic synovectomy is a safe and effective method.

Arthroscopic synovectomy of the knee has major potential advantages over open surgical techniques, including improved visualization of the knee joint, a more complete synovectomy, less postoperative pain, decreased postoperative knee stiffness/arthrofibrosis, decreased postoperative hemarthrosis, shorter hospitalization, lower surgical site morbidity, the surgery is performed through arthroscopic portals (thus the division of the quadriceps is avoided), better preservation of the menisci, and lastly, revision surgery, if required, is less complicated. The major arthroscopic disadvantage is that it may be a more technically challenging operation to perform, and for some diffuse and malignant conditions, it is contraindicated.

Indications

- Plica syndrome
- Pigmented villonodular synovitis (PVNS)
- Synovial chondromatosis/osteochondromatosis
- Synovial hemangioma
- Popliteal (Baker's) cyst
- Hemophilia
- Seronegative and seropositive arthropathies
- Infection
- Arthrofibrosis

Sgaglione NA, Lubowitz JH, Provencher MT, eds. *The Knee: AANA Advanced Arthroscopic Surgical Techniques* (pp 23-36).

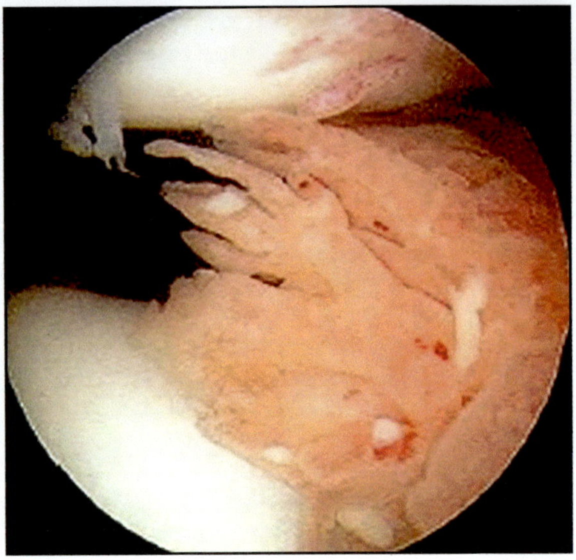

Figure 2-1. Arthroscopic photograph of focal PVNS within the patellofemoral articulation of the anterior compartment of the knee.

Arthroscopic synovectomy is indicated for a variety of conditions in patients who have been disabled for at least 6 months by pain and swelling and have not responded to conservative treatment. An established diagnosis of a synovial disorder is essential. In some instances, a histologic diagnosis should be made preoperatively.

Plica Syndrome

The medial knee plica can be found in approximately 70% of patients and may become hypersensitive after direct trauma to a flexed knee. It can also be sensitized from overuse. The lateral knee plica, when it exists, is rarely symptomatic. The clinical presentation is often similar to that of other conditions of the knee, including meniscal tear and patellar tendinitis, among others. There may be a snapping sensation along the medial knee during flexion on physical examination. Therefore, the diagnosis of plica syndrome is often clinical and a diagnosis of exclusion.[1] Magnetic resonance imaging (MRI) has been demonstrated to be of limited value in plica syndrome.[2] Arthroscopic resection of a symptomatic plica should be considered after a failed course of anti-inflammatory medication, consideration of steroids, and physical therapy. Diagnostic arthroscopic evaluation typically reveals an inflamed or hypertrophied medial plica. Postoperatively, mobilization and physical therapy is initiated immediately. In properly selected patients, good-to-excellent results can be expected after arthroscopic plica resection, with a success rate greater than 80% in one study.[3,4]

Pigmented Villonodular Synovitis

PVNS is a slowly progressing, locally invasive, and benign tumor of the synovium. It is characterized by the presence of hypertrophy and inflammation of the synovium with lobular, pedunculated lesions. Hemosiderin deposits within the synovium give it a classic brownish-red appearance (Figure 2-1). It is typically a monoarticular process, with the knee being most often affected. PVNS is subdivided into the following 2 entities: diffuse PVNS (DPVNS) and localized PVNS (LPVNS), with the diffuse form being the more common. LPVNS lesions typically originate at the meniscocapsular junction and are localized to the anterior compartment of the knee.

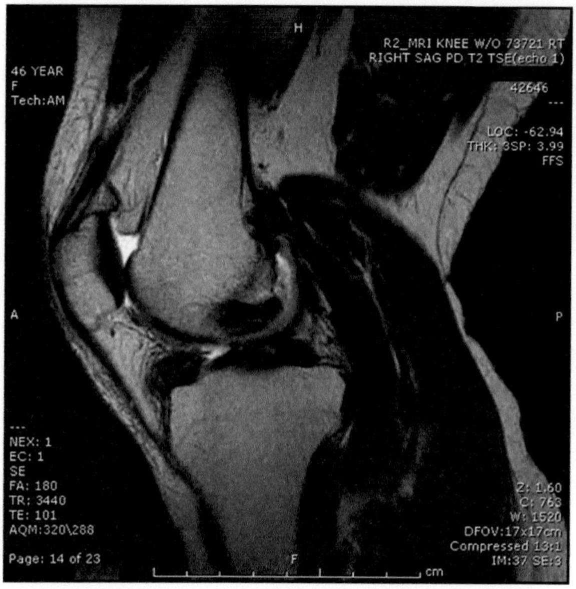

Figure 2-2. Proton density T2 sagittal MRI of PVNS.

Clinically, patients often present with symptoms similar to meniscal pathology as the synovium surrounding the anterior horn of the medial meniscus is most commonly affected. However, other localized areas of the knee, including the anterior horn of the lateral meniscus, medial/lateral recess, suprapatellar pouch, intercondylar notch, and suprapatellar fat pad, have been described. Due to its location, patients often present with symptoms such as pain, swelling, instability, locking, and catching.[5] LPVNS will typically present with more rapid onset of pain and swelling, which is in contrast to DPVNS, which is characterized by an insidious, slow progression of pain, swelling, and stiffness of the knee. Plain x-rays may demonstrate findings similar to that of a joint effusion or soft tissue swelling. These are present in less than 30% of PVNS cases. Thus, plain x-rays are not sensitive or specific enough to establish a correct diagnosis. On computed tomography (CT) scan, PVNS appears as a soft tissue mass with increased density compared to the muscle, and adjacent bony erosions and subchondral cysts may be seen. MRI currently remains the most useful diagnostic tool for PVNS (Figure 2-2). It allows the surgeon to better determine the extent of the lesions, especially in areas that are not easily accessible arthroscopically. High signal intensity regions may be present on T1 images (corresponding to fat deposition or hemorrhage) or T2 images (corresponding to joint effusion or synovial inflammation). Synovial fluid aspiration of the knee is not a reliable diagnostic tool as it typically yields brown or bloody fluid that may be seen in a variety of conditions and is not specific to PVNS.

Surgical resection is the treatment of choice for both LPVNS and DPVNS. Recurrence following excision of LPVNS is rare and after total synovectomy of DPVNS can be as low as 9%.[6] Malignant transformation and metastasis in patients with PVNS are rare, with a reported mortality rate of 50%.[7] Arthroscopic synovectomy is an effective treatment modality for PVNS, especially the localized form.[8] It has been associated with better functional results and lower rates of postoperative stiffness than open synovectomy as it allows for optimal visualization of lesions, especially in areas not easily accessible via an open technique, such as the posterior compartment. When compared to open synovectomy, arthroscopic synovectomy is associated with a shorter hospital stay and a shorter rehabilitation period. Flandry et al[6] demonstrated that rates of postoperative stiffness following open synovectomy were as high as 24% with the need for further manipulation. Nevertheless, improper use of this arthroscopic technique and an incomplete synovectomy may result in unacceptable recurrence rates. Arthroscopic synovectomy carries a risk of incomplete resection in DPVNS, as well as the theoretical risk of portal/joint seeding. In DPVNS, complete

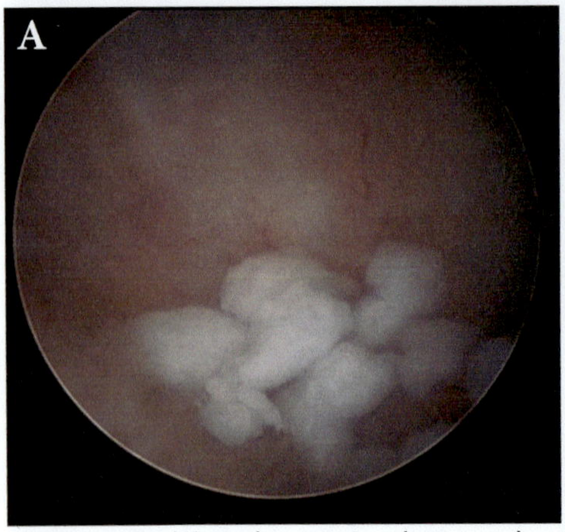

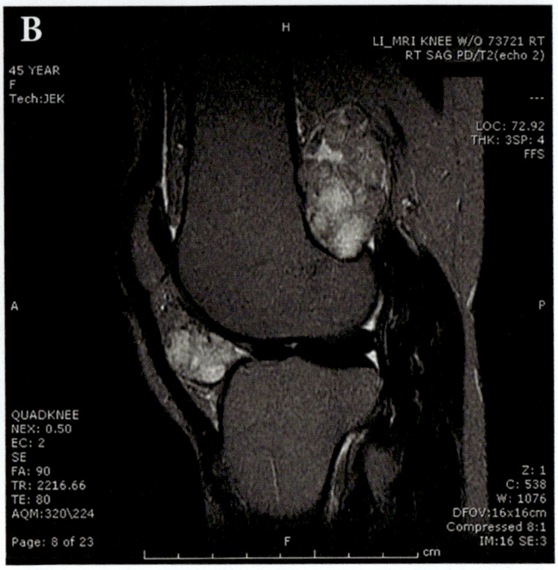

Figure 2-3. (A) Arthroscopic photograph of synovial chondromatosis. (B) T2-weighted sagittal MRI of synovial chondromatosis.

synovectomy is associated with better results and a substantially lower recurrence rate than partial excision.[9] However, complete arthroscopic synovectomy is technically demanding as the posterior compartment is almost always affected in DPVNS and recurrence rates are still significant.[8,10] Therefore, the surgeon must be comfortable working through posteromedial and posterolateral portals. With regard to the treatment of PVNS with invasion into the subchondral bone, open and arthroscopic techniques are reported to have a poor prognosis. Although radiation therapy has been used as an alternative treatment modality for invasive PVNS, results are mixed.[11,12] The combination of arthroscopic and open synovectomy for DPVNS shows promise and showed good results in recent studies with lower recurrence rates when compared to either modality alone.[11,13]

Synovial Chondromatosis/Osteochondromatosis

Synovial chondromatosis is a rare and benign metaplasia of the synovium in which numerous clusters of intra-articular cartilaginous and/or osteocartilaginous bodies are formed (Figure 2-3A). This condition most commonly occurs in middle-aged men and is often a monoarticular process, with more than 50% of cases presenting in the knee joint. It occurs in a primary or secondary form. Primary synovial chondromatosis occurs spontaneously with no preexisting identifiable joint pathology, whereas the secondary form presents in the setting of a preexistent, underlying disease, such as osteoarthritis, rheumatoid arthritis (RA), osteochondritis dissecans, etc. On presentation, patients will have pain, swelling, and possibly mechanical symptoms. The loose bodies are not typically revealed on plain x-rays in the absence of calcification. Therefore, CT scan is only useful for identifying calcified loose bodies. The usefulness of MRI depends on the degree of synovial proliferation and amount of calcification within these bodies. The cartilaginous nodules have intermediate signal intensity on T1-weighted images and high signal intensity on T2-weighted images (Figure 2-3B). MRI with intra-articular gadolinium contrast increases the sensitivity for detecting lesions.

Operative intervention is indicated for patients with recurrent painful effusions or mechanical symptoms. Although open treatment has been long described, arthroscopic synovectomy with removal of loose bodies has proven to be a safe and effective treatment for this disease.[14] The postoperative prognosis after excision is generally good, with low rates of recurrence and malignant transformation. Recurrence rates between arthroscopic and open synovectomy are equivalent, ranging from 0% to 31%. However, open treatment is associated with a higher incidence of prolonged rehabilitation and increased postoperative knee stiffness.

Synovial Hemangioma

Synovial hemangioma is a benign, vascular tumor that typically occurs in the knee. It is a rare condition and is more frequently seen in children and young adults. It presents as a recurrent, painful, monoarticular hemarthrosis. Patients will complain of pain, limited range of motion (ROM), and stiffness, with no history of prior trauma. An associated cutaneous hemangioma is seen in 40% of patients with a synovial hemangioma. On physical examination, a palpable, spongy, compressible mass may be present. Hemangiomas of the knee have been described in the following 3 forms: synovial, juxta-articular, or intermediate (containing both synovial and juxta-articular components). The intermediate form is often diffuse and considered unresectable. X-rays may reveal a soft tissue mass, calcified phleboliths, and/or hemophilia-like arthropathy with epiphyseal enlargement. On MRI, there is typically a lobulated, intra-articular mass with intermediate signal intensity on T1-weighted images and both high and low intensity areas on T2-weighted images. On the T2-weighted images, the high intensity areas represent pooling of blood in vascular spaces and the low intensity areas represent the fibrous septae of the vascular channel. MRI is essential to determine the location and extent of the lesion, thereby aiding in preoperative planning.[15]

Complete surgical excision of the mass is the definitive treatment, with preoperative embolization of the lesion often necessary to help reduce intra- and postoperative bleeding. Use of intraoperative coagulation/ablation during resection has also been shown to help reduce surgical bleeding.[16] For localized lesions, resection of the lesion with partial arthroscopic synovectomy is effective. For diffuse lesions, a complete synovectomy is required. Complete synovectomy is the only proven definitive treatment and is associated with a low recurrence rate. Successful complete arthroscopic synovectomy has been reported.

Popliteal (Baker's) Cyst

The popliteal (Baker's) cyst was first described by Lindgren as a continuous capsular fold of the posteromedial capsule and the gastrocnemius-semimembranosus bursa within which there is unidirectional flow as a result of a valvular mechanism.[17] This results in recurrent bursal effusions. The majority of popliteal cysts can be treated conservatively and, if symptomatic, are amenable to ultrasound-guided drainage. In children, they have a tendency to completely resolve over time with no treatment.[18] Reported recurrence rates after open resection of isolated popliteal cysts are high.[19] They are often associated with some other underlying intra-articular knee pathology, such as meniscal tear or degenerative joint disease. Often, arthroscopic management of a meniscal tear or early degenerative joint disease will resolve the symptomatic Baker's cyst. However, arthroscopic treatment of a popliteal cyst performed concurrently with other arthroscopic treatment of associated conditions may be considered. Effective treatment, both open and arthroscopic, involves the excision or obliteration of the slit-like valve that forms the channel between the knee joint and the bursal sack. Arthroscopic treatment techniques include an approach through the anteromedial portal,[20] a cystectomy through a posteromedial cystic portal, and all-inside suturing of the valve-like structure.[21] Regardless of the arthroscopic treatment technique chosen, all underlying associated intra-articular disorders must be addressed to minimize recurrence.

Hemophilia

Hemophilia is a group of genetic bleeding disorders characterized by a deficiency of factor VIII (hemophilia A) or factor IX (hemophilia B). Hemarthrosis is the most common and most disabling musculoskeletal manifestation of the disease, leading to arthropathy, capsular fibrosis, and joint contracture. Arthroscopic synovectomy is indicated in patients with recurrent hemarthroses that have failed conservative treatment for at least 6 months. Nevertheless, the presence of bony deformities, osteophytes, and joint destruction makes this procedure technically demanding. It has been shown to decrease the frequency of hemarthrosis, decrease the need for factor replacement, and improve pain and ROM.[22-24] The outcome following treatment is often correlated with the degree of joint destruction seen arthroscopically and on imaging.

An emphasis on maximizing factor replacement preoperatively is critical to prevent perioperative bleeding. Coordination with a hematologist is recommended for managing perioperative coagulation factor levels. Placement of a monitored drain and use of a compressive dressing postoperatively is recommended. Patients are typically admitted to the hospital for physical therapy, factor replacement, and monitoring. Postoperatively, use of a continuous passive motion machine will help facilitate early motion, and cryotherapy with ice packs can be used to improve pain and reduce swelling.

Seropositive Arthropathy

RA affects people predominantly between the ages of 35 and 50 years, with a 75% female predominance. Patients will present with pain and stiffness due to inflammation and, in severe cases, with hemorrhage and effusions, resulting in joint destruction over time. MRI will show enhancement in areas of bony erosion and cartilage loss.

New disease-modifying antirheumatic drugs (DMARDs) have revolutionized the treatment for RA. However, evidence supports that arthroscopic synovectomy can reduce joint destruction in younger patients who do not respond adequately to DMARDs, with the theoretical benefit of eliminating a major source of inflammatory chemokines and cytokines.[25] Although more technically demanding, complete arthroscopic synovectomy has advantages over conventional open synovectomy in that it is less invasive and, therefore, the preferred treatment in rheumatoid patients, who are at increased risk for postoperative infection and often have friable skin.[26] When compared to open treatment, complete arthroscopic synovectomy has also been shown to reduce intraoperative blood loss, hospital stay, and return to function.[27] However, one study showed a high recurrence rate when compared with open synovectomy.[28]

Seronegative Arthropathy

Seronegative arthropathy is a term used to describe a broad array of musculoskeletal conditions that share similar clinical and immunologic characteristics, including juvenile idiopathic arthritis, ankylosing spondylitis, psoriatic arthritis, and Reiter's syndrome. There is a genetic predisposition linked to the human leukocyte antigen genes, such as HLA-B27; therefore, it tends to run in families. Early in the disease process, patients typically present with generalized myalgia. As the disease progresses, patients go on to develop asymmetric joint pain and stiffness that worsens with inactivity and low back pain in addition to various nonmusculoskeletal symptoms, including constitutional symptoms, uveitis, urethritis, and gastrointestinal symptoms. Plain x-rays may show no abnormalities early in the disease, followed by progressive asymmetric oligoarticular joint involvement, juxta-articular osteoporosis, and a distinctive spinal pattern in the case of sacroiliitis and ankylosing spondylitis.

Treatment for seronegative arthritis starts with medication and physical therapy. In older patients with advanced disease and joint destruction, arthroplasty is the preferred definitive treatment, whereas synovectomy may serve as a prophylactic treatment measure in the growing child. Dell'Era et al reported results after synovectomy in children with juvenile idiopathic arthritis and found that arthroscopic synovectomy results in adequate postoperative knee ROM with shorter hospital stay when compared to open synovectomy.[29]

Contraindications/Controversial Indications

Absolute

- Intra-articular malignant conditions (eg, synovial sarcoma)
  - Treatment for such conditions is often radical excision with chemotherapy and/or radiation

Relative

- Surgeon lack of experience/proficiency
  - Performing a thorough synovectomy requires excellent technical skills and proficiency in arthroscopy. Inadequate/incomplete performance may lead to local recurrence and/or poor outcomes. Therefore, arthroscopic synovectomy is not recommended if the surgeon does not feel confident in his or her ability to perform a complete and adequate arthroscopic synovectomy. If this is the case, a traditional open approach should be utilized or the patient should be referred to an experienced arthroscopist.
- Severe arthritic changes/deformity/contractures
  - Such conditions may include advanced osteoarthritis, RA, seronegative arthritis, and hemophilia. In such cases, total knee arthroplasty is the definitive treatment of choice.

Pertinent Physical Findings

- Thorough history and physical exam
  - Document neurovascular status and discuss risk to posterior neurovascular structures when obtaining informed consent
- Effusion
  - Aspiration often performed to obtain synovial fluid analysis for diagnostic purposes, and in some cases provide temporary pain relief
- Reduced ROM and/or pain with passive ROM
- Tenderness to palpation, often diffuse in cases of inflammatory arthropathy
- Mechanical symptoms of clicking, catching, or locking

Preoperative Pertinent Imaging

- Standard knee x-rays to evaluate status of joint (eg, periarticular erosions in RA) and overall alignment/presence of any deformity
- MRI in evaluation of PVNS, synovial chondromatosis, hemangioma, and inflammatory arthropathies to evaluate synovium, extent of disease, and rule out other intra-articular lesions
- MRI in PVNS classically demonstrates low T1 and low T2 signal (due to hemosiderin deposits) and is useful in determining extent of intra- and extra-articular disease
- CT in cases of synovial chondromatosis is only useful when loose, calcific bodies are present

Operative Planning

X-rays and MRI images should be reviewed and accessible in the operating room prior to the start of the procedure. The authors recommend the use of a light general anesthetic. Consideration of local or regional nerve blocks may aid in the reduction of postoperative pain if needed. After the induction of general anesthesia, an examination under anesthesia should be performed, evaluating both the ROM and stability of the knee and compared to the contralateral knee. The incidence of infections with arthroscopy is very low. Nevertheless, the authors agree with the recent recommendations for patient weight-based dosing of cefazolin or clindamycin for true penicillin allergies, within 1 hour of incision or tourniquet inflation.

Equipment

The use of a well-padded thigh tourniquet may be considered as a more complete synovectomy may result in increased bleeding that can make visibility during arthroscopy difficult. In most cases, a 30-degree arthroscope is used for the majority of the procedure. Nevertheless, for adequate visualization of the posterior compartment, a 70-degree arthroscope is often necessary and should be available for the entire procedure. Initially, the inflow pump should be set at a low setting to reduce knee distention and fluid extravasation intraoperatively. It can be adjusted throughout the procedure accordingly. Although choice of shaver depends on the anatomy of the patient and the location of the synovectomy, a variety of shaver sizes should also be available. A 5.5-mm full-radius synovectomy blade is effective in the anterior compartment. A 3.5-mm full-radius synovectomy blade or a 4.5-mm curved synovial resector can be used in smaller knees or hard to reach areas, such as the posterior compartment and under the menisci.

Positioning and Portals

The patient is placed supine on the operative table. The authors' preference is that the operative leg be placed into a thigh-holding device 4 finger-breadths above the superior patella such that when the foot of the bed is lowered, the leg is allowed to hang free off the end of the table. This allows for deep flexion and varus/valgus stress of the knee without compromise of portal position. The well leg is placed into a well-leg holder. Alternatively, the procedure can be performed supine with knee flexed over the side of the table against a lateral post with the well leg placed supine on the flattened operative table. The operative extremity is then prepped and draped in the usual sterile technique.

Proper portal placement is critical for any arthroscopic procedure. Improper portal placement can lead to iatrogenic injury to the knee as well as inadequate synovectomy due to the difficulty of the procedure. It is often helpful to draw out the anatomy prior to obtaining the portals. A complete arthroscopic synovectomy of the knee can be performed through the use of a combination of 6 portals: anterolateral, anteromedial, lateral suprapatellar, medial suprapatellar, posterolateral, and posteromedial (Figure 2-4). In morbidly obese patients, direct visualization intra-articularly may be necessary when establishing the anterolateral and anteromedial portals in order to ensure proper portal placement. Palpation of bony landmarks is often precluded by excessive adipose tissue. Therefore, it may be helpful to establish a lateral suprapatellar or medial suprapatellar portal first in order to establish an anterolateral portal under direct visualization through which an anteromedial portal can then also be establish under direct visualization.

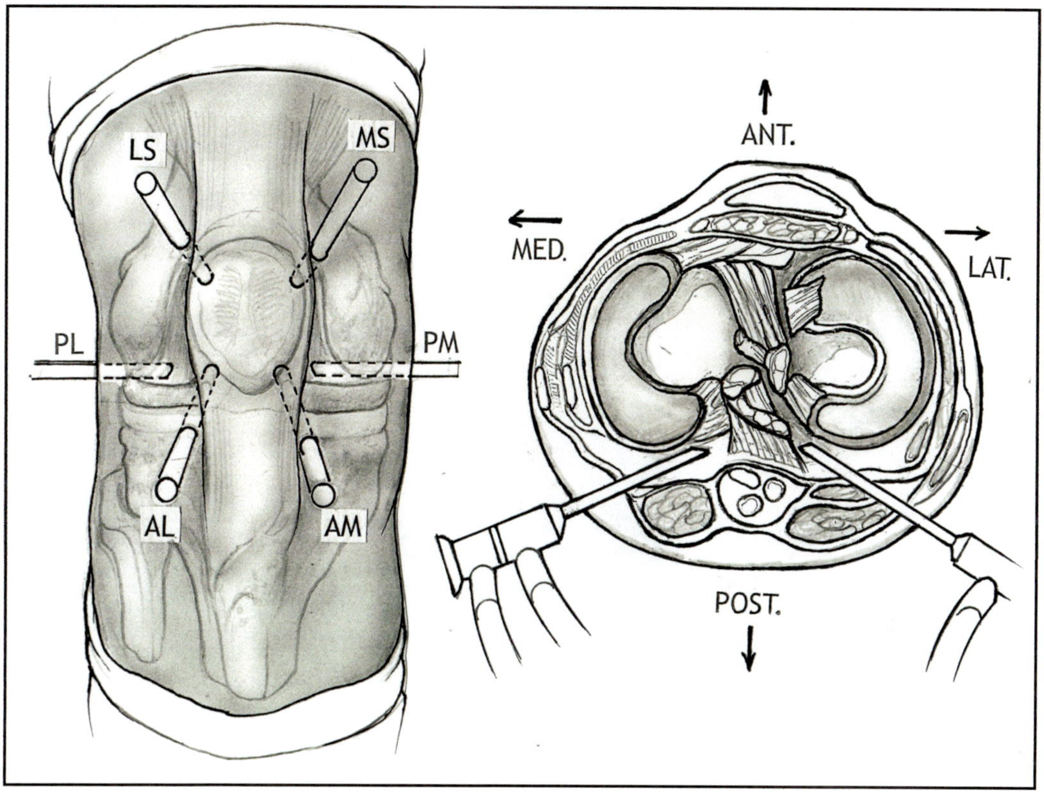

Figure 2-4. Illustration of the 6 arthroscopic portals used in a complete arthroscopic synovectomy of the knee.

Step-by-Step Description of the Procedure

Step-by-Step

- Supine position, well-padded thigh tourniquet, thigh-holding device 4-finger breadths above the superior patella, well leg placed in well-leg holder
- Operative leg prepped and draped in usual sterile fashion
- Mark out bony landmarks for eventual portal placement
- Inflate tourniquet
- Establish anterolateral and anteromedial portals in routine fashion
- Perform standard diagnostic arthroscopy
- With camera in suprapatellar pouch, establish lateral suprapatellar and medial suprapatellar portals
- Perform synovectomy as indicated, utilizing triangulation to gain access to the gutters, anterior compartment, and intercondylar notch
- Visualize the posterior compartments with the knee flexed 70 to 90 degrees
- Establish posteromedial and posterolateral portals under direct visualization
- Utilize 70-degree arthroscope to perform synovectomies of the posteromedial and posterolateral compartments in systematic fashion

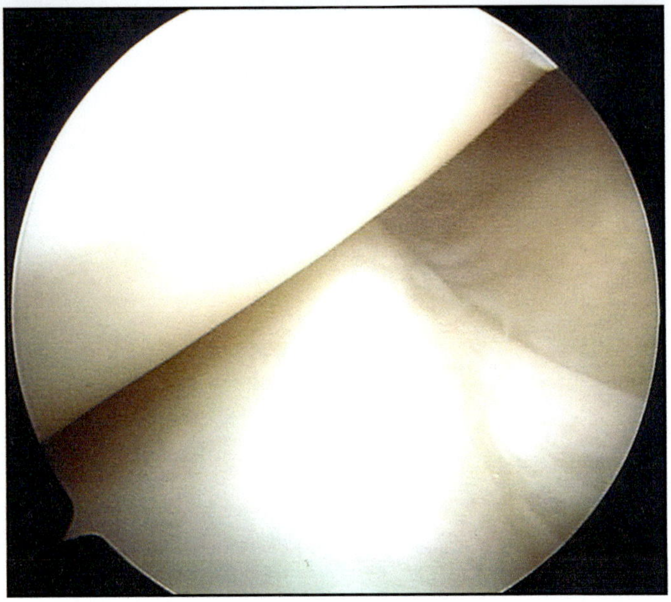

Figure 2-5. Arthroscopic view of the posteromedial compartment of the knee using the Gillquist maneuver.

Description of the Procedure

After the anterolateral and anteromedial portals are established, a standard diagnostic arthroscopy is performed, visualizing and probing the suprapatellar pouch, medial and lateral gutters, trochlear groove, undersurface of the patella, medial and lateral compartments, including the mensci, intercondylar notch, and cruciate ligaments. Any concurrent intra-articular pathology seen during diagnostic arthroscopy, such as meniscal or chondral injury, can be addressed throughout the procedure. In cases in which a pathologic specimen is required, an arthroscopic biter may then be used through the anteromedial portal to obtain a synovial tissue sample from an area of significant pathology. Alternatively, an arthroscopic trap may be placed in the suction tubing of the shaver to obtain significant quantities of resected synovium.

With the camera looking into the suprapatellar pouch, the lateral suprapatellar and medial suprapatellar portals are established under direct visualization approximately 1 cm above and 1 cm lateral (for lateral suprapatellar) or medial (for medial suprapatellar) to the corner of the patella. The 5.5- or 4.5-mm full-radius synovectomy blade can be used through these portals to resect the synovium in the suprapatellar pouch and the upper lateral and medial gutters and to access any portion of a hypertrophic anterior fat pad. Synovial resection is adequate when the shiny capsular layer that lies directly beneath is seen. The lower portions of the lateral and medial gutters can be accessed for resection by alternating the camera through the lateral and medial suprapatellar portals and using the shavers through the anterolateral and anteromedial portals. Next, synovectomy in the anterior compartment and intercondylar notch can be achieved by triangulation of the arthroscope and shaver through the anteromedial and anterolateral portals. The lower lateral and medial gutters can also be visualized and resected through these 2 portals.

There is a 15- to 28-mm safe zone between the posterior cruciate ligament and the popliteal neurovascular bundle for safe arthroscopy of the posterior knee.[30] By holding the knee flexed at 70 to 90 degrees, one can gain better access to the posterior compartment as the intercondylar notch is widened and the neurovascular bundle falls more posteriorly. A 70-degree arthroscope is then used for visualization of the posterior compartment. Furthermore, this allows the posterior neurovascular bundle to fall posteriorly. A modified Gillquist maneuver is performed with the arthroscope through the anterolateral portal and advanced under the posterior cruciate ligament in order to establish a posteromedial portal under direct visualization (Figure 2-5). Palpation of

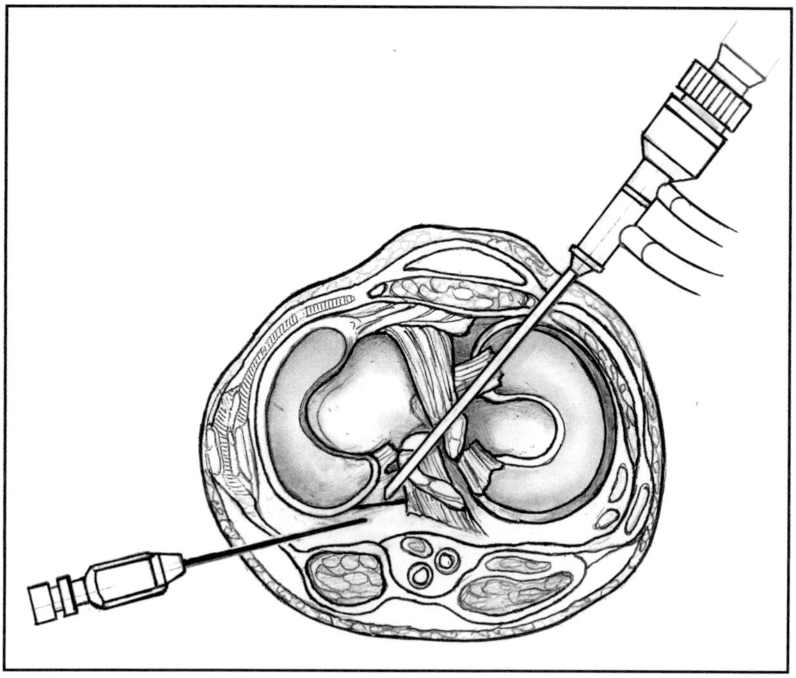

Figure 2-6. Illustration showing the arthroscopic technique for obtaining a posteromedial portal. A spinal needle is introduced into the posteromedial corner of the knee joint aiming anteriorly under direct visualization.

the posteromedial knee is performed under visualization to better localize portal placement. At this time, a spinal needle is introduced into the posteromedial corner of the knee joint aiming anteriorly (Figure 2-6). Dimming of the overhead and room lights and transillumination using the arthroscopy may also aid in introduction of the spinal needle. The posteromedial portal is the then established, and a blunt cannula is introduced via this portal. The cannula is best introduced over a switching stick to allow for easier and more accurate cannula placement. Caution must be exercised when introducing any instrument into the joint in this location with an emphasis on aiming slightly anteriorly to avoid iatrogenic injury to the posterior neurovascular bundle. The posteromedial portal is typically placed 16 to 35 mm from the saphenous vein.[30] Synovectomy of the posteromedial knee is then performed through this portal with a 4.5-mm shaver systematically from the periphery to the center. One must be mindful of the suction during this part of the procedure to avoid drawing the posterior capsule into the shaver, thereby risking accidental iatrogenic injury to vital posterior structures.

Lastly, the lateral portion of the posterior compartment is then accessed similarly by switching the arthroscope to the anteromedial portal. Holding the knee flexed at 90 degrees will allow the common peroneal nerve to fall further posteriorly behind the biceps femoris tendon. A spinal needle is introduced anterior to the biceps femoris tendon, 1 cm above the joint line and 1 cm posterior to the femoral condyle. The posterolateral portal is established and then cannulated like the posteromedial portal. The posterolateral portal is typically placed 40 to 52 mm from the peroneal nerve.[30] Synovectomy of the posterolateral knee is then performed similar to the posteromedial side in a systematic fashion.

Postoperative Protocol

Depending on the extent of synovectomy performed, a drain may be placed and monitored for at least 1 day prior to removal to reduce postoperative hemarthrosis. Nevertheless, this may not be needed if the bleeding is not significant at the conclusion of the case. A compressive dressing is applied to the knee. Patients can be made partial weightbearing with crutches for assistance and are typically discharged the same day or on the first postoperative day. Cryotherapy with ice packs can aid in postoperative reduction in pain and swelling. Oral pain medication should be prescribed, and physical therapy should start early to ensure rapid restoration of normal gait, ROM, and strength. Patients should be provided with written home instructions to begin immediate postoperative home therapy with a focus on active ROM and quadriceps strengthening. Although not critical, the use of a continuous passive motion machine to facilitate early motion is reasonable. The majority of patients approach near normal activity level by the fourth postoperative week.

Potential Complications

Complications resulting from arthroscopic synovectomy are similar to those of any arthroscopic procedure, including anesthesia concerns, infection, bleeding, deep venous thrombosis, arthrofibrosis, and iatrogenic injury to articular cartilage or neurovascular structures. Caution must be taken during the procedure to maneuver the arthroscope or instruments to avoid excessive pressure on the articular cartilage and to direct instruments away from vulnerable posterior structures when using the posterolateral and posteromedial portals, namely the neurovascular bundle, saphenous vein and nerve, and the common peroneal nerve. Other complications specific to arthroscopic synovectomy include hemarthrosis resulting in pain and stiffness, postoperative arthrofibrosis requiring a manipulation or arthroscopic lysis of adhesions, reflex sympathetic dystrophy, or incomplete resection resulting in recurrence or persistence of the synovial pathology, thereby requiring additional surgery.

Top Technical Pearls for the Procedure

1. Proper portal placement is paramount to achieve an adequate synovectomy and to avoid iatrogenic injury to articular cartilage and vital structures. Establishment of portals under direct visualization through an already obtained portal can aid in proper portal placement and facilitate the surgeon's ability to thoroughly access and remove all areas of pathologic synovium.
2. A modified Gillquist maneuver is performed with the knee flexed at 90 degrees and a 70-degree arthroscope through the anterolateral portal. It is advanced under the posterior cruciate ligament in order to access the posteromedial compartment. Through palpation under direct visualization, dimming of the operating room lights, and use of a spinal needle, proper posteromedial portal placement is achieved. The posterolateral portal is established in similar fashion.
3. A 5.5-mm full-radius shaver is effective in the anterior compartment and is often the workhorse for most of the procedure, whereas a 3.5-mm full-radius shaver or a 4.5-mm curved synovial resector can be used in smaller knees or hard to reach areas, such as the posterior compartment and under the menisci.
4. Synovectomy of the posterior knee is performed through the posterolateral and posteromedial portals with a 4.5-mm shaver, working systematically from the periphery to the center, alternating portals as needed.
5. Caution must be exercised when introducing any instrument into the posterior compartment of the knee, with an emphasis on aiming anteriorly to avoid iatrogenic injury to the posterior neurovascular bundle.

References

1. Shetty VD, Vowler SL, Krishnamurthy S, Halliday AE. Clinical diagnosis of medial plica syndrome of the knee: a prospective study. *J Knee Surg.* 2007;20(4):277-280.
2. Monabang CZ, De Maeseneer M, Shahabpour M, Lenchik L, Pouliart N. MR imaging findings in patients with a surgically significant mediopatellar plica. *JBR-BRT.* 2007;90(5):384-387.
3. Weckström M, Niva MH, Lamminen A, Mattila VM, Pihlajamäki KH. Arthroscopic resection of medial plica of the knee in young adults. *Knee.* 2010;17(2):103-107.
4. Muse GL, Grana WA, Hollingsworth S. Arthroscopic treatment of medial shelf syndrome. *Arthroscopy.* 2010;26(3):391-392.
5. Dines JS, Bernadino TM, Wells JL, et al. Long-term follow-up of surgically treated localized pigmented villonodular synovitis of the knee. *Arthroscopy.* 2007;23(9):930-937.
6. Flandry FC, Hughston JC, Jacobson KE, Barrack RL, McCann SB, Kurtz DM. Surgical treatment of diffuse pigmented villonodular synovitis of the knee. *Clin Orthop Relat Res.* 1994;(300):183-192.
7. Bertoni F, Unni K, Beabout JW, Sim FH. Malignant giant cell tumor of the tendon sheaths and joints (malignant pigmented vilonodular synovitis). *Am J Surg Pathol.* 1997;21(2):153-163.
8. Jain JK, Vidyasagar JV, Sagar R, Patel H, Chetan ML, Bajaj A. Arthroscopic synovectomy in pigmented villonodular synovitis of the knee: clinical series and outcome. *Int Orthop.* 2013;37(12):2363-2369.
9. De Ponti A, Sansone V, Malcherè M. Result of arthroscopic treatment of pigmented villonodular synovitis of the knee. *Arthroscopy.* 2003;19(6):602-607.
10. Sharma V, Cheng EY. Outcomes after excision of pigmented villonodular synovitis of the knee. *Clin Orthop Relat Res.* 2009;467(11):2852-2858.
11. de Carvalho LH Jr, Soares LF, Goncalves MB, Temponi EF, de Melo Silva O Jr. Long-term success in the treatment of diffuse pigmented villonodular synovitis of the knee with subtotal synovectomy and radiotherapy. *Arthroscopy.* 2012;28(9):1271-1274.
12. Park G, Kim YS, Kim JH, et al. Low-dose external beam radiotherapy as a postoperative treatment for patients with diffuse pigmented villonodular synovitis of the knee: 4 recurrences in 23 patients followed for mean 9 years. *Acta Orthop.* 2012;83(3):256-260.
13. Colman MW, Ye J, Weiss KR, Goodman MA, McGough RL III. Does combined open and arthroscopic synovectomy for diffuse PVNS of the knee improve recurrence rates? *Clin Orthop Relat Res.* 2013;471(3):883-890.
14. Samson L, Mazurkiewicz S, Treder M, Wiśniewski P. Outcome in the arthroscopic treatment of synovial chondromatosis of the knee. *Orthop Traumatol Rehabil.* 2005;7(4):391-396.
15. Winzenberg T, Ma D, Taplin P, Parker A, Jones G. Synovial haemangioma of the knee: a case report. *Clin Rheumatol.* 2006;25(5):753-755.
16. Barakat MJ, Hirehal K, Hopkins JR, Gosal HS. Synovial hemangioma of the knee. *J Knee Surg.* 2007;20(4):296-298.
17. Lindgren PG: Gastrocnemio-semimembranosus bursa and its relation to the knee joint. III. Pressure measurements in joint and bursa. *Acta Radiol Diagn (Stockh).* 1978;19(2):377-388.
18. Akagi R, Saisu T, Segawa Y, et al. Natural history of popliteal cysts in the pediatric population. *J Pediatr Orthop.* 2013;33(3):262-268.
19. Takahashi M, Nagano A. Arthroscopic treatment of popliteal cyst and visualization of its cavity through the posterior portal of the knee. *Arthroscopy.* 2005;21(5):638.
20. Sansone V, DePonti A. Arthroscopic treatment of popliteal cyst and associated intra-articular knee disorders in adults. *Arthroscopy.* 1999;15(4):368-372.
21. Calvisi V, Lupparelli S, Giuliani P. Arthroscopic all-inside suture of symptomatic Baker's cysts: a technical option for surgical treatment in adults. *Knee Surg Sports Traumatol Arthrosc.* 2007;15(12):1452-1460.
22. Yoon KH, Bae DK, Kim HS, Song SJ. Arthroscopic synovectomy in haemophilic arthropathy of the knee. *Int Orthop.* 2005;29(5):296-300.
23. Verma N, Valentino LA, Chawla A. Arthroscopic synovectomy in haemophilia: indications, technique and results. *Haemophilia.* 2007;13(suppl 3):38-44.
24. de Almeida AM, de Rezende MU, Cordeiro FG, et al. Arthroscopic partial anterior synovectomy of the knee on patients with haemophilia [published online ahead of print October 12, 2013]. *Knee Surg Sport Traumatol Arthrosc.*

25. Ogawa H, Itokazu I, Ito Y, Fukata M, Shimizu K. The therapeutic outcome of minimally invasive synovectomy assisted with arthroscopy in the rheumatoid knee. *Mod Rheumatol.* 2006;16(6):360-363.
26. Kim SJ, Jung KA, Kwun JD, Kim JM. Arthroscopic synovectomy of the knee joint in rheumatoid arthritis: surgical steps for complete synovectomy. *Arthroscopy.* 2006;22(4)461.e1-461.e4.
27. Masłoń A, Witoński D, Pieszyński I, Grzegorzewski A, Snyder M. Early clinical results of open and arthroscopic synovectomy in knee inflammation. *Orthop Traumatol Rehabil.* 2007;9(5):520-526.
28. Chalmers PN, Sherman SL, Raphael BS, Su EP. Rheumatoid synovectomy: does the surgical approach matter? *Clin Orthop Relat Res.* 2011;469(7):2062-2071.
29. Dell'Era L, Facchini R, Corona F. Knee synovectomy in children with juvenile idiopathic arthritis. *J Pediatr Orthop B.* 2008;17(3):128-130.
30. Pace JL, Wahl CJ. Arthroscopy of the posterior knee compartments: neurovascular anatomic relationships during arthroscopic transverse capsulotomy. *Arthroscopy.* 2010;26(5):637-642.

Please see videos on the accompanying website at www.routledge.com/9781617119996

3

Arthroscopic Treatment of Popliteal Cysts

Julie A. Dodds, MD

Introduction

Popliteal cysts occur relatively commonly in patients older than 50 years. Anatomists have been aware of the presence of popliteal cysts for more than 150 years. Adams[1] first described popliteal cysts in 1840 as an "enlarged bursa that is normally situated beneath the inner head of the gastrocnemius and communicates with the joint by a species of valvular opening." In 1897, Baker[2] described the association of the cyst with the semimembranosus bursa and with this, his name became associated with the cyst, frequently now called "Baker's cyst." Most of the popliteal cysts occurring at the time of Adams and Baker were due to the inflammation and swelling associated with tuberculosis of the knee. Although there have been a few modifications to the descriptions of these cysts, the popliteal cyst is best defined as an enlargement of the gastrocnemius-semimembranosus bursa, which communicates with the knee joint via a valve-like structure.[3-6] It is the presence of this valve-like structure that allows the cysts to be successfully treated via arthroscopic surgery.

Previous surgical treatment of popliteal cysts via the open approach has been described by multiple authors.[6-8] Complications have included fistula formation, recurrence, abscess, and saphenous nerve injury.[6,8] Many of these complications can be avoided by using an arthroscopic approach. Arthroscopic treatment of popliteal cysts was first described by Sansone and De Ponti.[9] Their treatment consisted mainly of decompression of the cyst through a hole in the posterior capsule. With this, at 1 year, all patients showed reduction in the size of the cyst, with 95% of patients displaying "optimal or good clinical results" at 2 years postoperatively. This technique has been further refined[10-12] by taking down the capsular fold that has been consistently identified in nearly all patients with popliteal cysts.[13] Ahn et al defined clearly the location of the valvular capsular fold at the medial aspect of the medial head of the gastrocnemius and described the technique they used to resect the fold.[11] Also described by Ahn et al was a posteromedial cystic portal, which provides access to the cyst itself. This portal is located just superior to the posteromedial portal and is used for resection of cyst walls if indicated. Follow-up magnetic resonance imaging (MRI) at a minimum of 6 months showed complete disappearance or significant decrease in size

Sgaglione NA, Lubowitz JH, Provencher MT, eds. *The Knee: AANA Advanced Arthroscopic Surgical Techniques* (pp 37-52).

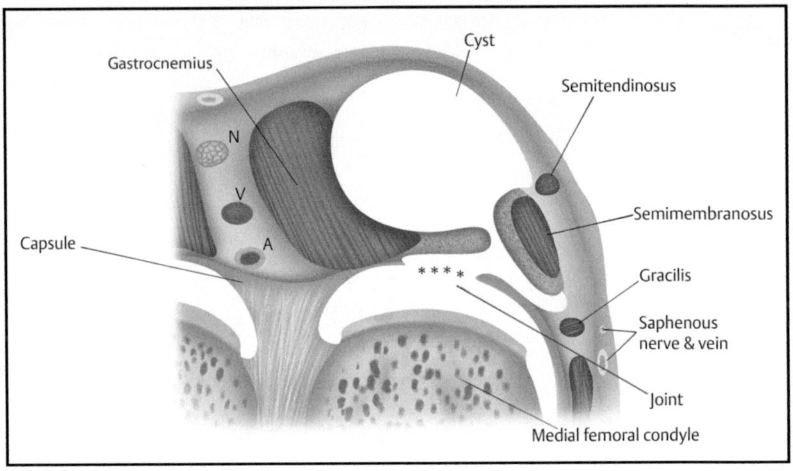

Figure 3-1. Cross-sectional anatomy of the location of a typical popliteal cyst. Note the superficial location of the tibial nerve (N) as compared to tibial vein (V) and artery (A). Asterisks (***) indicate the location of transverse synovial flap, which functions as one-way valve.

in all cysts and improved clinical outcomes in 94% of patients,[12] thus confirming the viability and value of arthroscopic treatment of popliteal cysts.

Popliteal cysts can be noted as incidental findings on MRI scan or can be severe enough to cause nerve and/or vascular complications. They have been noted in 30% of cadaver specimens[14] and have been identified on 5% of knee MRIs.[15] It is essential that the surgeon perform a precise history and physical examination to discern which popliteal cysts warrant treatment, surgical or nonsurgical. Pediatric popliteal cysts are usually asymptomatic and often resolve without treatment.[16]

Posteromedial knee mass and/or pain are the most common presenting symptoms of popliteal cysts. Cysts that exceed 5 cm are more likely to be symptomatic. Pain arising from the cyst itself is often difficult to discern from the posterior knee pain arising from associated intra-articular pathology, such as posterior horn medial meniscal tears. A sensation of fullness and the intermittent nature of the posteromedial pain as effusions and cyst distension occur tend to point toward a symptomatic cyst. Neurovascular compromise can also cause symptoms. Because of the more medial position of the nerve, most commonly seen are tibial nerve compression symptoms, including pain, gastrocnemius weakness and atrophy, burning sensations, and parasthesias. Tibial vein compromise can lead to pseudothrombophlebitic symptoms, including pain, swelling, and lymphedema. Arterial compromise is rare due to the medial and deep position of the tibial artery and its stiff walls (Figure 3-1). Rupture of a popliteal cyst has been known to cause acute compartment syndrome, necessitating acute fasciotomy.[17]

The accumulation and persistence of fluid within a popliteal cyst is proposed to be caused by 2 factors. The first is the overproduction of synovial fluid within the joint because of intra-articular pathology, synovitis, or both. Common intra-articular pathologies include chondromalacia, chondral debris, or meniscal tears. Systemic arthropathies, such as rheumatoid arthritis, gout, or chondrocalcinosis, can also cause persistent effusions. Increased synovial fluid within the joint is forced out through the posteromedial opening into the popliteal cyst, when present, and then becomes trapped within the cyst because of the 1-directional flow between the intra-articular cavity and the cyst due to the valvular mechanism.

Nonsurgical treatment has consisted of nonsteroidal anti-inflammatory drugs (NSAIDs), intra-articular corticosteroid injection,[18] and direct cyst aspiration with steroid injection. Aspiration of the cyst and injection with corticosteroid is felt to yield similar results to intra-articular corticosteroid injection.[19] NSAIDs may be effective if the knee effusion is caused by systemic arthropathy, such as rheumatoid arthritis. If intra-articular pathology exists, complete nonsurgical treatment may be less effective. Medial meniscal tears have been noted to be the most common pathology associated with popliteal cysts.[20] Addressing the intra-articular pathology, such as performing meniscectomy, may be adequate to allow the joint effusion to dissipate and the cyst may resolve on its own.[21] However, in patients with intra-articular pathology that cannot be corrected by arthroscopic means, such as high-grade chondral lesions (grades III and IV), the cyst often remains following arthroscopy, leading to poor patient satisfaction.[21] Symptomatic popliteal cysts in these patients are amenable to arthroscopic decompression of the cyst.

Indications

- Painful cyst (usually larger than 5 cm)
- Cyst causing neurovascular compromise
- Cyst occurring in the presence of grade III or IV chondromalacia or synovial disease
- Cyst not responding to conservative treatment

The most logical indication for arthroscopic treatment of popliteal cysts is a symptomatic cyst (usually larger than 5 cm), which occurs in a knee in which at least a portion of the intra-articular pathology will not be corrected by arthroscopic treatment (eg, grade III or IV chondromalacia). Also, arthroscopic treatment of the symptomatic cyst is indicated in knees without intra-articular pathology other than synovitis, such as seen in chondrocalcinosis or rheumatoid disease, in which conservative treatment (steroid injections, NSAIDs) has failed.

Loose bodies may also be present in popliteal cysts. These may cause continued fluid accumulation within the cyst, contributing to its inability to resorb, again necessitating arthroscopic treatment of the cyst itself.

Pertinent Physical Findings

- A mass can usually be palpated at or just below the joint line slightly medial to the midline in the popliteal fossa. Its medial position is due to the position of the cyst medial to the medial head of the gastrocnemius muscle and lateral to the semimembranosus muscle. Although most frequently extending distally to the joint line, the cyst can occasionally extend proximally, leading to fullness above the joint line and more central location, following the course proximally of the semimembranosus tendon.
- Ruptured cysts can cause acute compartment syndrome findings, such as pain with passive dorsiflexion of the foot.
- Venous compression can cause swelling and lymphedema.
- Tibial nerve compression can cause gastrocnemius atrophy and weakness.
- As mentioned previously, arterial compromise is rare.

Pertinent Imaging

- MRI is essential for preoperative planning prior to arthroscopic treatment of the cyst. Identifying the fluid collection as a true popliteal (Baker's) cyst can be best done by noting the surrounding structures on the MRI (Figure 3-2). The neck of the fluid collection must be present between the medial head of the gastrocnemius and the semimembranosus tendon for the pathology to be present, which is amenable to arthroscopic treatment. The valvular communication between the cyst and the joint is always present in this location. This is best identified on the axial sections. The cyst itself usually lies medial to the medial head of the

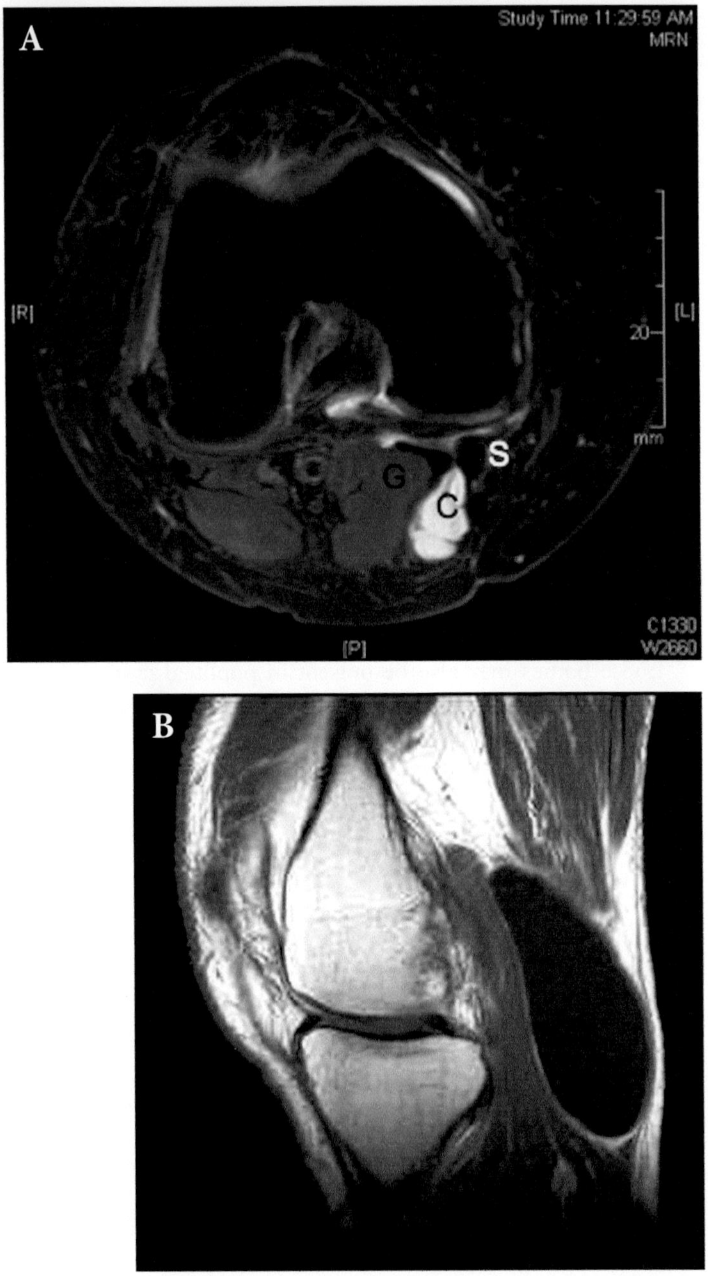

Figure 3-2. (A) Axial and (B) sagittal MRIs of a popliteal cyst (C). Note the location of the neck of the cyst between the medial head of the gastrocnemius muscle (G) and the semimembranosus tendon (S).

gastrocnemius. Locating the most superficial portion of the cyst on MRI is also important if cyst excision or loose body excision is to be performed. This can be best identified on the sagittal and coronal sections. If the cyst extends proximal to the joint line, it often follows the course of the semimembranosus tendon proximally, toward the midline of the popliteal fossa, often abutting the neurovascular bundle (Figure 3-3). This is essential to note if considering cystectomy. MRI may also help define other pathology that is to be addressed at the time of arthroscopy, such as meniscal tears and chondral injury, which are commonly associated with popliteal cysts.[20,21] MRI will also assist in diagnosing other popliteal masses that can present in a similar fashion. Although rare, popliteal artery aneurysms, synovial cell sarcomas, and

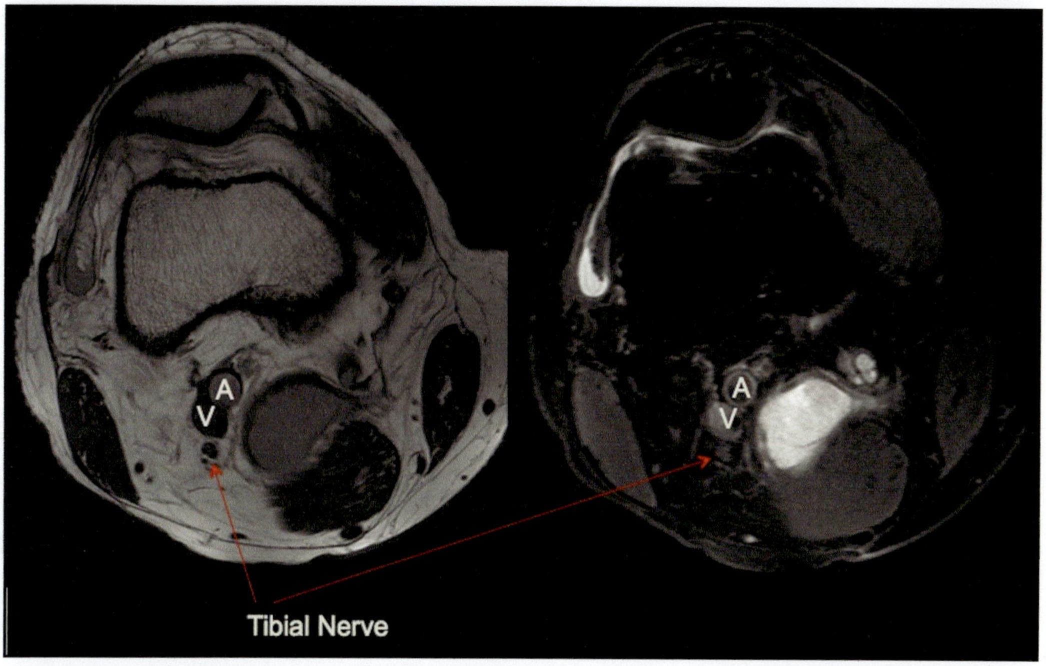

Figure 3-3. Axial MRI of a large popliteal cyst extending proximal to the joint line. Note the proximity of the cyst to the tibial nerve, vein (V), and artery (A).

hemangiomas can be mistaken for popliteal cysts on initial presentation. MRI findings for these entities differ greatly from popliteal cysts.

- Although ultrasound can also be used to diagnose and define a popliteal cyst, the surgeon must have an excellent understanding of the images and have the ability to identify surrounding structures. It is essential to have knowledge of the actual shape and position of the cyst.

Equipment

Standard arthroscopic equipment is required for arthroscopic decompression of popliteal cysts. In order to easily obtain access to the posteromedial aspect of the knee, a second arthroscopic sheath is recommended. An 18-gauge spinal needle is used for localization of portals. An arthroscopic shaver and biting baskets are often required for resection of the valvular mechanism, and arthroscopic graspers need to be available for loose bodies that may be encountered within the cyst. A 70-degree arthroscope is occasionally used to assist in visualization.

Positioning and Portals

The patient is placed in the supine position on the operating table. The operative knee is placed in a leg holder and flexed to 90 degrees over the end of the table. Care is taken to place the tourniquet and the leg holder high on the thigh, and the patient is brought as caudal as possible over the end of the table to allow better access to the posterior knee as needed. The well leg is placed in a flexed and abducted position in a well-leg holder to allow easier access to the medial aspect of the operative knee. It is recommended that gravity inflow only be used to minimize the chance of posterior fluid extravasation, possibly leading to compartment syndrome or venous compromise.

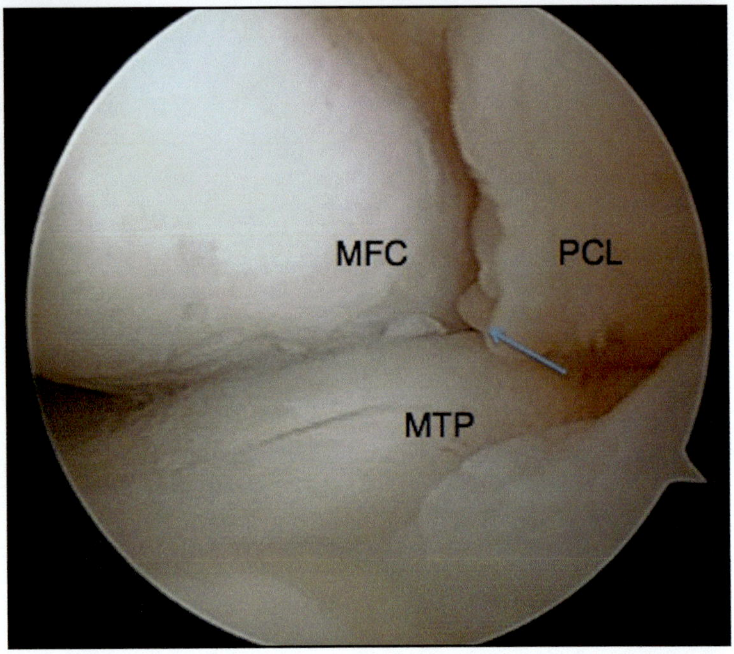

Figure 3-4. Arthroscopic image of the trifurcation location between the medial tibial plateau (MTP), MFC, and PCL for passage of the arthroscopic sheath into the posteromedial compartment.

Step-by-Step Description of the Procedure

After proper patient positioning, standard anteromedial and anterolateral portals are created. These portals are positioned close to the patellar tendon to allow passage through the notch into the posteromedial aspect of the knee. Intra-articular pathology is addressed in the standard fashion. The arthroscope is then passed into the posteromedial aspect of the knee. This is most easily performed under direct visualization. The arthroscope is transferred into the anteromedial portal and the "trifurcation" of the medial tibial plateau, medial femoral condyle (MFC), and the posterior cruciate ligament (PCL) is noted (Figure 3-4). An arthroscopic sheath is then passed from the anterolateral portal to the trifurcation and then guided between the PCL and the MFC into the posteromedial aspect of the knee. Due to the varying shape of the femoral condyle, the surgeon must be familiar with alternative methods. If the sheath does not pass easily, the passage can also be attempted from the anteromedial portal, visualizing from the anterolateral portal. If notch osteophytes are present, a burr may be needed to take down a small portion of the medial aspect of the MFC to allow the sheath to proceed past the condyle. It is also recommended that inflow be placed on the arthroscopic sheath to allow better distension of the compartment directly ahead of the arthroscope.

Once the sheath has been passed, the arthroscope is then transferred into the sheath to allow visualization of the posteromedial aspect of the knee. A spinal needle is used for localization of the posteromedial portal (Figure 3-5). The joint line is palpated, and the spinal needle is inserted percutaneously into the posteromedial knee under direct visualization (Figure 3-6). Transillumination can often be used to visualize and avoid the saphenous vein and the accompanying saphenous nerve. The spinal needle is also used for location of the valvular flap. This flap has been termed the *posterior transverse synovial infold (PoTSI) lesion*. It has been noted to be present on the majority of popliteal cysts (Figure 3-7). It is not always readily evident, and the spinal needle can be used to gently probe the posterior capsule to locate the PoTSI lesion. It is consistently located medial to the medial head of the gastrocnemius tendon at or just above the joint line. Upon moving the PoTSI lesion inferior, the opening into the cyst is often realized (Figure 3-8). The position of the spinal needle must be placed to allow resection of the flap with baskets and/or a shaver. If the PoTSI

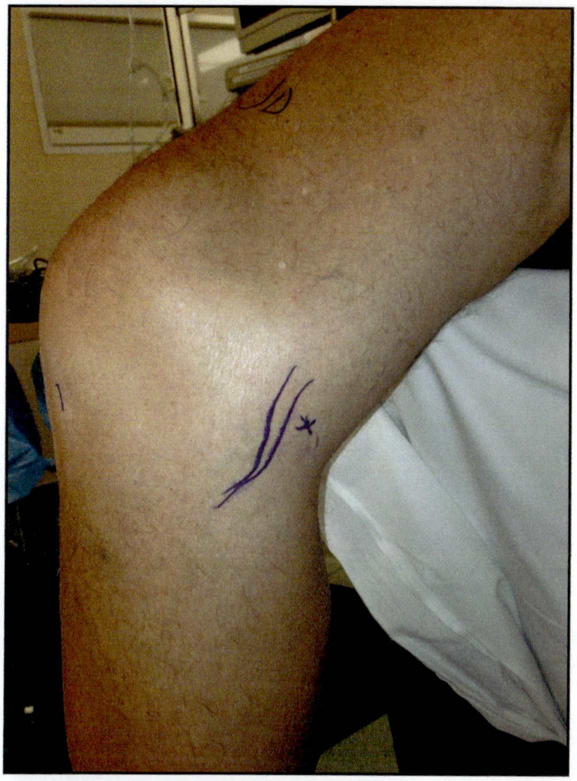

Figure 3-5. Photograph showing the usual location of the posteromedial portal (X) at the joint line, which often falls posterior to the saphenous nerve and vein.

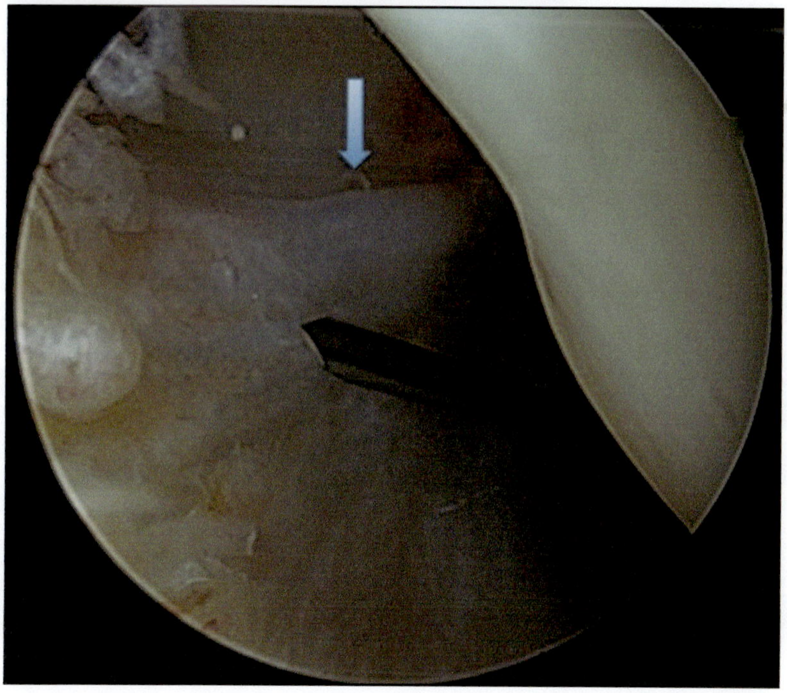

Figure 3-6. Spinal needle localization into the posteromedial portal under arthroscopic visualization. Note the location of the transverse synovial fold (arrow).

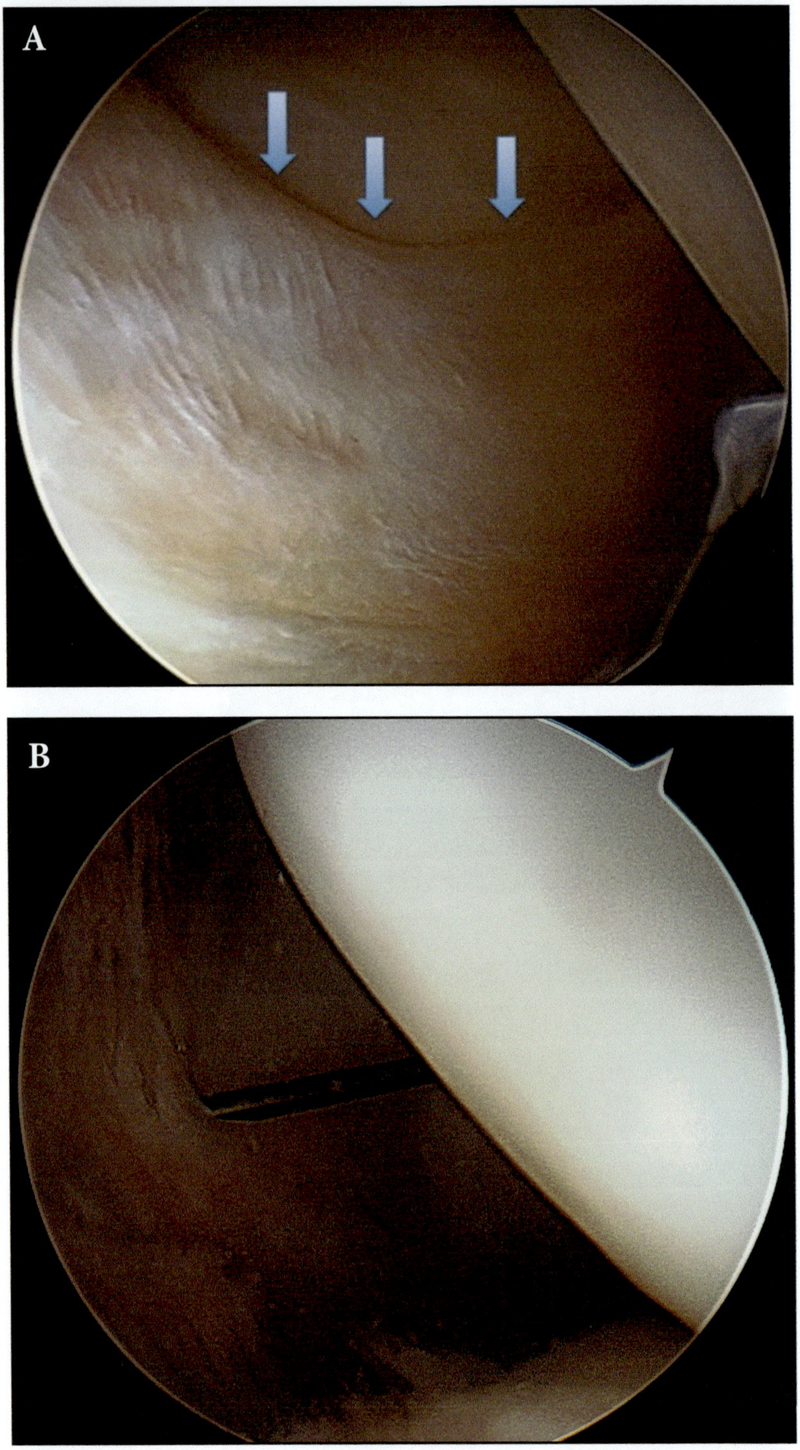

Figure 3-7. (A) Arthroscopic view of the posteromedial capsule showing a PoTSI lesion (arrows) and (B) view of the knee with no PoTSI lesion.

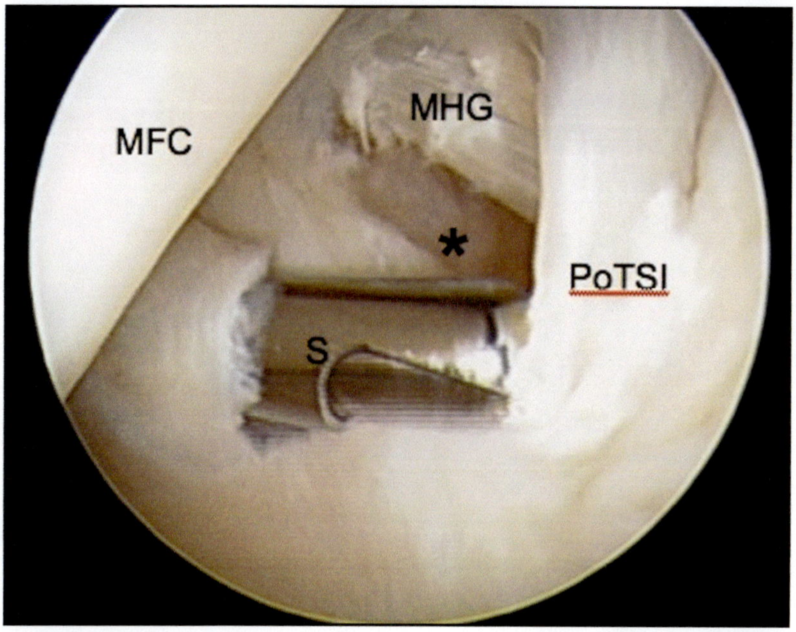

Figure 3-8. Arthroscopic view from the anterolateral portal showing the posteromedial compartment and the opening into a popliteal cyst. The shaver (S) is pulling inferior on the PoTSI lesion to reveal the medial head of gastrocnemius tendon (MHG) and cyst opening just medial to this (*).

lesion and/or the opening into the cyst is not easily identified, pressure on the posteromedial knee directly over the cyst can sometimes elicit a puff of fluid from the cyst through the opening into the knee. This fluid is usually more viscous and more yellowish than the synovial fluid and can be easily identified. Injection of the cyst with methylene blue pre- or intraoperatively can also help identify the opening, again with direct pressure on the cyst and intra-articular visualization. The preoperative MRI scan is helpful to identify the most superficial location of the cyst posteriorly to inject the dye.

Once the proper position for the posteromedial portal has been ascertained, a small longitudinal nick is created in the skin, and a cannula with a blunt trocar is passed under direct visualization into the posterior aspect of the knee. The PoTSI lesion is taken down with baskets and/or a shaver at the medial edge of the tendon of the medial head of the gastrocnemius, further revealing the opening into the popliteal cyst (Figure 3-9). An 8- to 10-mm opening is created in the PoTSI lesion to allow free flow of synovial fluid out of the cyst into the knee (Figure 3-10). The arthroscope is then transferred into the posteromedial portal to allow visualization of the interior of the cyst. Cyst walls are identified and often noted to be incompletely septated (Figure 3-11). Chondral or bony loose bodies are frequently encountered (Figure 3-12). These can sometimes be irrigated out or occasionally require a transcystic portal for removal. To irrigate the cyst, the arthroscopic sheath originally placed in the anteromedial or anterolateral portal is left in place in the posteromedial compartment while the arthroscope remains in the popliteal cyst via the posteromedial portal, allowing free flow of fluid out of the cyst into the sheath and out of the knee. Suction can also be placed on the anterior cannula while visualizing through the posteromedial portal to assist in irrigating out loose bodies.

In order to remove larger loose bodies from the cyst or resect the popliteal cyst, it is necessary to gain a working portal into the cyst. Prior to creating a transcystic portal, the MRI must be studied to assess the most subcutaneous location of the cyst (Figure 3-13). This is usually posterior, just medial to the midline, and below the joint line. The MRI will also be helpful to visualize any large subcutaneous veins that may lie between the cyst and the skin. Using transillumination from the arthroscope in the posteromedial portal, the planned location for the transcystic portal is first marked with a needle. Transillumination will often also outline any crossing veins. The needle is visualized in the cyst to ensure adequate access to the loose body or the cyst walls. A small nick is

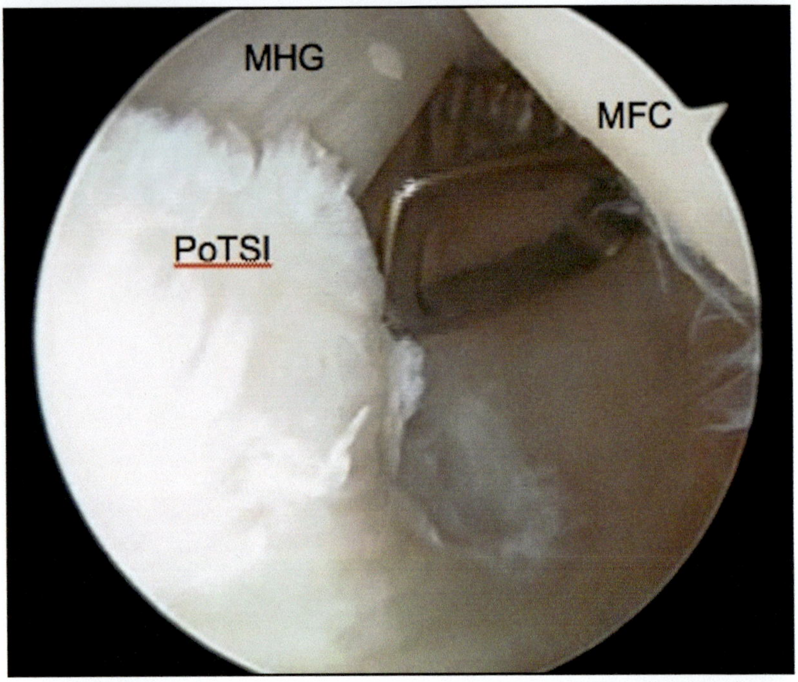

Figure 3-9. Arthroscopic view from anterolateral portal into the posteromedial compartment demonstrating resection of a PoTSI lesion with an arthroscopic basket punch. Note the relationship of the fold to the MFC and medial head of the gastrocnemius tendon (MHG).

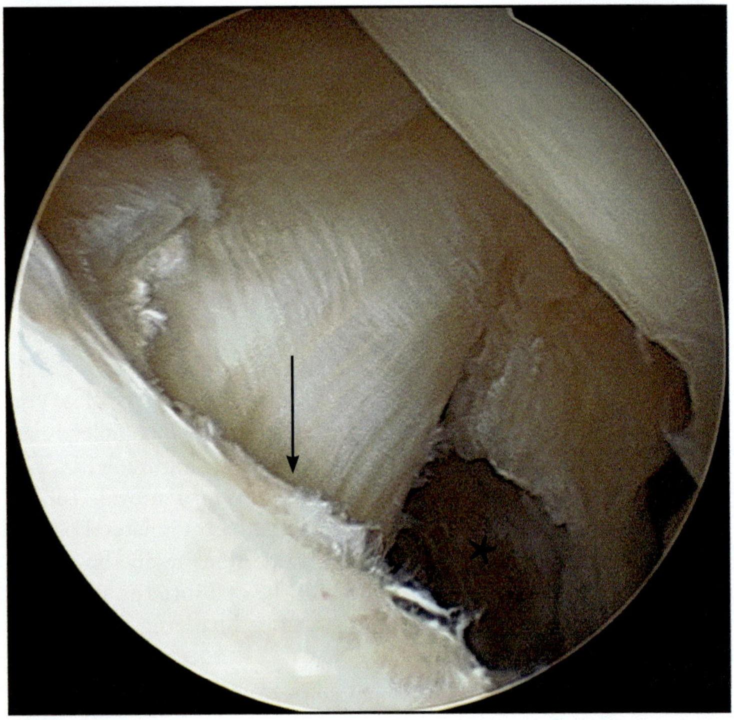

Figure 3-10. View from the anterolateral portal into the posteromedial compartment after resection of a portion of a PoTSI lesion (arrow) leaving an 8- to 10-mm opening from the knee joint into the popliteal cyst (*). The medial head of gastrocnemius tendon and MFC are also visible.

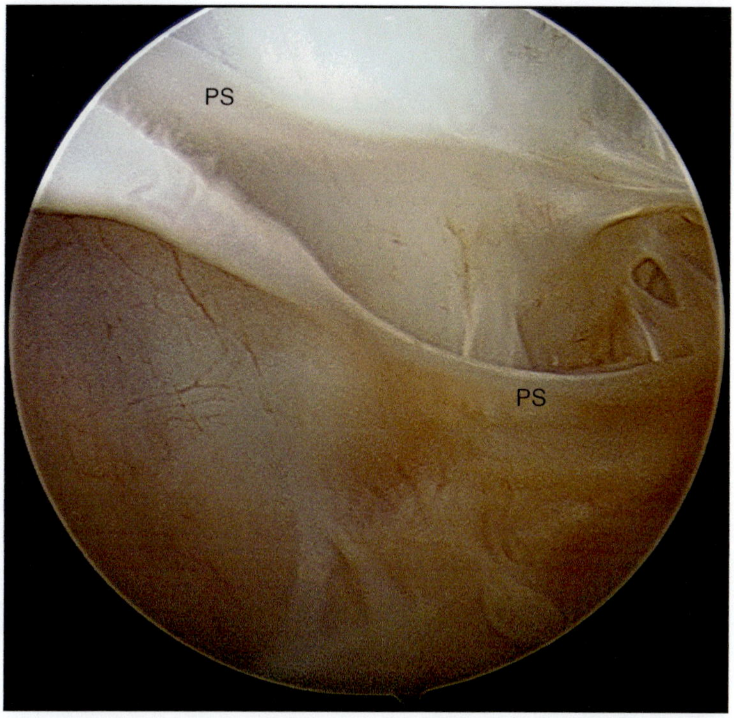

Figure 3-11. Interior view of a popliteal cyst from the posteromedial portal. Note the partial septations (PS).

created in the skin, and a blunt trocar and cannula are introduced into the cyst. Through this cannula, loose bodies can be removed or the cyst may be resected. Cyst resection is often not necessary as decompression of the cyst alone often leads to its resolution. Cyst excision can be performed similarly to a standard synovectomy, with extreme care to remove only the cyst lining and not wander lateral into the neurovascular structures. Cystectomy is performed in the case of recurrent cysts or if the cyst lining appears to consist of diseased synovium, such as that occasionally seen in rheumatoid or other systemic arthropathies.

Portals are closed with nonabsorbable sutures. It is important to close the posteromedial and transcystic portals as these may lead to cutaneous fistulas if they do not properly heal. These portals also tend to gap open more than the standard anterior arthroscopic portals. A compression dressing is placed over the posteromedial knee, with care not to compromise the mid portion of the popliteal fossa, in addition to the standard arthroscopic dressing. If cyst excision is performed, the patient is placed in intermittent pneumatic compression socks for 2 weeks to add additional compression to the proximal calf.

Postoperative Protocol

Full range of motion is allowed postoperatively. Leg elevation is essential to avoid knee and lower leg swelling. The patient is encouraged to bear weight as tolerated; discontinuing crutches as able and the performance of ankle pumps are advised to minimize risk of venous thrombosis. Gradual return to activities of daily living and sports activities, if applicable, is allowed. Patients usually return to all activities by 4 to 6 weeks postoperatively.

Recurrence rates, even with PoTSI flap excision only, have been rare in the literature and in the author's practice (Figure 3-14).[10,12]

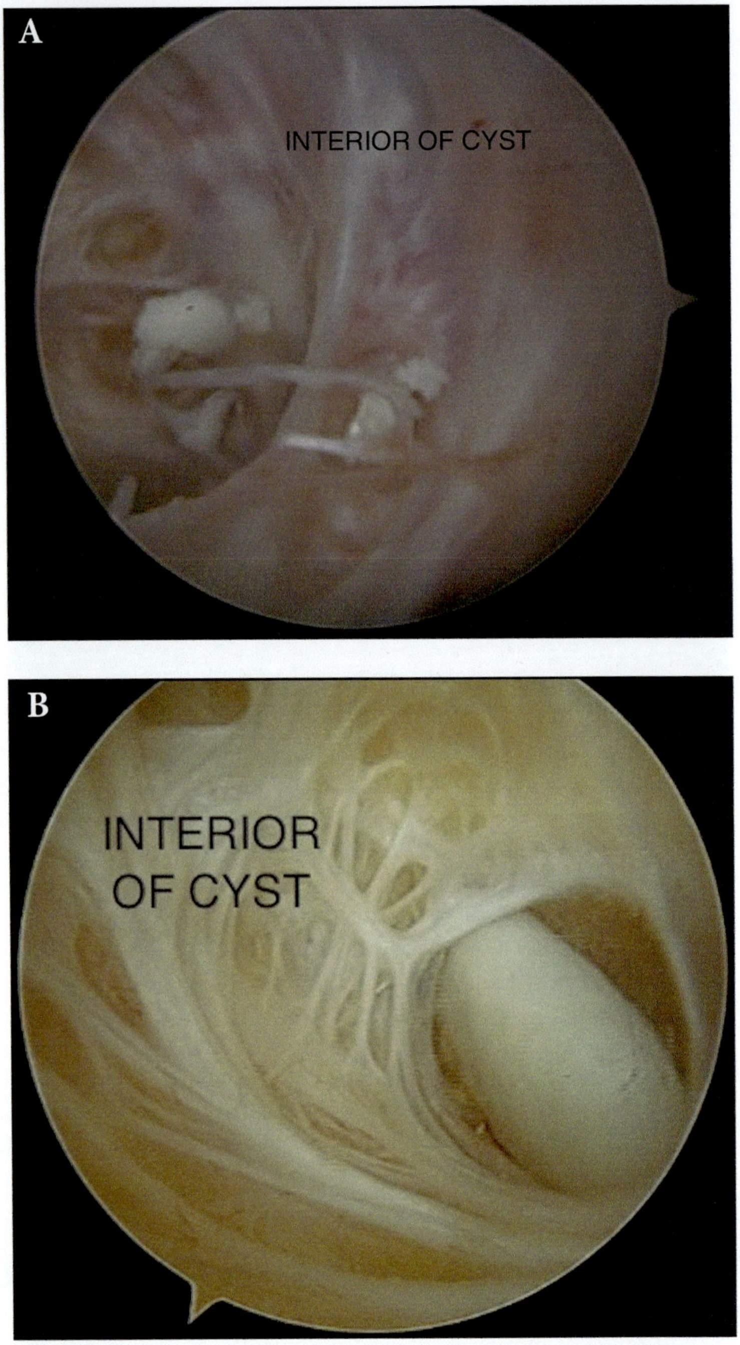

Figure 3-12. Interior view of popliteal cyst from the posteromedial portal with (A) chondral loose bodies and (B) bony loose body.

Potential Complications

Although minimal complications are usually associated with arthroscopic surgery, there are some circumstances with arthroscopic treatment of popliteal cysts that require special attention to avoid complications.

Popliteal cyst excision requires the creation of a posteromedial portal. This portal is placed along the medial joint line after localization with a spinal needle under direct arthroscopic visualization. Structures at risk when creating this portal include the saphenous nerve and the saphenous

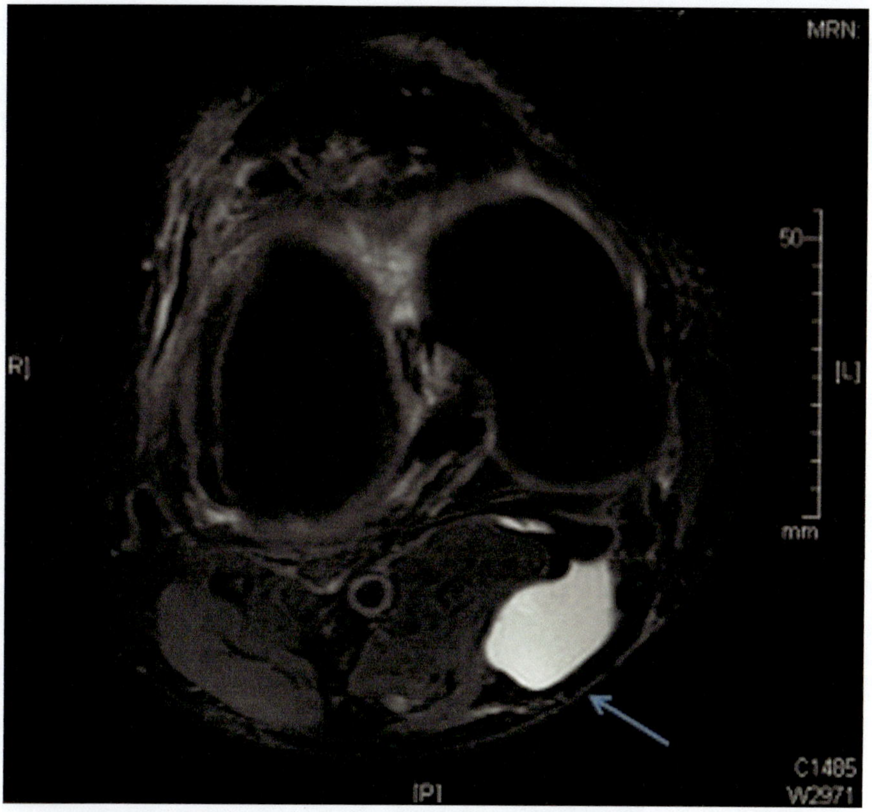

Figure 3-13. Axial MRI of a popliteal cyst demonstrating the most superficial position for the transcystic portal (arrow).

vein. Although these structures can sometimes be identified by transillumination prior to needle localization, this is not always possible due to the thickness of the subcutaneous tissue. After needle localization, a longitudinal nick is created in the skin only. Only blunt trocars should be used to introduce the posteromedial cannula. The smallest cannula possible should be used in this portal to minimize risk to the surrounding structures. A smooth cannula may also reduce this risk.

Also, when placing the posteromedial or anterior cannula into the posteromedial compartment, care must be taken not to plunge into the compartment. The popliteal artery, vein, and nerve can lie directly in the path of the cannula if placed too deep. Again, only blunt cannulas should be used when going into the posteromedial compartment.

The popliteal nerve, artery, and vein can also be at risk during the resection of the PoTSI lesion or of resection of the cyst itself. Resection of the PoTSI lesion should cause minimal risk as the lesion is located medial to the medial edge of the gastrocnemius tendon, with the neurovascular structures lying far more lateral between the 2 heads of the gastrocnemius. However, if one does not identify the medial head of the gastrocnemius upon entering the posterior compartment, the resection can be begun too laterally, putting the popliteal structures at risk. Upon resecting the cyst, if necessary, care must be taken to resect only the cyst lining. This plane can usually be easily identified. However, if the plane is not easily identified, especially when taking down the anterolateral portion of the cyst, it is better to leave this portion of the cyst in situ. In the author's experience, leaving a portion of the cyst in place does not necessarily lead to recurrence. Preoperative planning with the MRI scan will also help identify the proximity of the popliteal structures to the cyst as they are often completely shielded from the resection by the medial head of the gastrocnemius. Popliteal artery pseudoaneurysm after arthroscopic cystectomy has been reported.[22] Preoperative imaging confirmed the proximity of the cyst to the popliteal artery, with the concerning cysts often extending proximal and lateral to the usual cyst location.

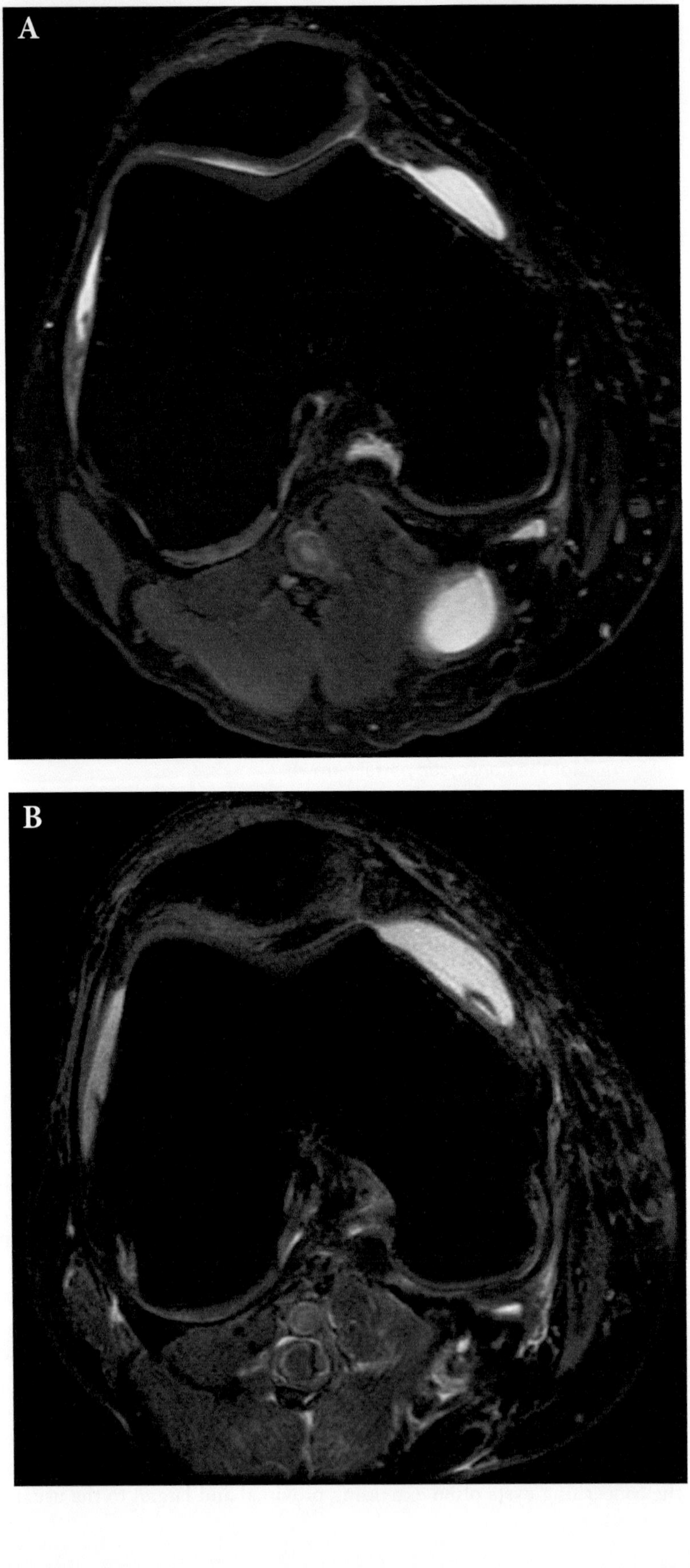

Figure 3-14. Axial MRI (A) pre- and (B) 3 weeks postoperatively showing complete resolution of a popliteal cyst with takedown of a PoTSI lesion and arthroscopic cyst irrigation only.

Venous thromboembolic (VTE) disease is uncommon in arthroscopic surgery. Although the author has seen no increased incidence of VTE with popliteal cyst decompression or excision, several precautions can be implemented to minimize the possibility of VTE. Gravity inflow only should be used when opening up, entering, or removing a popliteal cyst. Distension created with pump inflow can lead to cyst distention, possibly causing popliteal venous compression. Postoperative intermittent pneumatic calf compression devices are also recommended in patients with risk factors for VTE or extensive cyst resection. Elevation and weightbearing are encouraged postoperatively, also to minimize VTE occurrence.

Hematoma formation after popliteal cyst resection has been reported.[23] However, these often resolve with compression and rest. Compression dressing of the posteromedial knee is stressed following cyst resection or decompression, along with elevation, to try to minimize the chance of hematoma formation. The author has not encountered any postoperative hematomas that required aspiration or drainage or altered the normal postoperative course.

Theoretically, compartment syndrome after cyst excision is also a potential complication, although this has not be noted in the author's experience or been reported in the literature.

Conclusion

Arthroscopic treatment of popliteal cysts is a relatively straightforward procedure for treatment of symptomatic popliteal cysts. Cyst removal or decompression first requires location of the valve-like mechanism or PoTSI lesion at the medial edge of the medial head of the gastrocnemius tendon. The valve-like fold is then taken down through a posteromedial portal to allow free flow of fluid between the cyst and the intra-articular environment of the knee. Further work within the cyst requires placement of the arthroscope into the posteromedial portal and creation of a transcystic portal. Careful attention to the preoperative MRI and knowledge of anatomy can create a reproducible result with excellent patient satisfaction and low incidence of reoccurrence.

Top Technical Pearls for the Procedure

1. The surgeon must be familiar with the anatomy. Visualization of the cyst on preoperative MRI is essential to know the location of the cyst relative to the semimembranosus tendon, medial head of the gastrocnemius tendon, and tibial nerve, vein, and artery.
2. Arthroscopically, the surgeon must locate the PoTSI lesion at the medial head of the gastrocnemius tendon. This will lead to the opening of the cyst.
3. If when passing through the notch to get to the posteromedial compartment of the knee the scope sheath does not go easily, switch to visualizing through the anterolateral portal and pass the sheath through the anteromedial portal. A minimal MFC notchplasty is occasionally required.
4. Using a second arthroscopic sheath is helpful to allow direct visualization of the passage of the additional scope sheath into the posteromedial compartment via the trifurcation of the MFC, medial tibial plateau, and PCL.
5. Creation of the posteromedial portal should be localized first with a spinal needle, then created with a nick in the skin only, followed by a blunt trochar to avoid injury to the saphenous nerve.

References

1. Adams R. Chronic rheumatic arthritis of the knee joint. *Dublin J Med Sci.* 1840;17:520-522.
2. Baker WM. On the formation of the synovial cysts in the leg in connection with disease of the knee joint. *St Barth Hosp Rep.* 1877;13:245-261.
3. Gristina AG, Wilson PD. Popliteal cysts in adults and children. A review of 90 cases. *Arch Surg.* 1964;88:357-363.
4. Goldstein LA, Dickerson RC. *Atlas of Orthopedic Surgery.* Vol 2. St. Louis, MO: CV Mosby Co; 1974:762-763.
5. Lindgren PG, Willén R. Gastrocnemio-semimembranosus bursa and its relations to the knee joint. *Acta Radiol Diagn (Stockh).* 1977;18(5):497-512.
6. Rauschning W, Lindgren PG. Popliteal cysts (Baker's cysts) in adults. I: clinical and roentgenological results of operative excision. *Acta Orthop Scand.* 1979;50(5):583-591.
7. Hughston JC, Baker CL, Mello W. Popliteal cyst: a surgical approach. *Orthopedics.* 1991;14(2):147-150.
8. Vahvanen V. Popliteal cysts. A follow-up study on 42 operatively treated patients. *Acta Orthop Scand.* 1973;44(3):303-310.
9. Sansone V, De Ponti A. Arthrosopic treatment of popliteal cyst and associated intra-articular knee disorders in adults. *Arthroscopy.* 1999;15(4):368-372.
10. Ko S, Ahn J. Popliteal cystoscopic excisional debridement and removal of capsular fold of valvular mechanism of large recurrent popliteal cyst. *Arthroscopy.* 2004;20(1):37-44.
11. Ahn JH, Yoo JC, Lee SH, Lee YS. Arthroscopic cystectomy for popliteal cysts through the posteromedial cystic portal. *Arthroscopy.* 2007;23(5):559.e1-559.e4.
12. Ahn JH, Lee SH, Yoo JC, Chang MJ, Park YS. Arthroscopic treatment of popliteal cysts: clinical and magnetic resonance imaging results. *Arthroscopy.* 2010;26(10):1340-1347.
13. Kim KI, Lee SH, Ahn JH, Kim JS. Arthroscopic anatomic study of posteromedial joint capsule in knee joint associated with popliteal cyst. *Arch Orthop Trauma Surg.* 2014;134(7):979-984.
14. Guerra J Jr, Newell JD, Resnick D, Danzig LA. Pictorial essay: gastrocnemio-semimembranosus bursal region of the knee. *AJR Am J Roentgenol.* 1981;136(3):593-596.
15. Fielding JR, Franklin PD, Kustan J. Popliteal cysts: a reassessment using magnetic resonance imaging. *Skeletal Radiol.* 1991;20(6):433-435.
16. Akagi R, Saisu T, Segawa Y, et al. Natural history of popliteal cysts in the pediatric population. *J Pediatr Orthop.* 2013;33(3):262-268.
17. Sanchez JE, Conkling N, Labropoulos N. Compression syndromes of the popliteal neurovascular bundle due to Baker cyst. *J Vasc Surg.* 2011;54(6):1821-1829.
18. Acebes JC, Sánchez-Pernaute O, Díaz-Oca A, Herrero-Beaumont G. Ultrasonographic assessment of Baker's cysts after intra-articular corticosteroid injection in knee osteoarthritis. *J Clin Ultrasound.* 2006;34(3):113-117.
19. Di Sante L, Paoloni M, Ioppolo F, Dimaggio M, Di Renzo S, Santilli V. Ultrasound-guided aspiration and corticosteroid injection of Baker's cysts in knee osteoarthritis: a prospective observational study. *Am J Phys Med Rehabil.* 2010;89(12):970-975.
20. Stone KR, Stoller D, De Carli A, Day R, Richnak J. The frequency of Baker's cysts associated with meniscal tears. *Am J Sports Med.* 1996;24(5):670-671.
21. Rupp S, Seil R, Jochum P, Kohn D. Popliteal cysts in adults. Prevalence, associated intraarticular lesions, and results after arthroscopic treatment. *Am J Sports Med.* 2002;30(1):112-115.
22. Kp V, Yoon JR, Nha KW, Yang JH, Lee JH, Jegal H. Popliteal artery pseudoaneurysm after arthroscopic cystectomy of a popliteal cyst. *Arthroscopy.* 2009;25(9):1054-1057.
23. Cho JH. Clinical results of direct arthroscopic excision of popliteal cyst using a posteromedial portal. *Knee Surg Relat Res.* 2012;24(4):235-240.

Please see videos on the accompanying website at www.routledge.com/9781617119996

4

Arthroscopic Management of Tibial Plateau Fractures

Brian B. Gilmer, MD and James H. Lubowitz, MD

Introduction

Tibial plateau fractures typically present as a high-mechanism injury in a young patient, such as a car vs pedestrian or fall from height, or a low-energy fracture in elderly patients. Among athletes, they are common in skiers.[1,2]

The mechanism of injury is a combination of a varus or valgus deforming force and axial load resulting in a spectrum of shear and depression fracture patterns. The most common classification is the Schatzker system (Figure 4-1).

Several features of tibial plateau bony anatomy are critical for understanding and treating these injuries.[1]

- The lateral tibial plateau is convex and lies 2 to 3 mm proximal to the medial plateau. Raising depressed fragments of the lateral tibial plateau only to the level of the medial plateau will not result in anatomic restoration of the articular surface.
- Normally, the lateral condyle of the femur lies directly in line with the lateral rim of the tibial plateau and the medial condyle with the medial rim of the tibial plateau. Widening of the tibial plateau is a common feature of tibial plateau fractures, and failure to reduce the condylar width results in abnormal articular contact with the femoral condyles.
- On average, the proximal tibia has a posterior slope of 9 degrees. This observation is critical in obtaining proper fluoroscopic imaging during fixation to evaluate articular reduction.

Associated soft tissue injury with tibial plateau fracture is common. Frequency of lateral meniscal injury is frequently quoted as present in 42% to 45% of plateau fractures[3,4]; however, in one series, 91% of patients had evidence of lateral meniscal pathology and 77% had tear or avulsion of a cruciate or collateral ligament.[5] The menisci function as significant secondary stabilizers of the knee joint, and their treatment is related to outcomes. The clinical implications of associated cruciate and collateral ligament injury remain incompletely defined.

Arthroscopy has emerged as a useful tool for evaluating articular reduction and treating associated soft tissue pathology. Short-term results of arthroscopic reduction internal fixation

Sgaglione NA, Lubowitz JH, Provencher MT, eds. *The Knee: AANA Advanced Arthroscopic Surgical Techniques* (pp 53-62).

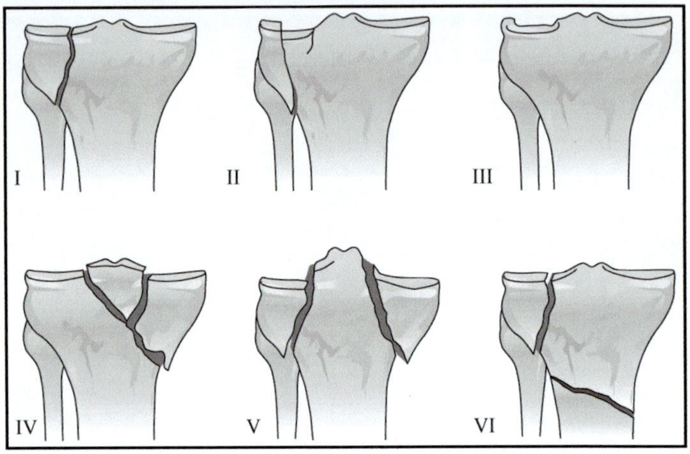

Figure 4-1. The Schatzker classification of tibial plateau fractures.

(ARIF) have been promising, with good and excellent results in greater than 90% of patients.[6-10] Medium-term results appear comparable to short-term results.[11,12] Not surprisingly, results of ARIF for more complex type V and VI fractures are less satisfactory but still approach 90% good and excellent.[13]

Tibial eminence avulsion fractures commonly occur in children and adolescents.[14] However, it is sometimes misunderstood that this condition occurs only in the young. Although less common, anterior cruciate ligament (ACL) avulsion also occurs in adults.[15,16]

Isolated intercondylar eminence fractures are avulsion fractures of the tibial insertion of the ACL. The most common classification system was initially described by Meyers and McKeever[17] (Figure 4-2). It is critical to understand that failure to completely reduce the displaced fragment alters the length-tension relationship of the ACL and results in functional cruciate instability. Several techniques have been described for fixation, and excellent outcomes have been reported.[18-22]

Indications

- Tibial plateau fractures
  - Articular depression and/or incongruity greater than 4 mm[1]
  - Schatzker type III and selected types I, II, and IV fractures
- Tibial eminence fractures
  - Meyers and McKeever type I fractures if associated with meniscal tears or concomitant pathology requiring arthroscopic treatment
  - Meyers and McKeever type II fractures typically require ARIF because of the high rate of incarceration of the anterior horn of the medial meniscus.
  - Most displaced Meyers and McKeever type III fractures

Controversial Indications

- Tibial plateau fractures
  - ARIF may be appropriate for types I, II, and IV, in which displacement of the split fragment is minimal

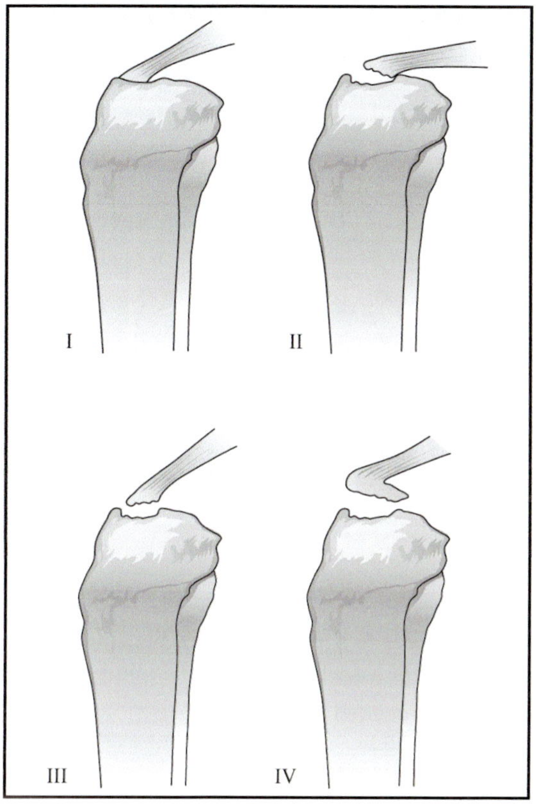

Figure 4-2. The Meyers and McKeever classification of ACL tibial spine avulsion injury.

  - Arthroscopically assisted open reduction and internal fixation is indicated for deformity effecting the mechanical axis of the limb.
  - Schatzker type V and VI fractures are best treated with arthroscopically assisted open reduction and internal fixation.
- Tibial eminence fractures
  - Some type IIIB fractures may be amenable to closed reduction because the large bony fragment can be reduced by the femoral condyles and soft tissue incarceration is less common.[14]

Pertinent Physical Findings

- Tibial plateau fractures
  - Compartmental pressures by serial clinical examination or Stryker needle examination
  - Elevated compartment pressures necessitate urgent fasciotomy and temporizing external fixation.
  - Vascular examination by palpable pulse, Doppler ultrasound, or ankle-brachial index
  - Ankle-brachial index less than 0.9 necessitates vascular surgery consultation
  - Evaluation of soft tissue envelope
  - Excessive swelling, blisters, or open wounds may require deferred or staged management with irrigation and debridement and temporizing external fixation.
  - Detailed physical examination should assess for associated injuries.

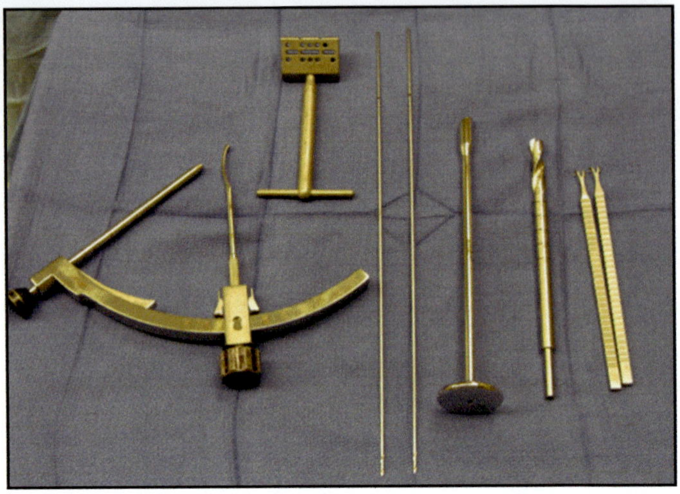

Figure 4-3. Equipment for ARIF of tibial plateau fractures, including angled guide, guide wires, cannulated tamp, cannulated drill, and meniscal retraction hooks.

- Tibial eminence fractures
  - Knee range of motion (ROM) should be evaluated to determine if fragment displacement is causing a mechanical block to motion or is preventing full knee extension.
  - Ligamentous examination is indicated to evaluate for associated soft tissue injury.
  - Detailed physical examination should assess for associated injuries.

Pertinent Imaging

- Tibial plateau fractures
  - Anteroposterior, lateral, and oblique x-rays reveal most tibial plateau fractures but can miss minimally displaced and joint depression fractures.
  - Noncontrast computed tomography (CT) scan is indicated for preoperative planning to evaluate fragment morphology, fracture pattern, and articular depression
  - Magnetic resonance imaging (MRI) is a useful adjunct to identify occult fractures and associated soft tissue pathology.[5,23]
- Tibial eminence fractures
  - Tibial eminence fractures are most frequently diagnosed with standard anteroposterior, lateral, and oblique knee x-rays.
  - Advanced imaging (CT or MRI) may be indicated when the classification or the size of the bony avulsion is uncertain and nonoperative treatment is being considered.[14]

Equipment

Equipment for ARIF of tibial plateau fractures includes standard arthroscopy equipment, ACL drill guide, guide wires, cannulated drill bits, and coring reamer, cannulated tamp, and large-diameter screws (Figure 4-3). Special equipment for tibial eminence fracture fixation includes standard arthroscopy equipment, ACL drill guide, guide wires, suture hook, nitinol wire loop, and high-strength suture material.

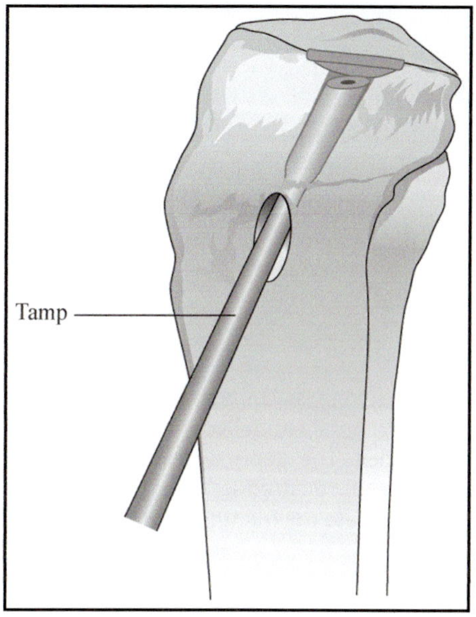

Figure 4-4. Cannulated, angled tamps reduce compression fracture elements via transtibial guide wires placed with an ACL guide and a modified, spoon-shaped marking hook.

Positioning and Portals

For tibial plateau ARIF, a standard operating table can be used with the patient supine. A circumferential leg holder and tourniquet are used with the leg resting at 90 degrees off the end of the table. The c-arm is inverted and brought in from the contralateral side so that the flat (image-acquiring) plate may be used as an operating table under the proximal tibia. Similarly, for tibial eminence fractures, the patient is positioned supine in a circumferential leg holder with the knee off the end of the table. Fluoroscopy is not routinely required.

Step-by-Step Description of the Procedure

Tibial Plateau Arthroscopic Reduction Internal Fixation

Our recommended technique for tibial plateau ARIF was inspired by Caspari et al,[24] Jennings,[25] and Buchko and Johnson.[26] Operative treatment must be tailored to specific fracture pattern.

If open plating is anticipated (ARIF without capsulotomy), the surgical dissection should be performed prior to arthroscopy to allow fluid to drain through the incision rather than into leg compartments. An initial arthroscopic lavage evacuates the hemarthrosis and allows arthroscopic assessment of the fracture. Diagnostic arthroscopy evaluates associated ligamentous and meniscal injuries.

For type I fractures, percutaneous, cannulated lag screws may be placed over guide wires after arthroscopic reduction is confirmed. In type II, III, and IV patterns, depressed fragments are first elevated using an angled tamp placed over a guide wire (Figure 4-4) before application of cannulated lag screws to prevent malreduction of the depressed fragments.

An ACL guide with a modified spoon-shaped tip to mimic the curve of the femoral condyle directs the guide pin in the center of the depressed fragments through a small incision in the proximal anteromedial tibial metaphysis. A coring reamer circumferentially penetrates the tibial cortex

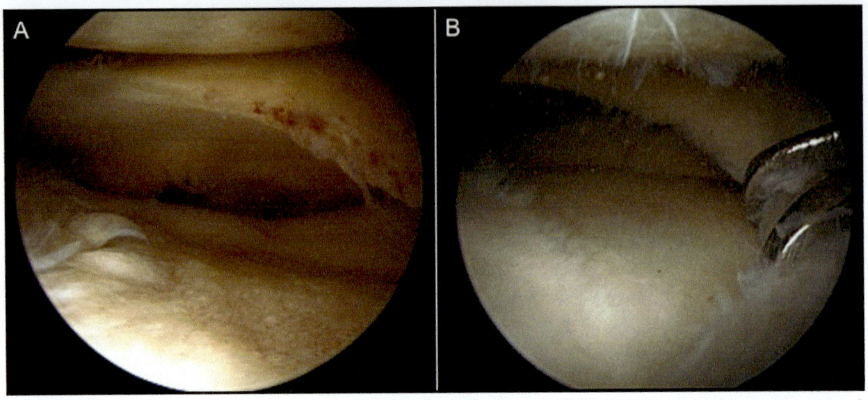

Figure 4-5. (A) Prereduction view of a Schatzker type III (lateral central compression) fracture viewed from an anterolateral portal in a left knee. The depressed articular surface results in widening of the lateral compartment. (B) Postreduction view of Schatzker type III fracture. A cannulated tamp is used to elevate the fracture site under arthroscopic visualization.

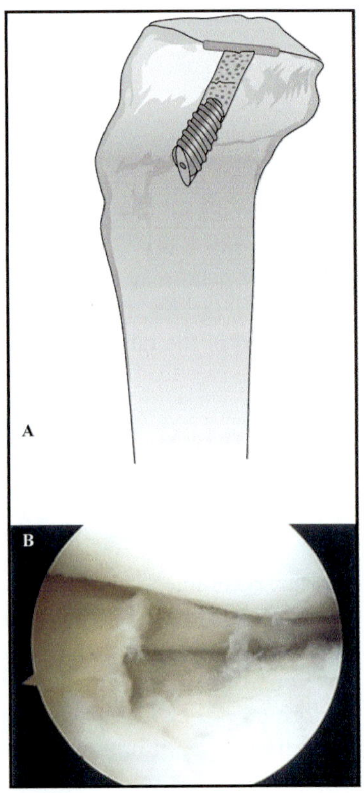

Figure 4-6. (A) A cannulated, bioabsorbable interference screw reduces and then buttresses the tibial plateau compression fracture via the metaphyseal window. (B) Arthroscopic view during screw insertion prevents excessive elevation and/or displacement of the articular fragment.

while removing as little bone as possible. The cannulated tamp is used to elevate the fracture site under arthroscopic visualization (Figure 4-5). The underlying metaphyseal bone and cortical disk serve as autograft. A calcium or hydroxyapatite-impregnated bioabsorbable cannulated interference screw of large diameter is then advanced through the cortical window to further elevate the fracture under direct arthroscopic visualization (Figure 4-6). The screw provides elevation of the fragment and rigid internal fixation of the fracture.

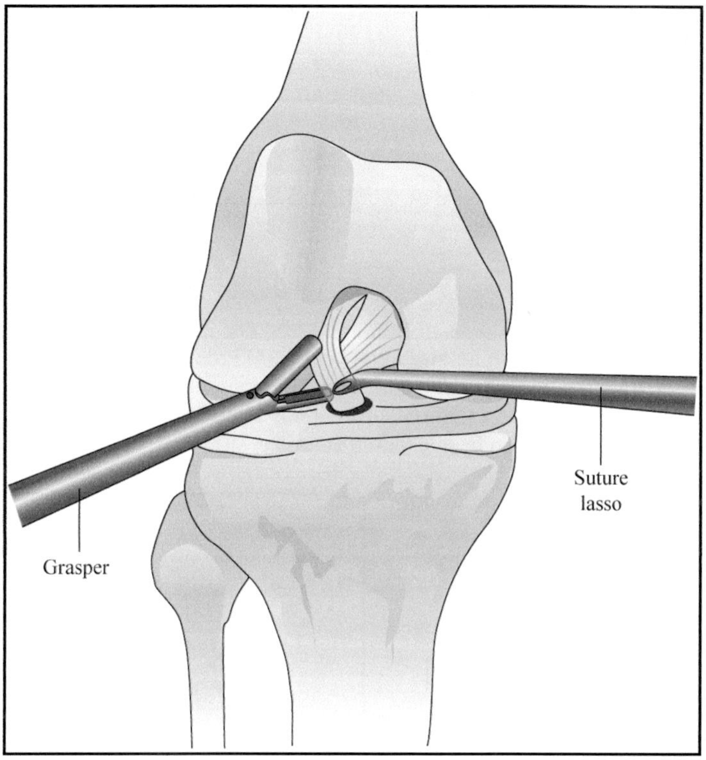

Figure 4-7. A 90-degree suture hook is placed through the fibers of the ACL. The wire loop within the hook is secured with an arthroscopic grasper.

For isolated or predominantly depression (type III) fractures, the screw obviates the need for percutaneous placement of subchondral, metal, cannulated buttress screws. For split depression (types II and IV) with significant metaphyseal displacement and more complex patterns (types V and VI) requiring open plating, major split fragments are reduced first, articular reduction is optimized and provisionally fixed with smooth K-wires. Finally, plate application can then compress the reduced articular surface, reduce condylar widening, and rigidly fix the fracture fragments.

Techniques for tibial plateau ARIF are demonstrated in the Video.

Tibial Eminence Arthroscopic Reduction Internal Fixation

ARIF of ACL avulsions with screws were described in 1993 by Lubowitz and Grauer,[27] but the authors now acknowledge disadvantages, including risks of comminution of the fracture fragment, posterior neurovascular injury, and the need for hardware removal. Because of these risks, ARIF using nonabsorbable sutures passed through drill holes and tied over the tibial tubercle is the authors' current preferred technique.

Initial lavage and diagnostic arthroscopy are performed. Standard anterolateral and anteromedial portals are used. Cannulas can be helpful in preventing soft tissue interposition during suture passage.

Early fracture callous, clot, and any entrapped meniscal tissue must be removed from the fracture bed before fracture reduction. A dental pick can be helpful for provisional stabilization during ensuing steps.

A 90-degree suture hook is introduced percutaneously and passed through the fibers of the ACL in its mid-coronal plane as close to the bony fragment (distal) as possible. The wire loop within the hook is secured with an arthroscopic grasper (Figure 4-7) and pulled via a cannula through either portal and loaded with a #2 high-strength suture. The high-strength suture is pulled back through the ligament fibers and out through the accessory portal.

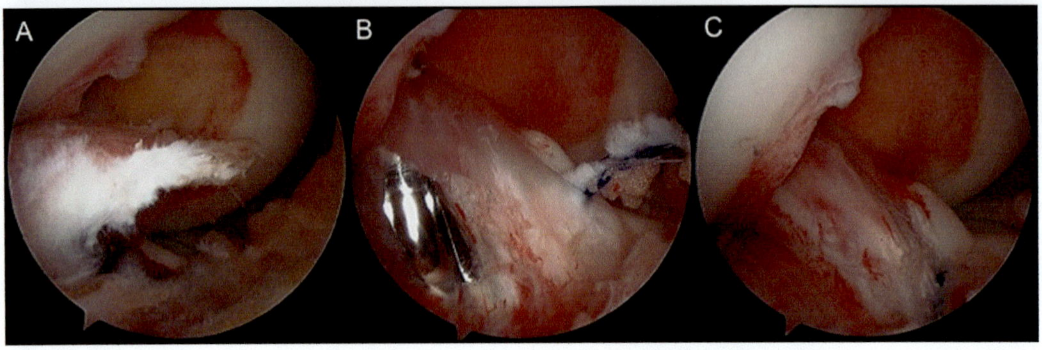

Figure 4-8. Arthroscopic view of a right knee from an anterolateral portal. (A) Preoperative view demonstrating elevated eminence avulsion fracture. (B) Drill enters lateral to the fragment, previously passed suture is visible medial to fragment. (C) Downward traction on suture limbs after final passing reduces elevated fracture fragment. (Reprinted with permission from Gregory Schmale, MD.)

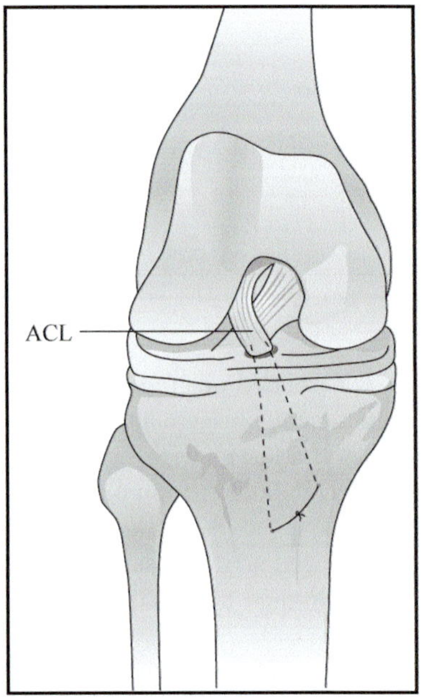

Figure 4-9. The fracture is reduced by pulling down on the suture ends, which are tied over the tibial tubercle.

An ACL guide is used to place medial and lateral drill holes on either side of the fragment through the intact bone adjacent to the fracture under arthroscopic visualization. A longitudinal incision is centered over the tibial tubercle, which allows subcutaneous access to the medial and lateral entry points. The medial pin enters the tibia just medial to the tubercle and the lateral pin just lateral.

A nitinol wire loop is passed up through the drill holes medially and laterally. Routine suture passage brings the suture ends out the medial and lateral drill holes. Distal traction on the suture ends reduces the fracture (Figure 4-8). The sutures are tied under tension while an assistant performs a reverse Lachman maneuver (Figure 4-9). Only one suture is required in most cases, but additional sutures can be added as described above.

Tibial eminence fractures, even after complete reduction and fixation, may demonstrate a few millimeters of superior displacement. Functional outcome remains excellent.[14]

Techniques for tibial eminence avulsion ARIF are demonstrated in the Video.

Postoperative Protocol

Patients are initially admitted for observation and pain control. ARIF provides rigid fixation and allows immediate early motion. Continuous passive motion can be a useful adjunct in the early postoperative period. Zero to 90 degrees of motion at 2 weeks and full ROM at 6 weeks is the goal. Weightbearing is delayed, generally for 12 weeks or until radiographic evidence of healing is present. Partial weightbearing is initiated and gradually advanced to full weightbearing over 4 weeks. A hinged knee bracing for 6 weeks is recommended for patients with associated collateral ligament injuries.

For intercondylar eminence avulsion fractures, the patient can be discharged on the day of surgery. Crutches are recommended, but patients are permitted to bear full weight with the knee locked in a brace in full extension. The brace is unlocked or removed for continuous passive motion. Early outpatient physical therapy is recommended to achieve 0 to 90 degrees of knee flexion at 2 weeks and full ROM by 6 weeks. Isometric quadriceps and hamstring strengthening with the knee locked in the brace is permitted during the first 6 weeks. After 6 weeks, the brace is discontinued and resistive exercises are introduced; however, terminal resisted extension is not allowed for 12 weeks.

Potential Complications

For ARIF, it is critical that calf compartments are continually palpated to ensure that fluid extravasation does not cause iatrogenic compartment syndrome.[28] Although intercondylar eminence avulsion fractures are contained injuries, they may be associated with capsular disruption and, thus, are not immune to this devastating complication. Dry arthroscopy whenever possible decreases fluid extravasation and risk of increased compartment pressure. Inadequate preoperative planning can result in unappreciated fracture lines that will displace if not appropriately reduced and rigidly fixed.

Top Technical Pearls for the Procedure

1. Preoperative planning should include careful assessment of fracture pattern and associated soft tissue injuries.
2. Careful fluid management and intraoperative monitoring for compartment syndrome is critical.
3. Major split fractures should be reduced first and then depressed fragments elevated before compression is applied.
4. In tibial eminence fractures, the fracture bed must be completely cleared of soft tissue, early callous, and clot prior to reduction.
5. Well-performed ARIF of tibial intercondylar eminence avulsion x-rays may show a few millimeters of fracture displacement. Functional outcomes are excellent.

References

1. Browner BD. *Skeletal Trauma*. 4th ed. Philadelphia, PA: Saunders; 2009.
2. Lubowitz JH, Elson WS, Guttmann D. Part I: arthroscopic management of tibial plateau fractures. *Arthroscopy*. 2004;20(10):1063-1070.
3. Mustonen AO, Koivikko MP, Lindahl J, Koskinen SK. MRI of acute meniscal injury associated with tibial plateau fractures: prevalence, type, and location. *AJR Am J Roentgenol*. 2008;191(4):1002-1009.

4. Colletti P, Greenberg H, Terk MR. MR findings in patients with acute tibial plateau fractures. *Comput Med Imaging Graph.* 1996;20(5):389-394.
5. Gardner MJ, Yacoubian S, Geller D, et al. The incidence of soft tissue injury in operative tibial plateau fractures: a magnetic resonance imaging analysis of 103 patients. *J Orthop Trauma.* 2005;19(2):79-84.
6. Tian M, Wang L, Zhang Y, Liu J. Curative effect of minimally invasive percutaneous plate osteosynthesis assisted by arthroscopy on 29 cases of tibial plateau fractures [in Chinese]. *Zhongguo Xiu Fu Chong Jian Wai Ke Za Zhi.* 2009;23(8):921-924.
7. Duan XJ, Yang L, Guo L, Chen GX, Dai G. Arthroscopically assisted treatment for Schatzker type I-V tibial plateau fractures. *Chin J Traumatol.* 2008;11(5):288-292.
8. Hung SS, Chao EK, Chan YS, et al. Arthroscopically assisted osteosynthesis for tibial plateau fractures. *J Trauma.* 2003;54(2):356-363.
9. Asik M, Cetik O, Talu U, Sozen YV. Arthroscopy-assisted operative management of tibial plateau fractures. *Knee Surg Sports Traumatol Arthrosc.* 2002;10(6):364-370.
10. Roerdink WH, Oskam J, Vierhout PA. Arthroscopically assisted osteosynthesis of tibial plateau fractures in patients older than 55 years. *Arthroscopy.* 2001;17(8):826-831.
11. Siegler J, Galissier B, Marcheix PS, Charissoux JL, Mabit C, Arnaud JP. Percutaneous fixation of tibial plateau fractures under arthroscopy: a medium term perspective. *Orthop Traumatol Surg Res.* 2011;97(1):44-50.
12. Scheerlinck T, Ng CS, Handelberg F, Casteleyn PP. Medium-term results of percutaneous, arthroscopically-assisted osteosynthesis of fractures of the tibial plateau. *J Bone Joint Surg Br.* 1998;80(6):959-964.
13. Chan YS. Arthroscopy- assisted surgery for tibial plateau fractures. *Chang Gung Med J.* 2011;34(3):239-247.
14. Lubowitz JH, Elson WS, Guttmann D. Part II: arthroscopic treatment of tibial plateau fractures: intercondylar eminence avulsion fractures. *Arthroscopy.* 2005;21(1)86-92.
15. Toye LR, Cummings DP, Armendariz G. Adult tibial intercondylar eminence fracture: evaluation with MR imaging. *Skeletal Radiol.* 2002;31(1):46-48.
16. Bonin N, Jeunet L, Obert L, Dejour D. Adult tibial eminence fracture fixation: arthroscopic procedure using K-wire folded fixation. *Knee Surg Sports Traumatol Arthrosc.* 2007;15(7):857-862.
17. Bucholz RW, Heckman JD, Court-Brown C, et al. *Rockwood and Green's Fractures in Adults.* 6th ed. Philadelphia, PA: Lippincott Williams & Wilkins; 2006.
18. Parr RR. Arthroscopic reduction and headless cannulated compression screw fixation of adults' tibial eminence fractures. *Am J Orthop (Belle Mead NJ).* 2006;35(12):558-561.
19. Lehman RA Jr, Murphy KP, Machen MS, Kuklo TR. Modified arthroscopic suture fixation of a displaced tibial eminence fracture. *Arthroscopy.* 2003;19(2):E6.
20. Hapa O, Barber FA, Süner G, et al. Biomechanical comparison of tibial eminence fracture fixation with high-strength suture, EndoButton, and suture anchor. *Arthroscopy.* 2012;28(5):681-687.
21. Senekovic V, Veselko M. Anterograde arthroscopic fixation of avulsion fractures of the tibial eminence with a cannulated screw: five-year results. *Arthroscopy.* 2003;19(1):54-61.
22. Kogan MG, Marks P, Amendola A. Technique for arthroscopic suture fixation of displaced tibial intercondylar eminence fractures. *Arthroscopy.* 1997;13(3):301-306.
23. Markhardt BK, Gross JM, Monu JU. Schatzker classification of tibial plateau fractures: use of CT and MR imaging improves assessment. *Radiographics.* 2009;29(2):585-597.
24. Caspari RB, Hutton PM, Whipple TL, Meyers JF. The role of arthroscopy in the management of tibial plateau fractures. *Arthroscopy.* 1985;1(2):76-82.
25. Jennings JE. Arthroscopic management of tibial plateau fractures. *Arthroscopy.* 1985;1(3):160-168.
26. Buchko GM, Johnson DH. Arthroscopy assisted operative management of tibial plateau fractures. *Clin Orthop Relat Res.* 1996;(332):29-36.
27. Lubowitz JH, Grauer JD. Arthroscopic treatment of anterior cruciate ligament avulsion. *Clin Orthop Relat Res.* 1993;(294):242-246.
28. Belanger M, Fadale P. Compartment syndrome of the leg after arthroscopic examination of a tibial plateau fracture. Case report and review of the literature. *Arthroscopy.* 1997;13(5):646-651.

Please see videos on the accompanying website at www.routledge.com/9781617119996

5

Arthroscopic Treatment of Arthrofibrosis

Sanjay Menon, MD and Leon (Lonnie) Paulos, MD

Introduction

Arthrofibrosis was described as the fibroplastic response of the joint to trauma in 1951.[1] In 1973, Enneking and Horowitz[2] demonstrated the intra-articular effects of immobilization in the knee, including progressive contracture of the capsule and pericapsular structures, encroachment of the joint by fibro-fatty connective tissue, and joint cavity obliteration. Further study yielded open techniques to manage the disorder and, in 1982, Sprague et al[3] described the first arthroscopic approach to the treatment of the stiff knee.

The physical changes noted by Enneking and Horowitz's classic article are identical to those observed with any kind of prolonged motion loss and must be addressed along with the underlying cause of the motion loss.

In general, a knee that has suffered hemarthrosis as a result of injury or surgery, which demonstrates persistent inflammation, decreased range of motion (ROM), and patella tightness, is indicated for intervention. However, the knee must be "cool" before any surgical intervention.

Indications

- Decreased ROM: Pain and decreased ROM after ligament reconstruction surgery, especially when performed during the acute phase and in combination with extra-articular procedures[4]
- Failure of nonoperative treatment or manipulation alone: Patients who have failed to regain full ROM within 4 to 6 weeks after surgery should be counseled regarding possible intervention for arthrofibrosis. If manipulation followed by judicious physical therapy, anti-inflammatory drugs, and hamstring stretching exercises between weeks 6 and 12 fails to bring about progress, then arthroscopic management is indicated typically between weeks 10 and 12.[5]

Sgaglione NA, Lubowitz JH, Provencher MT, eds. *The Knee: AANA Advanced Arthroscopic Surgical Techniques* (pp 63-73).

Controversial Indications

- Active inflammation: Surgical intervention should not be considered if the knee is still actively inflamed.
- Extensor lag: Surgery should be delayed when there is an extensor lag.[6] There should be full quad activation and strength prior to consideration of arthroscopic lysis of adhesions in the joint so as to maintain extension gains.

In summary, presurgical goals should include good quadriceps strength without lag and minimal swelling, warmth, and pain.

It is also imperative to consider the cause of the stiffness. Acute surgical intervention less than 21 days after injury[7,8] or prior to return of ROM and quad control[9] has been associated with development of arthrofibrosis. Prolonged postoperative immobilization, particularly in flexion, has also been implicated as a cause of chronic loss of motion.[10-12] Bleeding and inflammation can result in inability to regain ROM early.[13] Malposition of osseous elements, anterior placement of the tibial tunnel,[14,15] or overtensioning of ligamentous structures can cause disordered joint kinetics. Excessively aggressive physical therapy can potentially increase joint inflammation. Finally, patient factors, such as exuberant scar formation, can play a role.

In knee ligament surgery, there is potential for many of the above issues to occur as there can be nonisometric placement of grafts, fat pad trauma, notch impingement, and bleeding. These procedures are also typically followed by extensive and frequently aggressive physical therapy.

Pertinent Physical Findings

- Decreased ROM
- Decreased patellar glide from cranially to caudally (best test)
- Decreased patellar tilt
- Warmth and swelling with surrounding atrophy
- Flexed-knee gait
- Shelf sign (late finding)

Patients with arthrofibrosis present with persistent stiffness, pain, and typically a painful flexed-knee gait. Warmth and swelling will be present in the active phase, and there will commonly be surrounding atrophy. Notable physical findings include decreased ROM and decreased patellar glide. However, one must be aware that during the normal healing response, the patella will exhibit decreased mobility between weeks 4 and 12, with a gradual return of mobility as week 16 approaches (Video).

Knee motion loss can be graded based on deviation from normal flexion and extension[16] or by the pathoanatomy causing the motion loss. Del Pizzo et al[17] classified motion loss into the following 3 groups: Group 1 consisted of knees with extension less than 5 degrees and flexion greater than 110 degrees, group 2 had extension of 5 to 10 degrees with flexion between 90 and 110 degrees, and group 3 was limited to extension greater than 10 degrees or flexion less than 90 degrees. These were characterized as mild, moderate, and severe, respectively.

Arthrofibrosis has also been classified by its pathoanatomy. In the suprapatellar classification by Sprague et al,[3] group 1 consisted of discreet bands or a single sheet of adhesions traversing the suprapatellar pouch. Group 2 involved complete obliteration of the suprapatellar pouch and peripatellar gutters with masses of adhesions, and group 3 included the above with extracapsular involvement with bands of tissue from the proximal patella to anterior femur. Suprapatellar adhesions result in flexion loss only (Figure 5-1).

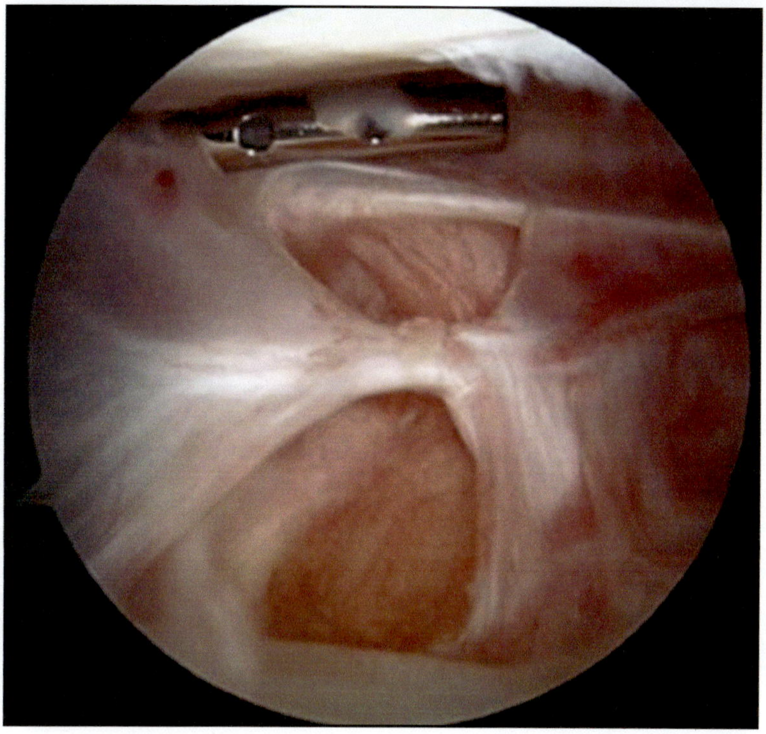

Figure 5-1. Adhesions in the suprapatellar pouch between the anterior femur and quadriceps muscle causing loss of flexion.

Infrapatellar entrapment may be associated with atypical pain, loss of extension and flexion, and sometimes patella infera (Video).[18] It can be classified as primary or secondary, such as entrapment caused by nonisometric graft placement. It can also be divided into 3 distinct stages. In stage I, the prodromal stage, there is periarticular inflammation and swelling combined with immobility and quadriceps weakness as demonstrated by an extension lag. Tenderness is noted about the patellar tendon and active ROM is painful. There is decreased excursion of patellar glide tests and patellar tilt, although not rigidly fixed in the early stage. In stage II, the active stage, there is essentially no patellar tilt, decreased medial to lateral glide, and loss of anterior tilt. There may be a positive shelf sign. A positive shelf sign is characterized by an increased slope between the inferior pole of the patella and the proximal tibia with the knee in extension (Figure 5-2). A positive shelf sign is typically a late finding that indicates significant chronicity and possible patella infera. Its appearance is due to the adhesion of the patella tendon to the anterior tibia. Stage III, the residual stage, is characterized by slightly more supple peripatellar and retinacular tissues but with more significant patellofemoral arthrosis as demonstrated by patellofemoral crepitation on examination and decreased joint space seen on x-rays. Patella infera is usually present.[19]

Infrapatellar entrapment combined with suprapatellar entrapment results in loss of extension and flexion. It is our opinion that loss of patellar mobility from cranially to caudally represents the most telling indicator on physical examination for recalcitrant arthrofibrosis.

Pertinent Imaging

Standard x-rays: Anteroposterior, bent knee posteroanterior, and Merchant view x-rays should be obtained, in addition to an excellent lateral image of the knee in 30 degrees of flexion. The lateral image is crucial to evaluate for patella infera, which can be measured using the modified Insall-Salvati method.[20] The length of the patella tendon is measured from its origin

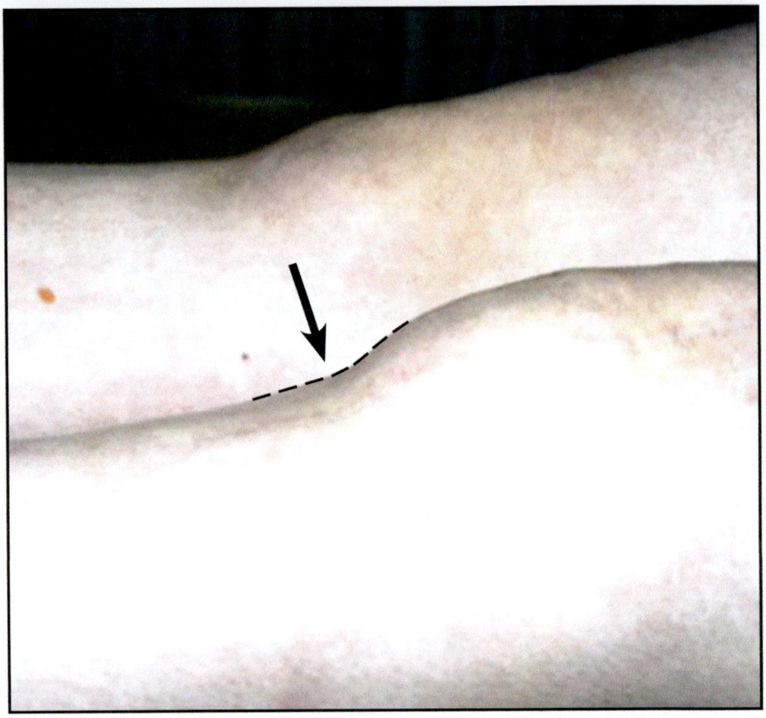

Figure 5-2. Positive shelf sign characterized by an increased slope between the inferior pole of the patella and the proximal tibia with the knee in extension. This occurs secondary to obliteration of the retropatella tendon bursa with adhesions to the anterior tibia.

from the inferior pole of the patella to its insertion at the proximal pole of the tibial tubercle. The length of the patella is then measured at its greatest diagonal length from its superior to inferior pole. The normal ratio of length of the patellar tendon:length of the patella should be approximately 1:1, with some minor gender variation. A ratio of less than 0.8 indicates patella infera (Figure 5-3).

Magnetic resonance imaging (MRI): MRI can be helpful to evaluate for causes of anterior impingement, including improper graft placement and exuberant scar formation anteriorly as well as the presence of a "pseudopatella tendon" (Figure 5-4).

Decision Making

Manipulation under anesthesia and manipulation under anesthesia with arthroscopic fibrinolysis have been shown to be effective treatments for postoperative motion loss.[15,21-23] In patients with arthrofibrosis who have good quadriceps strength with minimal pain, swelling, and warmth, the first question to be addressed is whether there is isolated flexion or extension loss or a combined problem (Figure 5-5).

In isolated contractures with positive inferior patellar tilt, manipulation alone should be performed prior to 4 months postoperatively. In more chronic situations, manipulation under anesthesia with arthroscopic lysis of adhesions is indicated to reduce risk of cartilage damage during manipulation. When inferior patellar tilt is obliterated, arthroscopic lysis of adhesions in addition to manipulation under anesthesia is indicated regardless of acuity or chronicity. If loss of patellar tilt persists, open treatment with possible interposition graft between the patella tendon and anterior tibia or correction of other anatomic issues must be considered (Figure 5-6).

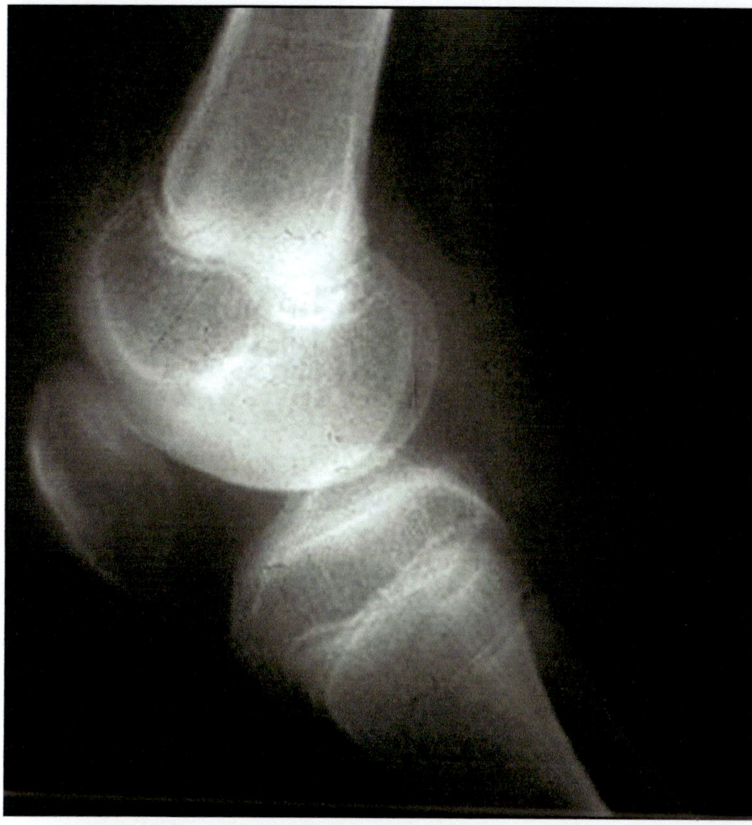

Figure 5-3. Lateral x-ray with the knee flexed 30 degrees demonstrating marked patella infera.

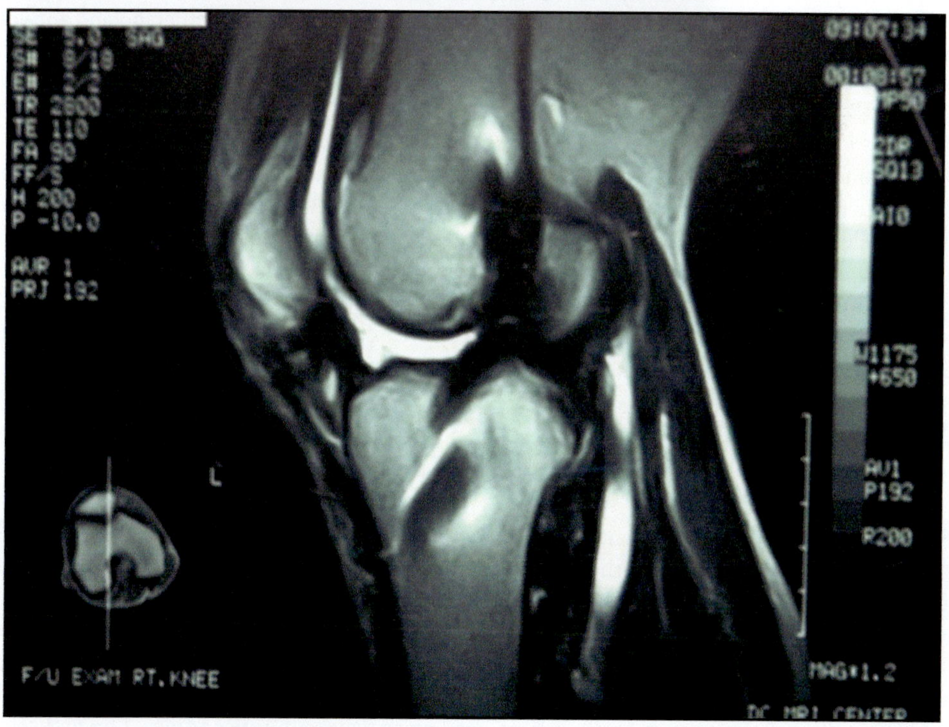

Figure 5-4. Sagittal MRI of a patient with advanced infrapatellar contraction syndrome. A prominent pseudotendon can be seen posterior to the patellar tendon. This represents fibrosis and remodeling of the fat pad.

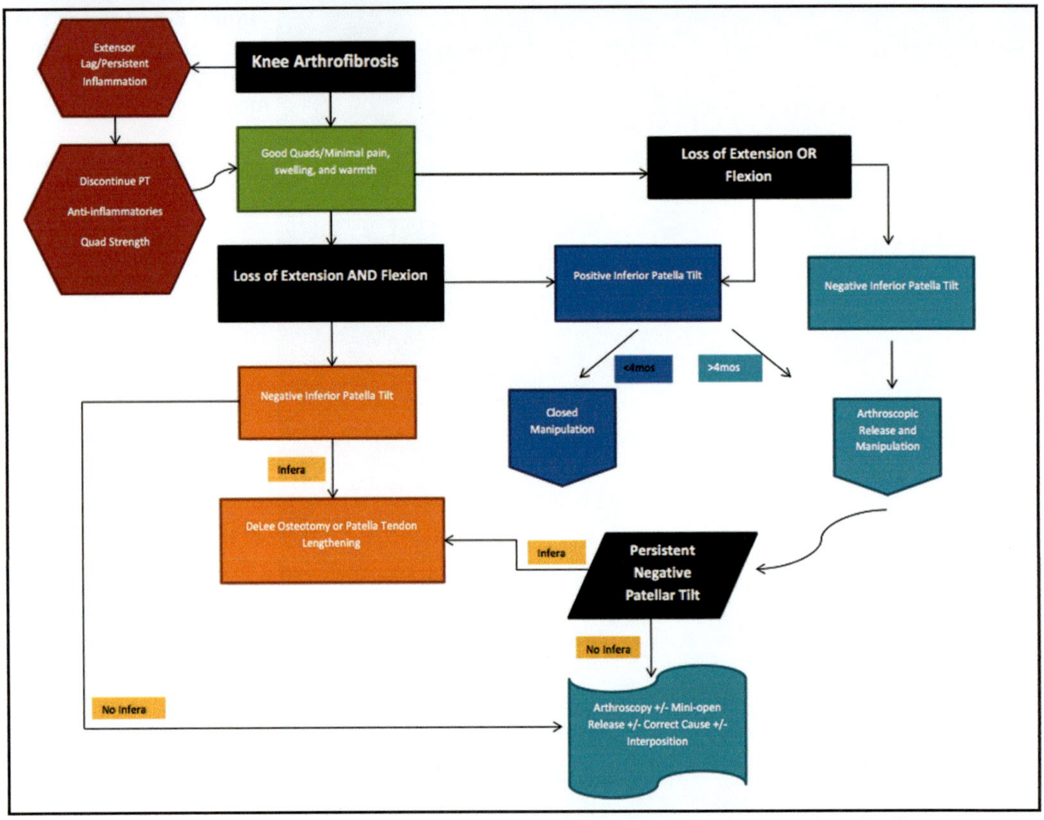

Figure 5-5. Algorithm for the management of knee stiffness. If extensor lag or signs of inflammation are present, discontinue aggressive ROM exercises and treat with quadriceps strengthening and anti-inflammatory drugs. When inflammation and strength improve, determine whether there is loss of flexion, extension, or both and then proceed accordingly.

In combined cases in which there is loss of flexion and extension, the height of the patella with respect to the joint line must be assessed. If there is loss of inferior patellar tilt and patella infera, a Delee osteotomy or other patella-lengthening procedure must be performed in addition to arthroscopic lysis of adhesions and manipulation under anesthesia (Figure 5-7). If the patellar height is normal in a combined contracture with loss of inferior patellar tilt, then arthroscopic lysis of adhesions should be performed with specific release of the distal patella and meniscal tibial interval.[24,25]

Equipment

Standard arthroscopy instruments are used. A 4.0- to 4.5-mm aggressive shaver can be used, but a radiofrequency ablation or other electrocautery-type device is preferred to maintain hemostasis while allowing for deliberate tissue dissection. Curved instruments, particularly a curved shaver, can also be helpful in order to address dense infrapatellar pathology when working toward the anterior portals. If an interposition graft is to be used, the authors typically use a Ventrio Hernia Patch (Bard) and have it available in the room for use. A pump should be used for fluid management, and an outflow cannula can be used at the surgeon's discretion. The arthroscopic fluid can be augmented with epinephrine to aid with visualization.

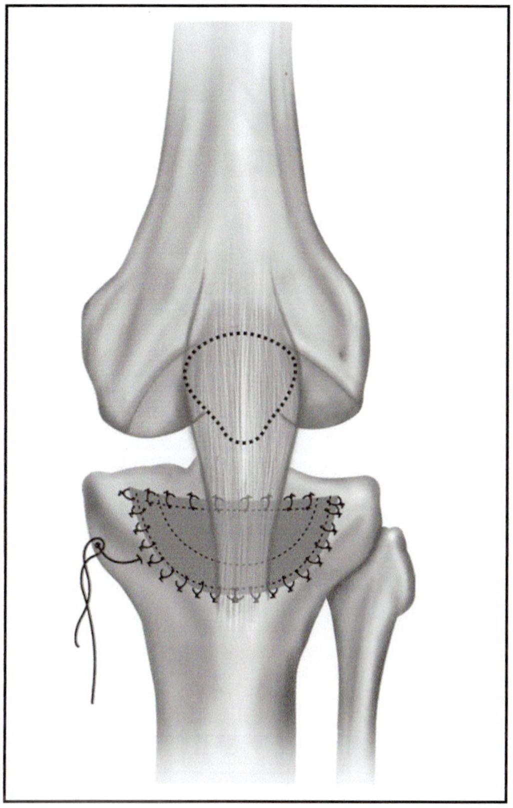

Figure 5-6. Illustration demonstrating placement of an interposition graft for severe infrapatellar contraction syndrome. The graft is placed to prevent adhesions between the patellar tendon and the anterior tibia. A nonreactive barrier is utilized or a hernia patch (Bard type) is used and cut to shape.

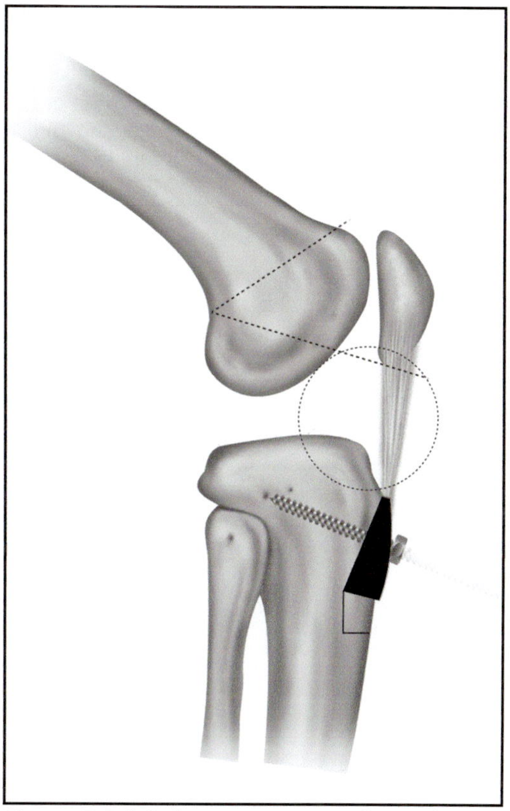

Figure 5-7. A Delee osteotomy can be performed in addition to arthroscopic lysis of adhesions in cases of patella infera with loss of inferior tilt. By moving the tubercle superiorly and anteriorly, the anterior interval and the normal patella position are restored.

Positioning and Portals

A standard arthroscopy setup is used, with the operative extremity in the Johnson leg holder and the end of the operating table fully flexed. The contralateral limb is placed in a limb holder with pneumatic compression for thrombosis prophylaxis. Care must be taken to ensure that the operative knee is placed well distal to the table break to allow for full flexion of the joint during the procedure. In addition, the leg holder must not impede access to the suprapatellar recess but must be distal enough to allow for sufficient varus and valgus stress to be placed on the joint (Figure 5-8). Alternately, the patient can be placed supine with a lateral post placed proximal to the lateral epicondyle of the femur. This is our preferred approach to allow unobstructed access proximally and unobstructed knee flexion. A tourniquet should be placed high on the thigh to allow for optimized hemostasis and visualization during the procedure.

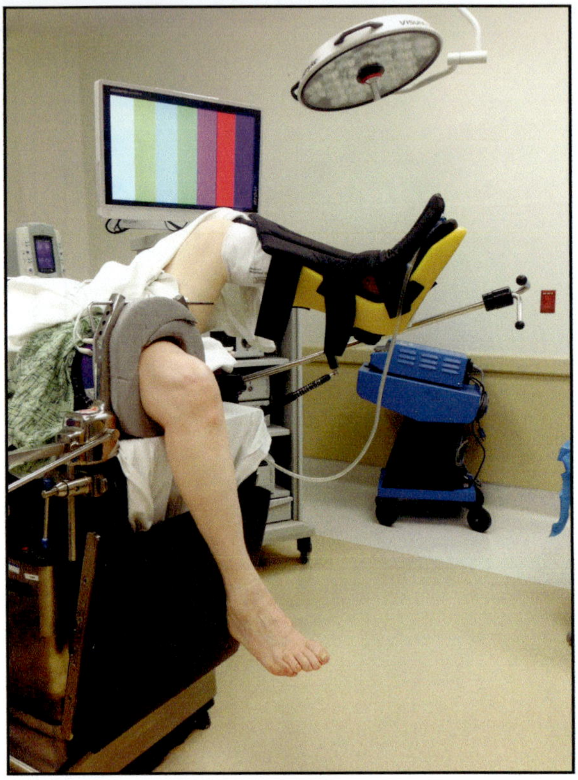

Figure 5-8. Appropriate intraoperative positioning must allow unobstructed access to the entire joint, including the suprapatellar recess, and must also allow for hyperflexion of the knee. A leg holder can be used, as shown here, or the patient can be placed supine with a lateral post.

Step-by-Step Description of the Procedure

The operative site is prescrubbed and marked in the preoperative holding area. The patient is then brought to the operating room and placed supine on the operating table. General anesthesia is administered, and regional anesthesia can be used to augment intra- and postoperative analgesia. In addition, a catheter can be placed to allow for continuous regional anesthesia postoperatively. An adductor canal block can provide excellent analgesia without quadriceps paralysis.

An examination is performed under anesthesia and the extremity is compared to the contralateral extremity. Degree of flexion and extension should be noted for both extremities, including description of the endpoints. Stability assessment should be performed. Patellar glides and patellar tilt should be evaluated and documented. The affected extremity is then prepped and draped in normal sterile fashion with positioning as described above. The limb is exsanguinated, and the tourniquet is inflated to 300 mm Hg, or at the surgeon's choice, 100 mm Hg greater than the systolic blood pressure.

A standard anterolateral arthroscopic portal is created using a #11 blade. It is not uncommon to encounter dense scar tissue at this site secondary to prior surgery. If this occurs and it is difficult to place the cannula and sheath or it is difficult to obtain excursion of these instruments, small scissors can be used to enlarge the lateral portal slightly superolaterally and inferiorly. The arthroscope can then be introduced into the notch and then into the suprapatellar area, taking the leg into extension.

The suprapatellar pouch may be obliterated with adhesions throughout the gutters as well as proximal to the patella. A second portal is established superolaterally. The cannula can be introduced and directed toward the bone, and then the retinaculum can be expanded with oscillating movements similar to establishment of a portal into the subacromial space of the shoulder. An arthroscopic shaver is introduced to clear the contents of the suprapatellar pouch until reasonable visualization can be obtained. The shaver is then substituted with a radiofrequency ablation device used to further expand and clear the suprapatellar pouch underneath the quadriceps tendon.

Looking medially from the anterolateral portal, a thickened plica may be identified and can be addressed with the ablation device from the superolateral portal. The entire medial gutter can then be released while viewing from this position. The ablation device can then be used from the superolateral portal to release the lateral gutter while viewing from the anterolateral portal.

The patella should then be reexamined. Medial and lateral glides should be improved, otherwise further release in the above manner is warranted. If the medial and lateral glides have improved but there is still restricted anterior tilt, the lateral compartment should be visualized to the intercondylar notch by bringing the scope from the lateral gutter into the compartment. There may be significant adhesions between the distal tip of the patella and the anterior tibia and intercondylar notch. Establish an anteromedial portal using a spinal needle with the knee in approximately 30 degrees of flexion to increase your working space anteriorly. It may be necessary to expand it sharply secondary to dense fibrotic tissue at the prior portal site. Gently debride the adhesions in the notch, taking care to avoid injury to the cruciate ligaments or cruciate grafts. After opening the notch, use the ablation device to further release the area behind the patellar tendon and release all tissue from the distal tip of the patella. Care should be taken to avoid injury to the patellar tendon and to avoid resection of the fat pad. Adhesions from the fat pad to the patella must be released, but the fat pad should be preserved. The fat pad should then be released from the tibia to allow exposure of the intermeniscal ligament. Again, using bipolar electrocautery, the interval between the tibia and anterior retinaculum of the knee is then resected, opening the interval and allowing more meniscal mobility.

At the completion of this step, the patella should be reevaluated. Medial and lateral glides and now anterior tilt of the patella should be improved. The remainder of the joint, including the menisci and any ligament grafts, should be visualized. There may be hypertrophic scar of the meniscus, which can be debrided with the shaver or radiofrequency device. The graft should be evaluated for a prominent bone block or for anterior impingement. If there is bone or fibrotic scar tissue from anterior impingement, it should be excised in its entirety and then the graft itself should be reevaluated. It can be thinned or lengthened by making small perpendicular incisions using a meniscal knife through the graft substance at multiple levels.

A final manipulation can then be performed, and then ROM, patellar glides, and patellar tilt can be retested. The instruments should be placed back into the joint after manipulation to evaluate the cruciate ligaments, as there can be partial or complete rupture of a fibrotic ligament with manipulation. Any torn tissue can be debrided at this time.

At the completion of the procedure, the fat pad and any ligament grafts should remain intact without excision. The patella should be mobile, and full ROM can be obtained. The knee is irrigated to remove any loose debris, the portals are closed using a nylon suture, and a soft, compressive dressing is applied. The tourniquet may be lowered prior to closure to evaluate hemostasis and/or a drain may be used at the surgeon's discretion.

Postoperative Protocol

The postoperative management of the patient must be criteria based, low force, essentially painless, and patient controlled. One must read the tissues and consider overall tissue injury, inflammation, and weakness, among other factors. Use of liberal analgesics as well as strong anti-inflammatory drugs, such as one or more Medrol (methylprednisolone) dose packs, can be used to aid with rehabilitation. Rest days must be allowed, and there should be no excessive manual pushing. The patient must actively perform ROM exercises. Rehabilitation should be directed toward regaining extension and quadriceps strength first, followed by flexion. After full passive and active extension are regained, arthroscopic lysis of adhesions with manipulation under anesthesia may be necessary to regain full flexion between 4 and 6 months postintervention.

Potential Complications

The most common complication after surgery for arthrofibrosis is inability to regain and maintain full joint ROM. Other reported complications have included skin tearing, unicortical fracture of the femoral condyle, superficial wound infection, deep wound infection, septic arthritis, peroneal nerve palsy, partial patellar ligament rupture, patellofemoral pain syndrome, and postoperative bleeding requiring reoperation. There is also a risk of recurrent patholaxity if ligament grafts or repairs are released during the procedure. Deep venous thrombosis is also a significant potential complication; therefore, these patients should be treated with mechanical and pharmacologic prophylaxis at the surgeon's discretion.

Top Technical Pearls for the Procedure

1. Premature manipulation of the knee or repeated surgeries invite more severe arthrofibrosis and infrapatellar contraction syndrome. Wait until the knee is less swollen and warm and there is less pain. The patient should have an active quadriceps contraction and no lag.
2. When treating arthrofibrosis that has been present for more than 16 weeks, it is best to precede the manipulation with an arthroscopic release. Arthroscopic release followed by manual manipulation is less damaging to other soft tissues and cartilage surfaces than manipulation alone.
3. The loss of an anterior patella tilt requires an arthroscopic or open release of the distal tip of the patella and retropatella tendon bursa without resection of the fat pad. Loss of the retropatella bursa invites repeated infrapatellar contraction syndrome and patella infera.
4. The most common cause of knee arthrofibrosis is knee ligament surgery. Excessive tension and/or ligament malposition will require ligament lengthening or resection.
5. The liberal use of postsurgical analgesics and anti-inflammatory drugs may be required. Conscientious postoperative guidance with the avoidance of painful and forced motion is the key to success.

References

1. Luck JV. Traumatic arthrofibrosis; the fibroplastic response of joints to trauma. *Bull Hosp Jt Dis.* 1951;12(2):394-403.
2. Enneking WF, Horowitz M. The intra-articular effects of immobilization on the human knee. *J Bone Joint Surg Am.* 1972;54(5):973-985.
3. Sprague NF III, O'Connor RL, Fox JM. Arthroscopic treatment of postoperative knee fibroarthrosis. *Clin Orthop Relat Res.* 1982;(166):165-172.
4. Harner CD, Irrgang JJ, Paul J, Dearwater S, Fu FH. Loss of motion after anterior cruciate ligament reconstruction. *Am J Sports Med.* 1992;20(5):499-506.

5. Cosgarea AJ, DeHaven KE, Lovelock JE. The surgical treatment of arthrofibrosis of the knee. *Am J Sports Med.* 1994;22(2):184-191.
6. Shelbourne KD, Patel DV. Treatment of limited motion after anterior cruciate ligament reconstruction. *Knee Surg Sports Traumatol Arthrosc.* 1999;7(2):85-92.
7. Shelbourne KD, Wilckens JH, Mollabashy A, DeCarlo M. Arthrofibrosis in acute anterior cruciate ligament reconstruction. The effect of timing of reconstruction and rehabilitation. *Am J Sports Med.* 1991;19(4):332-336.
8. Cosgarea AJ, Sebastianelli WJ, DeHaven KE. Prevention of arthrofibrosis after anterior cruciate ligament reconstruction using the central third patellar tendon autograft. *Am J Sports Med.* 1995;23(1):87-92.
9. Sterett WI, Hutton KS, Briggs KK, Steadman JR. Decreased range of motion following acute versus chronic anterior cruciate ligament reconstruction. *Orthopedics.* 2003;26(2):151-154.
10. Shelbourne KD, Johnson GE. Outpatient surgical management of arthrofibrosis after anterior cruciate ligament surgery. *Am J Sports Med.* 1994;22(2):192-197.
11. Noyes FR, Mangine RE, Barber SD. The early treatment of motion complications after reconstruction of the anterior cruciate ligament. *Clin Orthop Relat Res.* 1992;(277):217-228.
12. Noyes FR, Berrios-Torres S, Barber-Westin SD, Heckmann TP. Prevention of permanent arthrofibrosis after anterior cruciate ligament reconstruction alone or combined with associated procedures: a prospective study in 443 knees. *Knee Surg Sports Traumatol Arthrosc.* 2000;8(4):196-206.
13. Magit D, Wolff A, Sutton K, Medvecky MJ. Arthrofibrosis of the knee. *J Am Acad Orthop Surg.* 2007;15(11):682-694.
14. Yaru NC, Daniel DM, Penner D. The effect of tibial attachment site on graft impingement in an anterior cruciate ligament reconstruction. *Am J Sports Med.* 1992;20(2):217-220.
15. Romano VM, Graf BK, Keene JS, Lange RH. Anterior cruciate ligament reconstruction. The effect of tibial tunnel placement on range of motion. *Am J Sports Med.* 1993;21(3):415-418.
16. Shelbourne KD, Patel DV, Martini DJ. Classification and management of arthrofibrosis of the knee after anterior cruciate ligament reconstruction. *Am J Sports Med.* 1996;24(6):857-862.
17. Del Pizzo W, Fox JM, Friedman ML, et al. Operative arthroscopy for the treatment of arthrofibrosis of the knee. *Contemp Orthop.* 1985;10:67-72.
18. Paulos LE, Rosenberg TD, Drawbert J, Manning J, Abbott P. Infrapatellar contracture syndrome. An unrecognized cause of knee stiffness with patella entrapment and patella infera. *Am J Sports Med.* 1987;15(4):331-341.
19. Paulos LE, Wnorowski DC, Greenwald AE. Infrapatellar contracture syndrome. Diagnosis, treatment, and long term followup. *Am J Sports Med.* 1994;22(4):440-449.
20. Grelsamer RP, Meadows S. The modified Insall-Salvati ratio for assessment of patellar height. *Clin Orthop Relat Res.* 1992;(282):170-176.
21. Dodds JA, Keene JS, Graf BK, Lange RH. Results of knee manipulations after anterior cruciate ligament reconstructions. *Am J Sports Med.* 1991;19(3):283-287.
22. Fisher SE, Shelbourne KD. Arthroscopic treatment of symptomatic extension block complicating anterior cruciate ligament reconstruction. *Am J Sports Med.* 1993;21(4):558-564.
23. Klein W, Shah N, Gassen A. Arthroscopic management of postoperative arthrofibrosis of the knee joint: indication, technique, and results. *Arthroscopy.* 1994;10(6):591-597.
24. Steadman JR, Dragoo JL, Hines SL, Briggs KK. Arthroscopic release for symptomatic scarring of the anterior interval of the knee. *Am J Sports Med.* 2008;36(9):1763-1769.
25. Chen MR, Dragoo JL. Arthroscopic releases for arthrofibrosis of the knee. *J Am Acad Orthop Surg.* 2011;19(11):709-716.

Please see videos on the accompanying website at www.routledge.com/9781617119996

SECTION II

Meniscus

6

Arthroscopic Meniscal Resection

John C. Richmond, MD and Owen P. McGonigle, MD

Introduction

As the role of the arthroscope evolved in the 1970s, so did the diagnosis and treatment of meniscal tears. Whereas total meniscectomy was the norm in the era of open meniscal resection, the evolution to arthroscopic techniques demonstrated that partial meniscectomy was better than total meniscectomy. Despite these advances, meniscectomy, even partial, is associated with an increased risk of osteoarthritis.[1-3] Meniscal repair techniques have evolved over the past several decades in an attempt to improve outcomes. Unfortunately, the vast majority of meniscus tears cannot be treated with repair, and arthroscopic partial meniscectomy remains the best procedure in patients with symptomatic meniscal tears.

Arthroscopic partial meniscectomy is an outpatient procedure that can be done under a variety of anesthetic techniques (general, spinal, or regional with or without sedation). Prior to surgical intervention, nonoperative management is the mainstay of initial treatment in the majority of cases. Nonoperative management consists of ice, nonsteroidal anti-inflammatory drugs in patients in whom they are not contraindicated, physical therapy, activity modification, with the possible addition of intra-articular injection of steroids.

Indications

- Persistent pain despite conservative treatment
- Presence of mechanical symptoms
- Younger physiologic age
- Increased activity demands
- Failure of previous meniscal repair

Sgaglione NA, Lubowitz JH, Provencher MT, eds. *The Knee: AANA Advanced Arthroscopic Surgical Techniques* (pp 77-88).

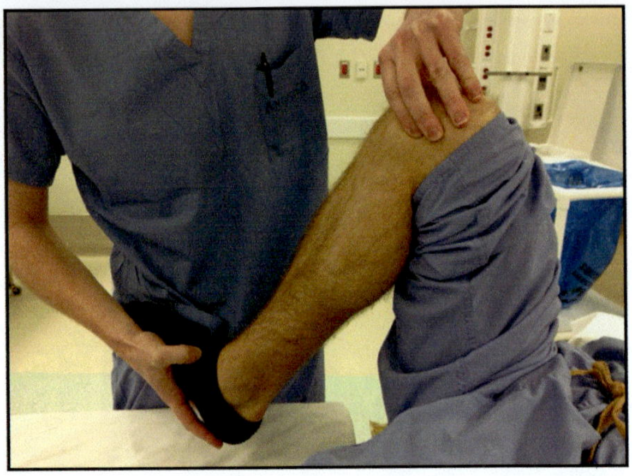

Figure 6-1. McMurray test for a meniscal tear.

Controversial Indications

- Tear amendable to repair
- Asymptomatic tear
- Stable tear (typically < 1.5 cm in length and incomplete, particularly in a patient with an anterior cruciate ligament [ACL]-deficient knee[4,5])
- Degenerative tear in patients with evidence of osteoarthritis (30% nonoperative failure rate requiring conversion to surgery[6])

Pertinent Physical Findings

Assessment of an injured knee always begins with a history. Meniscal tearing in a young patient is typically a relatively traumatic event. With age, meniscal tissue does degenerate, and tearing of the meniscus requires less force. Typically, a flexion rotation stress is associated with a tear, and when the tear is in the avascular portion of the meniscus, pain and swelling often take 24 hours or more to develop. In the middle-aged population, there may be no recollection of injury prior to the tear or simple activities, such as squatting down or kneeling, may be followed by increasing pain and swelling over a period of 24 hours or more associated with a tear. When history and physical examination are considered together, the overall sensitivity to diagnose a meniscal tear is 88% and specificity is 94%.[7]

- Effusion (acute injuries)
- Joint line tenderness (sensitivity of 86% for medial and 92% for lateral; specificity of 67% for medial and 97% for lateral)[8]
- McMurray test (Figure 6-1; with audible clunk sensitivity of 98% and specificity of 15%)[9]
- Steinman test
- Apley test

Pertinent Imaging

- Plain x-rays: Weightbearing anteroposterior and posteroanterior, lateral, and sunrise
- Magnetic resonance imaging (MRI)
- Ultrasound

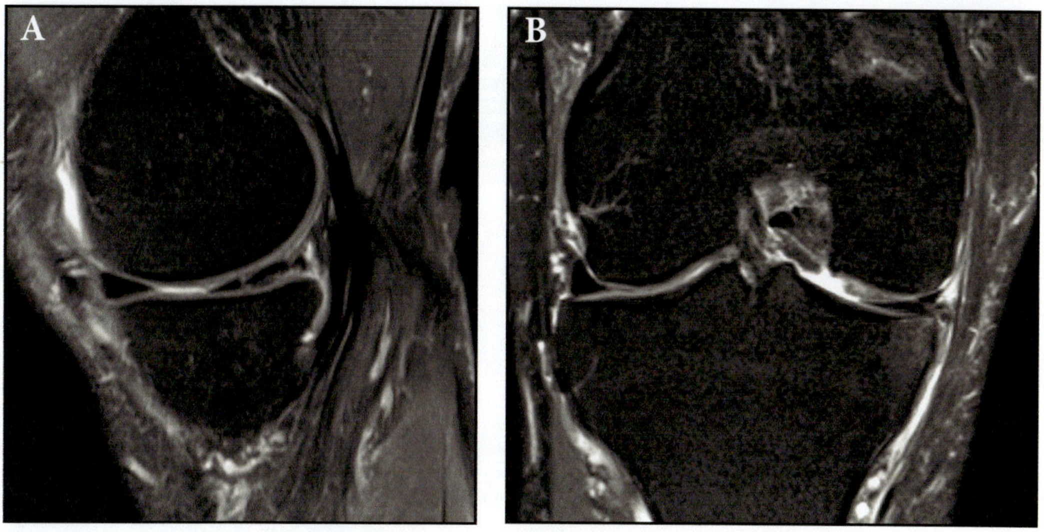

Figure 6-2. (A) Sagittal and (B) coronal MRIs of a complex, degenerative medial meniscal tear.

Plain x-rays, including bent knee posteroanterior (Rosenberg views),[10] are indicated to rule out other potential causes of a patient's symptoms (eg, loose body, osteoarthritis, osteochondritis dessicans). MRI is the gold standard for diagnostic imaging of meniscal tears (Figure 6-2). Diagnostic accuracy of MRI scanning for medial meniscal tears exceeds 90%[11]; due to the popliteal hiatus, it is somewhat less accurate for the lateral meniscus. Ultrasound has a sensitivity of 86.4%, a specificity of 69.2%, a positive predictive value of 82.6%, and a negative predictive value of 75% for detecting meniscal tears.[12] Use of ultrasound is limited due to a high level of operator dependence and low specificity.

Equipment

- Arthroscopic pump
- 30-degree arthroscope
- 70-degree arthroscope available
- Arthroscopic probe
- Array of arthroscopic punches (often termed *biters*; Figure 6-3)
- Motorized shaver 4.0 mm (3.5 or 3.0 mm for smaller or tighter knees)
- Arthroscopic knives (straight, banana, and back-cutting) may assist with meniscal resection

Positioning and Portals

The patient is positioned supine on the operating room table. A leg holder or a post is used to exert valgus and varus pressure during the procedure. There are multiple options for anesthesia for meniscectomy, but spinal or general anesthetics are generally preferred. The foot of the table can be left extended or dropped. If the foot is not dropped and a leg holder is used, it is important to have the leg holder positioned so the hip is flexed 30 degrees in order to keep the knee free and allow ready access for the arthroscopic instruments (Figure 6-4).

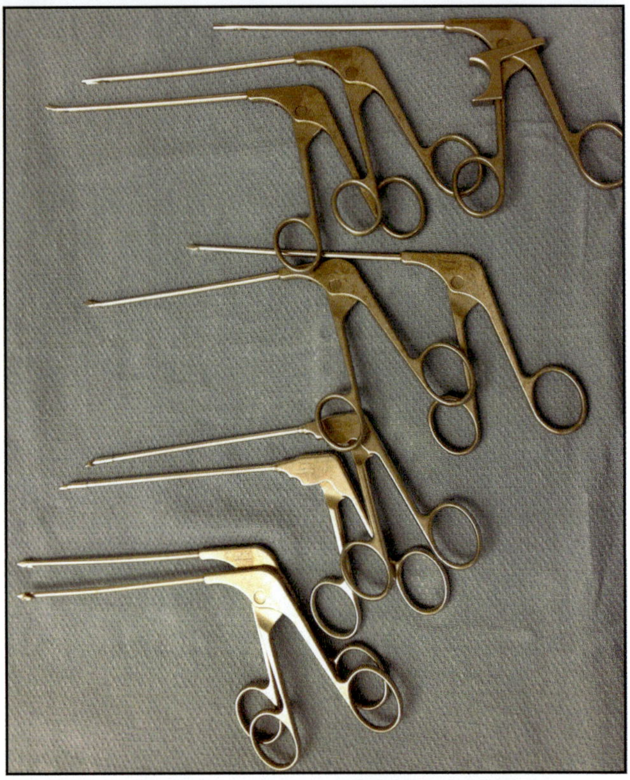

Figure 6-3. An array of punches facilitates resection of meniscal tears.

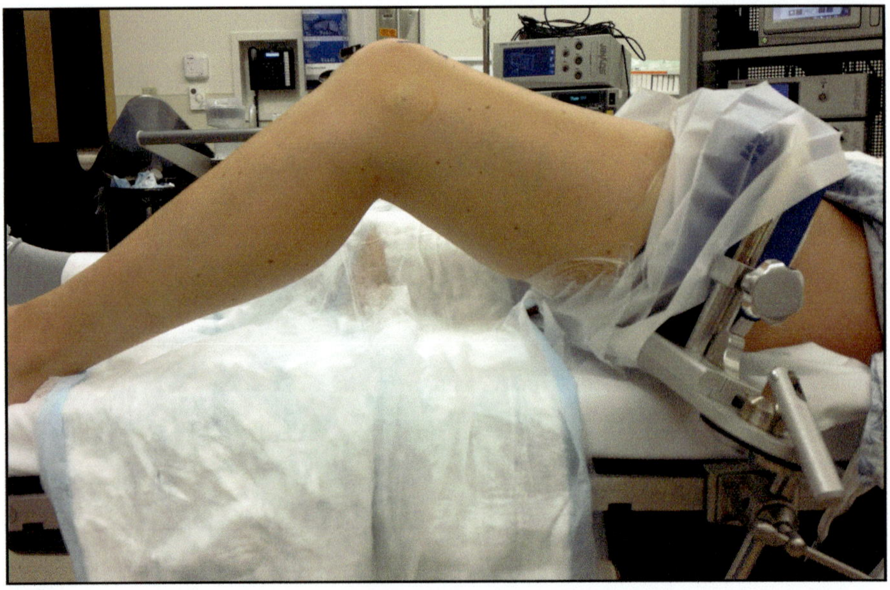

Figure 6-4. Photograph of the leg in a leg holder with the foot of the operating room table extended and the hip flexed 30 degrees to allow access to the knee.

Routine knee arthroscopy can be performed without the use of a tourniquet. This is facilitated by distending the joint prior to portal placement with a local anesthetic with epinephrine. (The senior author uses 50 cc of 1% Xylocaine (lidocaine) with epinephrine 1:100,000 sterilely injected prior to prepping and draping the leg.) Infiltration of the sites for portal placement with local

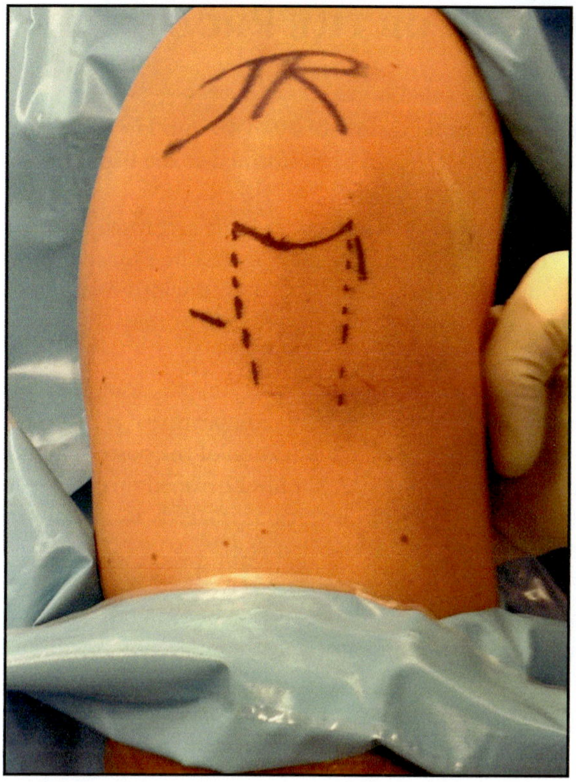

Figure 6-5. Portal sites for routine meniscectomy marked on a left knee. The lateral portal is relatively high, vertical, and just off the patellar tendon, which optimizes visualization and instrumentation. The medial portal is oblique for maximal flexibility.

anesthetic with epinephrine also facilitates knee arthroscopy without the use of a tourniquet. The senior author's preferred local anesthetic is 0.25% bupivacaine with epinephrine (1:200,000) for the portal sites.

There are multiple possible portals for arthroscopic meniscectomy. The senior author prefers a vertical portal just lateral to the proximal patellar tendon for the arthroscope and a relatively low oblique portal anteromedially for instrumentation (Figure 6-5).

The anterolateral portal should be developed with the knee flexed at least 50 degrees to protect the articular surfaces. Once the capsule and synovium have been penetrated using a blunt obturator, the knee is extended to facilitate positioning of the sheath in the suprapatellar pouch. The use of a spinal needle for localization of the anteromedial portal while visualizing from the anterolateral portal is often beneficial to optimize portal placement.

The surgeon should be prepared to use multiple other portals if necessary; specifically, the posteromedial or posterolateral portals may be helpful to remove a retained meniscal fragment that gets into the posterior compartment. These must be developed with the knee flexed to 90 degrees. Protection of the neurovascular structures when one of these portals is being established and used is paramount. The posterolateral portal must always be developed well anterior to the biceps tendon to avoid the peroneal nerve. These portals are most safely developed by initially using a spinal needle for localization. Placement of the cannula with a blunt obturator through the capsule should be done while directly visualizing the capsule.

Step-by-Step Description of the Procedure

The arthroscope is placed into the knee through the standard anterolateral portal with the use of a blunt obturator. With the use of a pump, a distension pressure of 30 to 40 mm Hg is typically all that is necessary. A complete diagnostic examination should be performed at the beginning of any arthroscopic knee procedure.

The anteromedial portal is next established as previously described, and the arthroscopic probe is introduced to inspect the menisci (Video). The medial meniscus should first be probed superiorly and inferiorly to identify any area of tearing and to define the length and width of any tear. Tear stability and proximity to the peripheral blood supply should be assessed as they are important aspects of the treatment decision.

The cruciates should be inspected after the medial compartment and, again, palpation is necessary not only to define anatomy but also the tension. Finally, the lateral compartment is inspected in the figure-4 position. Rotation of the 30-degree scope allows visualization of the posterior, mid, and anterior horns of the lateral meniscus in sequence. The offset should be aimed posteriorly to visualize the posterior horn and then carefully rotated as the inspection proceeds to lateral and anterior. Again, defining the extent and anatomy of the tear is the first step.

The classic arthroscopic surgical technique for resection of unstable longitudinal, flap, and parrot beak tears is termed the *cut and avulse technique*. In this technique, cutting or biting instruments are used to nearly completely detach the large unstable fragment from the remaining meniscus. Maintaining a few fibers intact prevents the formation of a free fragment that may float away. A grasping device is then used to grasp this large fragment and it is then avulsed, typically by repetitive rolling motions that wind up the stress to the small residual area of attachment.

Medial Meniscus Tears

Multiple tear patterns have been described in the medial meniscus. The more common ones are vertical longitudinal, horizontal cleavage, flap or parrot beak tear, radial tear, and complex tear. Complex tears incorporate at least 2 of the other tear patterns. Tears can also be broken down by their etiology (traumatic or degenerative). The goal of any meniscal resection is to remove the unstable and damaged meniscus substance while preserving as much normal or nearly normal meniscus as can be reasonably retained. The margins of the tear resection need to be carefully tapered such that there are no sharp transitions at the resection margin.

The first step in any meniscal resection is to define the anatomy of the tear. If the tear cannot be adequately visualized through the use of a post or leg holder and valgus stress, a relaxation technique of needling the medial collateral ligament (MCL) can be of benefit (Video). This can be done through the joint with an 18-gauge spinal needle or percutaneously with a 1.5-in needle with the bevel maintained perpendicular to the MCL fibers. Multiple perforations of the MCL are made just above the meniscus, then gentle to increasingly firm valgus stress is applied until the MCL releases adequately for visualization. This step is key in preventing damage to the articular cartilage during the performance of a meniscectomy. It is only necessary if there is inadequate space to visualize and instrument the meniscus without the release. Postoperatively, it leads to some increased pain in the medial compartment; the authors are careful to restrict any cutting or contact sports for at least 6 weeks following one of these releases.

Medial Tear Patterns

Vertical longitudinal tears typically occur in the posterior horn and may propagate along the circumferential fibers of the meniscus to the mid and anterior portion. Adequate valgus stress must be applied to facilitate visualization. External rotation of the leg may also assist in visualization by bringing the posterior tibia and attached medial meniscus forward in relationship to the femoral condyle. Attention is typically focused on the posterior lateral extent of the tear for the initial cut. Using scissors or a punch, the far lateral attachment of the unstable segment is cut such that there are only a few remaining fibers. Attention is then focused on the most medial or anterior locus of the tear, which should be completely released using a biter tapered into the axilla of the tear. The released portion of the meniscus can then be grasped and avulsed, typically by repetitive rolling motions. A small motorized shaver (3 to 4 mm) is then used to suction any debris from the release and then to smooth and balance the residual meniscus. If the vertical longitudinal tear extends too far anteriorly to be able to adequately begin the taper from the anteromedial portal, the anterior release is more easily fashioned with the arthroscope in the anteromedial portal and the cutting instrumented in the anterolateral portal (Video).

If a vertical longitudinal tear extends from the posterior horn anterior to the mid or anterior portion of the meniscus, it can be termed a *bucket handle tear* and may displace to lock the knee (Figure 6-6). The easiest way to resect a locked bucket handle tear is to reduce it by using valgus stress and a blunt obturator to manipulate it back into a reduced position. The authors recommend inspecting the peripheral rim to ascertain whether meniscal repair is an option prior to reducing the locked bucket handle tear. In a tight joint with a long-standing displaced segment, reduction of the displaced segment may not be possible. Using the needling technique described to relax the MCL can facilitate the reduction.

Flap tears of the posterior and mid portion of the medial meniscus are relatively common. They can result from a small vertical longitudinal tear that has propagated out through the free border of the meniscus. The resection technique for flap tears is identical to that of a vertical longitudinal tear, except if one is preferentially using the cut and avulse technique, there is only one attachment site and that should not be cut through completely. Tapering of the resection margins is crucial. Flap tears tend to occur more centrally located than the vertical longitudinal tears and are, therefore, in relatively softer, less dense meniscus tissue, which means they may often be readily resected by just the use of a shaver.

Horizontal cleavage tears typically occur in the older population and are more of a degenerative tear pattern. They can typically be thought of with central degeneration within the meniscus that propagates through to the undersurface through a rotation shear. They often cause pain but rarely mechanical symptoms. Typically, these tears are resected using a punch. Since the smaller leaflet is usually the inferior leaflet, that is the preferential one to remove. It is also technically more easily reached because the superior surface of the meniscus tends to ride up behind the condyle when there is a horizontal split. The leaflet that is selected to be removed should be resected back to the level such that there is no longer any pathologic motion between it and the remaining leaflet.

Complex tears are a result of a tear pattern that includes multiple planes (Figure 6-7). They are more common in older patients in whom the meniscus tissue is somewhat abnormal already. The meniscus should be probed and evaluated to identify the tear pattern as closely as possible prior to resection. Flap tears and vertical longitudinal tears are resected using the techniques previously identified. It is important to be certain that a flap is not left folded under the meniscus. This is typically the case if there is an undersurface flap that is located at the mid portion of the meniscus.

Lateral Meniscal Tears

The figure 4 position facilitates visualization and instrumentation of the lateral compartment. It is of benefit when anticipating a lateral meniscal tear that the anteromedial portal be slightly higher to facilitate crossing above the tibial spine to instrument the lateral meniscus. If one has a portal that is too low to readily accomplish this, the skin can be retracted somewhat proximally and a new capsular portal cut, allowing ready instrumentation of the lateral compartment.

Figure 6-6. (A) A displaced bucket handle tear of a left medial meniscus. The tear is too distant from the blood supply to have meniscal repair offer a reasonable chance of success. (B, C) Balanced, preserved meniscal rim following resection of the unstable segment for (A).

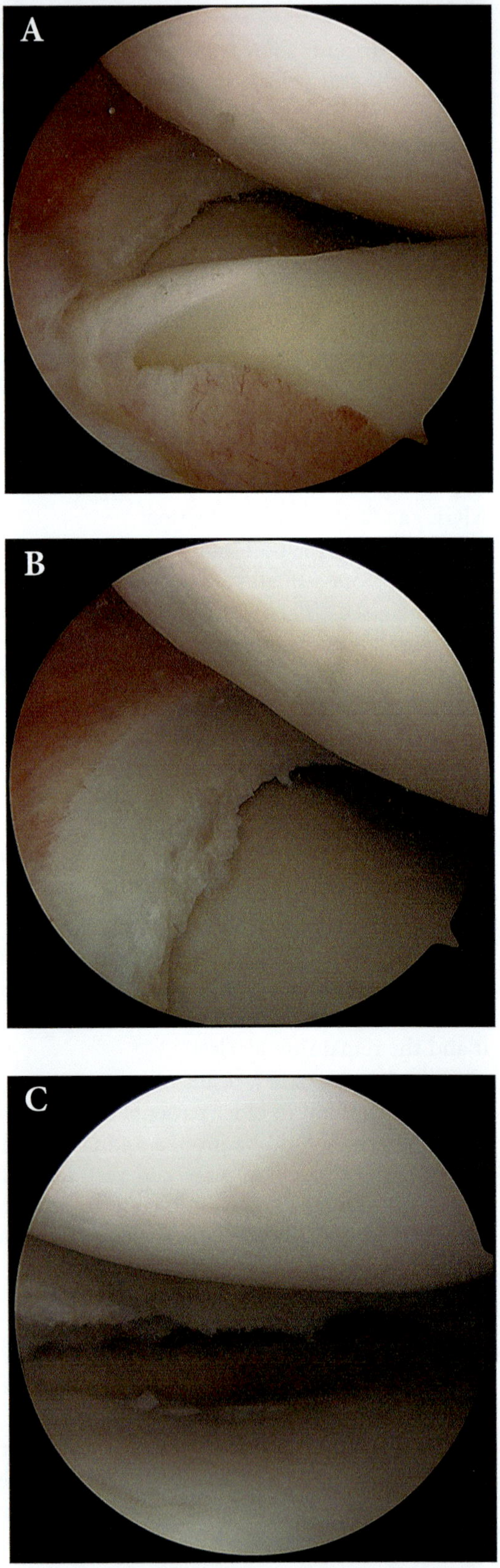

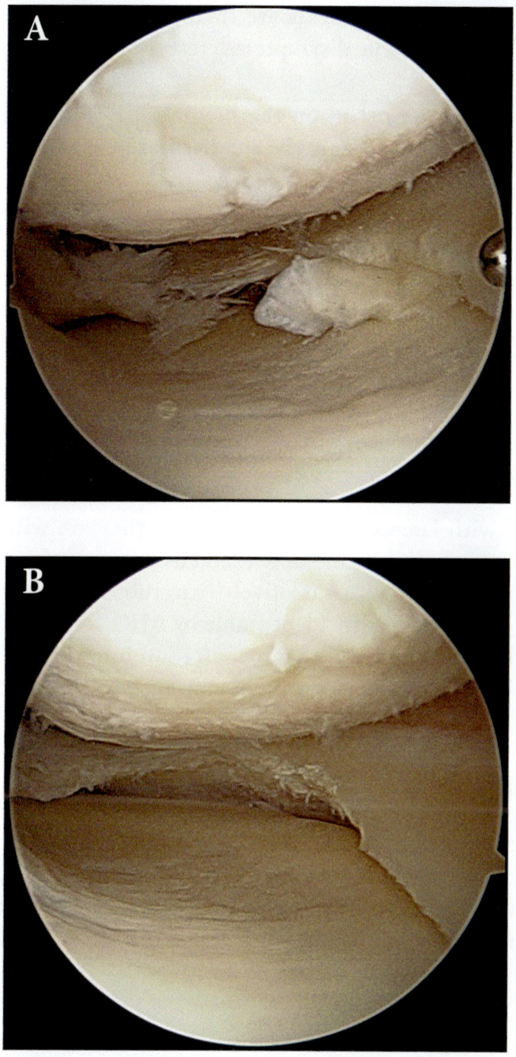

Figure 6-7. Complex tear (A) before and (B) after resection.

Lateral Tear Patterns

Different than the posterior horn medial meniscal tear, the vertical longitudinal tear in the posterior horn of the lateral meniscus may be asymptomatic. These should be probed and assessed. If they can be subluxed out from under the condyle anteriorly, they present an issue for recurrent symptoms. Shelbourne and Heinrich[13] demonstrated that if the tears are stable and behind the popliteus hiatus, they rarely cause symptoms and can be left in situ.

The cut and avulse technique remains appropriate for lateral meniscal resections. Because the arthroscope is typically located in the anterolateral portion for visualization of a lateral meniscal tear, attention to the more anterior axilla of the tear is readily accomplished with this position of the arthroscope, and the resection instrumentation is brought in from the anteromedial portal. It is technically difficult to release the posterior axilla of a vertical longitudinal tear in the lateral meniscus if the ACL is intact because the ACL will block access to this area when instruments are used through the anteromedial portal. In this case, it is optimal to switch portals with the arthroscope medial and instrumentation brought in laterally to facilitate an appropriate tapered release.

Flap tears of the lateral meniscus commonly have a flap at the posterior bony attachment of the meniscus. This is frequently associated with an ACL tear, and care must be taken that the bony attachment of the remaining meniscus stays intact. If these tears are small, resection is not necessary. If they are large and could potentially cause mechanical symptoms, resection should be accomplished.

Horizontal tears are less common in the lateral meniscus than on the medial side. This is a degenerative tear pattern, and resection should be based on removing the smaller leaflet as is done on the medial side.

Radial tears are common in the lateral meniscus. They are typically in the mid portion or slightly anterior to mid. If they extend out to the meniscosynovial junction in the vascular area of the meniscus, the deeper portions of these can be repaired with a complex repair. If they are entirely within the thin central portion of the meniscus, resection should be accomplished. The anterior leaflet can be done with the instruments brought in from the anteromedial portal using a side biter. The posterior leaflet can be accomplished through the same portal using a regular biter. Shaving to remove any site that may propagate is appropriate.

Lateral Meniscal Tear With a Meniscal Cyst

Meniscal cysts are more commonly associated with lateral meniscal tears than they are with medial tears. They are typically identified with a degenerative meniscal tear and usually arise from a tear that is just anterior to the mid meniscus. They present with a relatively firm rubbery nodule that may be painful and can be transilluminated. They are readily identifiable by MRI scan. The degenerative torn portion of the meniscus should be resected, and then penetration into the cyst with a small (3.0- to 3.5-mm) shaver is appropriate. One should open the entrance to this cyst adequately so that it will not reform.

Torn Discoid Lateral Meniscus

A discoid meniscus should not be resected unless it is causing mechanical symptoms. If the tear breaks through to the superior surface, it can be readily visualized. If the tear is entirely horizontal within the body of the meniscus or penetrates inferiorly, it can be difficult to visualize. Resection of a discoid meniscus should be carefully contoured to try to create as near a normal meniscus as can be accomplished.

Postoperative Protocol

With the use of supplementary local anesthesia into the portal sites and potentially into the joint, immediate postoperative pain from a partial meniscectomy is minimal. Closure of the incisions can be accomplished in several ways. The senior author's protocol is to use subcuticular sutures and adhesive strips followed by a bulky, gently wrapped, compressive dressing to help to minimize postoperative swelling. Cryotherapy can be of benefit in reducing the swelling during the postoperative period. The authors routinely instruct patients to use crutches until they can bear weight comfortably with a minimal limp. This is typically after several days. Range of motion exercises, quadriceps setting exercises, and straight leg lifts are appropriate early on to try to maintain quadriceps tone.

Deep vein thrombophlebitis (DVT), although uncommon after a routine meniscectomy, can occur. It is appropriate to take steps to minimize the chance of this. At the authors' institution, they routinely use elastic compression stockings as a mechanical means to reduce the risk of DVT. Chemoprophylaxis with 325 mg of aspirin once or twice a day for several weeks post knee arthroscopy is also reasonable.

At the first postoperative visit, one should be careful to assess for any signs of DVT. The authors consider referral to a physical therapist to regain strength and function in select patients. If they are capable of accomplishing this on their own, physical therapy is not a necessity following arthroscopic meniscectomy.[14]

Potential Complications

Iatrogenic injury to the articular surface is perhaps the most likely complication of meniscal surgery. Although not routinely reported, the surgeon must be vigilant in avoiding injury to the articular cartilage during instrumentation. Preventative measures, such as MCL relation technique, are important to limit damage. The risk of infection after arthroscopic partial meniscectomy is low; however, consequence of an infection can be devastating. The use of prophylactic antibiotics preoperatively is encouraged as a prophylactic measure. Serious neurovascular injuries, although rare, have been reported post meniscectomy. Vigilance must be maintained to avoid injury to the popliteal artery and tibial and peroneal nerves. Injury to the infrapatellar branch of the saphenous nerve during creation of the anterior arthroscopy portals is the most common neurologic injury. Sherman et al[15] reported a 22.2% incidence of sensory changes in this distribution after standard portals had been made. In some instances, injury can result in a painful neuroma in continuity or at the end of the transsection. This may be a significant problem and can result in complex regional pain syndrome in the rare patient. If a neuroma is encountered, desensitization massage is recommended.

Although injury to the MCL has been reported as a complication of knee arthroscopy due to the stress of trying to open a tight joint, the authors are strong advocates for the release of the MCL through needling techniques if the joint is at risk for significant articular surface injury. MCL injuries can be treated with brace protection against valgus stress in the immediate postoperative period.

Spontaneous osteonecrosis of the femoral condyle has been reported post meniscectomy with a variety of surgical techniques, including the use of laser, radiofrequency or plain electrocautery, and cold resections with the punch and shaver.[16] It is felt that this risk is higher with the use of laser or thermal devices; therefore, their use has been curtailed by many in routine meniscectomy. Spontaneous osteonecrosis post meniscectomy is an exceedingly uncommon event and typically occurs in middle-aged patients with early findings of osteoarthritis. It may relate to increased pressure upon an already damaged articular surface potentially exacerbated by the heat generated by the use of thermal devices.

Top Technical Pearls for the Procedure

1. Define the anatomy of the tear through careful review of the MRIs and probing during the arthroscopy to ascertain what tissue needs to be removed.
2. Resect only unstable and damaged tissue and preserve as much reasonable meniscal tissue as can be saved.
3. To avoid injury to the articular surfaces, have a low threshold to release the MCL, and always use the figure-4 position for the lateral meniscus.
4. Be prepared to switch instruments and arthroscopes to facilitate a taper of the meniscal resection.
5. Consider the use of a prophylactic antibiotics and the use of mechanical means and/or low-risk chemoprophylaxis for DVT.

References

1. Englund M, Roos EM, Lohmander LS. Impact of type of meniscal tear on radiographic and symptomatic knee osteoarthritis: a sixteen-year followup of meniscectomy with matched controls. *Arthritis Rheum.* 2003;48(8):2178-2187.
2. Englund M, Lohmander LS. Risk factors for symptomatic knee osteoarthritis fifteen to twenty-two years after meniscectomy. *Arthritis Rheum.* 2004;50(9):2811-2819.
3. Roos H, Laurén M, Adalberth T, Roos EM, Jonsson K, Lohmander LS. Knee osteoarthritis after meniscectomy: prevalence of radiographic changes after twenty-one years, compared with matched controls. *Arthritis Rheum.* 1998;41(4):687-693.
4. Neyret P, Donell ST, Dejour H. Results of partial meniscectomy related to the state of the anterior cruciate ligament. Review at 20 to 35 years. *J Bone Joint Surg Br.* 1993;75(1):36-40.
5. Allen CR, Wong EK, Livesay GA, Sakane M, Fu FH, Woo SL. Importance of the medial meniscus in the anterior cruciate ligament-deficient knee. *J Orthop Res.* 2000;18(1):109-115.
6. Katz JN, Brophy RH, Chaisson CE, et al. Surgery versus physical therapy for a meniscal tear and osteoarthritis. *N Engl J Med.* 2013;368(18):1675-1684.
7. Terry GC, Tagert BE, Young MJ. Reliability of the clinical assessment in predicting the cause of internal derangements of the knee. *Arthroscopy.* 1995;11(5):568-576.
8. Eren OT. The accuracy of joint line tenderness by physical examination in the diagnosis of meniscal tears. *Arthroscopy.* 2003;19(8):850-854.
9. Evans PJ, Bell GD, Frank C. Prospective evaluation of the McMurray test. *Am J Sports Med.* 1993;21(4):604-608.
10. Rosenberg TD, Paulos LE, Parker RD, Coward DB, Scott SM. The forty-five-degree posteroanterior flexion weight-bearing radiograph of the knee. *J Bone Joint Surg Am.* 1988;70(10):1479-1483.
11. Konan S, Rayan F, Haddad FS. Do physical diagnostic tests accurately detect meniscal tears? *Knee Surg Sports Traumatol Arthrosc.* 2009;17(7):806-811.
12. Shetty AA, Tindall AJ, James KD, Relwani J, Fernando KW. Accuracy of hand-held ultrasound scanning in detecting meniscal tears. *J Bone Joint Surg Br.* 2008;90(8):1045-1048.
13. Shelbourne KD, Heinrich J. The long-term evaluation of lateral meniscus tears left in situ at the time of anterior cruciate ligament reconstruction. *Arthroscopy.* 2004;20(4):346-351.
14. Goodwin PC, Morrissey MC, Omar RZ, Brown M, Southall K, McAuliffe TB. Effectiveness of supervised physical therapy in the early period after arthroscopic partial meniscectomy. *Phys Ther.* 2003;83(6):520-535.
15. Sherman OH, Fox JM, Snyder SJ, et al. Arthroscopy—"no-problem surgery." An analysis of complications in two thousand six hundred and 40 cases. *J Bone Joint Surg Am.* 1986;68(2):256-265.
16. Son IJ, Kim MK, Kim JY, Kim JG. Osteonecrosis of the knee after arthroscopic partial meniscectomy. *Knee Surg Relat Res.* 2013;25(3):150-154.

Please see videos on the accompanying website at www.routledge.com/9781617119996

7

Arthroscopic Meniscal Repair

Andrew D. Goodwillie, MD; Kevin R. Myers, MD; and Nicholas A. Sgaglione, MD

Introduction

Acute meniscal injury tends to occur following a traumatic compression-rotational injury of the knee as it moves from flexion into extension. Tears can be described by anatomic location within the knee (ie, posterior horn, body, anterior horn) or by the tear pattern (ie, horizontal, radial, longitudinal, bucket handle, oblique, or complex). Simple tear patterns tend to occur in younger patients following traumatic injury, whereas more complex tears involving multiple planes tend to occur in older individuals and are typically degenerative in nature. Complex degenerative tears may be acute or chronic in nature and tend to be irreparable.

Historically, the understanding of meniscal anatomy and its vascularity provided by the perimeniscal capillary plexus has dictated meniscal repair strategies. Cooper et al[1] divided the meniscus into 3 zones according to its vascularity, which was subsequently thought to correlate with the meniscus's intrinsic ability to heal. Meniscal repair was subsequently limited to peripheral tears within the red-red zone of the meniscus. However, there has been increased interest in the healing potential of tear patterns that were regarded by many as irreparable, including vertical tears within the red-white zone,[2] radial tears (Figure 7-1),[3] and horizontal cleavage tears (Figure 7-2).[4] Moreover, the improved ease of all-inside meniscal repair techniques outlined in this chapter have allowed surgeons to continue to push the boundaries of meniscal repair indications, especially for tears found in young adolescent athletes.[5] In addition, understanding the biology of the improved meniscal healing potential with concurrent anterior cruciate ligament (ACL) reconstruction has proposed the use of biologic augmentation to improve outcomes in isolated meniscal repairs.[6,7]

The reason to broaden the indications for surgical meniscus repair rests on the long-term outcomes of meniscectomized patients. The degree of meniscal resection has long been correlated with the increase of mean and peak contact stresses within the tibiofemoral compartment.[8] Long-term consequences of this include articular cartilage degeneration and risk of osteoarthrosis. For example, in a completely meniscectomized knee, tibiofemoral contact areas decrease 40% to 75% and peak local contact stresses can increase up to 235% of normal.[8] The importance of meniscal conservation cannot be overemphasized and provides a means to restore normal tibiofemoral contact pressures and limit the risk of osteoarthritis.[5,9]

Sgaglione NA, Lubowitz JH, Provencher MT, eds. *The Knee: AANA Advanced Arthroscopic Surgical Techniques* (pp 89-102).

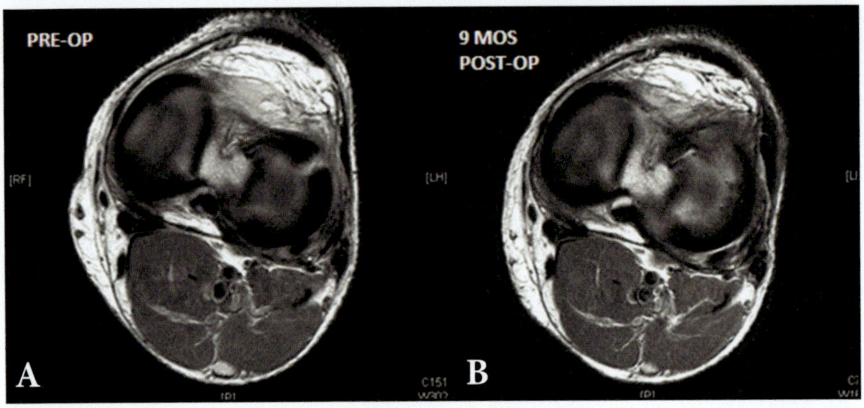

Figure 7-1. (A) Axial proton dense MRI sequences showing full-thickness radial tear anterior horn lateral meniscus in a 29-year-old athlete, and (B) evidence of healing after radial meniscal repair at 9 months postoperatively.

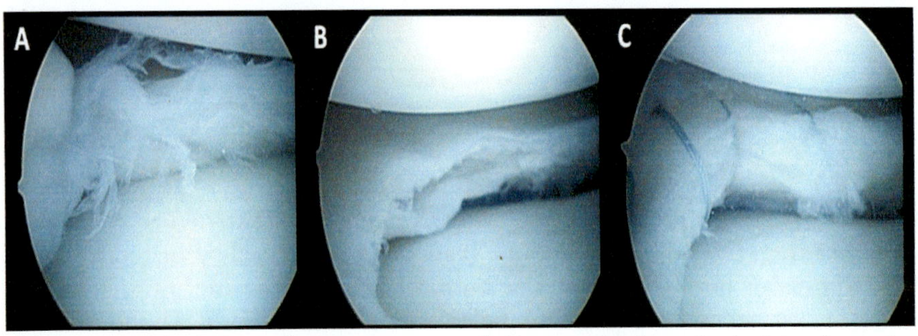

Figure 7-2. (A) Horizontal cleavage tear of the anterior horn-body lateral meniscus. (B) Cleavage tear following debridement and resection of a white-white zone. (C) Horizontal cleavage tear flowing repair with 3 all-inside vertical mattress sutures.

Indications

When indicating a patient for meniscal repair, tear location, pattern, vascularity, tissue viability, ability to hold repair sutures, and associated pathology should be evaluated. In addition, the surgeon should consider the patient's age, activity level, overall health, occupation, goals, expectations, and ability to comply with a strict postoperative rehabilitation protocol. A thorough history, including injury mechanism, activity-related pain, and the presence of mechanical symptoms (acute loss of motion, locking, catching, or instability), should also be obtained. After indication, a frank discussion should be had with the patient preoperatively outlining the long-term implications of an attempted repair over meniscectomy, including the potential risk of repair failure and the potential need for future surgical resection.

Acute surgical repair should be considered for any meniscus that is determined to be repairable at the time of diagnosis. If left untreated, a displaced tear can cause significant articular cartilage damage. In particular, any unstable tear that produces mechanical symptoms of locking or instability or a tear that is displaced or incarcerated within the joint should be repaired urgently. Repairable meniscal injuries in younger patients should also be considered for expeditious surgical repair. However, what constitutes a young patient can be hard to determine as there is currently no consensus regarding an age limit for attempted meniscal repair. What is known, however, is that the meniscal healing response and meniscal cellularity decrease with age.[10] However, successful repairs have been shown to be more than 85% in patients older than 40 years in medium-term follow-up studies.[11,12]

- Patient characteristics
  - Young athletic patients (younger than 40 years)
  - Acute traumatic meniscal injury with mechanical symptoms
  - Concomitant ACL reconstruction
  - Those willing to undergo postoperative rehabilitation
- Tear configuration
  - Unstable longitudinal/vertical tears longer than 1 cm
  - Bucket handle tears
- Tear location
  - Peripheral third red-red zone
  - Meniscal root injuries

Controversial Indications

- Patient characteristics
  - Older athletic patients (older than 40 years)
  - Chronic displaced tears with plastic deformity
- Tear configuration
  - Radial tears in young athletic patients
  - Horizontal cleavage tears in young athletic patients
- Tear location
  - Central red-white zone tears

Pertinent Physical Findings

Physical examination of the knee begins with observation of a patient's gait as he or she enters the examination room. A complete examination of the knee should then be performed and documented, including inspection, palpation, range of motion (ROM), stability testing, and provocative meniscal tests. Although there is no single physical examination finding that can reliably predict meniscal pathology, reproduction of the patient's symptoms with the examination techniques can be suggestive of intra-articular meniscal pathology. Pain with provocative testing may be considered a best test.

Examination Techniques

- Inspection of the joint visualizing effusion/localized joint line swelling
- Palpation of the joint line for focal medial or lateral joint line tenderness/parameniscal cyst formation
- Loss of full extension/flexion of the knee (ie, locking)
- Pain with ROM
  - Pain with deep knee flexion suggestive of posterior horn meniscal pathology
  - Pain with extension suggestive of anterior horn pathology
  - Reproducible catching during ROM with localized pain

- Positive meniscal provocative testing (best test)
  - McMurray test: Reproduced medial joint line pain when extending a flexed knee with a valgus and external rotation stress or lateral joint line pain when extending the knee with a varus and internal rotation stress
  - Apley test: Joint line pain with application of an axial load and internal/external rotation with the patient in a prone position. If a meniscus tear is the only pathology, relief will occur with distraction. No relief will occur if a concomitant collateral ligament injury is present.
  - Childress test: Reproduction of joint line pain with a squat/duck walk
  - Steinman test/Merkel sign: Pain with internal rotation of the tibia is consistent with a medial meniscus tear; pain with external rotation of the tibia is consistent with a lateral meniscus tear.

Pertinent Imaging

Radiographic imaging is obtained in any patient presenting with possible meniscal pathology and includes 4 standard x-ray views. Plain x-rays are used to evaluate for any concomitant bony pathology, extremity malalignment, arthritis, chondrocalcinosis, or findings consistent with any potential associated injuries (eg, loose bodies, osteochondral fractures/defects, osteochondritis dissecans lesions, Pellegrini-Stieda sign, and Segond sign).

Magnetic resonance imaging (MRI) is typically described as the gold standard in the diagnosis of meniscal pathology; however, it may not always be necessary. Its high sensitivity and specificity (96% and 97%, respectively)[13] typically confirms clinical suspicion of meniscal injury, delineates meniscal tear morphology, and evaluates for any additional articular cartilage or ligamentous injury. Contrast is not required for the diagnosis of meniscal pathology, although in the setting of prior meniscectomy, intra-articular gadolinium improves diagnostic sensitivity for new pathology.

- X-rays
  - 30- to 45-degree posteroanterior weightbearing flexion view
  - True lateral view
  - Notch view
  - Patella skyline view
- MRI without gadolinium
  - Increased signal intensity on T1- and intermediate-weighted images
  - Sequences include fast spin-echo proton density, fat-saturated fast-spin-echo T2, and T1

Equipment

- Arthroscopy tower
  - Light source
  - Monitor and recording device
  - 4-mm, 30-degree arthroscope with cannula (recommend having a 70-degree arthroscope available)
- Irrigation system
  - Inflow: Gravity inflow of lactated ringers solution vs high-pressure pump system
  - Outflow: To suction/pump

- Sterile knee arthroscopy pack
  - Drapes
  - Inflow/outflow tubing
- Instruments
  - Basic arthroscopy tray, including the following:
    - Arthroscopic probe
    - Various angled meniscal biters/graspers
    - Handheld motorized instrument (eg, 3.5-mm full-radius meniscal shaver)

Positioning and Portals

Positioning of the patient is typically performed with a lateral post or a knee holder. Regardless of the technique used, the key to positioning is verifying prior to draping that full access to the operative knee can be obtained. This includes ensuring full ROM, allowing for proper flexion angles, and adequate varus/valgus positioning of the knee. In addition, the contralateral extremity should be well padded with a sequential compression device applied to the calf. A tourniquet may also be used during the case if bleeding is suspected, such as in debridement of hypertrophic synovitis or a hypertrophic fat pad. However, to visualize vascularity of meniscal repair sites, the authors attempt to avoid tourniquet inflation during the case.

- Lateral post
  - The patient is positioned supine on the operating table with the operative leg positioned close to the lateral edge of the table.
  - The lateral post is placed mid-thigh and angled to enable a valgus force on the operative knee during arthroscopy.
  - The operative leg is placed into a figure-4 position to gain access to the lateral compartment, with gentle pressure placed by an assistant on the medial knee to provide a varus force.
- Knee holder (Figure 7-3)
  - The patient is positioned supine on the operating table with the operative leg positioned so that the femur is parallel to the floor and the patella is rotated toward the ceiling.
  - The knee holder is positioned approximately 2 to 3 in above the superior pole of the patella
  - The foot of the table is then dropped to 90 degrees to allow both legs to hang freely from the end of the table.

Step-by-Step Description of the Procedure

Anesthesia

- Most surgeons use general anesthesia with a laryngeal mask airway vs sedation in conjunction with local anesthesia.
- Our preference is to inject local anesthesia into the knee joint prior to arthroscopy, including a 30- to 40-cc intra-articular injection of a 50% mixture of 0.5% Marcaine (bupivacaine) and 1% lidocaine with epinephrine, with about 5 cc injected into each anticipated portal site.

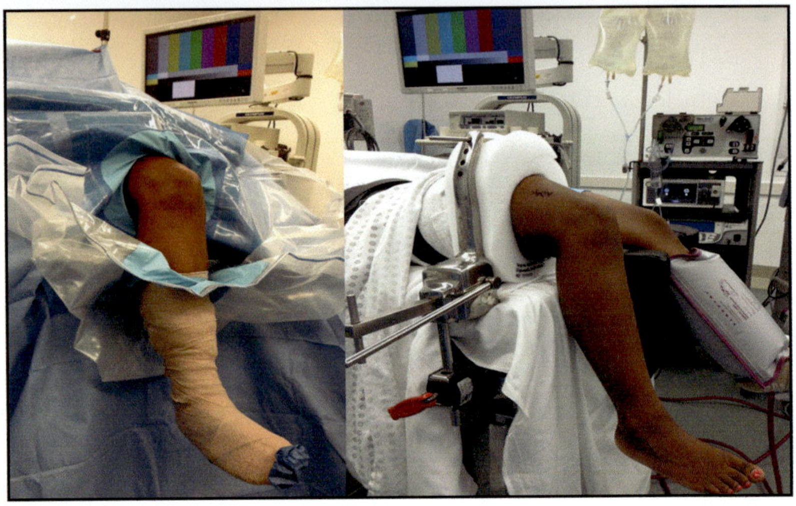

Figure 7-3. Standard arthroscopy setup and patient positioning for meniscal repair using a knee holder.

- Although still debated within the literature, in the authors' practice, a weight-based dose of a third-generation cephalosporin is given prior to anesthesia for preoperative antibiotics.
- Patients are also typically risk stratified for perioperative anticoagulation.
  - The authors' philosophy is that after risk stratification of the individual patient, if the patient is deemed high risk (prior history of deep vein thrombosis, clotting disorder etc), then the patient is given appropriate anticoagulation postoperatively.

Diagnostic Arthroscopy

- A time-out is performed, with the operative staff confirming that the surgical procedure and all surgical imaging/equipment has been made available and verified.
- With a #11 blade, an anterolateral viewing portal is created within the soft spot 1 cm lateral to the patellar tendon and adjacent to the inferior pole of the patella.
- With a valgus force directed on the knee, a working anteromedial portal is created under direct visualization within the medial soft spot 1 cm medial to the patellar tendon and 1 cm proximal to the joint line.

The working portal is localized arthroscopically with a spinal needle prior to portal placement.

  - When positioning the spinal needle anteromedially, confirm that the needle passes easily to the posterior horn of the medial meniscus without touching the medial femoral condyle. This ensures correct placement of the portal.
  - You may also use the concavity of the medial tibial plateau to ensure easy passage to the posterior horn of the meniscus.
  - Pie-crusting of the medial collateral ligament (MCL) using a 14-gauge needle can improve access to the medial compartment in overly tight knees (Figure 7-4).
- An optional accessory superomedial outflow portal can be made medial to the quadriceps at the superior pole of the patella directed obliquely into the joint.
- Perform a full diagnostic arthroscopy and evaluate the meniscal tear characteristics with the use of an arthroscopic probe.
  - Document the location, morphology, length, and tissue quality of the tear.
  - Document any chondral wear seen throughout the knee.

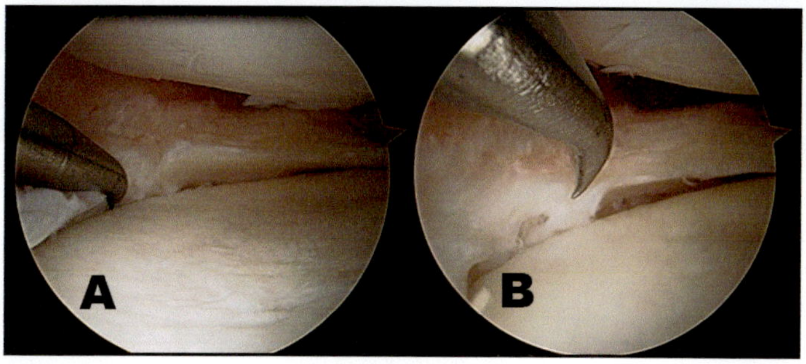

Figure 7-4. (A) Pre- and (B) post-MCL pie crusting.

Meniscal Preparation

- If amenable to repair, stimulate vascular in-growth at the edge of the tear with rasping or trephination.
  - Rasping may be performed by lightly abrading the fibrous tissue at the meniscal edges and the meniscosynovial junction with an arthroscopic shaver (with minimal suction) or meniscal rasp.
  - Trephination is performed by inserting a long 18- or 20-gauge needle percutaneously or through the arthroscopic portals across the meniscus tear to create vascular channels.
- Hold the meniscus reduced with use of a Mulberry knot (optional).
  - Pass a 0-Prolene suture through an 18-gauge needle passed from an outside-in technique and retrieve it arthroscopically from the working portal.
  - Tie multiple knots in the retrieved end of the suture and pull back into the joint; the meniscus will reduce to the periphery with continued traction.

Repair Techniques

Multiple techniques for meniscal repair have been described. Open repair techniques have been primarily replaced with inside-out, outside-in, and all-side techniques. Each arthroscopic technique is described in a stepwise fashion. Inside-out techniques are best used for middle or posterior horn tears. Outside-in techniques are typically used for tears of the anterior and middle third, as well as radial tears. All-inside techniques are used for most tear configurations and have evolved from nonsuture fixation that relied on reverse barbed fishhook designs (eg, Meniscus Arrow; ConMed Linvatec) to all-suture fixation techniques that have consistently shown to have superior results.[14-16]

Regardless of the technique chosen, the key to fixation is to achieve perpendicular compressive forces at the meniscocapsular junction. This may require the use of additional portals depending upon tear characteristics and may include the use of a superolateral, posteromedial, posterolateral, mid-patella, central, far medial, or far lateral portal. Slight elevation of the standard anterolateral or anteromedial portal may also provide improved access to the contralateral compartment for meniscal fixation.

Inside-Out Technique (Video)

- Posteromedial tears
  - Place the knee in 20 to 30 degrees of flexion to avoid tethering the capsule and avoid the saphenous nerve.
  - Make a 4- to 6-cm longitudinal incision along the posterior edge of the MCL, centered one-third above and two-thirds below the joint line (Figure 7-5A).

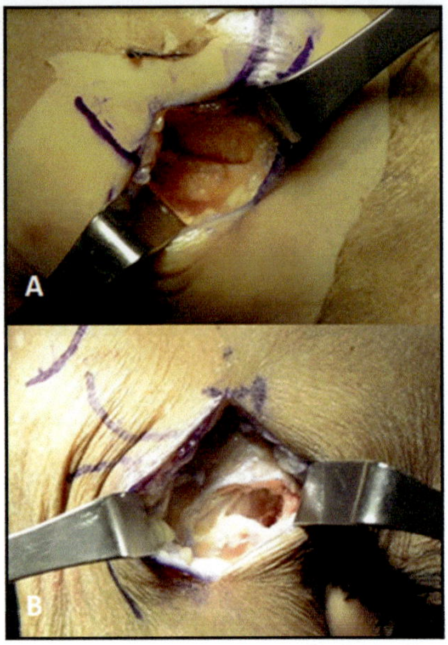

Figure 7-5. (A) Posteromedial inside-out incision. (B) Posterolateral inside-out incision.

  - ▹ Dissect anterior to the sartorius and semimembranosus musculature and retract posteriorly, exposing the medial head of the gastrocnemius that is retracted to expose the underlying capsule.
- ▸ Posterolateral tears
  - ▹ Place the knee in 90 degrees of flexion to allow the peroneal nerve, popliteus, and lateral inferior geniculate artery to fall posteriorly.
  - ▹ Make a 4- to 6-cm longitudinal incision at the posterior edge of the lateral collateral ligament and anterior to the biceps femoris tendon, centered one-third above and two-thirds below the joint line (Figure 7-5B).
  - ▹ Sharply dissect the fascial plane between the iliotibial band and the biceps tendon to expose the lateral head of the gastrocnemius.
  - ▹ Dissect deep and anterior to the lateral head of the gastrocnemius to expose the lateral capsule.
  - ▹ Place a popliteal retractor against the capsule to retract the gastrocnemius posteriorly to safely visualize, deflect, and capture the exiting repair needles.
- ▸ Pass a single- or double-lumen cannula arthroscopically through a working portal perpendicular to the tear.
- ▸ Pierce the meniscus above and below the tear site in a vertical mattress suture fashion with long flexible needles with high-strength, nonabsorbable 0 or 2-0 suture material by passing the needles through the cannula.
- ▸ Capture the needles separately through a posteromedial or posterolateral incision as previously described. Do not to pull either suture all the way through until both needles are passed.
- ▸ Tension each suture and tie down to the capsule while viewing the repair arthroscopically and confirming reduction and fixation of the meniscus.

Outside-In Technique

- ▸ Palpate the joint line and then pierce the joint line with an 18-gauge spinal needle, passing through the meniscocapsular junction, meniscal rim, and the torn fragment.

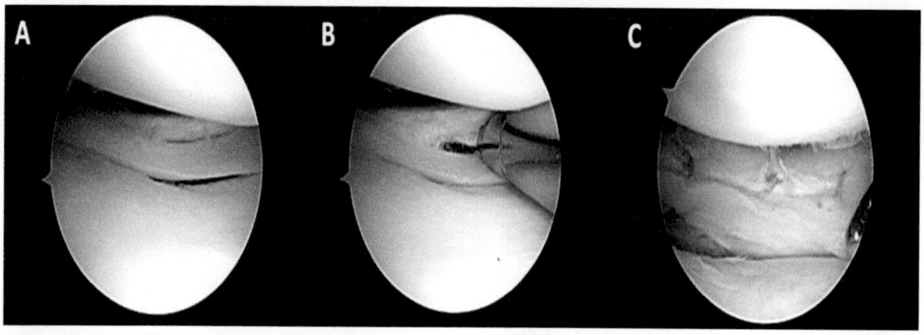

Figure 7-6. (A) Vertical tear of the posterior horn lateral meniscus. (B) Meniscal bed preparation with an arthroscopic shaver. (C) Vertical mattress suture configuration with reduction of a meniscal tear.

- Repierce the meniscus with another 18-gauge needle through the tear and pass a 0-Prolene suture through the working portal. Tie a 0 or 2-0 nonabsorbable, high-strength suture to the Prolene and shuttle through the meniscus.
- Repeat this procedure again through the meniscal tear to produce a vertical or horizontal mattress suture configuration by tying the free end of the 0 or 2-0 suture to the second pass of the Prolene suture. The needles should be spaced about 3 to 5 mm apart.
- A second outside-in technique is to use a proprietary meniscal device (ie, Meniscal Mender; Smith & Nephew) that includes a preloaded nitinol wire to allow easy passage of suture material without having to exit the joint (Video).
- After tensioning of the mattress suture, a small 1-cm skin incision is made between the suture strands, and blunt dissection is carried down to the capsule. An arthroscopic probe may be used to retrieve the sutures from within the incision, and the sutures are sequentially tied down to the capsule under direct visualization, taking care to avoid incarceration of any soft tissue (Video).

All-Inside Arthroscopic Technique (Video)

- Prior to using the insertion device, ensure that the chosen portal provides perpendicular access to the tear orientation. Creating a larger capsular incision through the portal can also aid in passage of the suture device and minimize soft tissue interference.
- Use a skid, sheath, or insertion cannula to facilitate arthroscopic access to the knee joint and protect chondral surfaces by serving as an arthroscopic retractor.
- Center the repair device at the center of the meniscal pathology to reduce the unstable tear fragment. Reduction of the tissue can be performed and maintained by the use of an outside-in stay suture (Mulberry knot), particularly of a displaced bucket handle tear, until the mattress sutures can be placed.
- Suture configuration can be horizontal or vertical; however, if possible, use vertical mattress suture configurations perpendicular to the tear to provide the strongest repair construct (Figure 7-6).[17]
- Use an arthroscopic knot pusher to manually assist in cinching down the knot. Avoid overtightening and puckering the repair. If this occurs, use a horizontal mattress suture configuration on the undersurface of the puckered area (Figure 7-7).
- Place subsequent all-inside sutures anteriorly and posteriorly at 4- to 5-mm intervals to avoid gapping, puckering, and tissue incongruence.

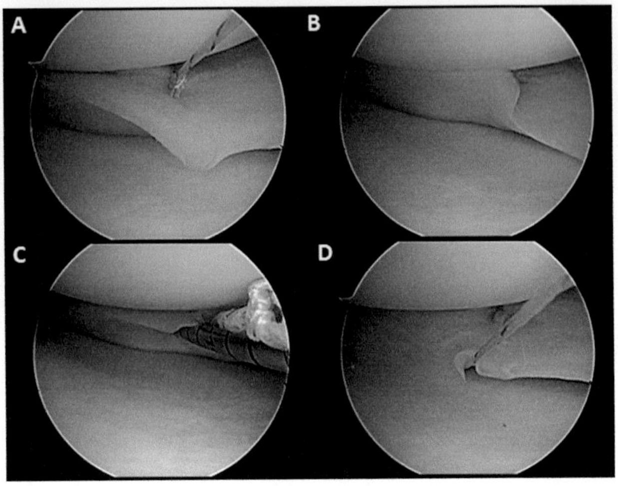

Figure 7-7. (A) Placement of a vertical mattress suture in a vertical posterior horn medial meniscus tear. (B) Meniscal puckering following placement of a vertical mattress suture. (C) Undersurface horizontal mattress suture placement. (D) Subsequent reduction of the meniscus.

Augmentation Techniques

Considering the poor vascularity of meniscal tissue, adjunct techniques can assist meniscal healing and improve clinical results.[7] Attempts to improve vascularity at the repair site are performed by the creation of vascular access channels through the use of meniscal debridement, rasping, excoriation, and trephination as previously described.[18] Newer biologic augmentation techniques have evolved in an attempt to recreate the enhanced meniscal healing seen during concomitant ACL reconstruction.[19]

Various arthroscopic techniques try to recreate this biologic advantage. Shaving or perforating the bone surface of the notch using a microfracture technique has been described as a practical and cost-effective method for creating a hemarthrosis and releasing growth factors and cytokines (Figure 7-8).[20] More recent technologies have promoted the use of a fibrin clot[21] or platelet-rich fibrin matrix[22] in an attempt to deliver biologically active factors directly to a meniscal repair site. The fibrin clot provides a chemotactic and mitogenic stimulus to the reparative process as well as a scaffold where fibrous tissue may form (Figure 7-9).[19] Platelet-rich fibrin matrix technique is a variant of platelet-rich plasma (PRP) delivery. The technique is performed by obtaining a sample of autologous blood intraoperatively (about 10 mL) and placing it in a centrifuge. After centrifugation is completed, the fibrin clotting cascade is activated with an agent such as calcium chloride, and the sample is placed through a second centrifuge step. This process minimizes platelet activation and traps inactivated platelets in the fibrin matrix, allowing sustained release of cytokines.[23] The matrix is then placed into the meniscal repair site. Proprietary technology is available to perform this method.

PRP has yet to be fully understood with meniscal repair techniques, and there are currently no randomized controlled trials investigating PRP usage and meniscal repair. Yet, the theoretical advantage of growth factors within platelets (transforming growth factor beta and platelet-derived, vascular endothelial, fibroblast, and epidermal growth factors) still exists. More information is required before they can be routinely used in meniscal repair surgery.

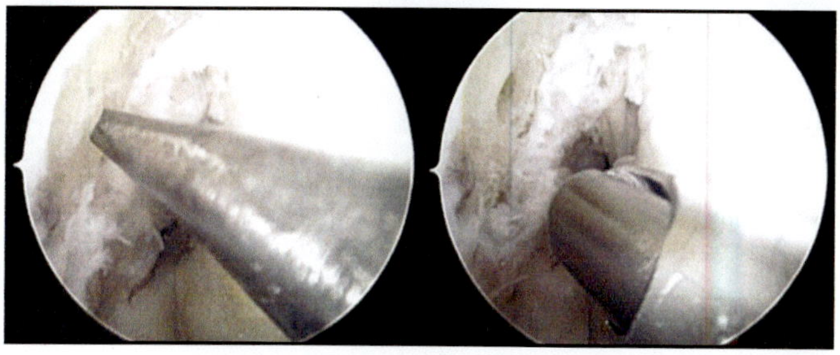

Figure 7-8. Microfracture of the femoral notch to aid meniscal healing.

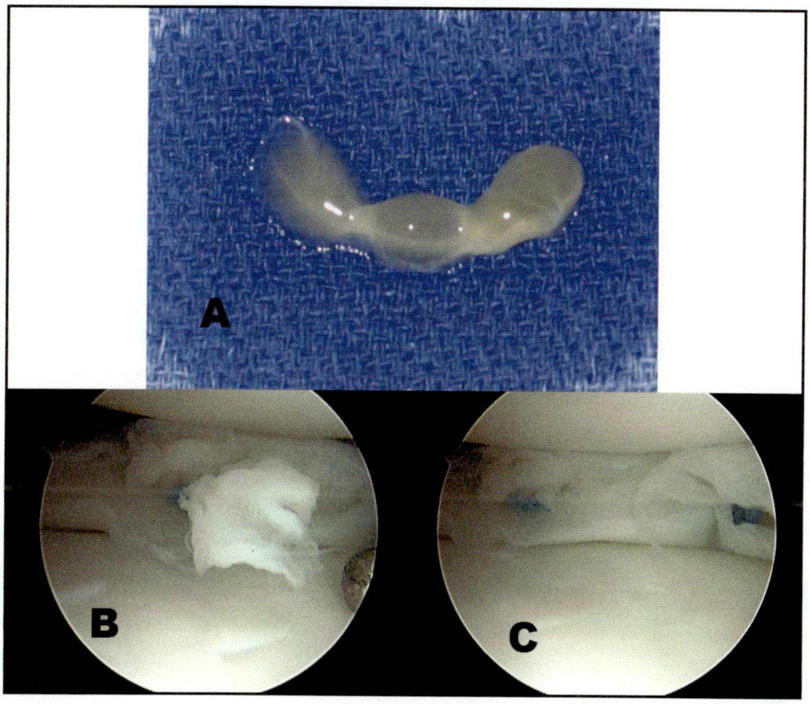

Figure 7-9. (A) A prepared fibrin clot. (B) The fibrin clot during insertion. (C) Final insertion position.

Postoperative Protocol

Postoperative care is individualized based on tear geometry, repair construct strength, associated surgical procedures, and surgeon preference. The authors prefer that the patient is placed into a hinged knee brace in the operating room locked in extension. Early passive ROM and early weightbearing with crutches is promoted; however, in the case of a radial repair, weightbearing is restricted for 6 to 8 weeks. Weightbearing ROM is restricted to 90 degrees for the first 3 weeks for nondisplaced meniscal tears and 4 to 6 weeks for displaced bucket handle tears. Bracing and crutch use are discontinued when the patient shows good quadriceps control and no antalgia. Return to pivoting sports ranges from 4 to 6 months or when the patient has no point tenderness or effusion and can show full extension and painless terminal flexion.

Potential Complications

Arthroscopic knee surgery has consistently been found to be a safe procedure. The overall incidence of complication has ranged from 0.56% to 8.2%.[24] Meniscus repair surgery is associated with a higher complication rate than meniscus resection, with reports as high as 18%.[25] The complications associated with meniscal repair and their incidence include infection (0.23% to 0.42%),[26] deep vein thrombosis (1.8% to 41.2%; average 6.8%),[27] and vascular (0.54% to 1.0%)[28] and neurologic complications (0.06% to 2.0%).[29]

The rate of infection is related to operative time, use of intraoperative corticosteroid injection, extended tourniquet use, medical comorbidities, and a history of prior surgery.[30] If a postoperative infection is suspected or diagnosed following a repair, it is appropriate to leave the implant or sutures in place during an urgent irrigation and debridement of the joint. However, the associated failure rate is higher.

Neurovascular injury, although rare, can be devastating for the patient. Vascular complications can include popliteal artery injury, pseudoaneurysm, and arteriovenous fistula formation. Neurologic injury can include direct or indirect nerve injury or complex regional pain syndrome. A systematic review by Grant et al[31] reported a 9% incidence of nerve irritation/injury with the inside-out technique vs 2% for all-inside techniques, including first-generation devices.

The most common pitfall in arthroscopic meniscal repair procedures is implant-related complications. Even newest-generation, all-inside fixators have all been associated with chondral damage secondary to implant abrasion.[31] If not used properly, the devices have a tendency to misfire, launch inaccurately, or break. This may lead to excessive chondral loss or a loose body/fragment within the joint. Other implant complications include inflammation superficial to the subcutaneous anchor, especially medially overlying the MCL, and cyst formation.

Top Technical Pearls for the Procedure

1. Prepare.
2. Reduce anatomically and provisionally stabilize using an outside-in PDS stitch.
3. Use high-strength femoral and tibial double vertical mattress sutures.
4. Consider hybrid techniques combining suture methodologies.
5. Individualize postoperative rehabilitation protocols.

References

1. Cooper DE, Arnoczky SP, Warren RF. Arthroscopic meniscal repair. *Clin Sports Med.* 1990;9(3):589-607.
2. Barber-Westin SD, Noyes FR. Clinical healing rates of meniscus repairs of tears in the central-third (red-white) zone. *Arthroscopy.* 2014;30(1):134-146.
3. Ra HJ, Ha JK, Jang SH, Lee DW, Kim JG. Arthroscopic inside-out repair of complete radial tears of the meniscus with a fibrin clot. *Knee Surg Sports Traumatol Arthrosc.* 2013;21(9):2126-2130.
4. Pujol N, Bohu Y, Boisrenoult P, Macdes A, Beaufils P. Clinical outcomes of open meniscal repair of horizontal meniscal tears in young patients. *Knee Surg Sports Traumatol Arthrosc.* 2013;21(7):1530-1533.
5. Vanderhave KL, Moravek JE, Sekiya JK, Wojtys EM. Meniscus tears in the young athlete: results of arthroscopic repair. *J Pediatr Orthop.* 2011;31(5):496-500.

6. Wasserstein D, Dwyer T, Gandhi R, Austin PC, Mahomed N, Ogilvie-Harris D. A matched-cohort population study of reoperation after meniscal repair with and without concomitant anterior cruciate ligament reconstruction. *Am J Sports Med.* 2013;41(2):349-355.
7. Anz AW, Rodkey WG. Biological enhancement of meniscus repair and replacement. *Sports Med Arthrosc.* 2012;20(2):115-120.
8. Baratz ME, Fu FH, Mengato R. Meniscal tears: the effect of meniscectomy and of repair on intraarticular contact areas and stress in the human knee. A preliminary report. *Am J Sports Med.* 1986;14(4):270-275.
9. Muriuki MG, Tuason DA, Tucker BG, Harner CD. Changes in tibiofemoral contact mechanics following radial split and vertical tears of the medial meniscus an in vitro investigation of the efficacy of arthroscopic repair. *J Bone Joint Surg Am.* 2011;93(12):1089-1095.
10. Mesiha M, Zurakowski D, Soriano J, Nielson JH, Zarins B, Murray MM. Pathologic characteristics of the torn human meniscus. *Am J Sports Med.* 2007;35(1):103-122.
11. Barrett GR, Field MH, Treacy SH, Ruff CG. Clinical results of meniscus repair in patients 40 years and older. *Arthroscopy.* 1998;14(8):824-829.
12. Noyes FR, Barber-Westin SD. Arthroscopic repair of meniscus tears extending into the avascular zone with or without anterior cruciate ligament reconstruction in patients 40 years of age and older. *Arthroscopy.* 2000;16(8):822-829.
13. Magee T, Williams D. 3.0-T MRI of meniscal tears. *AJR Am J Roentgenol.* 2006;187(2):371-375.
14. Kurzweil PR, Tifford CD, Ignacio EM. Unsatisfactory clinical results of meniscal repair using the Meniscus Arrow. *Arthroscopy.* 2005;21(8):905.e1-905.e7.
15. Lee GP, Diduch DR. Deteriorating outcomes after meniscal repair using the Meniscus Arrow in knees undergoing concurrent anterior cruciate ligament reconstruction: increased failure with long-term follow-up. *Am J Sports Med.* 2005;33(8):1138-1141.
16. Spindler KP, McCarty EC, Warren TA, Devin C, Connor JT. Prospective comparison of arthroscopic medial meniscal repair technique: inside-out suture versus entirely arthroscopic arrows. *Am J Sports Med.* 2003;31(6):929-934.
17. Becker R, Stärke C, Heymann M, Nebelung W. Biomechanical properties under cyclic loading of seven meniscus repair techniques. *Clin Orthop Relat Res.* 2002;(400):236-245.
18. Zhang Z, Arnold JA, Williams T, McCann B. Repairs by trephination and suturing of longitudinal injuries in the avascular area of the meniscus in goats. *Am J Sports Med.* 1995;23(1):35-41.
19. Scordino LE, Deberardino TM. Biologic enhancement of meniscus repair. *Clin Sports Med.* 2012;31(1):91-100.
20. Freedman KB, Nho SJ, Cole BJ. Marrow stimulating technique to augment meniscus repair. *Arthroscopy.* 2003;19(7):794-798.
21. Sethi PM, Cooper A, Jokl P. Technical tips in orthopaedics: meniscal repair with use of an in situ fibrin clot. *Arthroscopy.* 2003;19(5):E44.
22. Kwak HS, Nam J, Lee JH, Kim HJ, Yoo JJ. Meniscal repair in vivo using human chondrocyte-seeded PLGA mesh scaffold pretreated with platelet-rich plasma [published online ahead of print June 19, 2014]. *J Tissue Eng Regen Med.*
23. Rodeo SA, Delos D, Williams RJ, Adler RS, Pearle A, Warren RF. The effect of platelet-rich fibrin matrix on rotator cuff tendon healing: a prospective, randomized clinical trial. *Am J Sports Med.* 2012;40(6):1234-1241.
24. Small NC. Complications in arthroscopic surgery performed by experienced arthroscopists. *Arthroscopy.* 1988;4(3):215-221.
25. Sherman OH, Fox JM, Snyder SJ, et al. Arthroscopy—"no-problem surgery." An analysis of complications in two thousand six hundred and forty cases. *J Bone Joint Surg Am.* 1986;68(2):256-265.
26. Armstrong RW, Bolding F, Joseph R. Septic arthritis following arthroscopy: clinical syndromes and analysis of risk factors. *Arthroscopy.* 1992;8(2):213-223.
27. Sun Y, Chen D, Xu Z, et al. Deep venous thrombosis after knee arthroscopy: a systematic review and meta-analysis. *Arthroscopy.* 2014;30(3):406-412.
28. Kim T, Savino RM, McFarland EG, Cosgarea AJ. Neurovascular complications of knee arthroscopy. *Am J Sports Med.* 2002;30(4):619-629.
29. Rodeo SA, Forster RA, Weiland AJ. Neurological complications due to arthroscopy. *J Bone Joint Surg Am.* 1993;75(6):917-926.

30. Montgomery SC, Campbell J. Septic arthritis following arthroscopy and intra-articular steroids. *J Bone Joint Surg Br.* 1989;71(3):540.
31. Grant JA, Wilde J, Miller BS, Bedi A. Comparison of inside-out and all-inside techniques for the repair of isolated meniscal tears: a systematic review. *Am J Sports Med.* 2012;40(2):459-468.

Please see videos on the accompanying website at www.routledge.com/9781617119996

8

Arthroscopic Repair of Meniscal Root Avulsions

Amanda L. Weller, MD and Christopher D. Harner, MD

Introduction

The importance of the meniscal roots has been thoroughly described in the orthopedic literature. An injury to the lateral or medial posterior roots results in a loss of hoop stresses in the medial and lateral compartments, abnormal contact forces, a significant increase in tibiofemoral contact pressures, altered knee joint kinematics, and resultant degenerative joint disease.[1-11] On the medial side, a meniscal root tear has similar biomechanical consequences as a total medial meniscectomy.[1,2,6,12] Laterally, the effects of a root tear are significant but not as extreme.[10,13] Properly diagnosing and treating these injuries is critical to the health and integrity of knee articular cartilage.

In the past, these injuries have been difficult to consistently diagnose, especially on the medial side.[14-16] Advanced imaging and the identification of certain risk factors for the development of root tears have allowed surgeons and radiologists to better delineate patients with this detrimental injury. Risk factors for posterior medial root tears include increased age, female sex, varus mechanical axis, increased body mass index, higher Kellgren-Lawrence grade, and decreased sports activity.[2,4,9,16,17] The most common risk factor for a posterior lateral meniscal root tear is a concurrent anterior cruciate ligament (ACL) tear.[10] Because of the serious biomechanical consequences of root tears, these injuries must be addressed timely and appropriately. This chapter focuses primarily on the technique involved in the repair of medial and lateral root avulsions off of their bony insertions.

Indications

Posterior Medial Meniscal Root Tear

- Failure of nonoperative treatment, including nonsteroidal anti-inflammatory drugs, physical therapy, bracing, activity modifications, and injections[1,2,7,18]

Sgaglione NA, Lubowitz JH, Provencher MT, eds. *The Knee: AANA Advanced Arthroscopic Surgical Techniques* (pp 103-113).

- Pain with activities of daily living
- Repair is indicated in the setting of acute injury, minimal cartilage wear (less than Kellgren-Lawrence grade 3), normal/symmetric mechanical axis alignment, reducible tear with minimal extrusion, and good tissue quality.[2,7,19]

Contraindications

Contraindications for meniscal root repair include greater than or equal to grade 3 articular cartilage changes, poor root tissue quality (ie, cannot hold a suture), and/or irreducible root to the insertion site. In this setting, arthroscopic debridement may give temporary benefit.

Posterior Lateral Meniscal Root Tear

- Typically repaired in the setting of an ACL tear undergoing reconstruction[1,5,16,19]
- Partial avulsions may be left in situ if the meniscofemoral ligament is intact.[10,13,20]

Pertinent Physical Findings

Medial[2,19,21]

- Primarily occur as isolated injuries (approximately 90%)
- Load-dependent pain
- May present with a history of a pop with acute onset of pain
- Posteromedial knee pain (not joint line; most common symptom/best indicator of root tear)
- Pain with increased knee flexion (squatting, stairs)
- Minimal (if any) joint line tenderness (pain in posterior medial)

Lateral

- Usually (90% or greater) associated with an ACL tear and in the multiple-ligament–injured knee[5]
- Very rarely occurs as an isolated tear
- High-grade pivot shift (grade 3 or higher) in the setting of ACL tear[19]

Pertinent Imaging

- X-rays: Bilateral posteroanterior flexion weightbearing, lateral, and Merchant views (look carefully on the full weightbearing views for joint space narrowing and lateral tibial femoral subluxation)
- Long-leg cassette (medial meniscal root tear)
- Magnetic resonance imaging (MRI)[2,5,18,19,21-24]: "Ghost sign" (sagittal), vertical linear defect (coronal), radial linear defect (axial), meniscal extrusion greater than 3 mm (coronal)
- Assess articular cartilage changes in all 3 compartments (greater than grade 3 changes and/or tricompartmental changes should be documented and are contraindications to root repair)

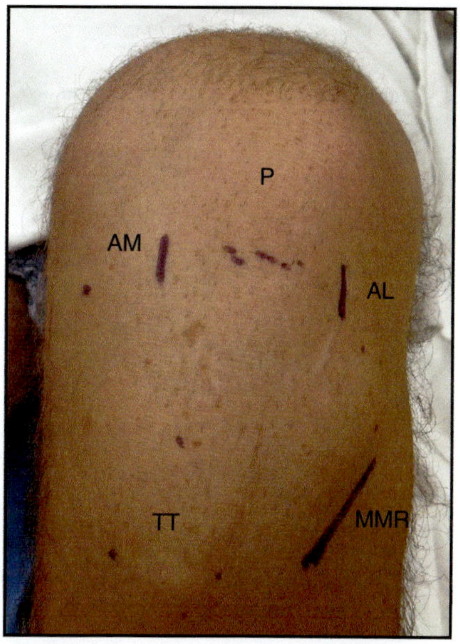

Figure 8-1. Incisions are marked in preparation for a medial meniscus root repair. AL, anterolateral portal; AM, anteromedial portal; MMR, incision for suture retrieval for medial meniscus root repair; P, patella; TT; tibial tubercle.

Equipment

- 30- and 70-degree arthroscopes
- 4.5-mm full-radius resector (straight and curved)
- ACL drill guide with guide pin (3/32-in K-wire)
- Meniscal rasp (used to roughen bony insertion)
- 70-degree upbend suture shuttle device
- Arthroscopic knot pusher
- Hewson suture passer
- 8-mm clear cannula
- #2 nonabsorbable braided suture
- 4.5-mm cancellous screw with washer

Positioning and Portals

The patient is positioned supine on an operating table. General anesthesia with a regional nerve block is typically used for this procedure. Preoperative intravenous antibiotics are administered. A post is placed alongside the thigh of the operative leg to aid in applying valgus stress for visualization. A bump is placed under the hip of the operative knee to reduce external rotation of the limb. A bar is secured to the bed with a clamp so the knee is positioned in 90 degrees of flexion when the foot is resting on the bar. The senior author does not use a tourniquet for this procedure. An examination under anesthesia is performed on both knees, including range of motion, ligamentous testing, and evaluation for effusion. Prior to prepping and draping, portal incisions and the medial or lateral tibial incisions are marked out and injected with 0.25% Marcaine (bupivacaine) with epinephrine (Figure 8-1).

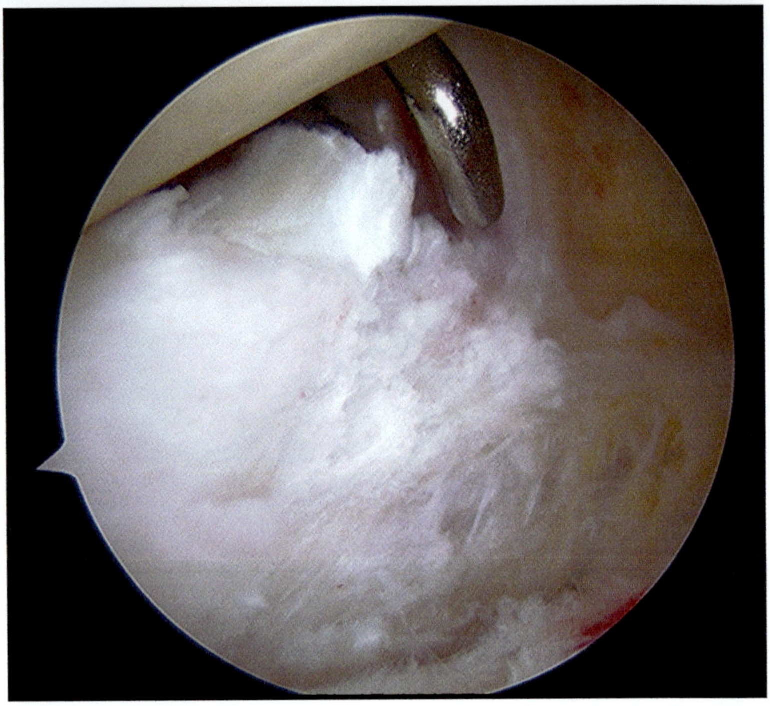

Figure 8-2. View of the medial meniscus root tear after placing the arthroscope through the intercondylar notch by using the Gillquist maneuver. The probe is entering the joint through the posteromedial portal.

Step-by-Step Description of the Procedure

Posterior Medial Meniscus Root Avulsion Repair

The repair begins by establishing the anterolateral and anteromedial portals after identifying the following important landmarks: the inferior pole of the patella, patellar tendon, and medial and lateral joint lines. A superolateral outflow portal is also used. The arthroscope is introduced into the anterolateral portal, and a diagnostic arthroscopy is performed. All 3 compartments of the knee are thoroughly evaluated in regard to chondral integrity. Any other associated injuries are identified. The medial meniscus can be evaluated by applying a valgus force to the extended knee and externally rotating the foot. The root of the medial meniscus is better visualized by positioning the arthroscope along the lateral aspect of the medial femoral condyle and under the posteromedial bundle of the posterior cruciate ligament, known as the Gillquist maneuver (Figure 8-2). At this juncture, the root can be probed and visualized to determine whether the tear is repairable or not.

After deciding to repair the root, a posteromedial portal can be established to aid in the repair. The knee is placed in 90 degrees of flexion, and the posteromedial capsule is visualized using the Gillquist view. An 18-gauge spinal needle is used for localization and placed approximately 1 cm proximal to the medial joint line and 5 mm posterior to the posterior edge of the medial femoral condyle. Once the needle is in the appropriate position confirmed under direct visualization, it is removed, and a #11 blade scalpel is used to incise the skin and soft tissues, also entering the capsule under direct visualization. The arthroscope can then be placed in the portal using a switching stick so that the anterolateral portal can be used for instrumentation.

A reverse notchplasty is performed for better exposure and visualization of the root. This is done using a 4.5-mm full-radius resector to remove 3 to 5 mm of articular cartilage from the posteroinferior aspect of the medial femoral condyle. This allows for more room to access the native insertion site of the root for preparation and tunnel placement. A meniscal rasp or curved shaver is then used to create a bleeding bone bed at the anatomic insertion site to promote healing of the repair.

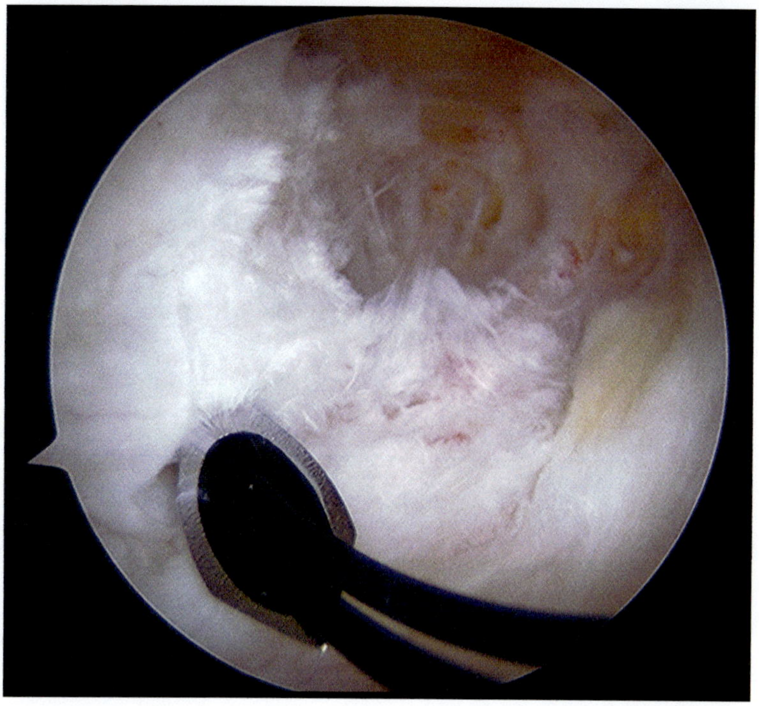

Figure 8-3. The suture shuttle device pierces the medial root, and the monofilament loop is passed.

An 8-mm clear cannula is placed in the anterolateral portal in preparation for suture passage. With the scope in the posteromedial portal, a suture shuttle device is used through the anterolateral portal to pierce the meniscal root in an inferior to superior direction (Figure 8-3). The monofilament loop is then passed and retrieved through the anterolateral portal. A braided suture loop is shuttled through the meniscus and out of the anterolateral portal so the free ends of the suture can be pulled through the loop, creating a loop stitch around the meniscus once the suture is cinched down through the anterolateral portal (Figure 8-4). This can be done by using an arthroscopic knot pusher. A second loop stitch should be attempted if possible for added strength.

To establish the tunnel for the sutures, an ACL drill tip guide is inserted through the anterolateral portal through the intercondylar notch and placed at the anatomic root insertion site. The drill sleeve is used to localize an incision site over the anterolateral tibia. This is a 3- to 4-cm oblique incision typically located at the anterolateral flare of the proximal tibia, distal to Gerdy's tubercle but overlying the very proximal extent of the tibialis anterior. The fascia of the tibialis anterior is incised and the muscle is gently elevated off the bone using a lap sponge and elevator or osteotome. The drill sleeve is then placed onto the tibia once the tip position is confirmed to be on the root insertion site. A 3/32-in guide pin is then drilled just to the tip of the ACL drill guide but not completely through the posterior cortex of the tibia. The tunnel is completed by gently tapping the pin through the posterior cortex with a mallet under direct visualization to avoid injury to the popliteal neurovascular bundle. The guide pin is then removed, and a Hewson suture passer is inserted into the tunnel in its place. The Hewson loop is removed through the anterolateral portal, and the suture ends are passed through the loop (Figure 8-5). The suture is then shuttled down through the tunnel. Suture passage is facilitated by using the ice tongs to create a pulley at the tunnel apex, thereby improving the angle of suture entry into the tunnel. The sutures are tied over a 4.5-mm cancellous screw with washer inserted into the anterolateral tibia. The sutures are tensioned with the knee in 30 degrees of flexion, and reduction of the root is visualized arthroscopically (Figure 8-6). After the sutures are secured, the tibialis anterior fascia is repaired using a 0-Vicryl suture, and the skin is closed in a layered fashion using 2-0 Vicryl and 4-0 Caprosyn sutures.

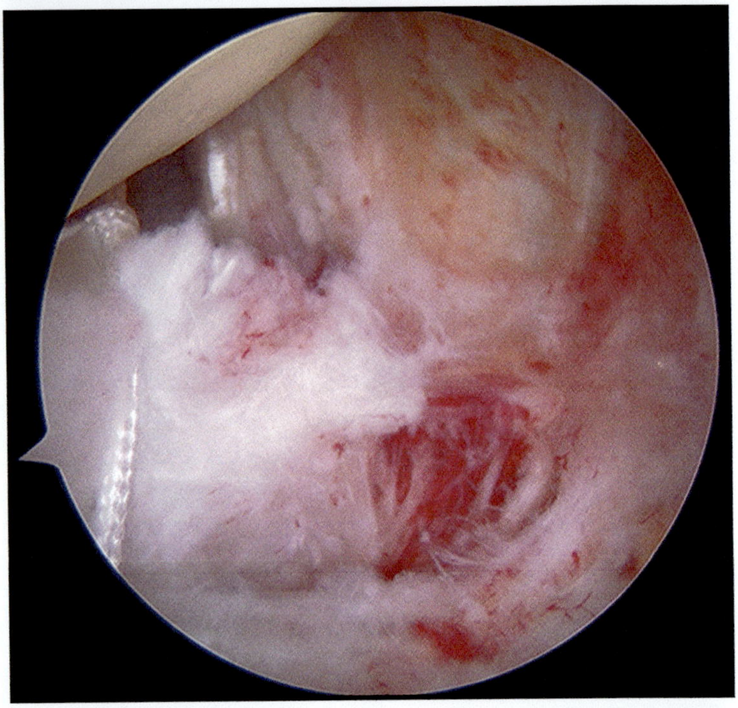

Figure 8-4. A loop stitch is placed through the medial root.

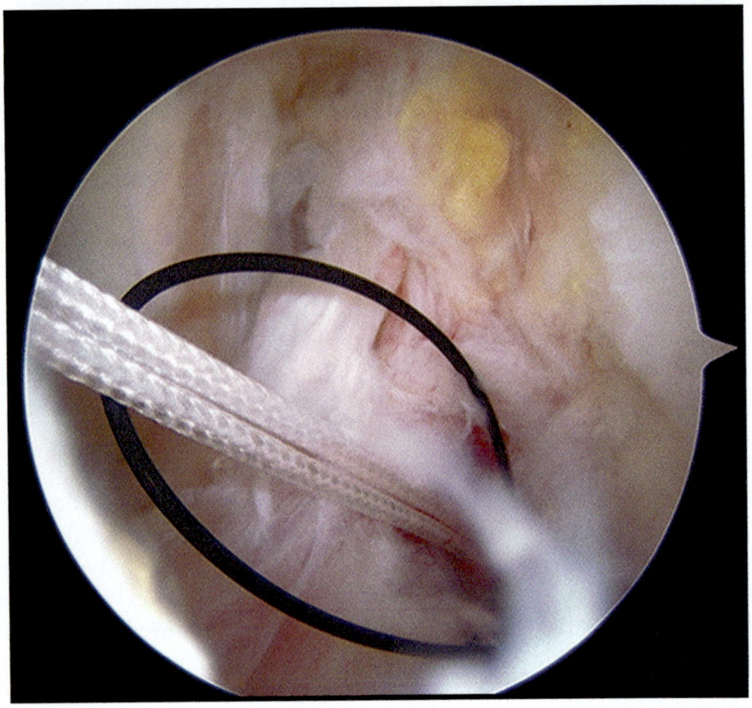

Figure 8-5. A Hewson suture passer is used to bring the suture ends from the loop stitch through the tibial tunnel and out the anterolateral cortex of the tibia.

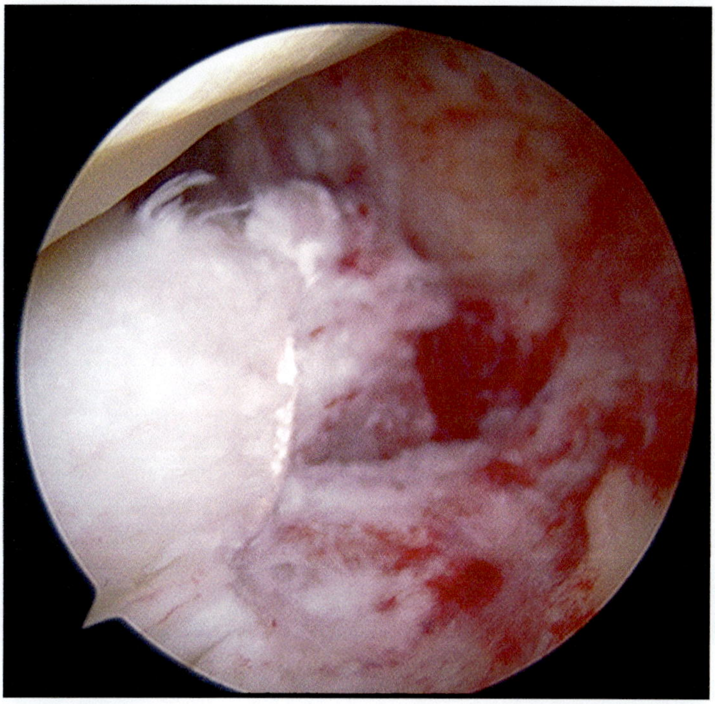

Figure 8-6. The sutures are tensioned, and the meniscus is reduced.

Posterior Lateral Meniscus Root Repair

This repair is performed in a similar manner as a medial-sided repair; however, a lateral root tear is typically encountered in conjunction with an ACL tear. The repair is therefore done after graft harvest and debridement of the torn ACL. This allows much easier visualization of the lateral root compared to the medial root.

The leg is placed in a figure-4 position to allow access to the lateral compartment with the arthroscope in the anterolateral portal. The anatomic root insertion site is identified and prepared using a shaver and meniscal rasp to create a bleeding bone bed (Figure 8-7). An ACL tip guide is introduced through the anteromedial portal and positioned at the insertion site (Figure 8-8). The drill sleeve is used to localize the skin incision typically made medial to the tibial tubercle. The incision starts just proximal to the level of the patellar tendon insertion and extends distally approximately 4 cm. A 3/32-in guide pin is then inserted using the same technique as for a medial repair. This tunnel is usually placed posterior and lateral to the tunnel for the ACL reconstruction. With the guide pin left in place, an 8-mm clear cannula can be inserted into the anteromedial portal, and a suture shuttle device is used to pierce the lateral meniscus for passage of a loop stitch using the same technique as previously described. Similarly, 2 loop stitches should be attempted for a stronger repair (Figure 8-9). The guide pin is then removed, and a Hewson suture passer is placed in the tunnel. The free ends of the suture are passed through the tunnel and pulled out of the anteromedial proximal tibia.

The sutures are secured over a 4.5-mm cancellous screw and washer with the knee positioned in 30 degrees of flexion. This is done after ACL graft passage but before ACL graft tensioning. Alternatively, the meniscal sutures for medial or lateral suture repair can be tied over a button on the tibial cortex.

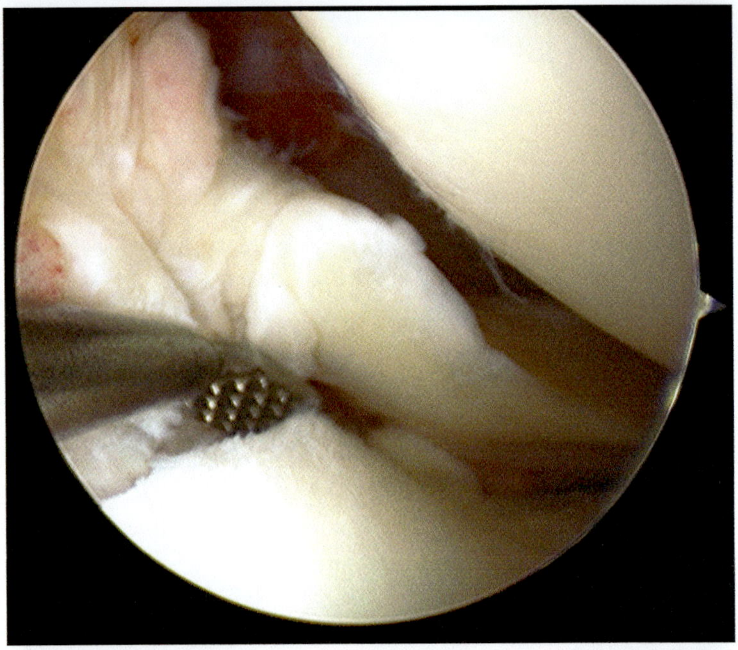

Figure 8-7. The insertion site of the lateral root is rasped aggressively to create a bleeding bone bed for better healing.

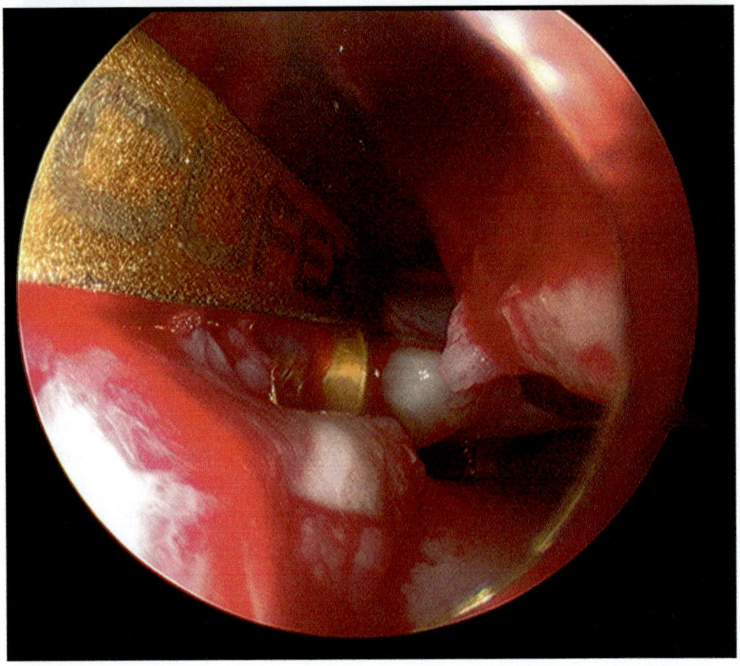

Figure 8-8. An ACL tip drill guide is positioned at the anatomic insertion site of the lateral root.

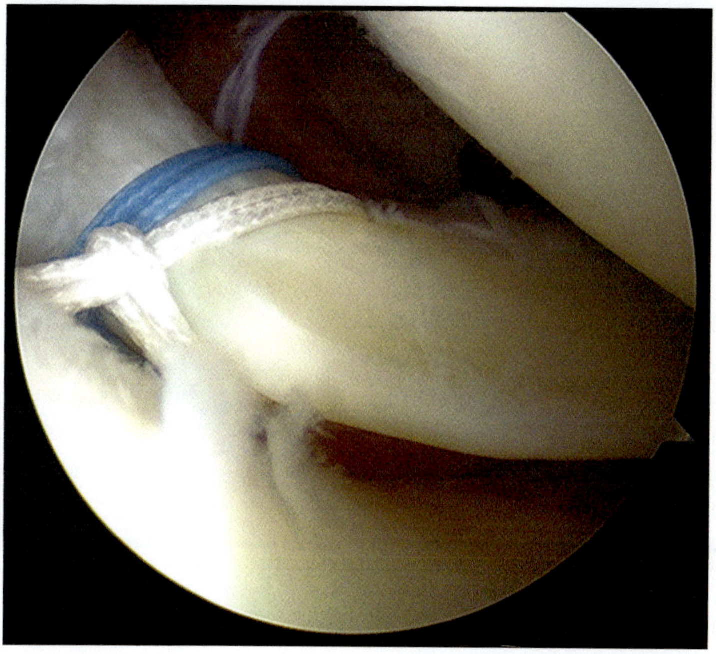

Figure 8-9. The lateral root avulsion is repaired with 2 loop stitches, and the suture ends are passed through the tibial tunnel.

Postoperative Protocol

In the immediate postoperative period, the knee is placed in a hinged brace locked at 20 degrees of flexion and the patient is made nonweightbearing. The patient is progressed to full weightbearing over the following 8 weeks. Initially, range of motion is restricted from 0 to 90 degrees and achieved using a continuous passive motion machine. The patient is allowed to perform quadriceps sets, calf pumps, straight leg raises, and heel slides in the immediate postoperative period. He or she is advanced to supervised physical therapy and more functional exercises once full weightbearing is allowed and achieved. Full return to activity can typically be achieved by 4 months in an isolated meniscal root repair.

Potential Complications

Complications include iatrogenic damage to the meniscus due to multiple passes of the suture shuttle device as well as iatrogenic damage to the cruciate ligaments from passage of instruments through the intercondylar notch. Nonanatomic repair, especially of the medial meniscus root, can lead to progression of osteoarthritic changes.[25] Damage to the popliteal neurovascular structures is possible with careless passage of the guide pin. Specific complications related to the above technique include interfering with tunnel placement for concurrent ACL reconstruction, suture abrasion in the bone tunnel, and suture creep.[2] Complications associated with knee arthroscopy but not specifically with root repair include deep vein thrombosis, infection, and arthrofibrosis.

Top Technical Pearls for the Procedure

1. Use an accessory posteromedial portal for better visualization of the medial meniscal root insertion.
2. For medial root repair, a reverse notchplasty allows for better access to the insertion site, which allows easier bed preparation, suture passage, and tunnel placement.
3. Bed preparation is crucial to aid in healing of the root back down to the insertion site and should be performed with a rasp and a shaver to create a sufficiently bleeding bone bed.
4. Two loop stitches are preferable to one; however, in the case of degenerative tissue, take care to avoid multiple passes through the meniscus as this will lead to further damage to the remaining root tissue.
5. The window for an anatomic repair is narrow, so identifying the anatomic insertion site is critical to optimal restoration of the function of the menisci.

References

1. Vyas D, Harner CD. Meniscus root repair. *Sports Med Arthrosc.* 2012;20(2):86-94.
2. Bhatia S, LaPrade CM, Ellman MB, LaPrade RF. Meniscal root tears: significance, diagnosis, and treatment. *Am J Sports Med.* 2014;42(12):3016-3030.
3. Henry S, Mascarenhas R, Kowalchuk D, Forsythe B, Irrgang JJ, Harner CD. Medial meniscus tear morphology and chondral degeneration of the knee: is there a relationship? *Arthroscopy.* 2012;28(8):1124.e2-1134.e2.
4. Guermazi A, Hayashi D, Jarraya M, et al. Medial posterior meniscal root tears are associated with development or worsening of medial tibiofemoral cartilage damage: the multicenter osteoarthritis study. *Radiology.* 2013;268(3):814-821.
5. Koenig JH, Ranawat AS, Umans HR, DiFelice GS. Meniscal root tears: diagnosis and treatment. *Arthroscopy.* 2009;25(9):1025-1032.
6. Wang KH, Hwang DH, Cho JH, Changale SD, Woo SJ, Nha KW. Arthroscopic direct repair for a complete radial tear of the posterior root of the medial meniscus. *Clin Orthop Surg.* 2011;3(4):332-335.
7. Jung YH, Choi NH, Oh JS, Victoroff BN. All-inside repair for a root tear of the medial meniscus using a suture anchor. *Am J Sports Med.* 2012;40(6):1406-1411.
8. Seo JH, Li G, Shetty GM, et al. Effect of repair of radial tears at the root of the posterior horn of the medial meniscus with the pullout suture technique: a biomechanical study using porcine knees. *Arthroscopy.* 2009;25(11):1281-1287.
9. Ozkoc G, Circi E, Gonc U, Irgit K, Pourbagher A, Tandogan RN. Radial tears in the root of the posterior horn of the medial meniscus. *Knee Surg Sports Traumatol Arthrosc.* 2008;16(9):849-854.
10. Bao HR, Zhu D, Gong H, Gu GS. The effect of complete radial lateral meniscus posterior root tear on the knee contact mechanics: a finite element analysis. *J Orthop Sci.* 2013;18(2):256-263.
11. Stärke C, Kopf S, Lippisch R, Lohmann C, Becker R. Tensile forces on repaired meniscal root tears. *Arthroscopy.* 2013;29(2):205-212.
12. Allaire R, Muriuki M, Gilbertson L, Harner CD. Biomechanical consequences of a tear of the posterior root of the medial meniscus. Similar to total meniscectomy. *J Bone Joint Surg Am.* 2008;90(9):1922-1931.
13. Forkel P, Herbort M, Schulze M, et al. Biomechanical consequences of a posterior root tear of the lateral meniscus: stabilizing effect of the meniscofemoral ligament. *Arch Orthop Trauma Surg.* 2013;133(5):621-626.
14. Casagranda BU, Leeman J, Costello JM, Rafiee B, Harner CD. Coronal oblique imaging of the knee: can it increase radiologists' confidence in diagnosing posterior root meniscal tears? *Clin Radiol.* 2013;68(6):e316-e322.
15. Wilson BF, Johnson DL. Posterior horn medial meniscal root repair with cruciate ligament/medial collateral ligament combined injuries. *Orthopedics.* 2011;34(12):986-988.

16. Matheny LM, Ockuly AC, Steadman JR, LaPrade RF. Posterior meniscus root tears: associated pathologies to assist as diagnostic tools [published online ahead of pring May 28, 2014]. *Knee Surg Sports Traumatol Arthrosc.*
17. Hwang BY, Kim SJ, Lee SW, et al. Risk factors for medial meniscus posterior root tear. *Am J Sports Med.* 2012;40(7):1606-1610.
18. Lee JH, Lim YJ, Kim KB, Kim KH, Song JH. Arthroscopic pullout suture repair of posterior root tear of the medial meniscus: radiographic and clinical results with a 2-year follow-up. *Arthroscopy.* 2009;25(9):951-958.
19. Peterson W, Forkel P, Feucht MJ, Zantop T, Imhoff AB, Brucker PU. Posterior root tear of the medial and lateral meniscus. *Arch Orthop Trauma Surg.* 2014;134(2):237-255.
20. Shelbourne KD, Roberson TA, Gray T. Long-term evaluation of posterior lateral meniscus root tears left in situ at the time of anterior cruciate ligament reconstruction. *Am J Sports Med.* 2011;39(7):1439-1443.
21. Lee YG, Shim JC, Choi YS, Kim JG, Lee GJ, Kim HK. Magnetic resonance imaging findings of surgically proven medial meniscus root tear: tear configuration and associated knee abnormalities. *J Comput Assist Tomogr.* 2008;32(3):452-457.
22. Lee SY, Jee WH, Kim JM. Radial tear of the medial meniscal root: reliability and accuracy of MRI for diagnosis. *AJR Am J Roentgenol.* 2008;191(1):81-85.
23. Choi SH, Bae S, Ji SK, Chang MJ. The MRI findings of meniscal root tear of the medial meniscus: emphasis on coronal, sagittal and axial images. *Knee Surg Sports Traumatol Arthrosc.* 2012;20(10):2098-2103.
24. Kim SB, Ha KJ, Lee SW, et al. Medial meniscus root tear refixation: comparison of clinical, radiologic, and arthroscopic findings with medial meniscectomy. *Arthroscopy.* 2011;27(3):346-354.
25. Stärke C, Kopf S, Gröbel KH, Becker R. The effect of nonanatomic repair of the meniscal horn attachment on meniscal tension: a biomechanical study. *Arthroscopy.* 2010;26(3):358-365.

Please see videos on the accompanying website at www.routledge.com/9781617119996

9

Arthroscopically Assisted Meniscal Transplantation

Thomas Carter, MD

Introduction

The meniscus plays a vital role in preserving normal knee function, including shock absorption, load transmission, stability, joint lubrication, and nutrition.[1,2] Thus, subtotal removal of the meniscus enhances the rate of degenerative arthritis in the knee.[3] Although preservation of the meniscus should be the standard of care, most tears are treated with excision. To recreate the function of the meniscus, many methods and materials have been explored. Meniscal allograft transplantation is the one proven option to treat those who have become symptomatic from excision of the meniscus (Figure 9-1).[4]

Since the first isolated meniscal transplant was performed in 1984, surgical techniques have continued to improve and have transitioned from open procedures to arthroscopic-assisted procedures.[5,6] Although some authors have reported good outcomes with only soft tissue fixation of the meniscus to the host, biomechanical studies show that if the horn attachments are secured with bone, the allograft more closely replicates the normal meniscus.[7] Thus, although it may be technically more difficult, it is currently recommended to use bone graft to bone tunnel fixation. The most commonly performed techniques to secure the horns through bone fixation are the bone bridge and bone plug methods.

Although several bone bridge variations have been described, the dovetail technique is the author's procedure of choice. It has the advantage of providing a bone slot that provides press-fit fixation and, therefore, does not require additional screws or sutures, as do the other bone bridge techniques. Although the bone bridge methods can be used for lateral and medial grafts, it is the author's preference to use the dovetail for lateral grafts and the double-bone plugs for the medial side. The distance between the lateral horn attachments is only a centimeter, whereas on the medial side, the distance is 2.5 cm or greater. In addition, the anterior horn attachment of the medial meniscus has been found to be of great variation.[8] By having the horns separate, one can modify the attachments to accommodate any graft-host mismatch. Conversely, the bone plug technique is not recommended on the lateral side. With the close proximity of the horn attachments, the 2 drill holes carry a significant risk of disrupting the bone between the holes and losing fixation.

Sgaglione NA, Lubowitz JH, Provencher MT, eds. *The Knee: AANA Advanced Arthroscopic Surgical Techniques* (pp 115-131).

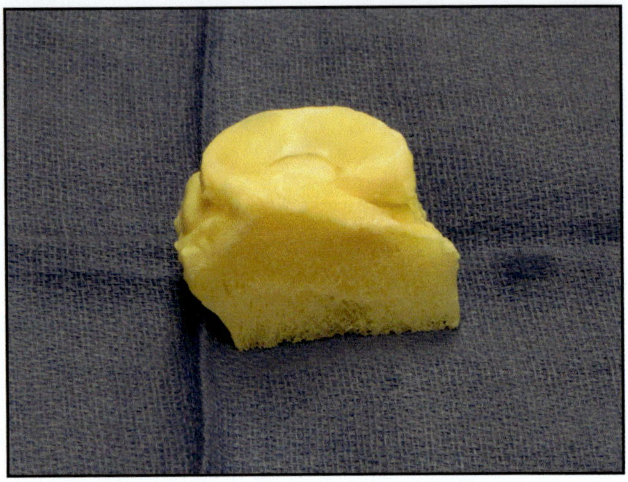

Figure 9-1. Fresh-frozen lateral meniscal allograft as provided by a tissue bank.

Indications

A thorough history is of vital importance and should include information regarding previous knee injuries, specific symptoms, and prior treatments and surgical procedures. For consideration of meniscal allograft transplantation, the patient should have pain localized to the meniscus-deficient compartment, although joint effusions can result in some generalized discomfort. Particular emphasis should also be paid to any chondral lesions, limb alignment, and ligament stability. An effort should be made to obtain operative reports and intraoperative photographs, which can be useful in determining the amount of meniscus remaining and the condition of the articular cartilage.

Meniscal transplant should be performed with the goal of reducing pain with the ability to increase activity level secondary.[9,10] Because of the lack of evidence, patients should not be told to expect the procedure to delay or prevent the progression of osteoarthritis.[11,12] Meniscal transplantation should be considered only when nonsurgical measures to control pain have been exhausted and/or there is evidence that the involved compartment is degenerating. In general, a patient should have a history of symptoms localized to the meniscus-deficient compartment and not have advanced arthritic changes. Grade IV chondromalacia is a contraindication unless a defect is focal and can be treated with a cartilage repair/replacement method. It is commonly recommended that patients should be younger than 50 to 55 years; however, this is controversial, and age restrictions should also be based on a patient's physiologic age.

- Majority of meniscus excised
- Pain in the meniscus-deficient compartment
- Chondromalacia no greater than grade III
- Knee without ligament laxity
- Age typically younger than 55 years

Controversial Indications

Although not absolute contraindications, patients with ligament laxity, limb malalignment, and full-thickness chondral defects need to have these addressed to be considered. It is well known that the medial meniscus is an important secondary stabilizer in patients with an anterior cruciate ligament (ACL)-deficient knee. In addition, chronically ACL-deficient knees have been shown to be associated with increased rates of meniscal tears. Thus, patients with ACL-deficient knees require reconstruction before the meniscus is replaced or, more commonly, at the same time as the meniscus.

Limb alignment is another circumstance that can substantially affect the outcome of meniscal allograft transplantation. Although it is not uniformly agreed upon, many surgeons will perform an osteotomy to unload the involved compartment if the mechanical axis is a few degrees greater than the contralateral knee. The extent of the correction is typically to have the mechanical axis pass through the contralateral tibial spine rather than the more extensive correction recommended for arthritic knees. The procedure can be staged or performed at the same time as the meniscus, which is what the author prefers.

Full-thickness cartilage defects have previously been considered to be a contraindication for meniscal allograft transplantation. However, if the defect is isolated and can be corrected with a cartilage repair or restoration procedure, it is not contraindicated. A systematic review of studies that reported the results of meniscus alone or combined meniscal allograft transplantation with cartilage repair procedures found similar results in 4 of the 6 studies.[13] Noyes et al[14] examined concomitant procedures, such as osteochondral autograft and ACL reconstruction in 40 meniscal transplantations and reported no increase in complications among patients who received concomitant procedures.

- Isolated full-thickness chondral defect
- Limb malalignment
- Age older than 55 years

The primary contraindication to meniscal allograft transplantation is advanced arthritis. A history of infection, inflammatory arthropathy, synovial disease, and morbid obesity represent other contraindications.

Pertinent Physical Findings

Physical examination should first focus on determining the location of pain and ruling out other possible pain generators. Palpation of the joint line usually elicits tenderness over the involved compartment. In addition, an effusion may be present depending on the patient's recent activity level. The physical examination should also seek to identify any potential ligamentous instability and malalignment that might need to be addressed at the time of surgery. Generally, range of motion (ROM) tends to be well preserved. One should not forget to evaluate the entire leg, contralateral limb, and core strength when evaluating for other possible contributing factors.

- Pain localized to the area of meniscus excision (best test)
- Inspection for joint effusion
- No ligament laxity
- No significant limb malalignment

Pertinent Imaging

A complete set of x-rays must be obtained for full evaluation of the knee. Not only should the joint space be assessed, but also spurring and flattening of the condyles, which may indicate that the knee is more arthritic than the joint space alone would indicate.

Views to obtain include the following:

- Weightbearing anteroposterior (AP) in full extension
- Weightbearing posteroanterior in 45 degrees of flexion, lateral with no rotation, and axial view of the patellofemoral joint

If x-rays are to be used for meniscal allograft sizing, a magnification marker should be placed on the cassette for 2 orthogonal views of the joint line. Any question of limb malalignment or gait abnormalities should necessitate long-leg alignment films.

- Magnetic resonance imaging (MRI) scans are typically obtained to determine if other pathology is present and is useful to evaluate for stress reaction in the bone.

Equipment

- Meniscal allograft
  - Sized match graft (plain x-rays are typically sufficient)
  - Fresh-frozen allograft preferred
- Arthroscopy tower and equipment for standard knee arthroscopy
- Meniscus repair devices (surgeon's preference)
- Long-length, open-ended meniscus suturing needles
- Lateral meniscal allograft
  - Dovetail instrumentation
  - Oscillating saw
- Medial meniscal allograft
  - ACL guide and drill system
  - 0.062 K-wire
  - Coring reamer (8 mm)
  - Small motorized burr
  - Polyethylene button or low-profile screw

Meniscal Allograft Sizing

The clinical outcomes following meniscal transplantation are dependent on matching the size of the allograft to the native meniscus. Allografts that are oversized lead to greater forces across the articular cartilage, whereas undersized allografts lead to normal forces across the articular cartilage but greater stress across the meniscus repair.[15] Sizing of meniscal allografts can be done by using plain x-rays, computed tomography (CT), or MRI. Sizing based on plain x-rays is most common with the Pollard method often followed and has been shown to correlate well with actual anatomical measurements.[16,17] The meniscal width can be determined by measuring the distance from the peak of the tibial eminence to the edge of the tibial plateau on the AP x-ray. Meniscal length can be obtained by measuring the sagittal length of the tibial plateau on the lateral x-ray. The medial and lateral meniscus length equals 80% and 70% of the tibial plateau, respectively. Although CT and MRI scans are more precise, they add additional cost with questionable benefit. A 5% difference in size is commonly stated as acceptable and able to be obtained with proper technique with plain x-rays.[18] Although not uniformly agreed, it is probably better to err on the graft being bigger in size because shrinkage of the graft is common and shown to be on average of 7% shrinkage in one of the author's studies.[19]

Meniscal Allograft Preservation

Four methods of preserving meniscal allografts are available and include fresh, cryopreserved, fresh frozen, and freeze dried (lyophilization).[20] Fresh grafts carry an increased risk of infection and immune load. Cryopreservation adds an increased cost and has not shown to be of improved results. Lyophilization alters the meniscal properties of the meniscus and is not recommended.

Thus, fresh-frozen grafts are the most commonly used allograft preservation method today. It is vital that the allografts are obtained from American Association of Tissue Banks–certified tissue banks, which require stringent procurement and processing methods to prevent contamination and infection of the grafts.

Additional concerns have been raised regarding the age of donors for meniscal allografts and the viability and tensile strength of the grafts. Current recommendations are for the transplantation of meniscal allografts from donors younger than 45 years. The tensile strength of meniscal tissue and the proteoglycan and collagen content have been shown to not vary with age among grafts examined from donors aged 15 to 44 years.[21]

Positioning and Portals

The patient is placed in the supine position on a standard operating room table. After anesthesia is induced, a thorough examination of the knee under anesthesia should be performed to evaluate ROM and knee stability. A tourniquet is placed on the thigh but often not used until the arthrotomy is made to insert the graft. Fluid extravasation can be significant and done under dry conditions, which can result in bleeding and impede visualization. Depending on the surgeon's preference, the leg may be left unsupported in the supine position or placed into a cushioned leg holder. Regardless of the technique, the posteromedial and posterolateral corners of the knee should be readily accessible for inside-out meniscal repair.

Step-by-Step Description of the Procedure

Portals, Incisions, and Arthroscopic Preparation

Once the patient is prepped and draped, the arthroscopic portal opposite of the involved compartment should be made first. A spinal needle is used to make certain that the working portal is directly in line with the horn attachments and ease in making the channel straight rather than have some obliquity. The arthrotomy will incorporate this portal in the later stages of the procedure. Diagnostic arthroscopy is then performed to evaluate the status of the articular cartilage, cruciate ligaments, and confirm meniscal deficiency (Figure 9-2). The meniscal allograft should not be opened until the patient is confirmed to be an appropriate candidate. Any meniscus remaining should be debrided to an outer rim of 1 to 2 mm, leaving a vascular source for healing and a reference for graft position. If possible, the anterior and posterior horn attachments should be preserved to serve as guides for the drilling of the tunnels/channel. A limited notchplasty should be performed if there is any difficulty with visualization of the posterior attachment.

For passage of the graft, a mini-arthrotomy is performed adjacent to the patellar tendon on the affected side and in line with the insertion sites of the anterior and posterior horns. An additional posteromedial or posterolateral incision is necessary for retrieval of sutures.

Lateral: Dovetail Technique

Recipient Bed Preparation

The dovetail technique is preferred for lateral meniscus transplantation. Initial preparation is the same whether medial or lateral as well as dovetail or bone plug. Complete visualization of the meniscal remnant and horn attachments are necessary, and a small notchplasty may be needed to see the entire posterior root. Anatomic placement of the bony bridge is imperative to prevent extrusion of the meniscal allograft.[22] Once the attachments are identified, a 4-mm burr

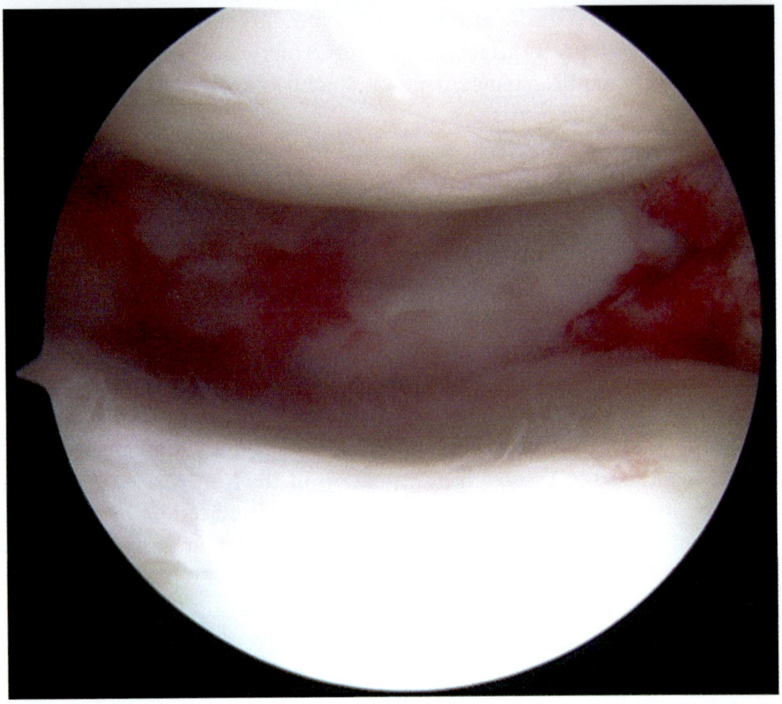

Figure 9-2. Meniscal-deficient lateral compartment.

is used to make a shallow (1- to 2-mm) trough directly in line with the anterior and posterior horns of the meniscus. This initial trough functions as a path for placement of an osteotome in the sagittal plane. A referencing depth line on the osteotome helps to maintain proper orientation as the tibial plateau slopes inferiorly when advancing from anterior to posterior. The osteotome should be advanced under direct visualization until it contacts the posterior tibial cortex. A 6-mm drill guide is fit over the osteotome, and the drill advanced. The guide enables the drill to be seen arthroscopically at all times, which helps maintain proper height and avoid breaking through the distal cortex (Figure 9-3). A second jig to accommodate a 7-mm drill at a height of 3 mm lower than the initial jig is then attached. The second drill is also seen at all times and is used to deepen the channel to 10 mm and expand the inferior aspect. A semitrapezoidal rasp is used to complete the dovetail slot (Figure 9-4). It is important that the rasp should follow the AP slope of the tibia, and the top of the rasps should remain flush with articular surface. The channel should be cleared of all remaining bone debris, and the channel sizer should be used to ensure the channel preparation is complete (Figure 9-5). A posterolateral incision should then be made using the interval between the iliotibial band and the anterior margin of the biceps femoris tendon for access to the capsule. Although staying in front of the biceps femoris should prevent injury to the peroneal nerve, formal exposure of the nerve can always been made.

Allograft Preparation

The meniscal allograft is typically sent by the tissue bank as a hemitibial plateau with the meniscus. It is imperative to see the entire horn attachments for proper bone cuts; thus, any excess soft tissue should be removed. The allograft bone should then be cut in an AP plane to the ends of the attachments. The end of the channel rasp is used to mark an outline of the desired dovetail design onto the ends of the bone as a reference for placing the graft in an upside-down position in the holding device (Figure 9-6). Three cutting jigs and an oscillating saw are used to complete the graft preparation. The first is a vertical cut on the medial aspect of the graft (Figure 9-7A). Often, this is already precut during the meniscal allograft processing. Next, the inferior cut is made in orientation to match the depth of the slot (Figure 9-7B). Finally, the third cutting guide is used to

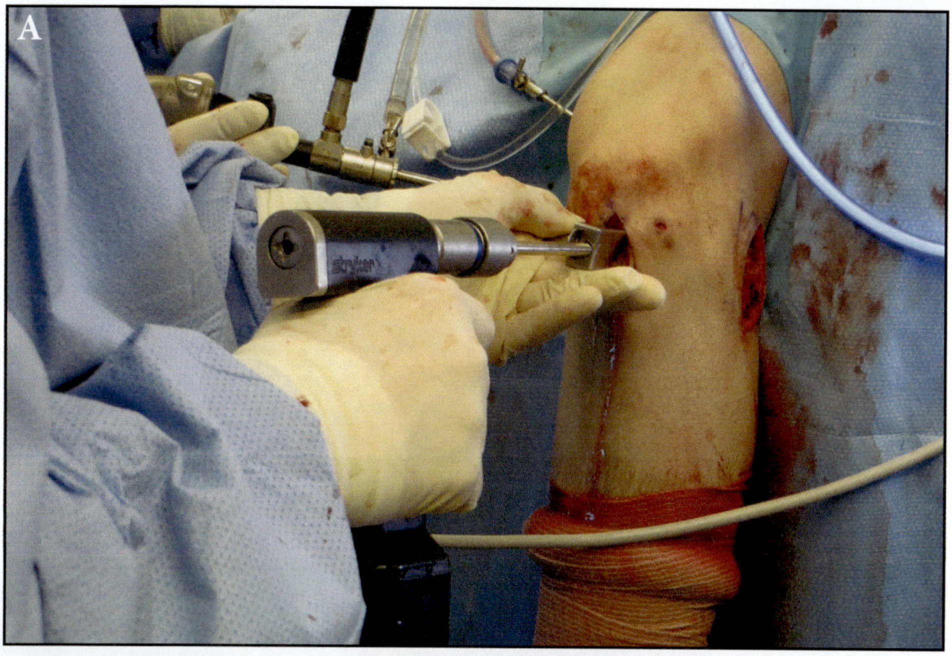

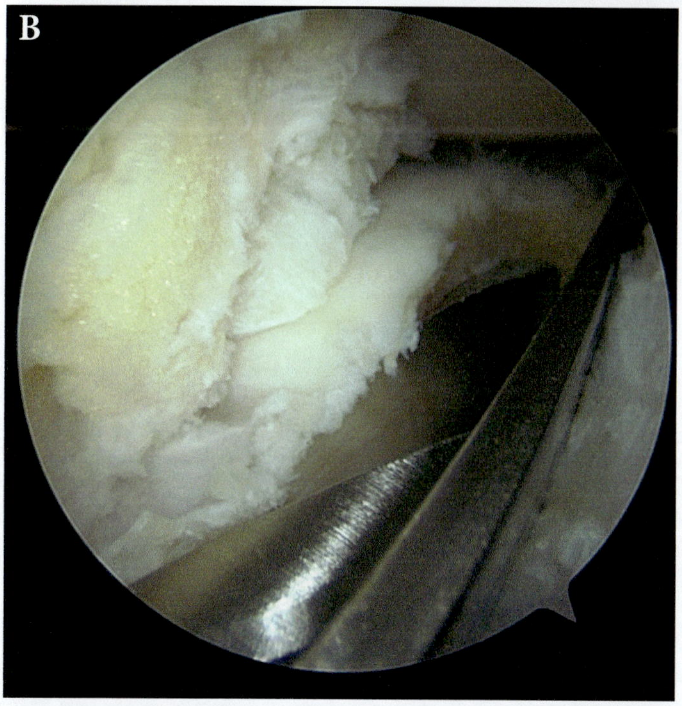

Figure 9-3. (A) The dovetail drill guide attached to the osteotome. (B) Arthroscopic view of the initial drilling of the channel.

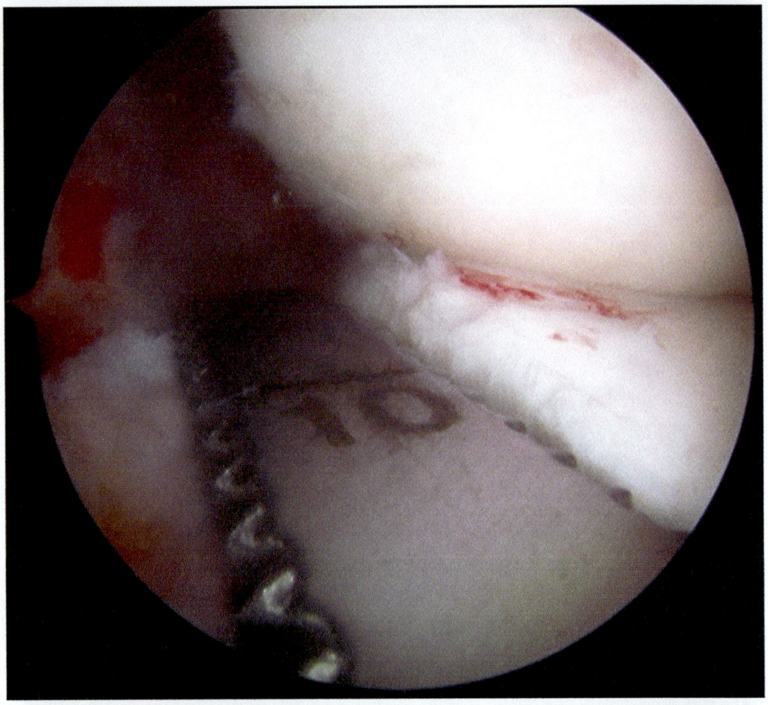

Figure 9-4. Rasp used to complete the tibia preparation.

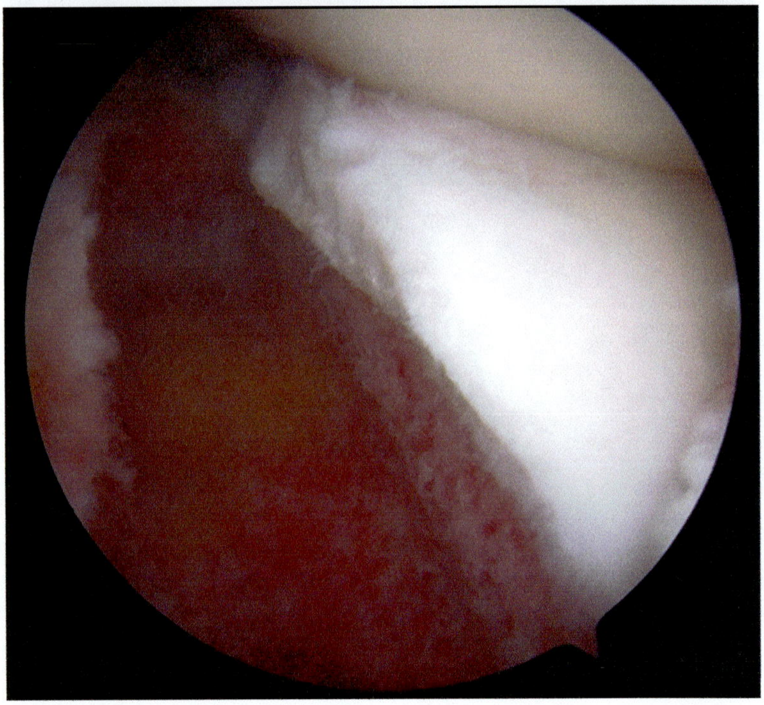

Figure 9-5. The channel is finished and ready for graft insertion.

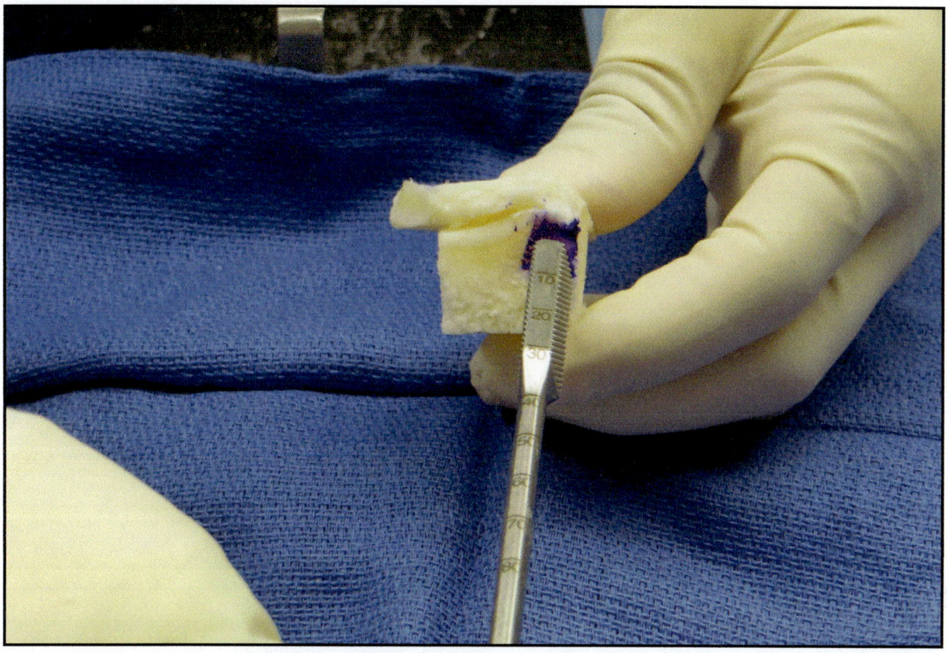

Figure 9-6. Dovetail outline on graft for reference of cuts.

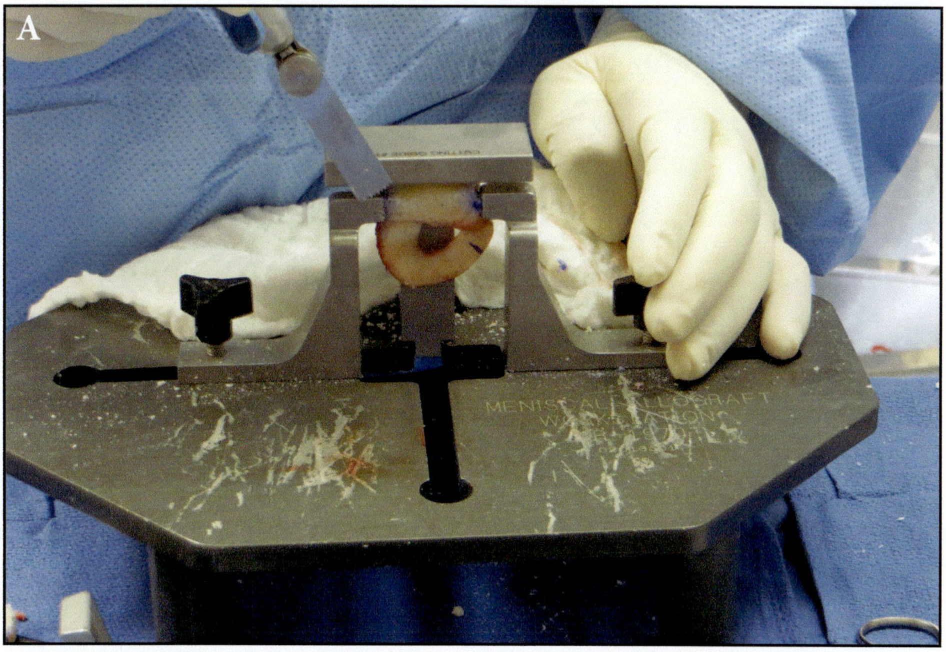

Figure 9-7. (A) Meniscus in a cutting jig with vertical cuts for dovetail preparation. *(continued)*

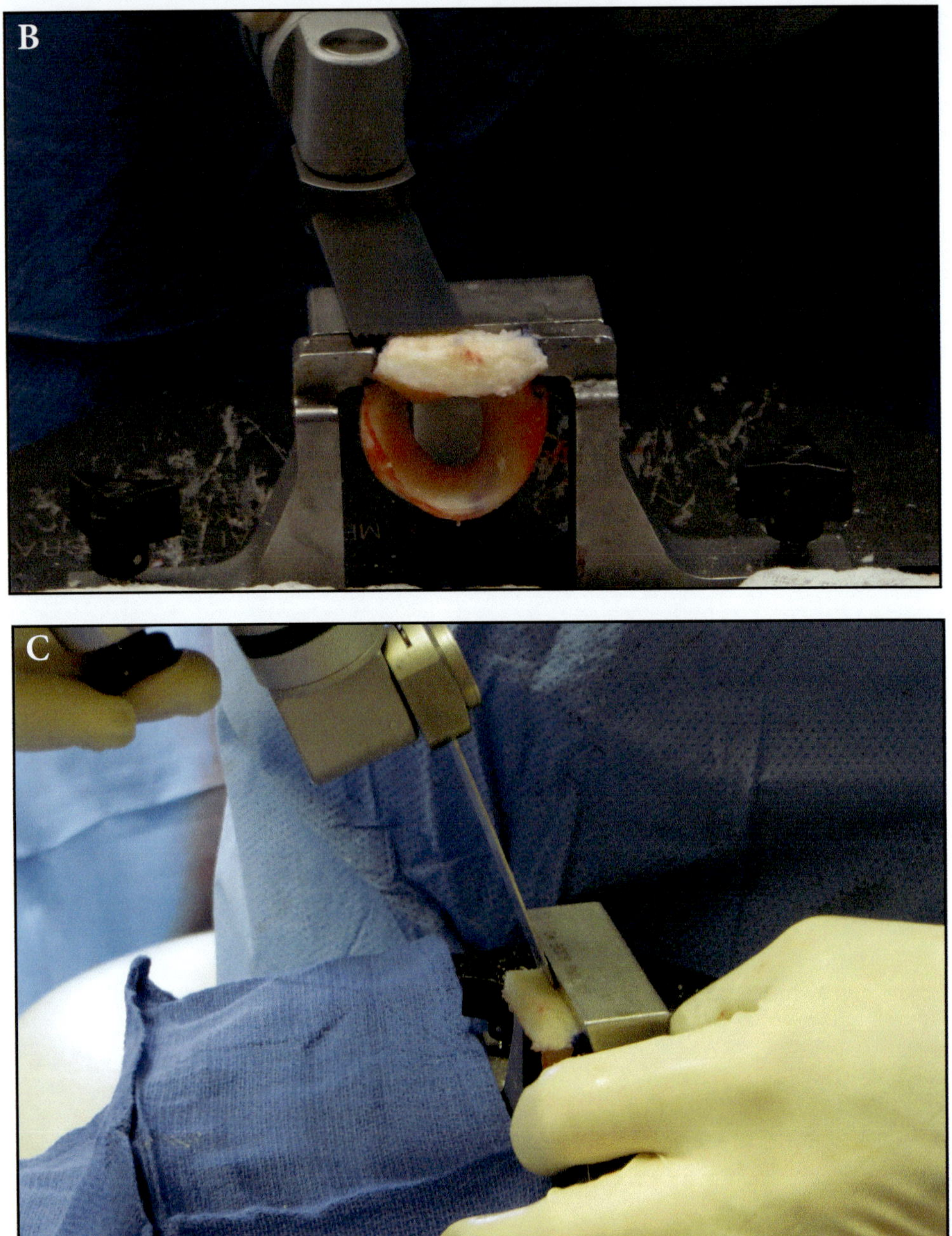

Figure 9-7 (continued). Meniscus in a cutting jig with (B) horizontal and (C) oblique cuts for dovetail preparation.

make the angled cut on the lateral aspect of the graft (Figure 9-7C). Once all cuts are complete, the sizing block is used to confirm it will allow a press fit, but the graft should also slide through smoothly (Figure 9-8). Any adjustments should be made at this time rather than trying to force the graft into the prepared channel. A 2-0 polydioxanone suture to be used as a reduction suture is placed through the posterior segment to complete the graft preparation.

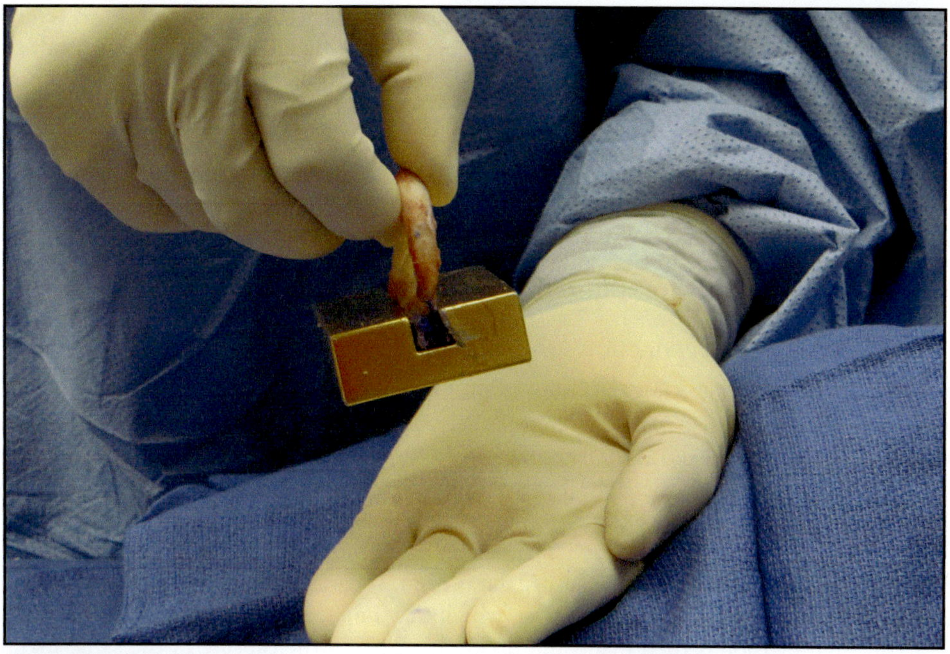

Figure 9-8. Completed graft in sizing block to confirm proper size and press-fit.

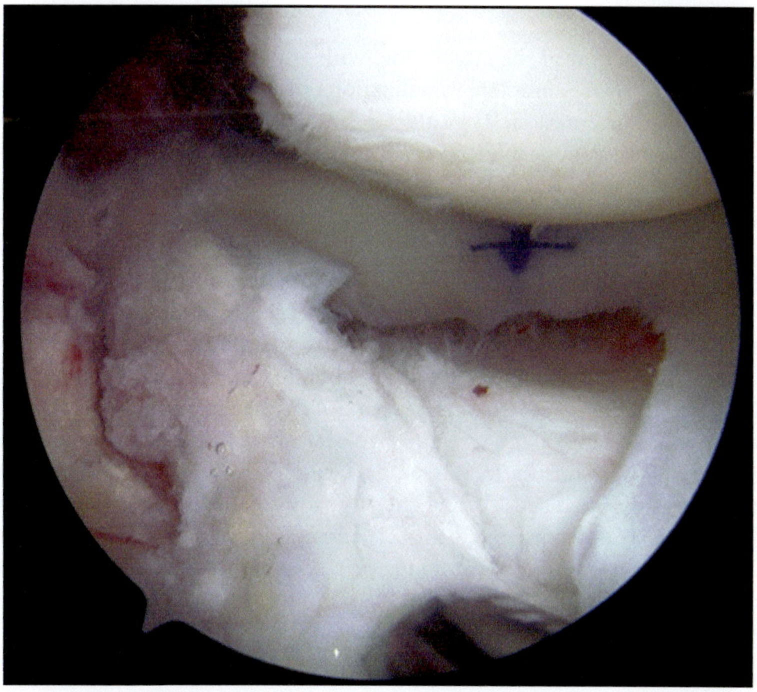

Figure 9-9. Reduced graft with a reduction suture seen.

Meniscus Implantation

The reduction suture is passed out through the posterolateral incision for application of gentle traction once the graft is inserted into the tibial channel. If needed, a bone tamp can be used to gently push the bone block further into the knee until contact with the posterior wall of the tibia (Figure 9-9). At this point, the anterior arthrotomy is closed to prevent fluid extravasation, and the rest of the meniscus sutured. Various techniques can be used, but the surgeon's preference for repairing a bucket handle meniscus tear is common. If only all-inside technique is used, special attention needs to be made to ensure that the graft is not extruded outward when tightening the fixation device. The author's preference is inside-out sutures for the posterior and middle horns and outside-in for the anterior horn. All-inside sutures will be used at the most posterior aspect if additional fixation near the root is needed. Absorbable and nonabsorbable sutures can be used, as second-look arthroscopies have shown that healing of the graft has not been a common problem. Usually, 8 to 10 sutures are required to completely secure the graft.

Medial: Double Bone Plug Technique (Video)

Recipient Bed Preparation

An ACL guide set at 60 degrees is used to place a guide pin into the anatomic posterior horn insertion of the old meniscus. A steep angle is selected to assist in reducing the plug, similar in reason to the tibial tunnel during posterior cruciate ligament surgery. The tibial tunnel is then drilled to a diameter of 7 mm, with the 1-mm difference allowing easy placement of the bone plug. A shuttle suture is passed up the tibial tunnel, retrieved, and brought out of the knee. Although the suture can be removed through the scope portal, the author has found it easy to make the anterior arthrotomy prior to bringing the suture out. Often, soft tissue can be entrapped between the suture and a subsequent arthrotomy incision, which may impede bringing the graft into the knee. A posteromedial incision is then made and dissected down to the capsule in the same manner as one would for a medial meniscus repair using inside-out sutures.

Allograft Preparation

Initial graft preparation is similar to that of the lateral side, with any remaining capsular tissue attached to the meniscus removed to ensure complete visualization of the horn attachments. They are then marked for size and planned orientation. Typically, an 8-mm coring reamer will encompass the horn attachment. The posterior bone plug is performed first, with a 0.062-in K-wire passed to enter the center of the attachment at a roughly a 60-degree angle to mimic the angle of the tibial tunnel. A collared pin is placed into the pilot hole, and the 8-mm coring reamer is used to create a bone plug. The bone plug end is then trimmed to be 6 mm in diameter and 8 mm in length. The size has been found to sufficiently secure the attachment but not be too large to impede reduction of the plug. Although a 6-mm coring reamer can be used, the author has found it easier to use the slightly larger corer to ensure fully encompassing the attachment and that it is less likely to damage the plug during harvest. The anterior horn is obtained in a similar fashion, but the plug is maintained at an 8-mm diameter and 10-mm length because reduction is not difficult. To insert and secure the posterior bone plug, a 2-0 nonabsorbable suture is passed up through the bone plug, sutured through the meniscal horn attachment, and brought back down the plug. It is imperative to include the edge of the meniscus during the suturing to add additional strength to the suture because the bone plug can be disrupted if pulled forcefully by itself. The anterior bone plug can be secured using the same suturing technique or placed in press-fit means, which are described later. As with the dovetail technique, a polydioxanone suture is placed through the meniscus to function as a reduction suture (Figure 9-10).

Meniscus Implantation

The meniscus reduction sutures are passed into the knee and retrieved through the posteromedial incision using open-ended needles and inside-out technique. The posterior bone plug suture is placed through the tibial tunnel suture and subsequently brings the bone plug suture out the tibial tunnel entrance. The surgeon applies gently on the bone plug suture and uses his or her index finger to carefully reduce the plug and bring the meniscus into the knee. At the same time, an assistant uses light tension on the reduction suture to help bring the meniscus into the knee, which also prevents the graft from flipping over.

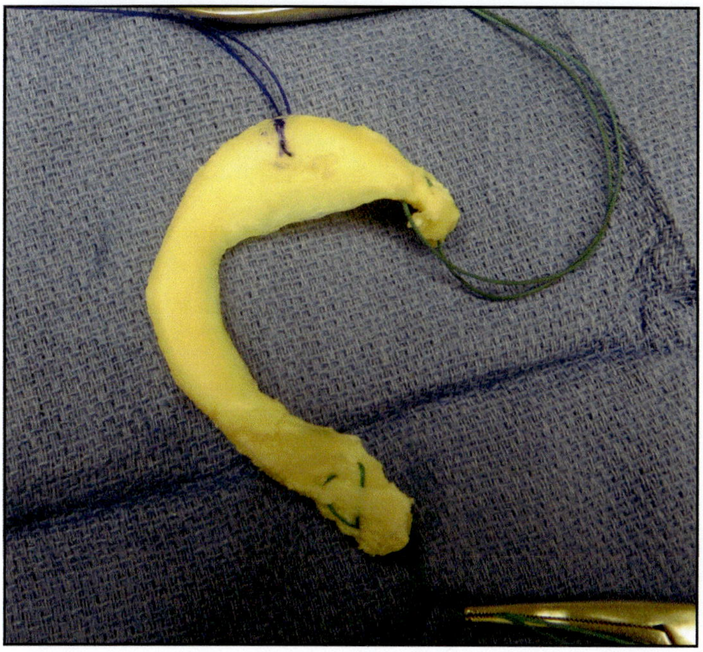

Figure 9-10. Completed double bone plug of a medial allograft.

Although the anterior plug can be placed right after the posterior plug, it is the author's preference to place a posterior then medial suture for initial fixation before securing the anterior horn. The author has found that by suturing the graft in this manner, the graft position is more adaptable to any differences between the graft and host (Figure 9-11). For example, if the anterior plug is secured first and the placement is incorrect, the difference needs to be made when suturing the remaining meniscus. It can thus result in a graft that is extruded outward or one in which there may be excess tension on the repair. If the preliminary fixation is done posterior then middle, it is much easier to make adjustments for the anterior bone plug placement.

Once the anterior bone plug site is determined, a guide pin is placed and overreamed with an 8-mm drill to a depth of 1 cm. The anterior bone plug can be secured with a suture or can be press-fit. Until experience is gained, it is wise to use a suture because ensuring a secure press-fit has a learning curve. If the graft is to be secured with a bone plug stitch, a small hole to accommodate a suture-passing device is made in the anterior tibia and the plug sutures brought down reducing the plug into the socket. The sutures from the 2 plugs are then tied to one another for fixation. With the press-fit method, the tibia socket is made 1 to 2 mm less deep, and a tamp is used to compress the plug into the socket. The suture for the posterior plug is tied down at tibia opening once it has been reduced. The author has found that a simple, inexpensive polyethylene button serves just as well as a more expensive fixation device. Subsequent suturing of the meniscus is the same as previously described for the dovetail method.

Concomitant Procedures

Combined Anterior Cruciate Ligament Reconstruction and Meniscal Transplantation

The main concern when reconstructing an ACL in conjunction with a meniscal allograft is the tibial tunnels/channel preparation. If a bone bridge technique is used on the medial side, there can be a small area of overlap with the channel and the tibial ACL tunnel. Therefore, all bone preparation should be completed prior to either graft placement. If there is any overlap, the

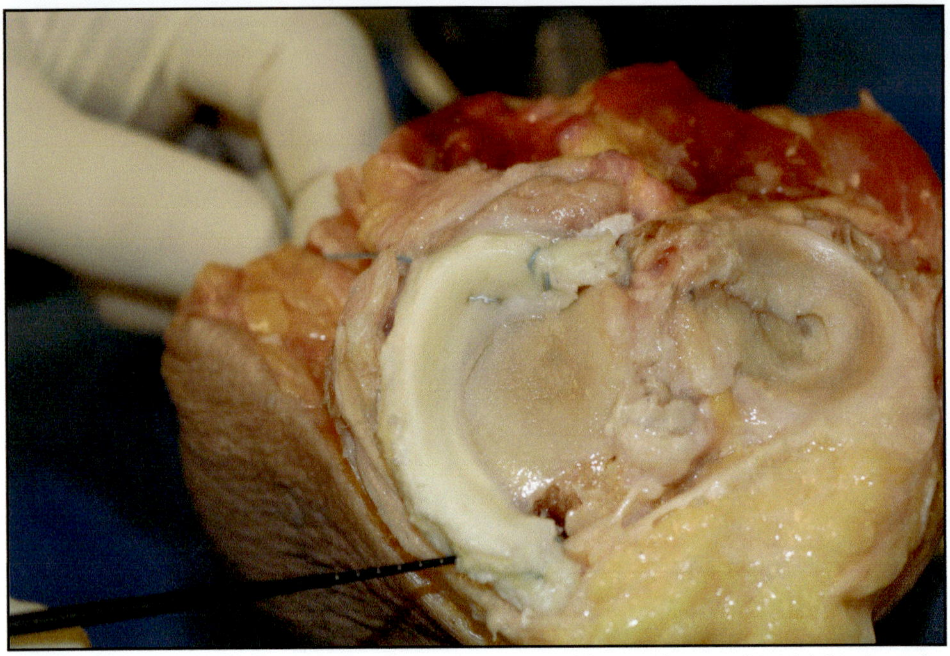

Figure 9-11. Tibial plateau demonstrating placement of bone plugs and initial fixation of a medial graft. Note the significant difference in distance between the medial and lateral horn attachments.

meniscal allograft is placed first. The drill can then be inserted up the ACL tunnel and carefully used to remove bone that would prevent the ACL from passing. Conversely, if one tried to place the ACL graft first, it would prevent reduction of the bone bridge into the slot or cause damage to the ACL graft.

If the double bone plug technique is used in conjunction with an ACL, overlap of tunnels should not occur if proper technique is used. Some tips can help to further limit the risk. If the tibia is small, then the meniscus tunnel is drilled more midline and the ACL slightly more medial than usual to enable more cortical bone between the drill holes. If the ACL tunnel appears to be in close proximity to the anterior horn attachment, the plug socket can be drilled at a slight lateral angle to have it directed away from the tibia tunnel.

For lateral meniscal allografts, overlap of the ACL tunnel of bone channel should not occur if placed properly. In the event an error occurs, it should be addressed in the same manner as noted for a bone bridge graft placed on the medial side.

High Tibial Osteotomy and Meniscal Transplantation

Osteotomies are typically performed when the mechanical alignment is toward the involved compartment by more than a few degrees greater than the contralateral knee. All aspects of the meniscal portion of the procedure, except placement of the graft, are completed prior to the osteotomy and its fixation. When performing a bone bridge allograft, if the osteotomy is made as inferior on the tibia as possible, the plate and screws should be distal enough to not have overlap with the channel. If the bone plug technique is used, the posterior tunnel should be drilled as steep of an angle on the tibia as possible. It helps keep the tunnel more posterior and decreases the risk of overlap with the osteotomy screws. If there is a concern of overlap, keep the drill for the meniscus inserted in the bone tunnel to identify its location when the osteotomy screws are placed.

Articular Cartilage Repair and Meniscal Transplantation

As noted under Indications, if there is an isolated defect that can be addressed with a cartilage repair/restoration procedure, the patient may still be a candidate for a meniscal allograft. Typically, they are performed in conjunction with one another. Because many of the cartilage techniques have fixation methods that are not initially durable and are thus at risk for disruption, the meniscal allograft is commonly completed first.

Postoperative Protocol

The initial postoperative care is to control pain, limit swelling, and obtain full extension. Weightbearing is limited for the initial 4 weeks. A postoperative ROM brace is worn during this period, with flexion limited to 90 degrees to minimize the meniscus translation and subsequent stress on the posterior repair.

At 4 weeks, patients are allowed full weightbearing and unrestricted ROM. Stationary biking with low resistance and straight leg swimming are also started at that time. Progressive, low-impact strengthening is implemented when the gait pattern has returned to normal. Most surgeons recommend waiting until 4 months to allow jogging, although the author has found no detriment if it is allowed as early as 12 weeks. Regardless of the time, patients with moderate arthritis are strongly discouraged to avoid high impact activities permanently.

From 4 to 6 months, leg strengthening is progressed as comfortable, with core and balance exercises stressed. Patients are released at 6 months if strength and endurance are comparable to the contralateral leg and agility testing is normal. Regardless of the degree of chondromalacia, patients' expectations should not be to return to unlimited high-impact or contact sports.

Potential Complications

The reported complication rates vary widely, with initial series as high as 50%. However, as experience and indications have been refined, the rates have dropped significantly (Figure 9-12).[23,24] In a meta-analysis of 44 studies, Elattar et al[25] found an overall complication rate of 21.3%. The most common complication was tearing of the graft. In a systematic review of the literature on meniscal transplantation, Matava[26] noted 45 tears in 547 patients for a tear rate of 8.2%. The mean follow-up of the 15 studies reviewed was 55 months (range, 6 months to 14.5 years). In a long-term series of 100 patients, Verdonk et al[27] reported that the cumulative survival rates following transplantation at 10 years for medial meniscal allografts were 74.2% and 69.8% for the lateral meniscus.

Whenever discussing allografts, infection and immune reaction are expressed as a concern. Because fresh-frozen meniscal grafts are acellular, significant immune reactions are rare, with review articles typically stating an occurrence of 1%. To date, no reports of HIV transmission have been described from the use of meniscal allografts. The prevalence of infection is no higher than standard meniscus repair procedures.

As with any meniscal repair method, a major concern for complication is neurovascular injury. Arthrofibrosis is another possible complication that may be overlooked. If only the capsule is remaining to suture the graft, the capsule can become entrapped if care is not taken to ensure the posterior sutures are not overtightened. In addition, arthrofibrosis is of greater concern for meniscal allografts than standard meniscus repairs because the arthrotomy and extensive anterior horn suturing can result in more anterior compartment scarring.

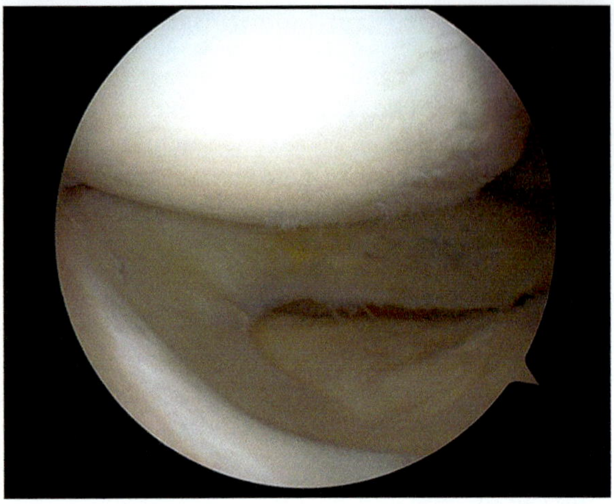

Figure 9-12. Second-look arthroscopy at 6 months showing that the allograft is well healed.

Top Technical Pearls for the Procedure

1. The working portal should not be the first portal made. The contralateral portal is made first, and a spinal needle is used to make certain the working portal will be directly in line with the meniscal horn attachments.
2. Make certain that the horn attachments to the bone are fully seen. If not, the bone cuts or coring reamer can easily disrupt the attachments from the bone.
3. The reduction suture should not be in the middle segment of the graft. If so, it will tend to pull the graft outward rather than posterior and, in the process, ironically prevent reduction.
4. Although the anterior bone plug can easily be placed right after the posterior plug is reduced, it should not be unless the graft is a perfect match. The posterior and middle segments should be positioned first because the anterior segment is more amenable to graft position adjustments.
5. The initial few sutures should be on the upper aspect of the meniscus to ensure it is opposed directly to the capsule. If the sutures are inferior, they have a tendency to put the graft outward and result in overlap with the capsule.

References

1. Renström P, Johnson RJ. Anatomy and biomechanics of the menisci. *Clin Sports Med.* 1990;9(3):523-538.
2. Baratz ME, Fu FH, Mengato R. Mensical tears: the effect of meniscectomy and of repair on intraarticular contact areas and stress in the human knee. A preliminary report. *Am J Sports Med.* 1986;14(4):270-275.
3. Allen PR, Denham RA, Swan AV. Late degenerative changes after meniscectomy. Factors affecting the knee after operation. *J Bone Joint Sur Br.* 1984;66(5):666-671.
4. Brophy RH, Matava MJ. Surgical options for meniscal replacement. *J Am Acad Orthop Surg.* 2012;20(5):265-272.
5. Garrett JC. Meniscal transplantation: a review of 43 cases with two to seven year follow-up. *Sports Med Arthrosc Rev.* 1993;2:164-167.
6. Cole BJ, Carter TR, Rodeo SA. Allograft meniscal transplantation: background, techniques, and results. *Instr Course Lect.* 2003;52:383-396.

7. Abat F, Gelber PE, Erquicia JI, Pelfort X, Gonzalez-Lucena G, Monllau JC. Suture-only fixation technique leads to a higher degree of extrusion than bony fixation in meniscal allograft transplantation. *Am J Sports Med.* 2012;40(7):1591-1596.
8. Berlet GC, Fowler PJ. The anterior horn of the medial meniscus. An anatomic study of its insertion. *Am J Sports Med.* 1998;26(4):540-543.
9. Carter TR, Rabago M. Meniscal allograft transplantation: ten-year follow-up. *Arthroscopy.* 2012;28(suppl 1);e17-e18.
10. LaPrade RF, Willis NJ, Spiridonov SI, Perkinson S. A prospective outcomes study of meniscal allograft transplantation. *Am J Sports Med.* 2010;38(9):1804-1812.
11. Kim JG, Lee YS, Bae TS, et al. Tibiofemoral contact mechanics following posterior root of the medial meniscus tear, repair, meniscectomy, and allograft transplantation. *Knee Surg Traumatol Arthrosc.* 2013;21(9):2121-2125.
12. Vundelinckx B, Vanlauwe J, Bellemans J. Long-term subjective, clinical, and radiographic outcome evaluation of meniscal allograft transplantation in the knee. *Am J Sports Med.* 2014;42(7):1592-1599.
13. Harris JD, Cavo M, Brophy R, Siston R, Flanigan D. Biological knee reconstruction: a systematic review of combined meniscal allograft transplantation and cartilage repair or restoration. *Arthroscopy.* 2011;27(3):409-418.
14. Noyes FR, Barber-Westin SD, Rankin M. Meniscal transplantation in symptomatic patients less than fifty years old. *J Bone Joint Surg Am.* 2004;86(7):1392-1404.
15. Huang A, Hull ML, Howell SM. The level of compressive load affects conclusions from statistical analyses to determine whether a lateral meniscus allograft restores tibial contact pressure to normal: a study in human cadaveric knees. *J Orthop Res.* 2003;21(3):459-464.
16. Pollard ME, Kang Q, Berg EE. Radiographic sizing for meniscal transplantation. *Arthroscopy.* 1995;11(6):684-687.
17. Yoon YR, Kim TS, Lim HC, Lim HT, Yang JH. Is radiographic measurement of bony landmarks reliable for lateral meniscal sizing? *Am J Sports Med.* 2011;39(3):582-589.
18. McDermott ID, Sharifi F, Bull AM, Gupte CM, Thomas RW, Amis AA. An anatomical study of meniscal allograft sizing. *Knee Surg Sports Traumatol Arthrosc.* 2004;12(2):130-135.
19. Carter T, Economopoulos KJ. Meniscal allograft shrinkage—MRI evaluation. *J Knee Surg.* 2013;26(3):167-171.
20. Rijk PC. Menisal allograft transplantation—part I: background, results, graft selection and preservation, and surgical considerations. *Arthroscopy.* 2004;20(7):728-743.
21. Bursac P, York A, Kuznia P, Brown LM, Arnoczky SP. Influence of donor age on the biomechanical and biochemical properties of human meniscal allografts. *Am J Sports Med.* 2009;37(5):884-889.
22. Choi NH, Yoo SY, Victoroff BN. Position of the bony bridge of lateral meniscal transplants can affect meniscal extrusion. *Am J Sports Med.* 2011;39(9):1955-1959.
23. Hutchinson ID, Moran CJ, Potter HG, Warren RF, Rodeo SA. Restoration of the meniscus: form and function. *Am J Sports Med.* 2014;42(4):987-998.
24. Wirth CJ, Peters G, Milachowski KA, Weismeier KG, Kohn D. Long-term results of meniscal allograft transplantation. *Am J Sports Med.* 2002;30(2):174-181.
25. Elattar M, Dhollander A, Verdonk R, Almqvist KF, Verdonk P. Twenty-six years of meniscal allograft transplantation: is it still experimental? A meta-analysis of 44 trials. *Knee Surg Sports Traumatol Arthrosc.* 2011;19(12):147-157.
26. Matava MJ. Meniscal allograft transplantation: a systematic review. *Clin Orthop Relat Res.* 2007;(455):142-157.
27. Verdonk PC, Demurie A, Almqvist KF, Veys EM, Verbruggen G, Verdonk R. Transplantation of viable meniscal allograft. Survivorship analysis and clinical outcome of one hundred cases. *J Bone Joint Surg Am.* 2005;87(4):715-724.

Please see videos on the accompanying website at www.routledge.com/9781617119996

SECTION III

Patella

10

Arthroscopic Treatment of Patellar Tendinopathy (Jumper's Knee)

Jason L. Koh, MD and Neil C. Dunleavy, MD

Introduction

Patellar tendinopathy is widely recognized as a degenerative process of the patellar tendon, occurring with increased frequency in jumping athletes. In 1973, Blazina et al[1] coined the term *jumper's knee* to describe the condition, which has a strong predilection for affecting athletes involved in intense repetitive jumping activity, such as basketball and volleyball. Lian et al[2] showed an overall prevalence of jumper's knee in 613 elite athletes of 14.2%, with the highest prevalence in volleyball (44.6%) and basketball (31.9%) players.

Although first viewed as an inflammatory condition and often referred to as patellar tendinitis, it is now understood from histopathological study that the condition is mostly degenerative and multifactorial, likely involving a complex cascade of events resulting in damaged, painful tissue. Excessive or repetitive loading during jumping has been implicated as a cause.[3-5] Some evidence has found a longer distal nonarticular facet in patients with patellar tendinopathy,[6] but others have not identified significant differences that could contribute to impingement as a cause of patellar tendinopathy.[7] The proximal posterior degenerated tendon tissue has shown evidence of neoinnervation and neovascularity in addition to collagenous disorganization.[8,9] In addition, Hoffa's fat pad has been implicated for impinging on a protruded inferior pole of the patella and developing sensitive pain receptors as part of the disease process.[10]

Treatments have varied greatly in nature and success. A trial of nonoperative treatment is well supported in the literature, with most authors recommending at least 3 to 6 months of conservative measures prior to considering surgical intervention.[11-13] Most clinicians advocate a short period of discontinuation from the offending activity and a structured physical therapy program focusing on eccentric quadriceps strengthening exercises and knee range of motion (ROM). Other nonoperative measures have included a short course of nonsteroidal anti-inflammatory drugs, cryotherapy, platelet-rich plasma injections, and low-energy radial extracorporeal shock wave therapy.[14-16]

When conservative measures fail to provide adequate relief of symptoms, surgical management is considered. Traditionally, open surgical methods have been applied with success, with the goal of removing the degenerated area of patellar tendon while often excising the protruded inferior

Sgaglione NA, Lubowitz JH, Provencher MT, eds. *The Knee: AANA Advanced Arthroscopic Surgical Techniques* (pp 135-143).

pole of the patella.[17-19] In recent years, open surgery has increasingly been replaced by arthroscopic techniques. Support for arthroscopy comes not only from its minimally invasive nature but also its proposed ability to address the complex nature of the degenerative process in a more reliable and complete manner, including excision of the protruded inferior pole of the patella without harming intact tendon tissue, resection of the proximal posterior painful fat pad, direct resection of affected tendon tissue, cauterization of tendon neovasculature, and the possible use of more accelerated rehabilitation.[20-26]

Multiple studies support open and arthroscopic procedures as successful management strategies for chronic patellar tendinopathy unresponsive to conservative treatment,[21] with a recent trend favoring arthroscopy. In a recent systematic review, Marcheggiani Muccioli et al[20] found that satisfactory results were achieved in 92.4% of arthroscopically treated patients and in 87.2% of patients treated with open surgery. Return to sport rates also favored arthroscopy (84.2% vs 76.6%).[20] However, evidence is limited, and no randomized controlled prospective trials have compared open vs arthroscopic treatment. Arthroscopic treatment has been demonstrated to be superior to sclerosing injections in one randomized trial.[27]

Indications

Arthroscopic debridement is indicated for the treatment of an established, chronic patellar tendinopathy that has failed at least 3 to 6 months of nonsurgical management that includes eccentric strengthening exercises for the knee extensor mechanism.[12,22] It has been described for the treatment of proximal to mid-tendon lesions; arthroscopic debridement of patella tendinopathy at the insertion of the tendon to the tibial tubercle is technically difficult to perform due to challenges in the visualization of this area.

- Chronic patellar tendinopathy
- Failed 3 to 6 months of nonsurgical treatment, including eccentric strengthening
- Proximal to mid-tendon lesions

Controversial Indications

No significant controversy exists with regard to proceeding to surgical management after failure of nonsurgical treatment. No clear data support arthroscopic compared to open surgical treatment[20] or distal pole resection of the patella in addition to tendon debridement alone.[12]

- Has not failed eccentric strengthening of the extensor mechanism
- Distal lesion

Pertinent Physical Findings

Tenderness is usually located at the junction of the distal pole of the patella and the proximal patellar tendon.

- Best test: Point tenderness at the attachment of the patellar tendon to the inferior pole of the patella
- Pain with squatting or jumping
- Soft tissue swelling at the inferior pole of the patella/patellar tendon
- Mild warmth at the patella tendon

Pertinent Imaging

- X-rays: Anteroposterior, lateral, and sunrise views; usually normal but may show enthesophyte (traction spur) at the inferior patella
- Ultrasound: May show a hypoechoic region in the patellar tendon or a thickened tendon in areas of degeneration. Color Doppler ultrasound may show increased vascularity[23]
- Magnetic resonance imaging ([MRI] T1 and T2): May show increased signal in areas of degeneration; may show tendon thickening

Equipment

The following are required to perform this procedure: standard arthroscopy equipment; a spinal needle for portal localization; a 4-mm, high-definition, 30-degree arthroscope; an arthroscopic shaver; an arthroscopic burr; and a 90-degree arthroscopic radiofrequency ablation device.

Positioning and Portals

The patient should be placed supine with ability to flex the knee. Tourniquets, posts, or leg holders should be placed proximal enough to allow placement of a superior portal for viewing purposes.

Step-by-Step Description of the Procedure

Preoperatively, the size and location of the lesion can be identified on MRI or ultrasound. Axial views can provide information about the medial-lateral size and location of the tendon, and sagittal views can give the length of area. Prior to induction, the patient is examined and the area of maximal tenderness and discomfort is noted and marked. This provides a guide for the area of treatment.

The knee is prepped and draped to allow a superolateral portal, as well as the standard inferolateral and inferomedial portals. Placement of a thigh tourniquet is recommended, but it may not often require inflation. The inferior portals are made, and a thorough diagnostic arthroscopy is performed.

Following standard treatment and visualization through the inferolateral portal, a proximal superolateral portal is created (Figure 10-1). The scope is switched from the inferolateral to the superolateral portal (Figure 10-2) and is used to examine the inferior pole of the patella (Figure 10-3) and fat pad (Figure 10-4). A needle can be placed directly through the preoperatively marked area of the lesion into the joint (Figure 10-5), helping identify the area of damage intra-articularly. Once the needle can be seen, it is removed and a skin incision for a transpatellar tendon portal is created directly in line with the area of damage. A blunt trocar and cannula are introduced through the tendon and fat pad into the joint following the previously defined needle trajectory (Figure 10-6). An arthroscopic shaver or radiofrequency ablation device is used to resect the proximal aspect of Hoffa's fat pad (Figure 10-7). This will allow visualization of the degenerated patellar tendon and also allow for excision of a possible source of pain. Care is taken not to damage the tendon during this process. The entire fat pad need not typically be resected because the area of degeneration is typically focused to the proximal posterior aspect of the tendon. The undersurface of the patellar tendon and its fibers can be easily visualized at this point (Figure 10-8).

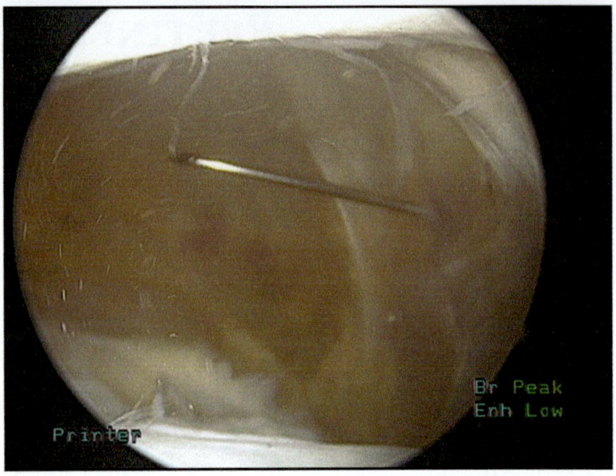

Figure 10-1. Identify the location of the superior portal with a spinal needle to ensure appropriate visualization.

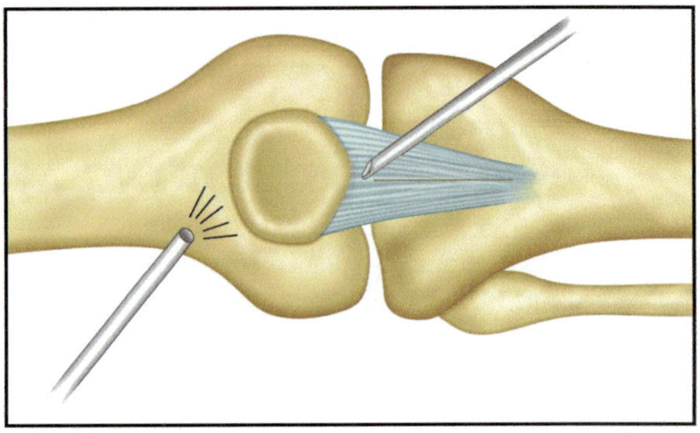

Figure 10-2. Diagram of the superior portal. The authors prefer the superolateral portal for ease of use and less trauma to the vastus medialis obliquus, which decreases quadriceps irritation.

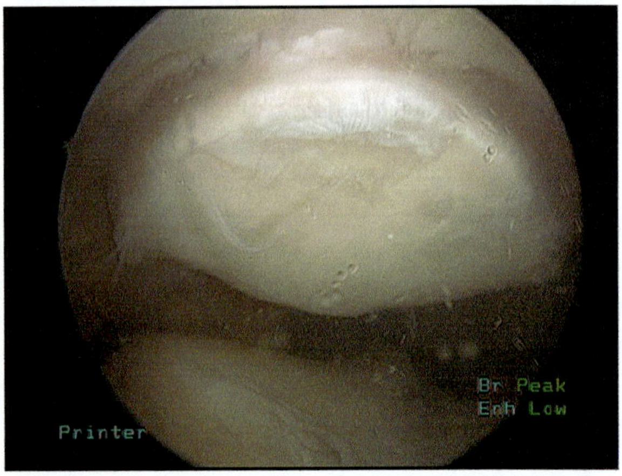

Figure 10-3. Typical view from the superior portal showing the patella and trochlea.

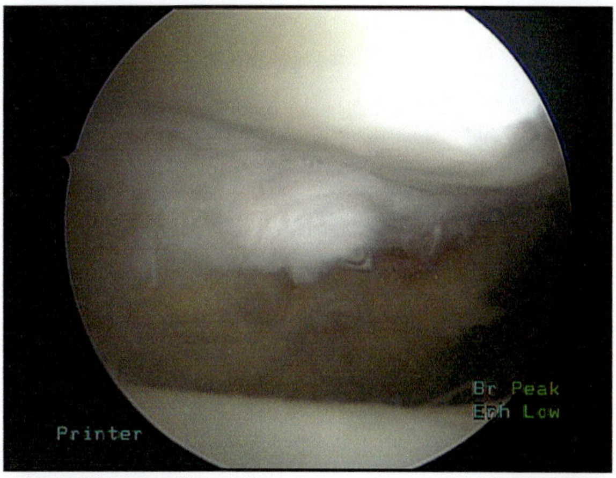

Figure 10-4. View of the infrapatellar fat pad at the inferior pole of the patella. Typically, the scope needs to be advanced distally to view this region.

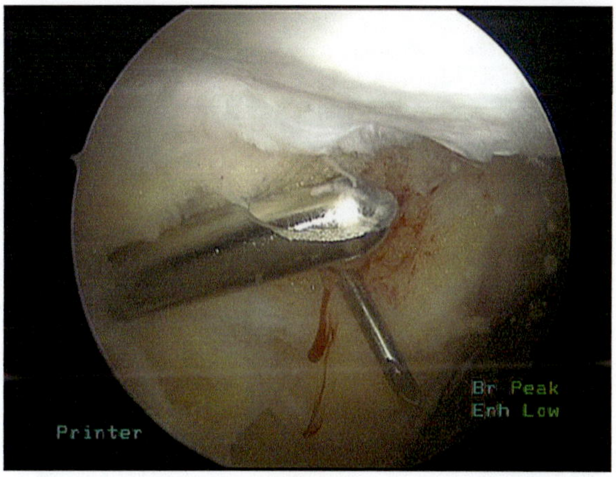

Figure 10-5. View showing the spinal needle through area of maximal tenderness of the patellar tendon and advanced through fat pad. This helps localize the lesion. If desired, a medial or lateral portal shaver can help clear away the fat pad.

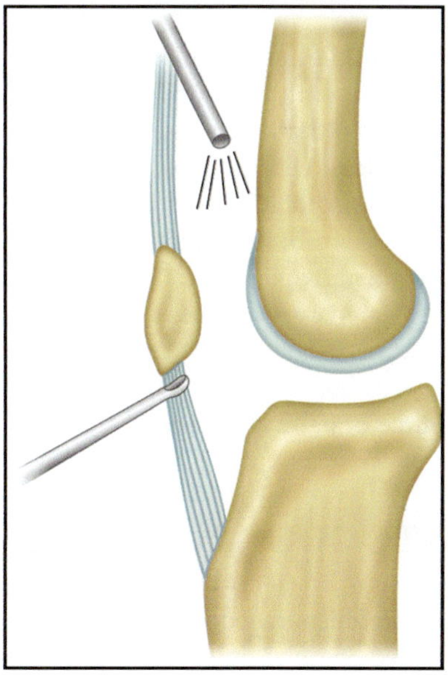

Figure 10-6. Diagram of relative location of the scope and transpatellar tendon portal.

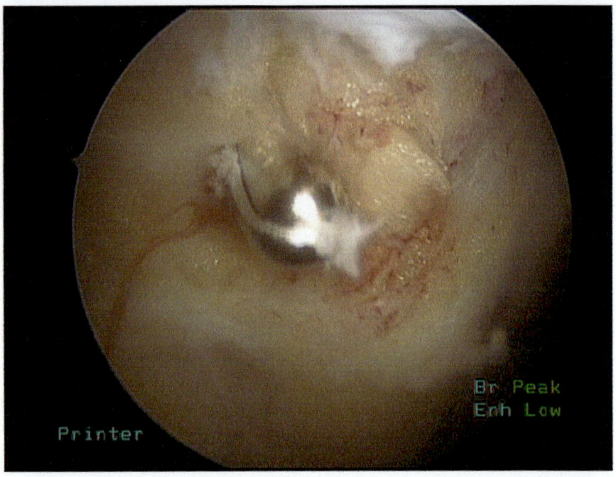

Figure 10-7. The infrapatellar fat pad is removed posterior to the tendon lesion.

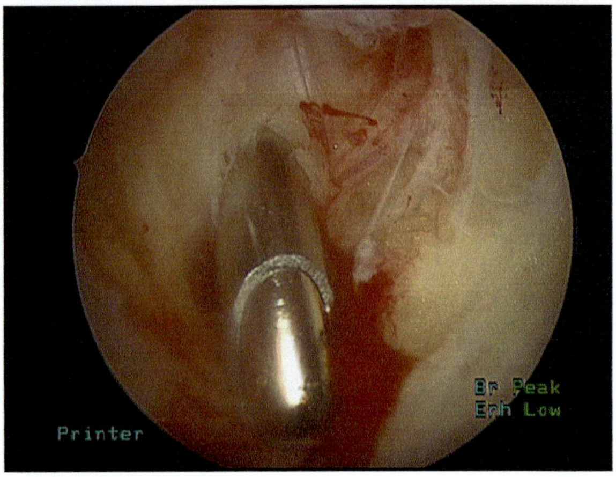

Figure 10-8. Tendon fibers (vertically oriented) are exposed.

The patellar tendon should be inspected completely to identify areas of mucoid degeneration or hypervascularity characteristic of chronic patellar tendinopathy. These degenerated areas should be resected with the arthroscopic shaver. Debridement of the damaged tissue can also be guided by preoperative imaging. Viewing from multiple portals is recommended to ensure thorough removal of degenerated tissue. Typically, an 8- to 10-mm wide segment of degenerative tendon at the central inferior pole of the patella is removed (Figure 10-9). Intact tendon tissue should be carefully protected and preserved. The adequacy of the debridement of degenerative tissue can be confirmed by placing the arthroscope into the central portal and inspecting the margins of the resection. Any neovessels found within the tendon should be cauterized. If felt necessary, an osteoplasty of the inferior patella is performed with an arthroscopic burr or bone-cutting shaver, to both enhance a healing response within the tendon and remove a potential source of painful impingement.

Postoperative Protocol

Postoperatively, early ROM and immediate weightbearing are encouraged to avoid stiffness and accelerate recovery of function. Eccentric strengthening closed chain exercises are initiated as quadriceps function returns. Running typically is allowed by 5 to 6 weeks postoperatively. Return to sport is guided by collaboration of the patient, the physician, and the physical therapist.

Return to sport is often accomplished by 10 to 12 weeks postoperatively.[24]

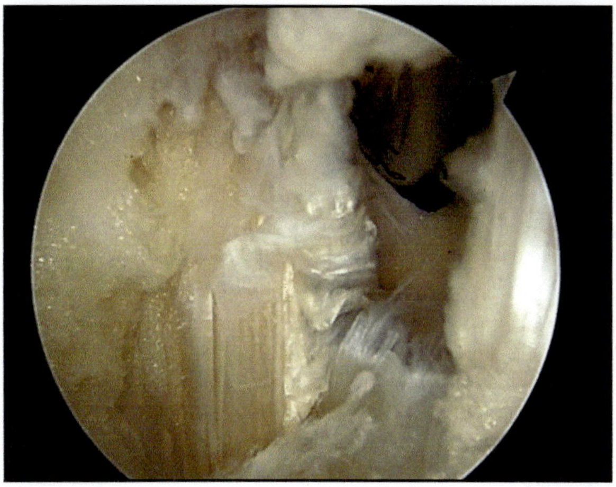

Figure 10-9. The patellar tendon is debrided at the area of abnormality.

Potential Complications

Although rare, vigorous resection of the patellar tendon can lead to partial or complete patellar tendon rupture. Inability to cauterize neovessels can theoretically lead to hematoma. Osteophytes at the site of the inferior patellar osteoplasty are occasionally found postoperatively but are often asymptomatic.

Top Technical Pearls for the Procedure

1. Establish a superior viewing portal (superolateral preferred) to visualize the fat pad.
2. Place a spinal needle through a preoperatively identified area of pathology (imaging, maximum tenderness to palpation).
3. Create a transpatellar tendon portal and place the shaver into the joint.
4. Obtain proper visualization of the degenerated patellar tendon by resecting an adequate amount of Hoffa's fat pad.
5. Resection margins can be assessed by placing the scope through the transpatellar tendon portal to see if residual degenerative tendon or neovessels remain.

References

1. Blazina ME, Kerlan RK, Jobe FW, Carter VS, Carlson GJ. Jumper's knee. *Orthop Clin North Am.* 1973;4(3):665-678.
2. Lian OB, Engebretsen L, Bahr R. Prevalence of jumper's knee among elite athletes from different sports: a cross-sectional study. *Am J Sports Med.* 2005;33(4):561-567.
3. Dillon EM, Erasmus PJ, Müller JH, Scheffer C, de Villiers RV. Differential forces within the proximal patellar tendon as an explanation for the characteristic lesion of patellar tendinopathy: an in vivo descriptive experimental study. *Am J Sports Med.* 2008;36(11):2119-2127.

4. Lavagnino M, Arnoczky SP, Elvin N, Dodds J. Patellar tendon strain is increased at the site of the jumper's knee lesion during knee flexion and tendon loading: results and cadaveric testing of a computational model. *Am J Sports Med.* 2008;36(11):2110-2118.
5. Bahr MA, Bahr R. Jump frequency may contribute to risk of jumper's knee: a study of interindividual and sex differences in a total of 11,943 jumps video recorded during training and matches in young elite volleyball players. *Br J Sports Med.* 2014;48(17):1322-1326.
6. Lorbach O, Diamantopoulos A, Kammerer KP, Paessler HH. The influence of the lower patellar pole in the pathogenesis of chronic patellar tendinopathy. *Knee Surg Sports Traumatol Arthrosc.* 2008;16(4):348-352.
7. Schmid MR, Hodler J, Cathrein P, Duewell S, Jacob HA, Romero J. Is impingement the cause of jumper's knee? Dynamic and static magnetic resonance imaging of patellar tendinitis in an open-configuration system. *Am J Sports Med.* 2002;30(3):388-395.
8. Maffulli N, Testa V, Capasso G, et al. Similar histopathological picture in males with Achilles and patellar tendinopathy. *Med Sci Sports Exerc.* 2004;36(9):1470-1475.
9. Khan KM, Bonar F, Desmond PM, et al. Patellar tendinosis (jumper's knee): findings at histopathologic examination, US, and MR imaging. Victorian Institute of Sport Tendon Study Group. *Radiology.* 1996;200(3):821-827.
10. Fredberg U. Tendinopathy—tendinitis or tendinosis? The question is still open. *Scand J Med Sci Sports.* 2004;14(4):270-272.
11. Bahr R, Fossan B, Løken S, Engebretsen L. Surgical treatment compared with eccentric training for patellar tendinopathy (jumper's knee). A randomized, controlled trial. *J Bone Joint Surg Am.* 2006;88(8):1689-1698.
12. Cucurulo T, Louis ML, Thaunat M, Franceschi JP. Surgical treatment of patellar tendinopathy in athletes. A retrospective multicentric study. *Orthop Traumatol Surg Res.* 2009;95(8 suppl 1):S78-S84.
13. Ferretti A, Conteduca F, Camerucci E, Morelli F. Patellar tendinosis: a follow-up study of surgical treatment. *J Bone Joint Surg Am.* 2002;84(12):2179-2185.
14. Larsson ME, Käll I, Nilsson-Helander K. Treatment of patellar tendinopathy—a systematic review of randomized controlled trials. *Knee Surg Sports Traumatol Arthrosc.* 2012;20(8):1632-1646.
15. Furia JP, Rompe JD, Cacchio A, Del Buono A, Maffulli N. A single application of low-energy radial extracorporeal shock wave therapy is effective for the management of chronic patellar tendinopathy. *Knee Surg Sports Traumatol Arthrosc.* 2012;21(2):346-350.
16. Charousset C, Zaoui A, Bellaiche L, Bouyer B. Are multiple platelet-rich plasma injections useful for treatment of chronic patellar tendinopathy in athletes? A prospective study. *Am J Sports Med.* 2014;42(4):906-911.
17. Kaeding CC, Pedroza AD, Powers BC. Surgical treatment of chronic patellar tendinosis: a systematic review. *Clin Orthop Relat Res.* 2007;(455):102-106.
18. Gill TJ, Carroll KM, Hariri S. Open patellar tendon debridement for treatment of recalcitrant patellar tendinopathy: indications, technique, and clinical outcomes after a 2-year minimum follow-up. *Sports Health.* 2013;5:276-280.
19. Shelbourne KD, Henne TD, Gray T. Recalcitrant patellar tendinosis in elite athletes: surgical treatment in conjunction with aggressive postoperative rehabilitation. *Am J Sports Med.* 2006;34(7):1141-1146.
20. Marcheggiani Muccioli GM, Zaffagnini S, Tsapralis K, et al. Open versus arthroscopic surgical treatment of chronic proximal patellar tendinopathy. A systematic review. *Knee Surg Sports Traumatol Arthrosc.* 2013;21(2):351-357.
21. Coleman BD, Khan KM, Kiss ZS, Bartlett J, Young DA, Wark JD. Open and arthroscopic patellar tenotomy for chronic patellar tendinopathy. A retrospective outcome study. Victorian Institute of Sport Tendon Study Group. *Am J Sports Med.* 2000;28(2):183-190.
22. Pascarella A, Alam M, Pascarella F, Latte C, Di Salvatore MG, Maffulli N. Arthroscopic management of chronic patellar tendinopathy. *Am J Sports Med.* 2011;39(9):1975-1983.
23. Willberg L, Sunding K, Ohberg L, Forssblad M, Alfredson H. Treatment of jumper's knee: promising short-term results in a pilot study using a new arthroscopic approach based on imaging findings. *Knee Surg Sports Traumatol Arthrosc.* 2007;15(5):676-681.
24. Alaseirlis DA, Konstantinidis GA, Malliaropoulos N, Nakou LS, Korompilias A, Maffulli N. Arthroscopic treatment of chronic patellar tendinopathy in high-level athletes. *Muscles Ligaments Tendons J.* 2013;2(4):267-272.

25. Lorbach O, Diamantopoulos A, Paessler HH. Arthroscopic resection of the lower patellar pole in patients with chronic patellar tendinosis. *Arthroscopy.* 2008;24(2):167-173.
26. Romeo AA, Larson RV. Arthroscopic treatment of infrapatellar tendonitis. *Arthroscopy.* 1999;15(3):341-345.
27. Willberg L, Sunding K, Forssblad M, Fahlström M, Alfredson H. Sclerosing polidocanol injections or arthroscopic shaving to treat patellar tendinopathy/jumper's knee? A randomised controlled study. *Br J Sports Med.* 2011;45(5):411-415.

Please see videos on the accompanying website at www.routledge.com/9781617119996

11

Arthroscopic Treatment of Patellar Instability

Jeffrey Halbrecht, MD

Introduction

There has been great emphasis recently on invasive methods of medial patellofemoral ligament (MPFL) reconstruction for patellar instability.[1-6] Although these techniques can be effective and appropriate for severe cases of instability caused by MPFL insufficiency, it is important to keep perspective on the appropriate indications for these techniques. MPFL reconstruction with a graft is indicated when the native MPFL is incompetent and the remaining native tissue is inadequate to be repaired or reefed primarily. A graft may also be considered in severe cases of trochlear dysplasia. However, in the great majority of cases with mild or moderate instability, a simple reefing of the MPFL is a highly successful procedure, whether done arthroscopically or by mini-open techniques, and is a less-invasive and less-expensive procedure.[7,8]

Numerous studies have been published documenting the effectiveness of arthroscopic patellar realignment (APR) for patellar instability, with success rates greater than 90% and no or minimal complications.[9-16] MPFL reconstruction, although effective, is an open invasive procedure fraught with potential complications in up to 26% of patients,[17,18] including patellar fracture, overtightening, and nonisometric placement of the graft resulting in pain, stiffness, and medial tracking.[17,18] These complications have not been reported with arthroscopic realignment.

Anatomic studies and clinical experience have shown that the MPFL heals in an elongated fashion following subluxation or dislocation.[19] Reefing of this lax MPFL is possible in a procedure similar to capsulorrhaphy of the shoulder for laxity of the glenohumeral ligaments and results in effective tightening of the native tissue.[7,8]

Indications

- Mild to moderate patella instability
- Lateral patella subluxation
- Pediatric patients with open growth plates

Sgaglione NA, Lubowitz JH, Provencher MT, eds. *The Knee: AANA Advanced Arthroscopic Surgical Techniques* (pp 145-160).

Candidates for isolated arthroscopic reefing include patients with lateral patellar subluxation or lateral dislocation with mild to moderate instability. These patients typically have good integrity of their native tissues and are amenable to reefing of this native tissue. In a typical community orthopedic practice, this represents the majority of patients with patellar instability. In addition, APR is an excellent choice for pediatric patients with open growth plates, whereas MPFL reconstruction with drill holes has increased risks.

In contrast, MPFL reconstruction with a graft would be recommended for patients with severe instability, which is often associated with significant underlying dysplasia and would have a higher risk for failure with an arthroscopic realignment. On physical examination, these more severe cases often have a severe J sign with 3- to 4-quadrant lateral translation of their patella easily demonstrated. In particular, patients with severe trochlear dysplasia place higher-than-normal forces on their MPFL due to the lack of bony constraint to the patella. For these patients, a formal MPFL reconstruction with a graft (possibly in conjunction with a tubercle osteotomy) is more appropriate because these patients require an extra strong MPFL in order to overcome the underlying dysplasia.[20] Finally, APR is contraindicated for patients with a previously failed reefing or poor native tissue for any reason, including old scarring, radiation, or collagen disorders, such as Ehlers-Danlos syndrome.

Controversial Indications

- Lateral patellofemoral compression syndrome
- Lateral patellofemoral arthritis

Patellar Pain and Arthrosis

Arthroscopic realignment can also be effective in treating lateral patellar femoral pain caused by patellar tilt (lateral patellofemoral compression syndrome) and early arthrosis of the lateral facet of the patella. In combination with a lateral retinacular release, an arthroscopic medial reefing can help further tilt and translate the patella medially enough to unload the lateral facet, relieving pain from lateral patellar femoral tilt and compression.

Contraindications

- Poor quality native tissue
- Revision surgery
- Severe trochlea dysplasia
- Acute MPFL avulsion

APR is contraindicated in patients with poor-quality native tissue. This will typically be in patients with severe recurring instability over many years, revision cases, or in patients with underlying collagen disease. APR is also contraindicated in patients with severe trochlear dysplasia, where an extra-strong MPFL is necessary to overcome extreme lateral translation forces caused by lack of bony congruity. Finally, patients with an acute avulsion of the MPFL following a recent dislocation that is clearly demonstrated on magnetic resonance imaging (MRI) will need an open reattachment of the MPFL if surgery is to performed within the first 6 weeks post injury. After 6 weeks, the MPFL is usually adequately reattached and, at this point, an APR may be undertaken if instability persists.

Relative Contraindications

- Inadequate arthroscopic skills
- Fluid extravasation
- Open procedure already being performed

Relative contraindications include lack of arthroscopic surgical skills to perform the procedure, fluid extravasation limiting the ability to complete the procedure, or in patients who may already require an open procedure for other reasons (eg, cartilage resurfacing).

Combination Procedures

Arthroscopic realignment can be effective in conjunction with other patellar instability procedures. In a patient undergoing a tibial tubercle realignment, who has associated mild MPFL laxity, the author has found the addition of APR an effective and less invasive method to supplement this procedure.

Pertinent Physical Findings

- Tilt
- Translation
- Q angle
- J sign

Patients will demonstrate increased lateral translation of the patella to manual stress with the knee in extension, which is often associated with apprehension. The amount of translation is typically increased compared to their normal knee and is typically 2 to 3 quadrants (50% to 75%). If the patella translates 4+ quadrants easily, this may indicate that the native MPFL is too damaged for an arthroscopic approach.

Often, the lateral retinaculum will be tight. This is particularly true for chronic subluxators and dislocators. There will often be a positive patellar tilt test, whereby the examiner will not be able to tilt the patella above the neutral plane with passive stress with the knee in extension. Patients with a tight lateral retinaculum may need to have this tissue released or lengthened as part of their procedure because an excessively tight lateral retinaculum will tether the patella, limiting its ability to be translated medially, even with a medial reefing. In less chronic cases of lateral instability, the lateral retinaculum is often not overly tight, and a lateral release should be avoided. When a lateral release is indicated, care should be taken to avoid extending the release too proximally into the vastus lateralis, and some authors suggest that a lengthening is preferable to a release.[21]

There will often be a positive J sign. The patella will form an inverted letter J as the patient is asked to extend the knee from 90 to 0 degrees. In severe cases of instability in which the patella jumps over laterally with active terminal extension, the instability may be too severe for an arthroscopic approach.

The Q angle should be evaluated in extension and 20 degrees of flexion. Although this test can be unreliable, if the Q angle is greater than 15 degrees, further studies need to be performed to make sure that the patient does not need a distal realignment procedure, possibly in conjunction with treatment of his or her MPFL. Although the Q angle is not always reliable, a high angle should be an indication to obtain an MRI or computed tomography (CT) scan to measure the tibial tubercle–trochlear groove (TT-TG) distance, which is a more accurate way of evaluating distal bony alignment.[22]

Pertinent Imaging

- X-ray Merchant view (congruity, tilt)
- X-ray lateral (alta, trochlea dysplasia)
- MRI (TT-TG distance, chondral defects, MPFL status)

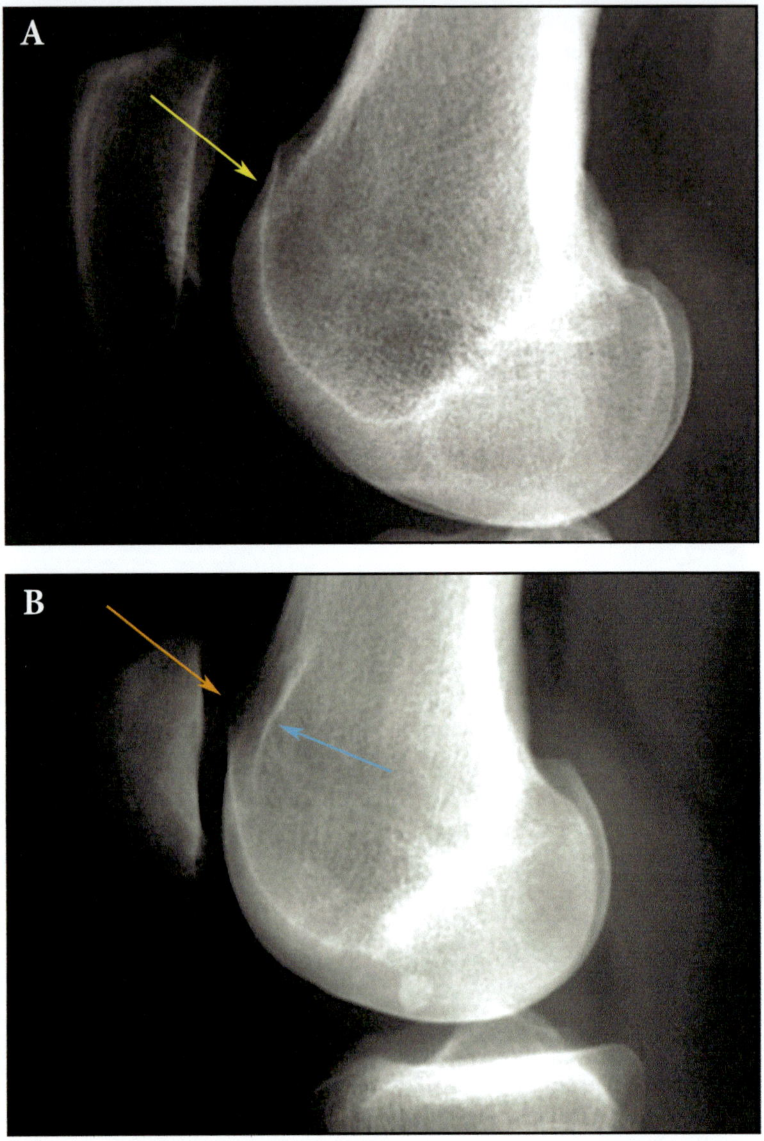

Figure 11-1. Lateral x-ray of the knee showing typical signs of severe trochlear dysplasia, including a crossing sign (yellow arrow), supratrochlear spur (orange arrow), and double contour (blue arrow) of the anterior cortex.

All patients should have preoperative Merchant and true lateral x-rays. The Merchant view is useful for assessing the amount of patellar tilt, patellar translation, and trochlear dysplasia and narrowing of the patellofemoral joint space from arthrosis. Medial bony avulsion fragments and marginal osteophytes can also be seen. The presence of an acute avulsion fracture of the MPFL would indicate the need for an open repair of this fragment or direct repair of the MPFL back to the patella. The presence of arthrosis would affect the outcome and treatment recommendations. If lateral arthrosis is present, arthroscopic stabilization is a viable option. If medial facet arthrosis is present, any medial tightening procedure, whether arthroscopic or open, may be contraindicated because this would compress the medial facet and likely increase pain and the progression of the arthrosis.

A true lateral view is useful for evaluating trochlear dysplasia. A crossing sign, supratrochlear spur, or a double contour of the anterior cortex indicates the presence of a shallow, dysplastic trochlea (Figure 11-1).[23] If these findings are present, a formal MPFL reconstruction with a graft

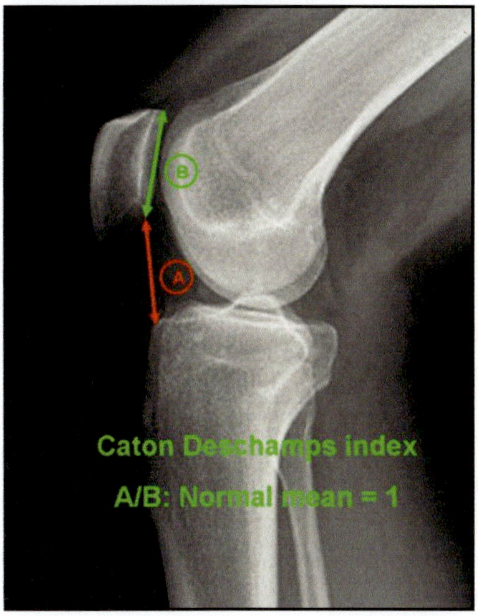

Figure 11-2. Measurement of patella alta is best measured on a lateral x-ray using the Caton-Deschamps ratio.

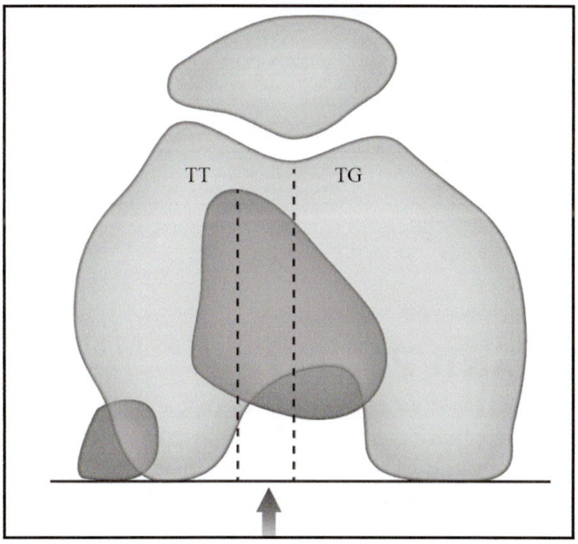

Figure 11-3. The TT-TG distance should be measured on preoperative CT scan or MRI. If the distance is greater than 20 mm, a tibial tubercle osteotomy should be considered.

is often indicated. Rarely, in patients with extreme trochlear dysplasia, particularly for revision surgery, a trochleoplasty may also be considered.

Patellar height should also be measured on the preoperative lateral view. Significant patella alta is an additional contributing factor for patellar instability.

Although various measurements have been described for this measurement, the author prefers the Caton-Deschamps ratio, which measures from the anterosuperior angle of the proximal tibia to the inferior pole of the patellar articular surface, divided by the articular length of the patella (Figure 11-2).[24] If this measurement is greater than 1.2, a distalization osteotomy of the patella may need to be considered as part of the operative procedure.

MRI is an essential part of the author's preoperative planning and can be used to measure the TT-TG.[22] This measurement is the accepted method for determining if the tubercle is malaligned. If the distance is greater than 20 mm, the addition of a distal realignment (tibial tubercle osteotomy) should be considered (Figure 11-3).[22,25,26]

MRI is also useful for the evaluation of chondral injuries. Acute chondral fractures and loose bodies are common with patellar dislocation, and one should look for them. Acute patellar dislocations often cause chondral fractures of the medial facet of the patella or the lateral aspect of the distal lateral trochlea. Chronic lateral patellar tracking can lead to degenerative chondral wear of the lateral facet of the patella or trochlea. The presence of a large chondral defect or significant arthrosis may affect surgical planning. For small grade 4 chondral defects, a microfracture is usually planned as part of the arthroscopic procedure. For large defects (> 2 cm), patients may require a 2-stage procedure, including an open implantation of cartilage (chondrocyte implantation or cartilage graft) that would preclude the sensibility of an arthroscopic realignment procedure. In rare cases of acute patellar dislocation, if a large osteochondral fragment is present, direct repair of the fragment using chondral darts or screws may be an option.

Equipment

This procedure can be performed with routine instruments typically found in most operating rooms and is inexpensive. The following items are necessary:

- 4.0-mm arthroscope
- 5.0-mm cannula
- A Touhy (epidural) needle (17- or 18-gauge) for suture passing (BD Perisafe Modified Tuohy Point Epidural Needle 17 G x 3 ½ in; Becton Dickinson)
- Arthroscopic knot pusher
- Arthroscopic suture retriever
- Arthroscopic suture cutter
- Ball tip rasp

Positioning and Portals

The patient is placed supine. A tourniquet is applied but rarely inflated. An arthroscopic leg holder is placed to assist with diagnostic arthroscopy and to stabilize the leg but should be placed high on the thigh to avoid interfering with the suture retrieval and tying from the supralateral portal (Figure 11-4). After diagnostic arthroscopy, much of the procedure is done with the leg in extension on a padded Mayo stand.

Step-by-Step Description of the Procedure

Examination Under Anesthesia

Examination under anesthesia is an important part of the procedure because patients with patellar instability are often apprehensive, and their examinations while awake can be limited. The involved knee should be compared to the opposite knee for patellar tilt and translation. Verify whether the patella can be fully dislocated with manual pressure or simply subluxated. Evaluate whether the patella subluxates or dislocates with passive range of motion (ROM) from 90 to 0 degrees (a passive J sign).

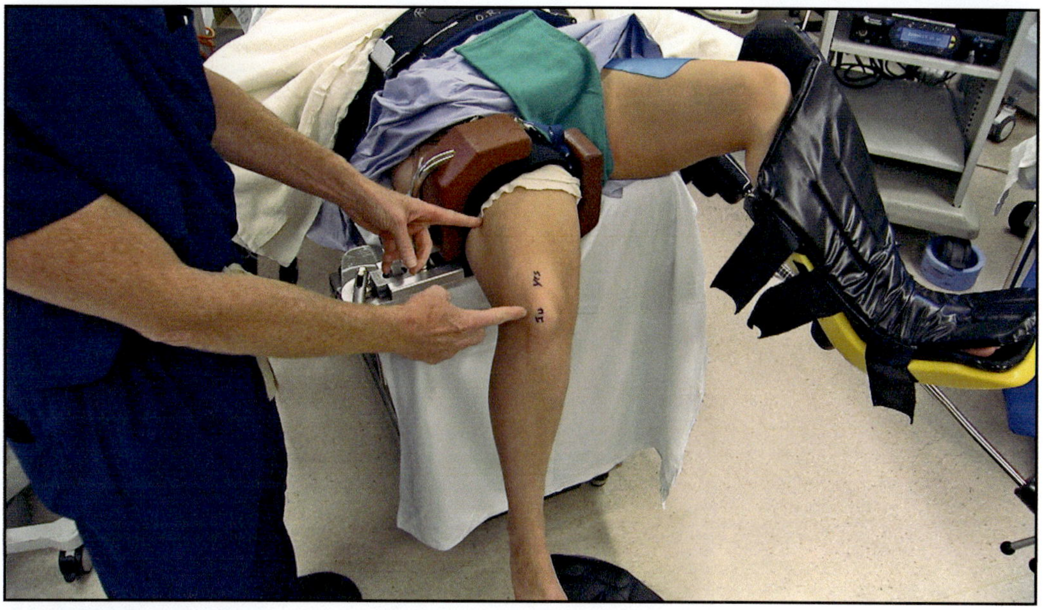

Figure 11-4. The leg holder should be placed high on the thigh to avoid interference with suture tying from the supralateral portal.

Diagnostic Arthroscopy

A diagnostic arthroscopy is performed. Evaluate the integrity of the articular cartilage and look for loose bodies, which are removed or fixed in rare cases. Acute chondral fractures are common with patellar dislocation. Treatment of chondral injuries should be performed prior to the stabilization procedure. Grade 4 chondral defects are typically treated with microfracture. Lesser degrees of chondromalacia should be debrided. Lateral facet osteophytes should be removed. The remainder of the knee is evaluated for any additional pathology that may require treatment. Patellar tracking is evaluated under direct visualization. Confirmation is made of patellar tilt and translation (Figure 11-5).

Create a Healing Response (Figure 11-6)

The medial retinaculum is abraded with an arthroscopic ball tip rasp in order to create a healing response to facilitate healing of the tissue to itself after reefing is performed. An arthroscopic whisker blade attached to the shaver can also be used.

Superolateral Cannula (Figure 11-7)

A cannula is inserted using a superolateral portal. This cannula should be placed approximately 1 cm proximal and 1 cm posterior to the lateral patella. The angle is important because this cannula is used for arthroscopic knot tying, and a more direct angle will facilitate knot tying. The angle should be checked with a spinal needle and should allow direct access beneath the patella to the medial retinaculum.

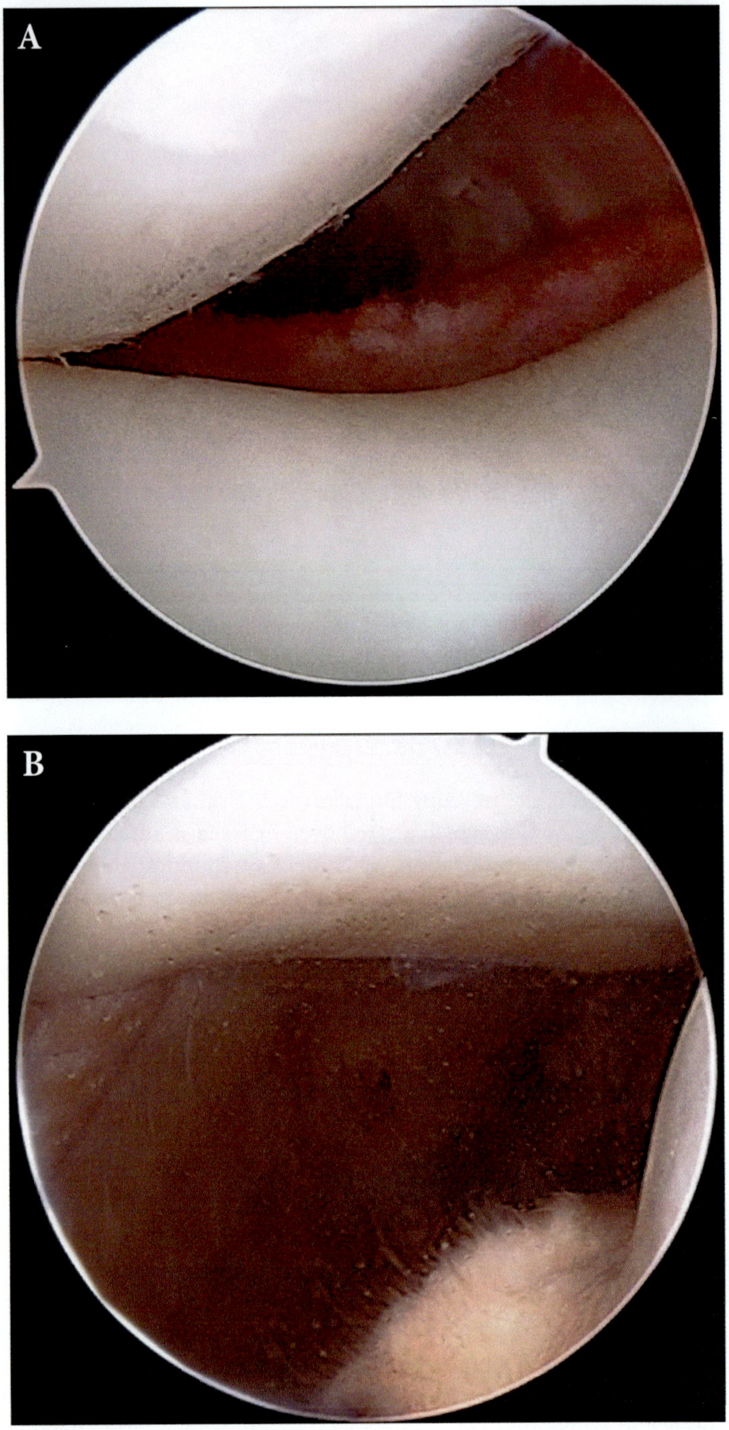

Figure 11-5. (A) Intraoperative verification of patellar tilt prior to a realignment procedure. (B) Intraoperative appearance of lateral patella translation prior to realignment.

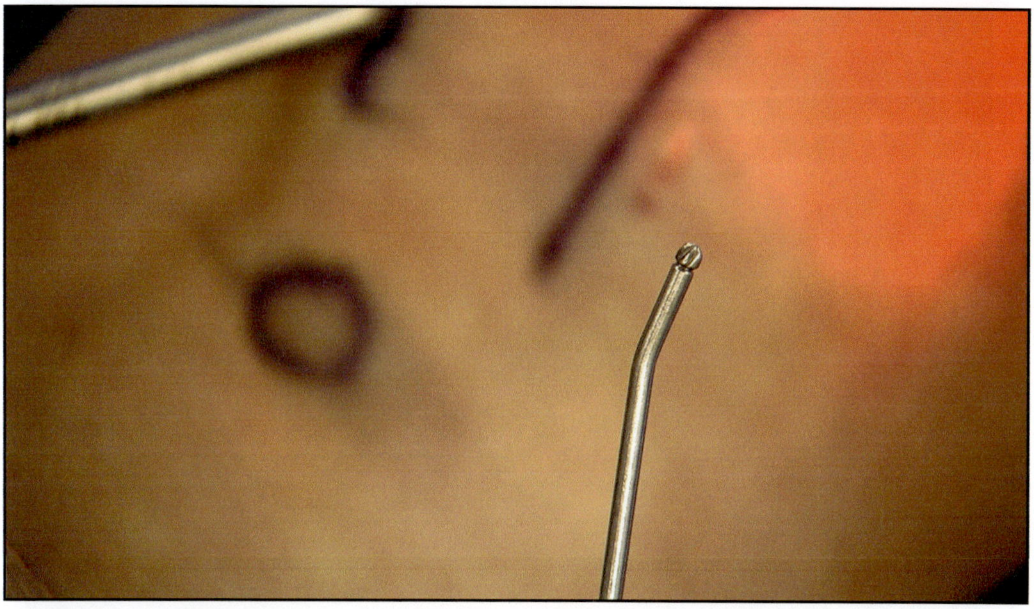

Figure 11-6. A healing response is created along the medial retinaculum with a ball tip rasp by abrading the synovium and capsule.

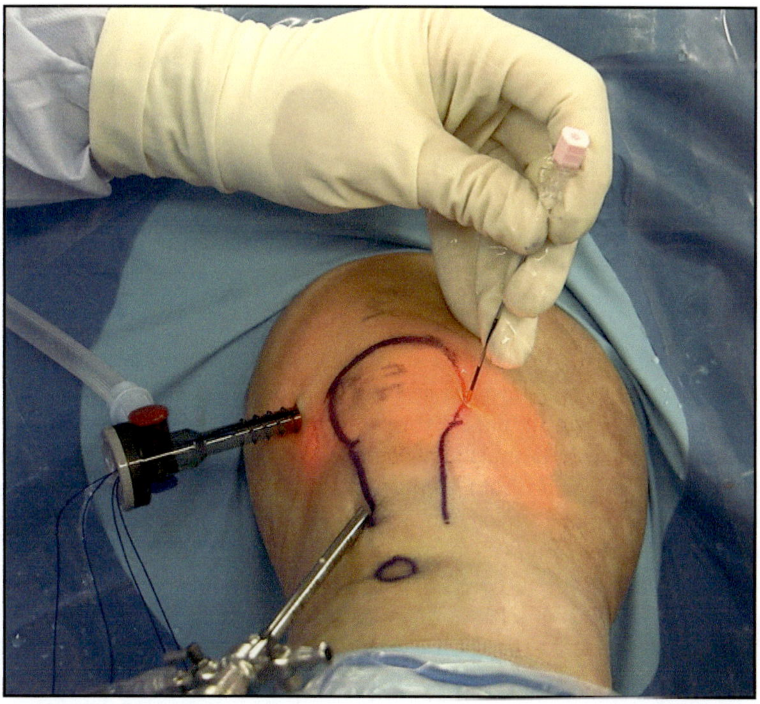

Figure 11-7. A superolateral cannula is inserted as a working cannula for suture retrieval and knot tying.

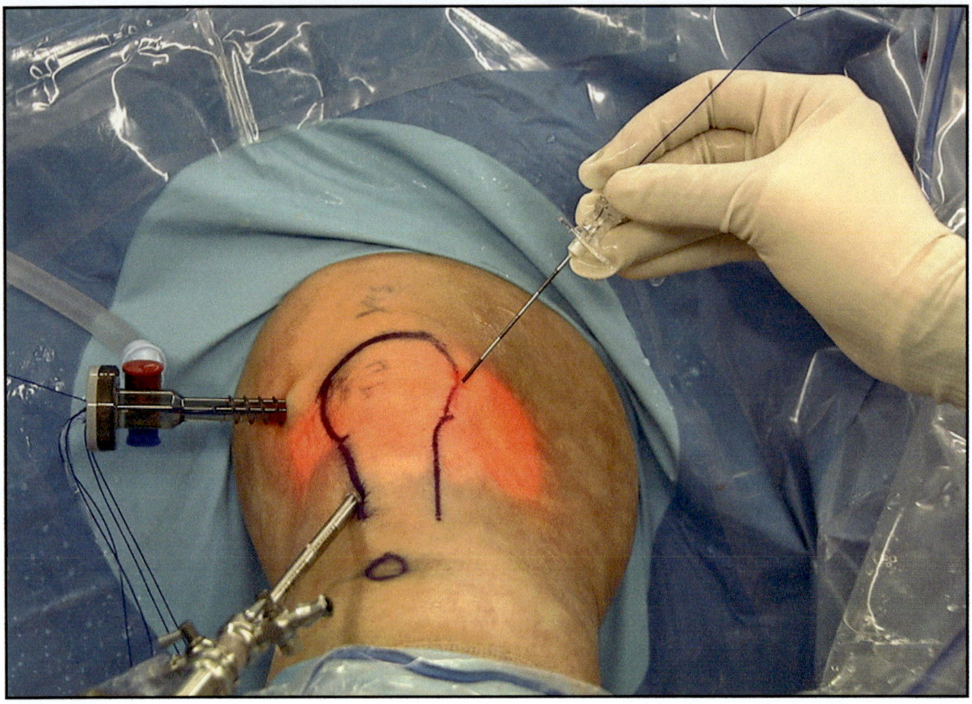

Figure 11-8. (A) Outside view of the suture being passed through a Tuohy epidural needle. *(continued)*

Passage of Sutures (Figure 11-8)

The scope is in the anterolateral portal for easiest viewing of the medial retinaculum. A Tuohy needle is then used to pass suture percutaneously along the medial retinaculum. Unlike a spinal needle, the Tuohy needle is an epidural needle with a distal curve and a beveled inner edge that prevents the suture from being inadvertently cut during passage. The average number of sutures used is 4 but can range from 3 to 6. Sutures are placed from proximal to distal beginning at the superior edge of the patella at 5- to 10-mm intervals. Anatomically, these sutures incorporate the MPFL as well as a portion of the medial patella tibial ligament. It is important to take adequate bites of tissue. The Tuohy needle is inserted just adjacent to the patella into the joint. A #1 polydioxanone (PDS) suture is manually passed through the needle (Figure 11-9A). The passed end is retrieved from the supralateral cannula and clamped. The needle is then withdrawn to the subcutaneous tissue and passed posteriorly 2 to 4 cm depending on the amount of tightening necessary for that particular patient (Figure 11-9B). The needle will appear back in the joint with a loop of suture. This loop is then retrieved out of the supralateral cannula, having now created an all-inside stitch. Both limbs of the PDS will now be clamped together for later tying (Figure 11-9C). Knot tying is usually performed using an arthroscopic knot pusher and multiple alternating half hitches, although a Duncan loop or other sliding knot can also be used. This procedure is repeated 3 to 6 times until the desired number of sutures have been placed (Figure 11-10). The author prefers using PDS sutures because of concerns about chronic knot irritation to the patient. The surgeon may choose to shuttle a permanent suture as an alternative.

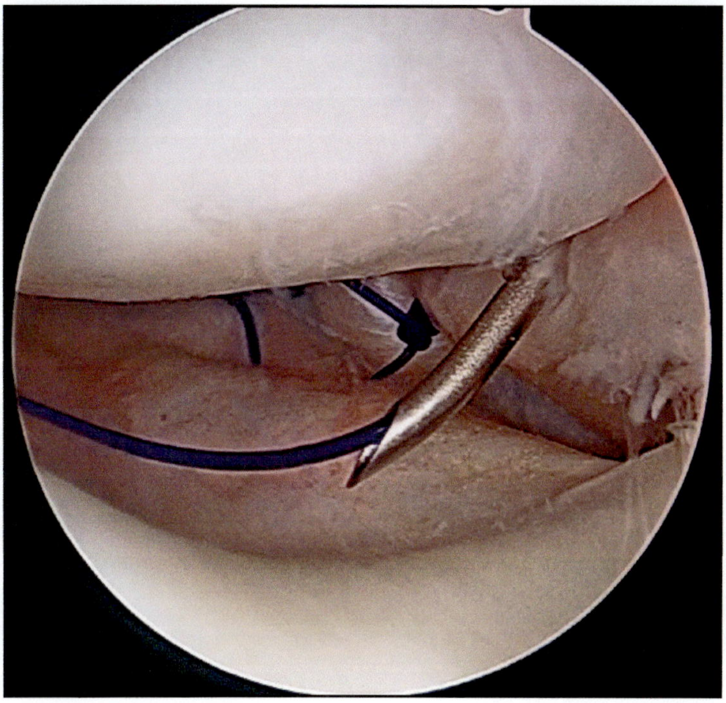

Figure 11-8 (continued). (B) Arthroscopic view of the suture being passed through a Tuohy epidural needle.

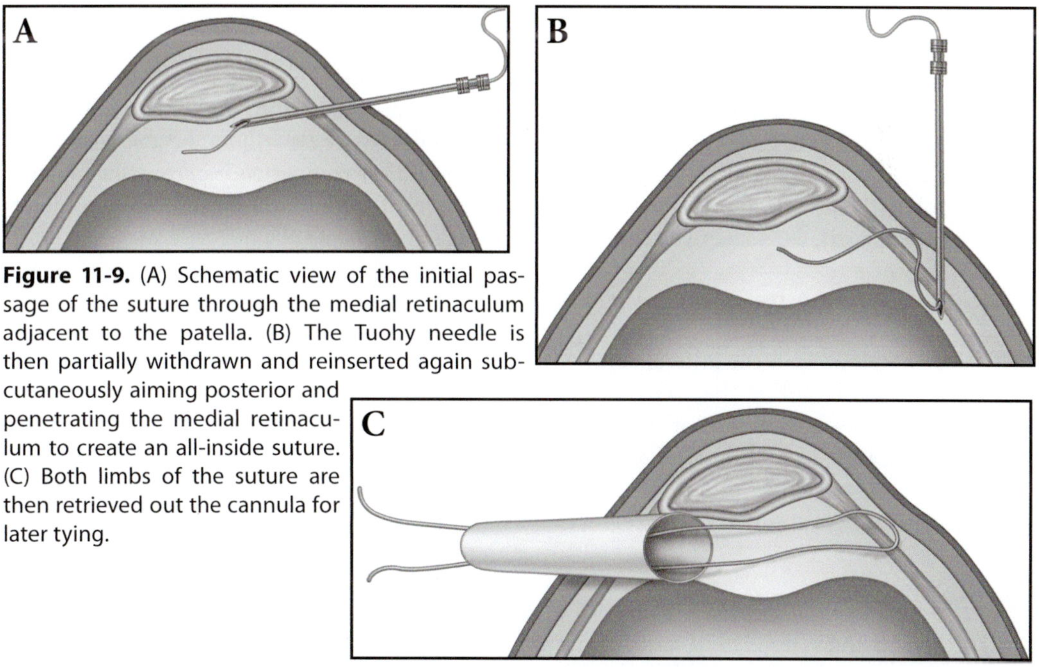

Figure 11-9. (A) Schematic view of the initial passage of the suture through the medial retinaculum adjacent to the patella. (B) The Tuohy needle is then partially withdrawn and reinserted again subcutaneously aiming posterior and penetrating the medial retinaculum to create an all-inside suture. (C) Both limbs of the suture are then retrieved out the cannula for later tying.

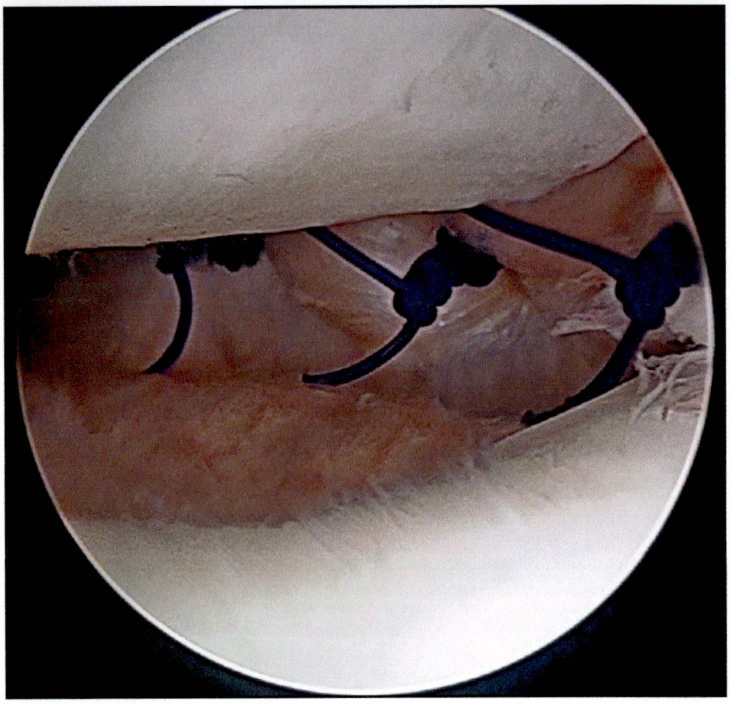

Figure 11-10. Final arthroscopic appearance of the tied medial sutures after completion of all-inside medial reefing.

Lateral Retinacular Release

A lateral release or lengthening may be performed at this time. The need for a lateral release is based on the presence of a tight retinaculum. In more chronic cases of instability, the lateral retinaculum is usually extremely tight and, unless it is released, the patella will not be able to translate medially, even with a medial reefing. In these cases, the author recommends performing a lateral release or lengthening. In more acute cases of instability, or if the lateral retinaculum is not felt to be tethering the patella, a lateral release is not necessary.

Knot Tying

The arthroscope is in the anterolateral portal. All sutures are currently located in the superolateral cannula. The author then retrieves the most inferior sets of sutures out through the anteromedial portal to get them out of the way, leaving just the most proximal of the sutures in the superolateral cannula. Arthroscopic knot tying is then performed of this suture. Simple sutures or a sliding knot (Duncan loop) may be used. The next most proximal suture is then retrieved back through the cannula and tied (Figure 11-11). This process is repeated until all sutures are tied.

Assessment

The knee is then flexed, and patellar tracking and stability are evaluated. The goal is to have the patella centered in the trochlear groove at 20 to 25 degrees of knee flexion (Figure 11-12). Verification is also made that lateral patella overhang has been eliminated (Figure 11-13). Gentle manual translation can also be checked to verify that the MPFL is snug and that all excess lateral translation has been eliminated. If necessary, additional sutures may be added at this time. One of the major advantages of this technique is that the medial reefing is titrated under direct arthroscopic vision. Only the necessary number of sutures are placed to achieve neutral tracking, which eliminates any risk of overcorrection.

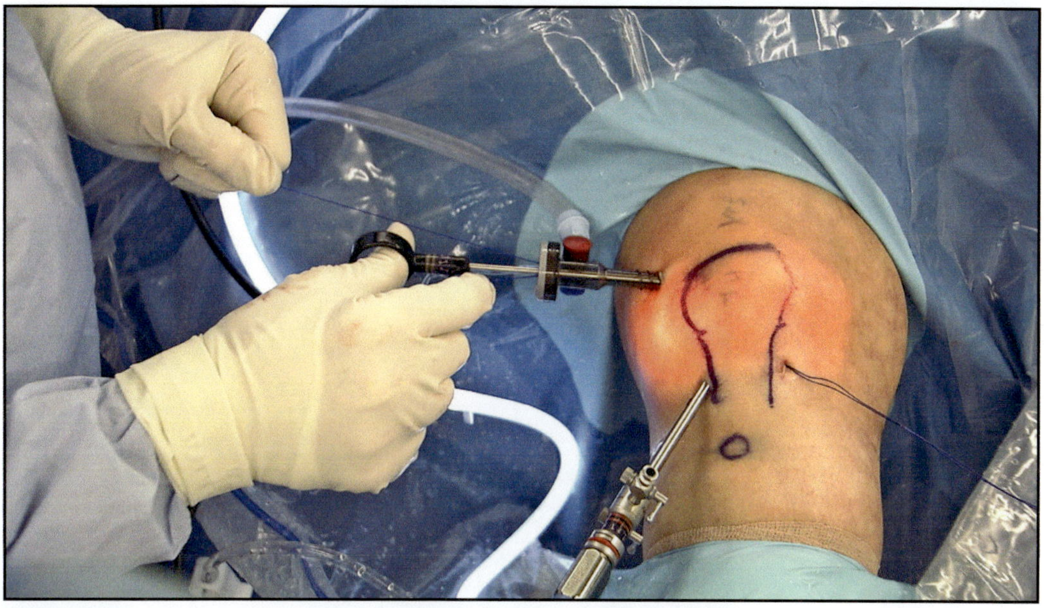

Figure 11-11. Outside view of arthroscopic knot tying of the most superior stitch performed through the supralateral cannula while the more inferior stitches are parked in the anteromedial portal for subsequent tying.

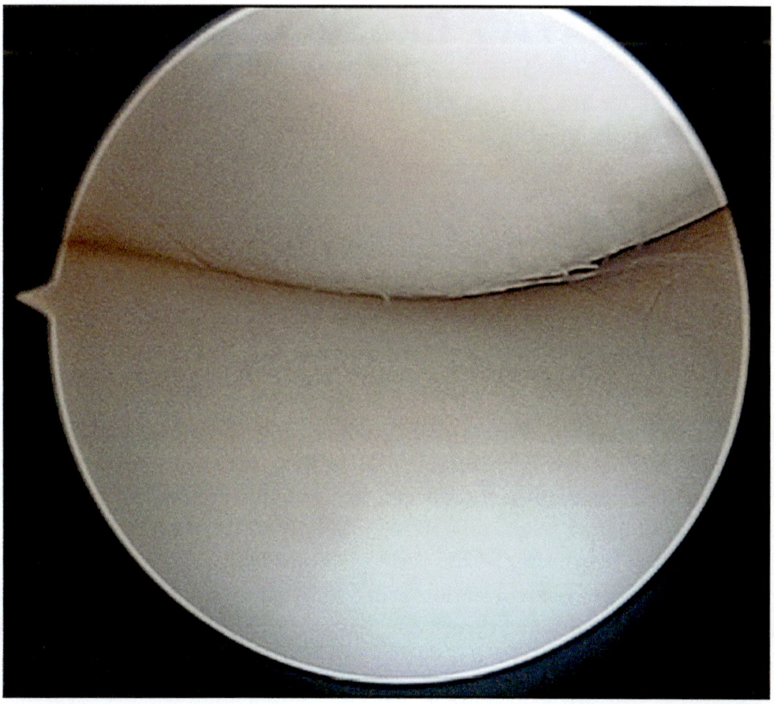

Figure 11-12. Final view of the patella, which is now well aligned in the center of the trochlear groove following arthroscopic realignment.

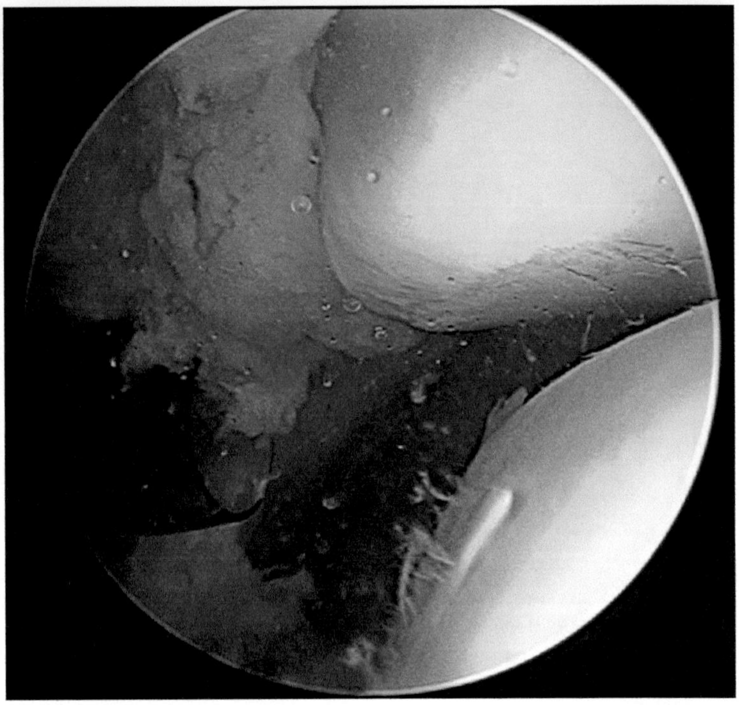

Figure 11-13. Arthroscopic appearance of corrected lateral overhang and translation of the patella relative to the trochlear edge.

Postoperative Protocol

The patient is placed in a hinged-knee brace that is locked in full extension. Partial weightbearing is permitted with crutches. Ankle ROM and isometric quadriceps contractions are allowed immediately. At 1 week, the patient returns for suture removal and is instructed in heel slides from 0 to 30 degrees. ROM is gradually increased to 90 degrees over the first 3 to 4 weeks. The brace is discontinued at 4 weeks, and ROM is increased to full. Patients can usually return to full sports participation at 4 months.

Potential Complications

One of the advantages of arthroscopic patellar stabilization is that complications are rare. Postoperative stiffness is possible but has not been seen in the author's patient population using the rehabilitation protocol described. Early on in the development of this procedure, the author immobilized the patients for 4 weeks before beginning ROM and had several patients with postoperative stiffness. The author advises beginning ROM early as described.

The author has experienced no cases of overcorrection using this technique. He thinks this is unlikely because the procedure is performed under direct visualization and the patella position can be titrated based on the number of sutures and the size of the tissue bite taken.

Recurring instability is possible with this procedure as with any other, although the incidence has been low.[9-16] Risk of recurrence can be minimized by proper patient selection and adherence to the technical details as outlined.

This procedure will not be effective if it is performed on a patient who needs bony realignment surgery for severe dysplasia or has inadequate integrity of his or her native MPFL tissue.

Top Technical Pearls for the Procedure

1. Create an adequate healing response.
2. Take adequate bites of tissue (larger bites for more severe instability).
3. Use the Tuohy epidural needle for suture passage.
4. Use more sutures if necessary (average of 4 sutures).
5. Add lateral release for patients with a significant tilt and tethered patella.

References

1. Bicos J, Fulkerson JP, Amis A. Current concepts review: the medial patellofemoral ligament. *Am J Sports Med.* 2007;35(3):484-492.
2. Buckens CF, Saris DB. Reconstruction of the medial patellofemoral ligament for treatment of patellofemoral instability: a systematic review. *Am J Sports Med.* 2010;38(1):181-188.
3. Ahmad CS, Brown GD, Stein BS. The docking technique for medial patellofemoral ligament reconstruction: surgical technique and clinical outcome. *Am J Sports Med.* 2009;37(10):2021-2027.
4. Christiansen SE, Jacobsen BW, Lund B, Lind M. Reconstruction of the medial patellofemoral ligament with gracilis tendon autograft in transverse patellar drill holes. *Arthroscopy.* 2008;24(1):82-87.
5. Drez DJ Jr, Edwards TB, Williams CS. Results of medial patellofemoral ligament reconstruction in the treatment of patellar dislocation. *Arthroscopy.* 2001;17(3):298-306.
6. Steiner TM, Torga-Spak R, Teitge RA. Medial patellofemoral ligament reconstruction in patients with lateral patellar instability and trochlear dysplasia. *Am J Sports Med.* 2006;34(8):1254-1261.
7. Ma LF, Wang F, Chen BC, Wang CH, Zhou JW, Wang HY. Medial retinaculum plasty versus medial patellofemoral ligament reconstruction for recurrent patellar instability in adults: a randomized controlled trial. *Arthroscopy.* 2013;29(5):891-897.
8. Harle D, Smith T, Loveday DT. Medial reefing versus medial patellofermoral ligament reconstruction for patellar instability. *Eur J Orthop Surg Traumatol.* 2010;20(7):547-551.
9. Henry JE, Pflum FA Jr. Arthroscopic proximal patella realignment and stabilization. *Arthroscopy.* 1995;11(4):424-425.
10. Small NC. Arthroscopically assisted proximal extensor mechanism realignment of the knee. *Arthroscopy.* 1993;9(1):63-67.
11. Yamamoto RK. Arthroscopic repair of the medial retinaculum and capsule in acute patellar dislocations. *Arthroscopy.* 1986;2(2):125-131.
12. Ahmad CS, Lee FY. An all-arthroscopic soft-tissue balancing technique for lateral patellar instability. *Arthroscopy.* 2001;17(5):555-557.
13. Halbrecht JL. Arthroscopic patella realignment: an all-inside technique. *Arthroscopy.* 2001;17(9):940-945.
14. Halbrecht JL. Arthroscopic management of patella instability. *Oper Tech Orthop.* 2007;17(4):211-215.
15. Haspl M, Cicak N, Klobucar H, Pecina M. Fully arthroscopic stabilization of the patella. *Arthroscopy.* 2002;18(1)E2.
16. Fukushima K, Horaguchi T, Okano T, Yoshimatsu T, Saito A, Ryu J. Patellar dislocation: arthroscopic patellar stabilization with anchor sutures. *Arthroscopy.* 2004;20(7):761-764.
17. Shah JN, Howard JS, Flanigan DC, Brophy RH, Carey JL, Lattermann C. A systematic review of complications and failures associated with medial patellofemoral ligament reconstruction for recurrent patellar dislocation. *Am J Sports Med.* 2012;40(8):1916-1923.
18. Parikh SN, Nathan ST, Wall EJ, Eismann EA. Complications of medial patellofemoral ligament reconstruction in young patients. *Am J Sports Med.* 2013;41(5):1030-1038.
19. Tom A, Fulkerson JP. Restoration of native medial patellofemoral support after patella dislocation. *Sports Med Arthrosc.* 2007;15(2):68-71.

20. Schöttle PB, Scheffler SU, Schwarck A, Weiler A. Arthroscopic medial retinacular repair after patellar dislocation with and without underlying trochlear dysplasia: a preliminary report. *Arthroscopy.* 2006;22(11):1192-1198.
21. Pagenstert G, Wolf N, Bachmann M, et al. Open lateral patellar retinacular lengthening versus open retinacular release in lateral patellar hypercompression syndrome: a prospective double-blinded comparative study on complications and outcome. *Arthroscopy.* 2012;28(6):788-797.
22. Schoettle PB, Zanetti M, Seifert B, Pfirrmann CW, Fucentese SF, Romero J. The tibial tuberosity-trochlear groove distance; a comparative study between CT and MRI scanning. *Knee.* 2006;13(1):26-31.
23. Dejour H, Walch G, Neyret P, Adeleine P. Dysplasia of the femoral trochlea [in French]. *Rev Chir Orthop Reparatrice Appar Mot.* 1990;76(1):45-54.
24. Caton JH, Dejour D. Tibial tubercle osteotomy in patello-femoral instability and in patellar height abnormality. *Int Orthop.* 2010;34(2):305-309.
25. Dejour H, Walch G, Nove-Josserand L, Guier C. Factors of patellar instability: an anatomic radiographic study. *Knee Surg Sports Traumatol Arthrosc.* 1994;2(1):19-26.
26. Dejour D, Coultre B. Osteotomies in patello-femoral instabilities. *Sports Med Arthrosc.* 2007;15(1):39-46.

Please see videos on the accompanying website at www.routledge.com/9781617119996

12

Reconstruction of the Medial Patellofemoral Ligament for Instability

Joseph Carney, MD; Matthew A. Pifer, MD;
Kentaro P. Suzuki, MD; and Donald C. Fithian, MD

Introduction

Patellofemoral instability as a clinical entity depends on factors of constraint, such as the ability of the patella to engage in the trochlea as well as the soft tissue restraints to patellar mobility. The medial patellofemoral ligament (MPFL) is the primary ligamentous restraint against lateral patellar displacement with the MPFL reported to provide between 50% and 60% of the medial soft tissue resistance to lateral dislocation of the patella.[1-3] Consequently, patellar dislocation often results in injury to the medial retinacular ligaments, including the MPFL, leading to increased lateral patellar mobility. Competency of the MPFL is necessary and sufficient to restore lateral patellar mobility to a normal range; consequently, surgical treatment should aim for restoration of a functional MPFL.[4]

Indications

Nonoperative treatment is typically indicated for acute, first-time dislocators without associated osteochondral fracture or loose bodies.

Surgical management is indicated for the following:

- Recurrent patellar instability (at least 2 documented instability events) and a confirmatory physical examination demonstrating excessive lateral patellar laxity[4-7]: For these recurrent dislocators, MPFL reconstruction is the current procedure of choice.
- Osteochondral fracture or a loose body that is potentially repairable or causing mechanical symptoms: Consideration must be given to the size and location of the donor fragment and the presence of adequate subchondral bone when considering fragment repair. In the presence of osteochondral injury being addressed surgically, one can perform concomitant MPFL reconstruction.
- Smaller, isolated chondral injuries: Surgery may be indicated if mechanical symptoms are present. Nonoperative treatment is appropriate in the absence of mechanical symptoms.

Sgaglione NA, Lubowitz JH, Provencher MT, eds. *The Knee: AANA Advanced Arthroscopic Surgical Techniques* (pp 161-172).

Pertinent Physical Findings

History (Important Component of Evaluation[8])

- Patellar instability event
- History of prior patellar instability events
- Presence or absence of mechanical symptoms (locking, catching, etc)
- Presence or absence of crepitus (if present, can indicate clinically significant mechanical symptoms possibly requiring surgical treatment)

Physical Examination

General

- Range of motion (ROM): Block to motion could indicate symptomatic loose body
- Size of effusion: Acute, traumatic instability events tend to lead to moderate/severe effusions, but consider osteochondral fracture if a large, tense effusion is present.
- A comprehensive physical examination is needed to assess for cruciate/collateral injury.

Medial Patellofemoral Ligament-Specific (Authors' Recommended Best Tests)

- Patellar translation: With the knee flexed to 30 degrees, lateral patellar translation greater than 2 quadrants (or approximately 10 mm) signifies increased laxity.
- Patellar apprehension: Patient apprehension when performing lateral translation further supports MPFL injury.

Other Signs Indicative of Medial Patellofemoral Ligament Injury

- Tenderness along the medial retinaculum
- Check-rein sign: Absence of endpoint to translation

Important Considerations

- Patient guarding can lead to a false-negative result.
- Intra-articular anesthetic can be used to assist with patient evaluation.
- If gross hemarthrosis is present on joint aspiration, consider magnetic resonance imaging (MRI) to evaluate for an osteochondral fracture/loose body.

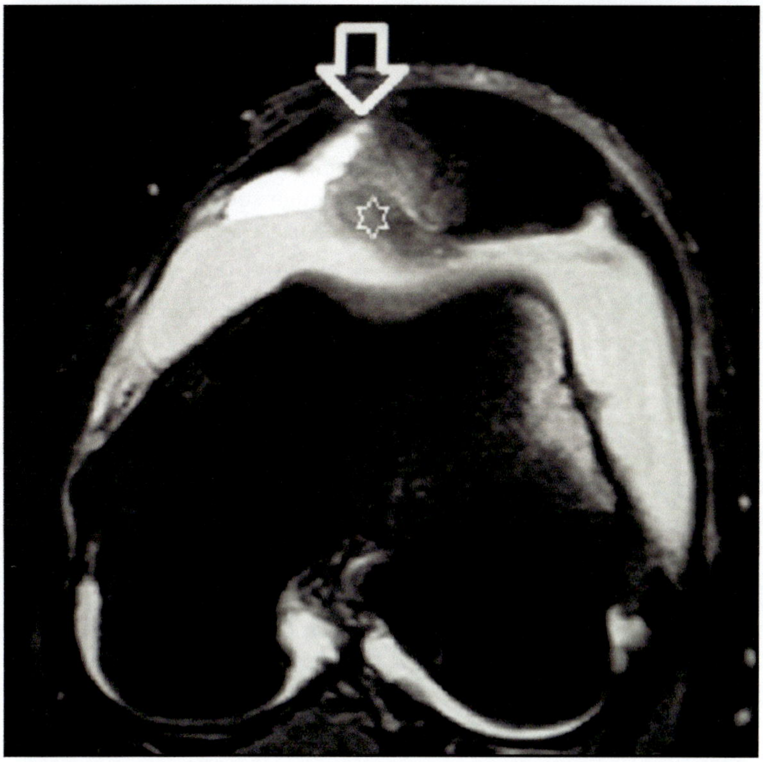

Figure 12-1. MRI axial image of a patient after a lateral patellar dislocation showing an osteochondral loose fragment (star) and injury to the MPFL (arrow). Note the large effusion, which is often seen when osteochondral injury occurs from lateral patellar subluxation or dislocation.

Pertinent Imaging

- Plain x-rays: Important for identifying avulsion fractures, loose bodies, patella alta, and trochlear dysplasia
  - Standing anteroposterior view
  - True lateral view with the knee flexed 30 degrees: Allows for measurement of patellar height and assessment of trochlear dysplasia
  - Axial patellar view at 30 or 45 degrees of flexion: Important for finding subluxation, dislocation, or avulsion fractures
- Computed tomography (CT): Can further identify and characterize avulsion or osteochondral fractures/loose bodies; evaluates trochlear dysplasia
- Stress radiography: With the knee flexed to 30 degrees, obtain an axial patellar view bilaterally with laterally directed force to the medial aspect of the patella. A side-to-side increase of 3.7 mm or more of lateral translation on the symptomatic vs asymptomatic side is considered abnormal.[9]
- MRI
  - Identifies the location and degree of medial soft tissue injury
  - Reported to be more accurate than arthroscopy in identifying MPFL injuries[10]
  - MPFL injuries occur commonly in the form of tears near the femoral attachment or avulsions off the femur but may also occur as midsubstance tears or avulsions off the patella. Injuries to multiple sites in the medial ligamentous complex can occur.[11]
  - Can identify osteochondral injuries on the patella and femur as well as loose bodies that may be missed on plain x-rays (Figure 12-1)

Important Imaging Considerations for Preoperative Planning

- Patellar height
  - Authors' preferred method of measurement is that of Caton and Deschamps (ie, the ratio between the distance from the lower edge of the patellar articular surface to the upper edge of the tibial plateau and the length of the patellar articular surface).[12]
  - A ratio of 1.2 or greater indicates patella alta, which predisposes the patient to patellar instability due to late engagement of the patella in the trochlea as the knee flexes.
  - If patella alta is present, tibial tubercle osteotomy and distalization should be considered as an additional procedure.
- Tibial tubercle–trochlear groove (TT-TG) distance
  - The TT-TG offset is the transverse distance between the anterior tibial tuberosity and the center of the trochlear groove.[13]
  - Distance can be measured on axial CT or MRI, although some argue that these imaging modalities are not interchangeable as MRI has been reported to underestimate the TT-TG offset when compared with CT.[14]
  - When lateral offset measures 20 mm or more, medialization of the tibial tubercle can be considered as an additional procedure to address patellofemoral instability.
- Trochlear morphology
  - Important consideration as severe cases of trochlear dysplasia can challenge the long-term success of MPFL reconstruction
  - Can be assessed on a true lateral x-ray (the posterior borders of both femoral condyles are strictly superimposed)
  - A crossing sign occurs when the floor of the trochlea crosses the anterior border of both femoral condyles, thus indicating trochlear dysplasia.[13]
  - A positive trochlear prominence (ie, the sagittal distance between the trochlear groove and the anterior femoral cortex) greater than 3 mm on the lateral view has been shown to correlate well with trochlear dysplasia.[11,13]
  - Axial MRI has been shown to more accurately classify trochlear groove anatomy (in comparison to axial x-rays or CT) when assessing trochlear dysplasia.[15]

Equipment

The following equipment is recommended in addition to standard soft tissue retractors for the authors' preferred method of MPFL reconstruction:

- Knee arthroscopy equipment if knee arthroscopy is to be performed prior to MPFL reconstruction
- Soft tissue tendon stripper for the harvest of semitendinosus graft (the authors prefer a closed tendon stripper)
- 4.5-mm drill with guide for drilling tunnels in the patella for each end of the semitendinosus tendon graft
- Small curved curette to clear the patellar tunnels of debris for graft passage
- 18-gauge steel wire to be fashioned to retrieve suture through the patellar tunnels. Alternative options include commercially produced curved suture passer devices.

- Smooth 2.4-mm guide wire pin (Beath pin equivalent) diameter, and if applicable, with eyelet for suture. This pin is used to drill into the center of the femoral MPFL footprint and guide the reamer for MPFL femoral tunnel creation. If the pin is too long, it can interfere with obtaining fluoroscopy to confirm anatomic positioning of the pin in the MPFL origin.
- Fluoroscopy for checking the position of the guide pin in the femoral footprint of the MPFL. The authors prefer to use a Mini-C arm equivalent.
- Cannulated reamers of various diameters from 5 to 8 mm for drilling the femoral tunnel
- Interference screws for fixation of grafts in the femoral tunnel. Typically, screws run from lengths of 20 to 25 mm and diameters of 5 to 8 mm.
- #0 or #1 absorbable suture
- #5 braided polyethylene suture
- #2 nonabsorbable sutures

Positioning and Portals

The patient is positioned supine. A small bump may be placed under the hip to prevent external rotation. A sterile bump may also be placed under the knee to maintain slight flexion. If performing knee arthroscopy prior to MPFL reconstruction, it is recommended to do so with the bed kept flat, allowing the knee to be flexed over the side of the bed in lieu of dropping the foot of the bed for knee flexion. Arthroscopy can be performed to stage or address articular cartilage lesions and rule out preexisting severe arthritis if there is any question about the cartilage health of the patellofemoral joint. Fluoroscopy can be brought in from the ipsilateral side of the bed when needed to obtain a lateral view of the distal femur to confirm anatomic placement of the guide pin in the MPFL femoral footprint.

Step-by-Step Description of the Procedure

Examination Under Anesthesia

- Perform an examination under anesthesia to confirm excessive lateral patellar mobility. Increased laxity is signified by more than 10 mm of lateral translation and the absence of an endpoint with the knee at 30 degrees of flexion.

Semitendinosus Tendon Graft Harvest and Preparation

- The sartorial fascia is exposed through a 2- to 3-cm skin incision made 2 cm medial and distal to the medial border of the tibial tubercle.
- The sartorial fascia is incised in line with the palpable gracilis tendon.
  - Avoid making this incision too deep to avoid injury to the underlying superficial medial collateral ligament.
- Identify and isolate the gracilis (proximal) and semitendinosus (distal) tendons from their deep aspect (ie, from within the bursal layer).
- Apply tension to the semitendinosus while freeing it from the crural fascia at the posteromedial corner with tissue scissors.
- Place stay sutures of #0 or #1 absorbable suture on a tapered needle, and then divide the tendon from the tibial insertion.

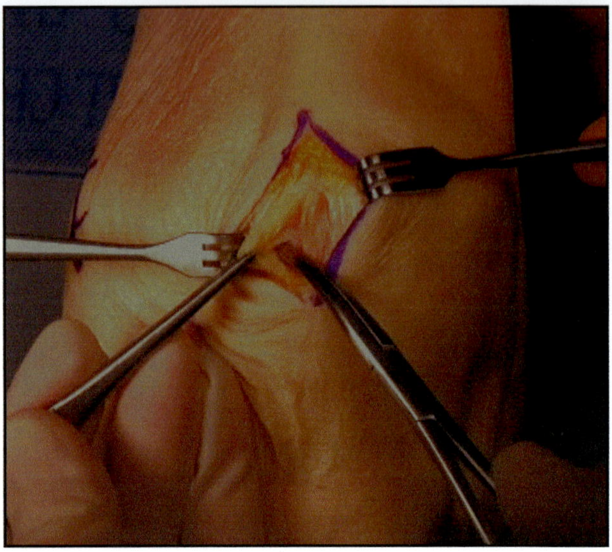

Figure 12-2. Dissection along patella to drill patella tunnels that extends medially and dorsally around the patella through layers 1 and 2, stopping after the transverse fibers of the native MPFL have been cut. Soft tissue tract overlying the capsule dissected toward femoral tunnel site.

- Once all tendinous slips have been freed, harvest the semitendinosus tendon using a closed (preferred) or open tendon stripper.
- Baseball stitches are placed on both free ends with #2 nonabsorbable suture for later graft passage through the 2 patellar tunnels.
- The graft is prepared on the back table by first sizing the graft to 240 mm and then folding it in half, leaving a doubled graft of 120 mm. It is recommended to make the doubled graft length no less than 120 mm to ensure adequate graft length.
- A #5 polyethylene suture is placed through the loop to be used for pulling the doubled graft into the blind femoral tunnel.
- A baseball stitch 25 mm in length with #0 or #1 absorbable suture is placed in the looped end of the graft to sew together the 2 graft strands that will be in the femoral tunnel.

Patellar Tunnel Placement

- A longitudinal incision the length of the patella is made at the junction of the medial and middle thirds of the patella (in line with the medial border of the patellar tendon at the distal patellar pole).
- The medial 8 to 10 mm of the patella is exposed by subperiosteal dissection with a #15 scalpel.
- The dissection extends medially and dorsally around the patella through layers 1 (longitudinal retinaculum) and 2 (native MPFL), stopping after the transverse fibers of the native MPFL have been cut. The capsule (layer 3) is left intact (Figure 12-2).
- A 4.5-mm drill hole is placed on the medial side of the upper pole of the patella adjacent to the articular margin (Figure 12-3).
  - A corresponding drill hole is placed on the anterior surface of the patella approximately 8 mm from the medial border. (This point corresponds to the lateral edge of the original retinacular dissection.)
  - The 2 drill holes are connected with a curved curette.

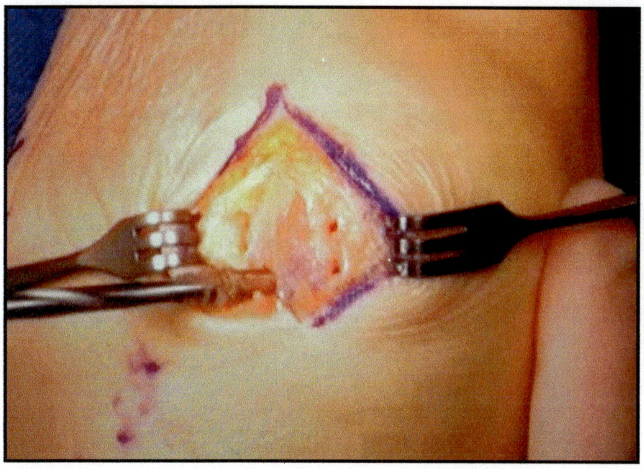

Figure 12-3. Medial to lateral tunnels in the patella tunnels drilled with a 4.5-mm drill on the medial side of the upper pole of the patella adjacent to the articular margin. Note that the patellar tunnel was drilled to intersect with the drill hole in anterior surface of the patella to allow graft passage through the tunnel and then back over itself.

- A second 4.5-mm drill hole is placed on the medial side of the patella at a point two-thirds down the length of the patella.
    - A corresponding drill hole is placed on the anterior surface of the patella about 8 mm from the medial border, and the 2 holes are connected with a curved curette.
- If the semitendinosus graft is more than 4.5 mm in diameter, the drill holes are enlarged slightly to facilitate graft passage.
- It is important to avoid placing the distal patellar tunnel distal to the native insertion of the MPFL to avoid constraining the distal pole of the patella.

Femoral Tunnel Placement and Checking Isometry

- A skin incision is made just anterior to the palpable ridge connecting the medial femoral epicondyle and the adductor tubercle.
    - The knee is flexed slightly to facilitate palpation of this landmark (flexion moves the hamstrings posteriorly away from the medial epicondyle).
    - If the landmarks are difficult to palpate, a small skin incision is made, and palpation is done through the wound to identify the ridge.
- The graft may be placed between layers 1 and 2 or between layers 2 and 3 (joint capsule) (ie, it may lie superficial or deep to the native MPFL).
    - Placing the graft between layers 2 and 3 is preferred because blind dissection superficial to the native MPFL may disrupt the insertion of the vastus medialis oblique into the anterior portion of the MPFL; in addition, by placing the graft deep to the native MPFL, the latter may be repaired to the graft during wound closure.
    - The graft should not be placed deep to the capsule because it should remain extra-articular to avoid graft abrasion and facilitate complete healing.
- Using a long, curved clamp, the selected interval is developed (preferably between layers 2 and 3) from the patellar incision anteriorly to the medial femoral epicondyle posteriorly (Figure 12-4).
- With the tip of the clamp overlying the ridge between the medial epicondyle and adductor tubercle, layers 1 and 2 are incised using a #15 blade.
- The tip of a Beath pin is placed at a point approximately 9 mm proximal and 5 mm posterior to the medial epicondyle; the pin is then passed toward the lateral side of the femur. Accuracy of pin placement should be confirmed by lateral fluoroscopic imaging, with ideal tunnel location approximately 1 mm anterior to the posterior cortex extension line, 2.5 mm distal to the

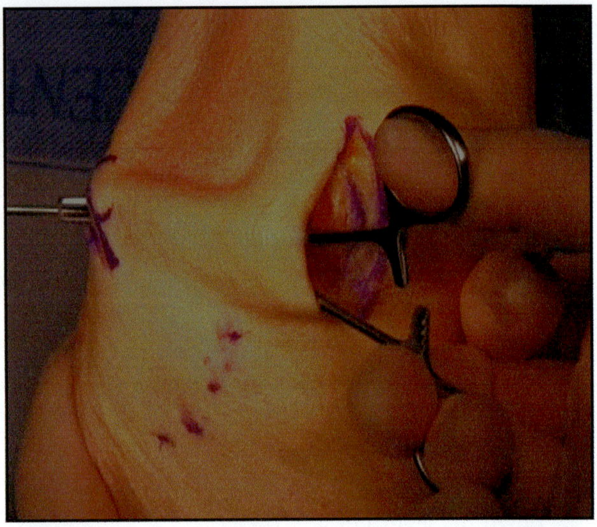

Figure 12-4. The soft tissue interval is developed between the patellar incision anterior to the femoral tunnel incision site posteriorly, preferentially between layers 2 and 3.

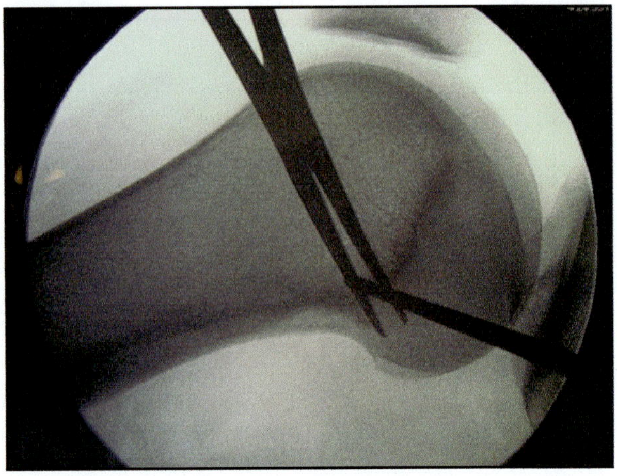

Figure 12-5. Lateral intraoperative fluoroscopic image of the distal femur with accurate pin placement approximately 1 mm anterior to the posterior cortex extension line, 2.5 mm distal to the posterior origin of the medial femoral condyle, and proximal to the level of the posterior point of the Blumensaat line on a lateral x-ray with both posterior condyles projected in the same plane.[16] A hemostat is clamped onto the guide pin at a point immediately adjacent to the cortical bone to allow identification of the point where the pin enters the distal femur, which will be the site of the drilled tunnel.

posterior origin of the medial femoral condyle, and proximal to the level of the posterior point of the Blumensaat line on a lateral x-ray with both posterior condyles projected in the same plane (Figure 12-5).[16]

- A loop of #5 braided polyethylene suture is passed around the Beath pin, through the dissected retinacular tunnel, and then through one of the patellar tunnels.
- The knee is taken through ROM to evaluate isometry while holding the suture at the anterior aspect of the patellar tunnel to evaluate for length changes of the suture during ROM (Figure 12-6).
  - If lengthening occurs in flexion, a second Beath pin is placed more distally toward the medial epicondyle. The first pin is left in place to facilitate repositioning while drilling the second Beath pin. The loop of #5 suture is passed around the second Beath pin, and the knee is put through ROM again. If isometry is acceptable, the first Beath pin is removed.
  - If lengthening occurs in extension, a second Beath pin is placed more proximally toward the adductor tubercle. The first pin is left in place to facilitate repositioning while drilling the second Beath pin. The loop of #5 suture is passed around the second Beath pin, and the knee is put through ROM again. If isometry is acceptable, the first Beath pin is removed.

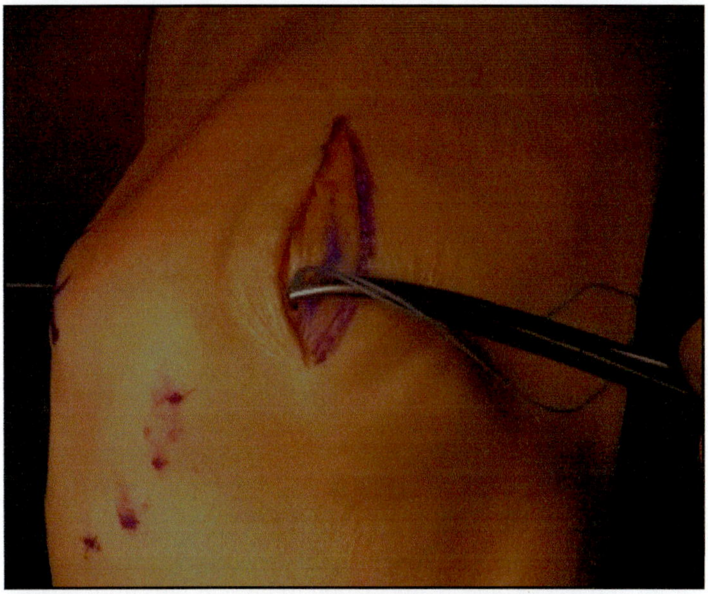

Figure 12-6. Evaluation for isometry of the femoral tunnel placement with suture passed around the pin at the anticipated femoral tunnel location, through the soft tissue tunnel, and into the patellar tunnel. The suture ends are held or secured with a clamp at the anterior aspect of the patellar tunnel to evaluate for length changes of the suture during ROM.

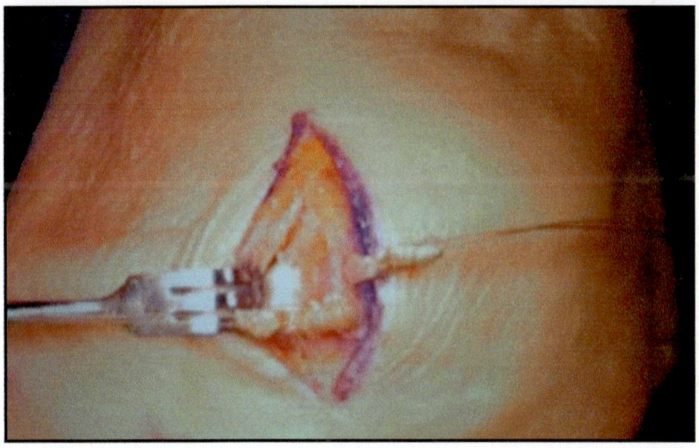

Figure 12-7. The graft arms individually enter the medial border of the patella through their respective tunnel and exit anteriorly, doubling back to be sutured to themselves.

- Once the femoral pin site is accepted, a blind tunnel is reamed into the femur the size of the doubled graft. For a semitendinosus graft, this usually is 6 to 7 mm in diameter.
- The femur is reamed to a depth of at least 20 mm, with a preferred depth of 25 mm.

Graft Passage and Fixation

- The #5 suture placed through the loop of the graft is passed through the Beath pin, and the pin is then advanced out the lateral femoral cortex to pass the graft into the femoral tunnel.
- Fixation to the femur may be achieved reliably with a 20- to 25-mm interference screw.
- The looped isometry suture, if left in place in the retinacular tunnel, may be used to pass the free ends of the graft through the retinacular interval created previously.
- The free graft arms are passed individually through their respective patellar tunnels using double 18-gauge stainless steel wire or a curved suture passer.
- The graft arms enter the medial border of the patella and exit anteriorly to be doubled over themselves for suture fixation (Figure 12-7).

- The free graft arms are doubled back and sutured on themselves just medial to the patella using 2 figure-8 mattress sutures of #2 nonabsorbable suture on a tapered needle.
- Patellar mobility is checked after the first suture is placed. There should be a good endpoint, or checkrein, with the knee in full extension and at 30 degrees of flexion, full knee ROM, and 7 to 9 mm of lateral patellar displacement from the centered position at 30 degrees of flexion.
- Excess graft is sharply removed.
- The native MPFL is sutured to the graft, and then the retinaculum is closed over the graft.
- The wounds are closed in standard fashion.

Postoperative Protocol

- Weightbearing as tolerated is allowed immediately postoperatively in a drop-lock or knee extension brace.
- Passive ROM and resisted closed chain exercises are started as soon as possible to restore ROM and quadriceps control. Preserving motion is key after MPFL surgery.
- Bracing may be continued for up to 6 weeks during ambulation to prevent falls until quadriceps control is restored. Circumferential measurement of quadriceps 10 cm above the superior pole of the patella can aid in evaluating restoration of the quadriceps.
- Patients are allowed to return to stressful activities, including sports, when they attain full ROM and have regained at least 80% of their quadriceps strength compared to the noninjured limb.
- If at least 90 degrees of flexion is not achieved by 6 postoperative weeks, then the intensity of the therapy program must be increased. Manipulation under anesthesia may be needed between 9 and 12 weeks postoperatively if stiffness does not resolve with therapy alone.

Potential Complications

- Inadequate graft length can occur if the total tendon length is less than 240 mm or in very large patients. Subsequently, the authors recommend getting consent from patients for potential allograft tendon use with an appropriately sized allograft on standby.
- Breakage of the patella bone bridge may occur during preparation of the 2 patellar tunnels or during passage of an oversized graft through a tight patellar tunnel. If this occurs, a second exit hole can be drilled more laterally on the anterior patellar surface. Another option is to drill the tunnel transversely across the patella, exiting at the lateral patellar margin. The graft can be secured by tying the sutures over a button or suturing the graft to the soft tissues on the lateral patellar border.
- Nonanatomic femoral tunnel placement will result in inappropriate graft behavior during ROM and reliably produce inadequate results.
- Excessive medial patellar constraint results in a painful, overconstrained patella.[17-19]
- It is imperative not to set the graft in tension but to instead ensure the MPFL graft is lax throughout a ROM becoming tight only when the patella is displaced laterally from its centered position.
- Symptomatic hardware can occur when the femoral tunnel interference screw is left proud outside of the femoral tunnel. Ensuring the screw is buried in the femoral tunnel can avoid this complication. Screw removal is acceptable, but it is recommended that the patient be fully

rehabilitated and back to unrestricted activities prior to this. Avoiding screw removal within 6 months after surgery is recommended. When removing the interference screw, careful attention should be paid to avoid violating the MPFL graft.

- Patellar fracture can occur after MPFL reconstruction, but it is the authors' opinion that patellar fracture is less likely using this technique because large implants and transverse bone tunnels are avoided. If patellar fracture occurs, treatment using standard AO techniques is recommended.
- Postoperative stiffness can occur if motion is not encouraged after MPFL reconstruction surgery. It is recommended that MPFL reconstruction be avoided with concomitant procedures that have competing postoperative rehabilitation protocols that require motion protection.

Top Technical Pearls for the Procedure

1. Indications
   - Surgical management is indicated for patients with at least 2 documented patellar instability events and a confirmatory physical examination demonstrating excessive lateral patellar laxity.
   - Perform examination under anesthesia to confirm excessive lateral patellar mobility.
2. Femoral tunnel placement is one of the most critical steps in the operation.
   - Adjust the tunnel placement to ensure appropriate graft behavior during flexion and extension, recreating isometry.
   - Check for accurate tunnel placement using fluoroscopy.[16]
3. Set the MPFL graft length without tension.
   - Center the patella in the patellar groove and ensure that the MPFL graft is lax throughout ROM, becoming tight only when the patella is displaced laterally from its centered position.
   - The patella should enter the trochlea from the lateral side as the knee is flexed.
   - The graft should not be tensioned because it serves as a checkrein. It should be set to a length that allows no excessive slack and no tension.
4. Avoid excessive medial constraint by ensuring the graft is not tight.
   - If the patella enters the trochlea from the medial side as the knee is flexed or if there is less than 5 mm of lateral patellar glide with gentle manual force at 30 degrees of knee flexion, then the graft is overtensioned. The sutures should be removed and the graft length set again.
5. Postoperative motion preservation is key after MPFL reconstruction.
   - Passive ROM and resisted closed chain exercises are started as soon as possible to restore ROM and quadriceps control.
   - Weightbearing as tolerated is allowed immediately postoperatively in a drop-lock or knee extension brace.

References

1. Conlan T, Garth WP Jr, Lemons JE. Evaluation of the medial soft-tissue restraints of the extensor mechanism of the knee. *J Bone Joint Surg Am.* 1993;75(5):682-693.
2. Panagiotopoulos E, Strzelczyk P, Herrmann M, Scuderi G. Cadaveric study on static medial patellar stabilizers: the dynamizing role of the vastus medialis obliquus on medial patellofemoral ligament. *Knee Surg Sports Traumatol Arthrosc.* 2006;14(1):7-12.
3. Hautamaa PV, Fithian DC, Kaufman KR, Daniel DM, Pohlmeyer AM. Medial soft tissue restraints in lateral patellar instability and repair. *Clin Orthop Rel Res.* 1998;(349):174-182.
4. Fithian DC, Gupta N. Patellar instability: principals of soft tissue repair and reconstruction. *Tech Knee Surg.* 2006;5:19-26.
5. Mäenpää H, Lehto MU. Patellar dislocation. The long-term results of nonoperative management in 100 patients. *Am J Sports Med.* 1997;25(2):213-217.
6. Nikku R, Nietosvaara Y, Aalto K, Kallio PE. Operative treatment of primary patellar dislocation does not improve medium-term outcome: a 7-year follow-up report and risk analysis of 127 randomized patients. *Acta Orthop.* 2005;76(5):699-704.
7. Nikku R, Nietosvaara Y, Kallio PE, Aalto K, Michelsson JE. Operative versus closed treatment of primary dislocation of the patella: similar 2-year results in 125 randomized patients. *Acta Orthop Scand.* 1997;68(5):419-423.
8. Fithian DC, Paxton WE, Stone ML, et al. Epidemiology and natural history of acute patellar dislocation. *Am J Sports Med.* 2004;32(5):1114-1121.
9. Teitge RA, Faerber WW, Des Madryl P, Matelic TM. Stress radiographs of the patellofemoral joint. *J Bone Joint Surg Am.* 1996;78(2):193-203.
10. Panagiotopoulos E, Strzelczyk P, Herrmann M, Scuderi G. Cadaveric study on static medial patellar stabilizers: the dynamizing role of the vastus medialis obliquus on medial patellofemoral ligament. *Knee Surg Sports Traumatol Arthrosc.* 2006;14(1):7-12.
11. Elias DA, White LM, Fithian DC. Acute lateral patellar dislocation at MR imaging: injury patterns of medial patellar soft-tissue restraints and osteochondral injuries of the inferomedial patella. *Radiology.* 2002;225(3):736-743.
12. Caton J, Deschamps G, Chambat P, Lerat JL, Dejour H. Patella infera. Apropos of 128 cases [in French]. *Rev Chir Orthop Reparatrice Appar Mot.* 1982;68(5):317-325.
13. Dejour H, Walch G, Nove-Josserand L, Guier C. Factors of patellar instability: an anatomic radiographic study. *Knee Surg Sports Traumatol Arthrosc.* 1994;2(1):19-26.
14. Camp CL, Stuart MJ, Krych AJ, et al. CT and MRI measurements of tibial tubercle-trochlear groove distances are not equivalent in patients with patellar instability. *Am J Sports Med.* 2013;41(8):1835-1840.
15. Salzmann GM, Weber TS, Spang JT, Imhoff AB, Schöttle PB. Comparison of native axial radiographs with axial MR imaging for determination of the trochlear morphology in patients with trochlear dysplasia. *Arch Orthop Trauma Surg.* 2010;130(3):335-340.
16. Schöttle PB, Schmeling A, Rosenstiel N, Weiler A. Radiographic landmarks for femoral tunnel placement in medial patellofemoral ligament reconstruction. *Am J Sports Med.* 2007;35(5):801-804.
17. Elias JJ, Cosgarea AJ. Technical errors during medial patellofemoral ligament reconstruction could overload medial patellofemoral cartilage: a computational analysis. *Am J Sports Med.* 2006;34(9):1478-1485.
18. Muneta T, Sekiya I, Tsuchiya M, Shinomiya K. A technique for reconstruction of the medial patellofemoral ligament. *Clin Orthop Rel Res.* 1999;(359):151-155.
19. Nomura E, Horiuchi Y, Kihara M. Medial patellofemoral ligament restraint in lateral patellar translation and reconstruction. *Knee.* 2000;7(2):121-127.

Please see videos on the accompanying website at www.routledge.com/9781617119996

13

Tibial Tubercle Transfer

Jeffrey T. Spang, MD; Benjamin R. Parker, MD; and
John P. Fulkerson, MD

Introduction

Patellofemoral pain and dysfunction is often caused by improper tracking and concomitant maldistribution of forces between the patella and the trochlear groove. In addition, patellar instability is a common problem that often requires surgical intervention. When performed on the appropriately selected patient, tibial tubercle transfer (TTT) is a powerful surgical technique for altering mechanical alignment, allowing redistribution of loads within the articular cartilage, and promoting patellar stability. Medialization and anteromedialization of the tibial tubercle are effective ways to dissipate loads on the lateral patellofemoral compartment.[1,2] The surgical procedure is clinically successful and allows patients to resume increasing levels of activity.[3]

Indications

- Patellofemoral instability, patellar and trochlear focal chondral lesions
- Lateral patellar compression syndrome and patellofemoral articular degeneration
- Procedure in conjunction with soft tissue patellar stabilization, chondral replacement therapies, and patellofemoral resurfacing
- Patellofemoral pain and/or instability associated with a poorly balanced patellar-trochlear articulation[4,5]
- Medialization with minimal anteriorization in patients for whom the major pathology is patellar instability[6]
- Patients with significant patellar tilt and significant articular degeneration in the lateral and inferior patellofemoral joint

Sgaglione NA, Lubowitz JH, Provencher MT, eds. *The Knee: AANA Advanced Arthroscopic Surgical Techniques* (pp 173-185).

Controversial Indications

- TTT-anteromedialize the tibial tubercle as an adjunct to autologous chondrocyte implantation procedures in the patellofemoral joint in an effort to redistribute the joint forces to protect the cartilage implantation.[7]
- Distalization procedures in patients with recurrent instability in the setting of patella alta. Distalization can be added in conjunction with a TTT.[6,8]

Contraindications

- Significant proximal pole arthritis or cartilage disease
- Significant medial trochlear cartilage disease
- Complex regional pain syndrome
- Medical or psychiatric disorders prohibiting surgical intervention[4,5]

Pertinent Physical Findings

- Evaluation in upright, sitting, and supine positions[9]
- Gait, muscle tone/core strength, patellar height, and general lower extremity alignment
- Knee effusion and mechanical symptoms suggesting focal chondral injury
- Tenderness and pain along the lateral retinaculum suggesting tight retinacular structures. Restricted patellar mobility can indicate fixed patellar tilt and increase contact pressures on the lateral patellofemoral articulation.[8,10]
- Examination of the medial patellofemoral ligament and retinacular patency
- Overall limb alignment, Q angle, femoral anteversion
- J sign refers to the inverted J path of the patella from 0 to 45 degrees as the patella begins to laterally subluxate and then suddenly shifts to engage with the trochlear groove. The sign indicates that the patella-trochlear articulation may have malalignment or that the medial soft tissues and ligamentous structures are deficient.[8]
- Pain associated with the patellofemoral grind test, the Clarke's test, or weightbearing knee flexion is an important finding, indicating increased patella-trochlear contact pressures.[11]

Best Test

- The best test for determining an optimal candidate for anteromedialization is the step down test (to establish that a distal patella articular lesion is likely causing pain) in which the patient has subpatellar pain upon stepping down with the contralateral leg. If this test reproduces the patient's symptom, and imaging and/or arthroscopic evidence documents tilt with a distal/lateral patella articular lesion, the patient is likely a candidate for anteromedialization once nonoperative measures have failed.

Pertinent Imaging

- Computed tomography and magnetic resonance imaging (MRI) examination are useful tools in evaluating the mechanical anatomy of the relationship of the patella to the trochlear groove (tibial tubercle to trochlear groove).[12-15]
- Standard anteroposterior, lateral, and axial views of the patella, in addition to full-length standing films, can give insight into overall alignment and articulation variations within the knee. Patellar height (Insall-Salvati ratio) can be assessed using the lateral position.

Equipment

Various guide systems are currently on the market for tibial tuberosity osteotomies. The Arthrex T3 AMZ system and DePuy Synthes Tracker AMZ Guide provide a guided system for creating a controlled osteotomy on the tibia while protecting soft tissue structures and controlling the degree of realignment of the extensor mechanism. Some surgeons, with experience and training, may be able to perform most tubercle transfer osteotomies without using a guide.

- Arthroscopy equipment
- Intraoperative fluoroscopy
- Sharp and dull soft tissue retractors
- Dissection scissors
- Wide and narrow sagittal bone cutting blades (osteotomes; one-half and one-quarter in)
- K-wires (2.1 and 2.4 mm)
- Small fragment or large fragment fixation sets (Synthes or Stryker)

Positioning and Portals

The patient is positioned in a supine position with a lateral post on a regular operating table. A small ipsilateral hip bump may be appropriate to help align the knee with the patella facing directly anterior. The patient should be prepped and draped in the usual sterile fashion with the arthroscopic setup that is comfortable for the operating surgeon. However, because tubercle transfer requires an exposure of the anterolateral tibia, draping may need to be adapted to allow access to all appropriate anatomical structures. If the lithotomy position with a leg holder is preferred, a Mayo stand can be used to support the leg after the arthroscopic portion of the case is completed. One should position the knee such that a full range of motion (ROM) may be performed to assess patellofemoral tracking arthroscopically after the osteotomy correction is performed.

Step-by-Step Description of the Procedure

Medialization

A complete examination under anesthesia should confirm significant patellar lateralization and possibly dislocation. A full diagnostic arthroscopy should be performed to assess the articular cartilage and view the trochlear/patellar interface throughout a ROM (Figure 13-1). If the lateral soft tissues appear to be tethering the patella, an arthroscopic lateral release can be performed at this stage. A longitudinal incision can be made beginning approximately 2 cm above the tibial

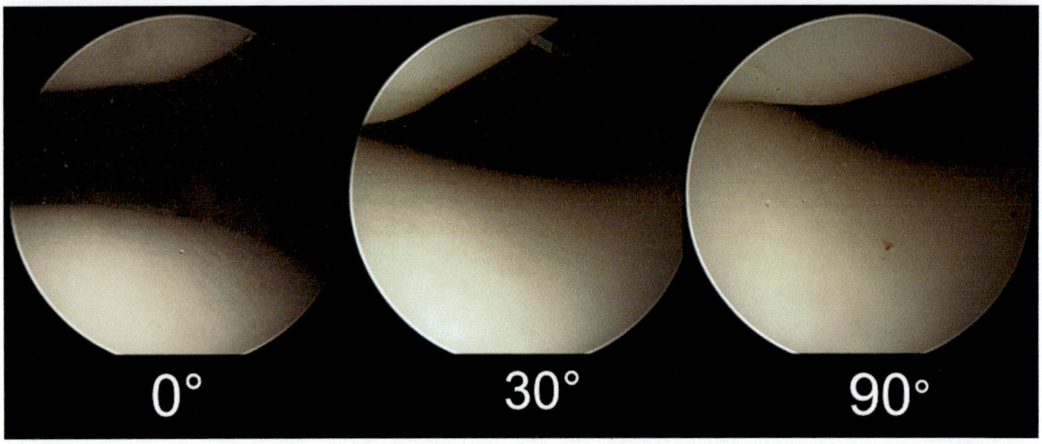

Figure 13-1. Arthroscopic views of the patellofemoral joint prior to procedure throughout the ROM. The patella has significant contact forces on the lateral trochlea, and there is significant patellar tilt secondary to weak medial soft tissues. (Reprinted with permission from Ganesh Kamath, MD.)

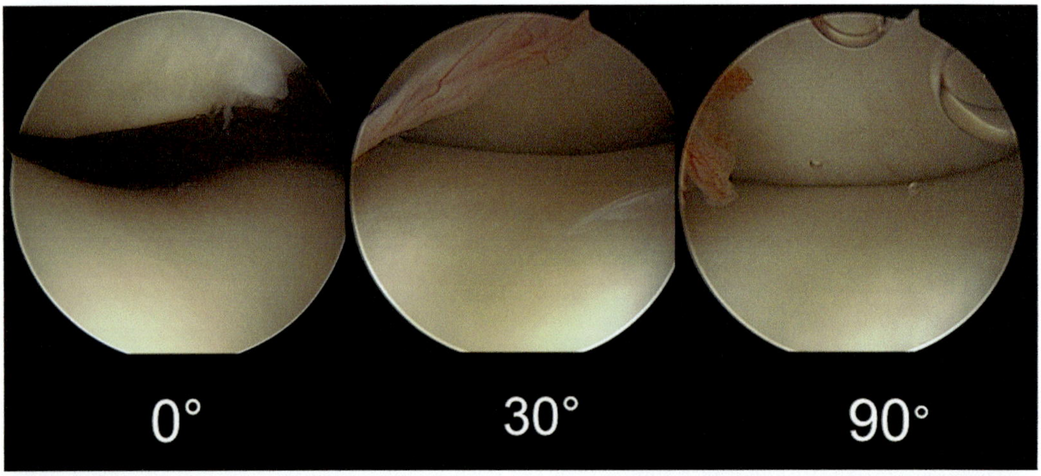

Figure 13-2. Arthroscopic view of the patellofemoral joint postoperatively throughout the ROM. The patella now reengages the trochlea in uniform alignment. (Reprinted with permission from Ganesh Kamath, MD.)

tubercle and carrying the incision approximately 6 cm distal to the tibial tubercle. Careful soft tissue dissection of the patellar tendon along its lateral and medial borders should increase mobilization (Figure 13-2). Often, the fat pad must be released from the posterior of the patellar tendon to allow sufficient mobilization and appropriate visualization (Figure 13-3). The tibialis anterior origin muscle fascia is released and reflected posteriorly using electrocautery and/or a Cobb elevator. The medial and lateral borders of the patellar tendon are clearly defined using blunt dissection and a retractor or a vessel loop is placed around the tendon (Figure 13-4).

Depending on surgeon preference, the osteotomy can begin with a cut transverse to the long axis of the tibia just proximal to the patellar tendon insertion. This can be done with small osteotomes or a small fine oscillating saw while protecting the patellar tendon. This transverse proximal cut may also be performed after the long sloping longitudinal cut (Figure 13-5).

With the patella oriented anteriorly, protective retractors are used retract the tibialis anterior and expose the entire proximal anterior tibia for the extent of the incision. A fine tooth oscillating saw blade is used to create an approximately 5- to 7-cm longitudinal osteotomy (Figure 13-6).

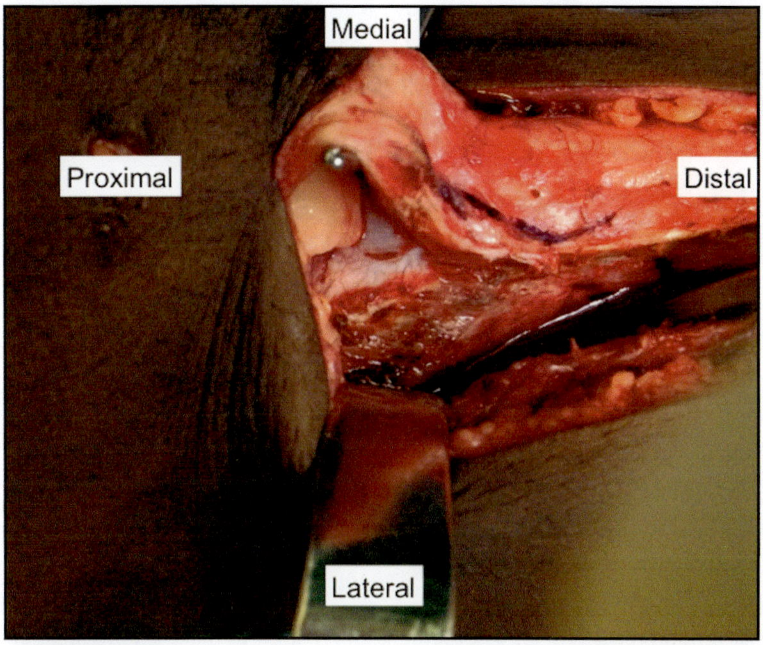

Figure 13-3. Lateral tibia exposure with appropriate removal of soft tissues. This allows for ideal soft tissue protector placement and protects the underlying vasculature. (Reprinted with permission from Ganesh Kamath, MD.)

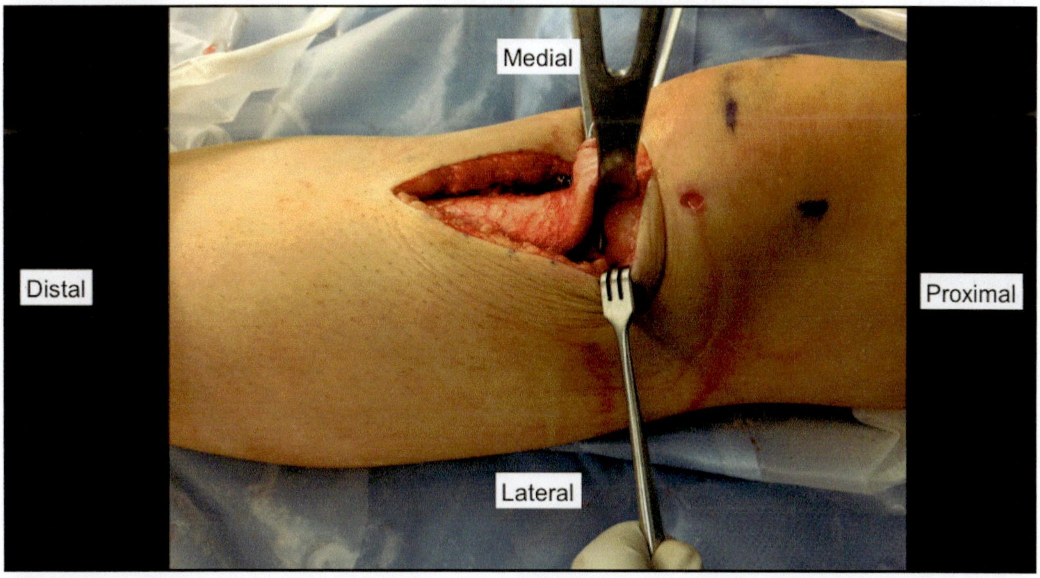

Figure 13-4. Lateral tibial exposure with appropriate identification and exposure of the patellar tendon. This is important for avoiding iatrogenic injury. (Reprinted with permission from Ganesh Kamath, MD.)

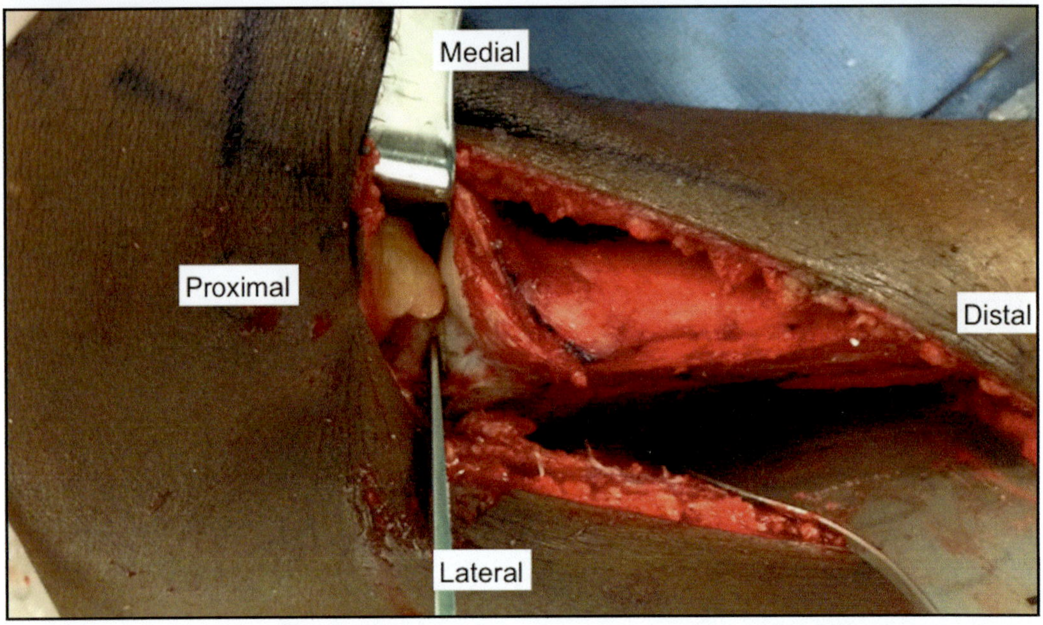

Figure 13-5. With the patellar tendon retracted, an osteotome is safely used to make a transverse cut through the tibia. (Reprinted with permission from Ganesh Kamath, MD.)

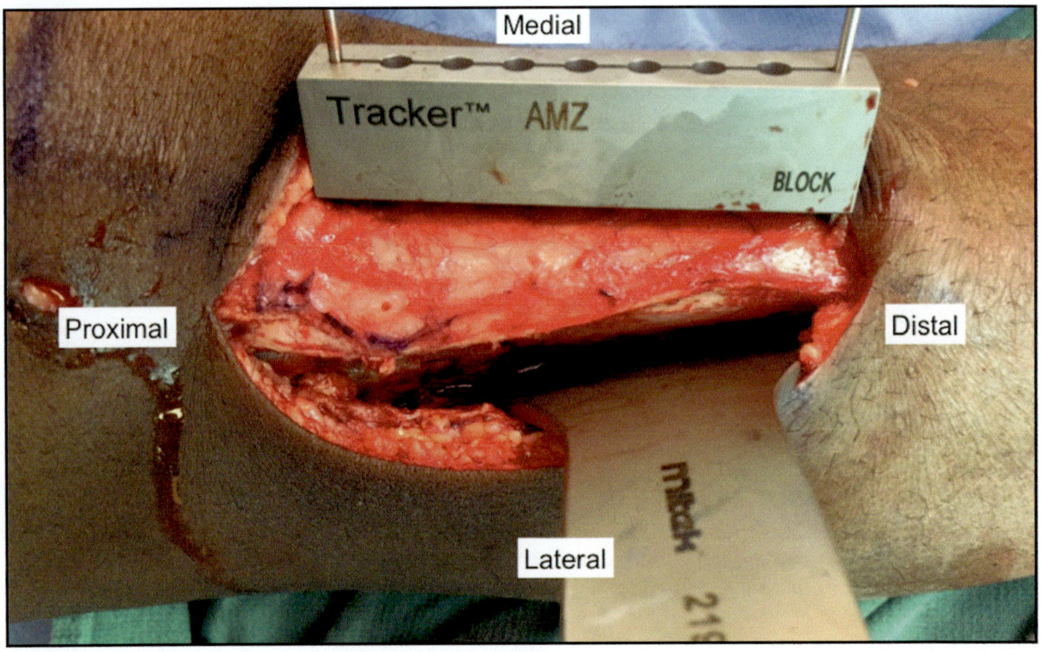

Figure 13-6. Once the exposure is complete, the AMZ Guide can be placed to reference the bone cut. (Reprinted with permission from Ganesh Kamath, MD.)

With the knee held in a straight anteroposterior orientation, the saw blade is placed about 5 mm behind the insertion of the medial patellar tendon into the tibial tuberosity, oriented in a transverse plane, and then rotated slightly such that the blade, upon making the cut, will move anteriorly as it proceeds distally. Place a target point approximately 5 cm distal to the tibial tuberosity directly at the anterior crest of the tibia. By raising the saw anteriorly, the steepness

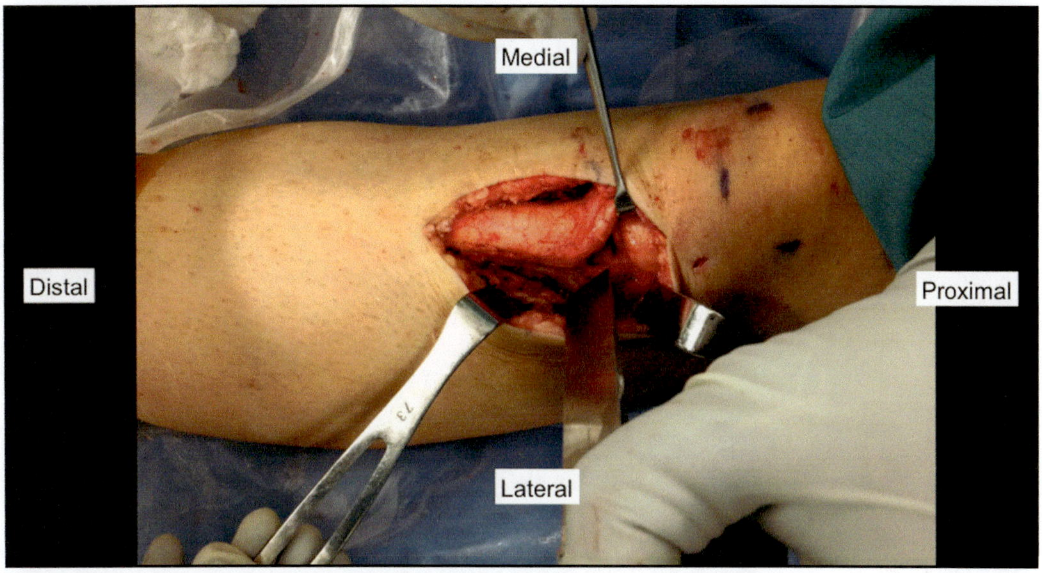

Figure 13-7. Lateral connecting osteotomy. An osteotome is used to connect the transverse tibial osteotomy to the main osteotomy. (Reprinted with permission from Ganesh Kamath, MD.)

(and thus the desired anteriorization of the tibial tubercle) can be adjusted. It is important to create the angle of the osteotomy anteriorly at its distal aspect to avoid creating an unnecessary stress fracture in the tibia by notching the tibia. The osteotomy should exit the tibia smoothly, leaving a small bone bridge (such that a simple greenstick fracture over the distal end is all that is needed to release the osteotomized fragment in a straight medial direction once all cuts are completed).

An oblique connecting cut is needed on the lateral side to connect the longitudinal and the transverse cuts to allow release of the osteotomized tubercle (Figure 13-7). The proximal cut above the patellar tendon insertion provides a shelf upon which the transferred osteotomy fragment may rest securely after transfer in the medial direction, supplementing screw fixation (Figure 13-8).

In many cases, the tibial tuberosity will be moved about 1 cm medially. The tibial tuberosity should be moved only as far medially as is necessary to create better tracking of the patella into the trochlea, avoiding excessive medialization (Figure 13-9).

Excessive medialization may lead to medial patellar instability, which is a serious postoperative complication. The goal is to recreate a more normal tracking pattern in which the patella goes slightly laterally in extension and then moves proximally into the center of the trochlea with knee flexion. A K-wire can be used to hold the osteotomy in place as patellar tracking is evaluated. Arthroscopic and open evaluation of patellar tracking can be used to evaluate dynamic patellar tracking (Figures 13-2, 13-9, and 13-10). Once proper tracking of the patella is established, two 4.5 screws or three 3.5 screws should be used to stabilize the transferred tibial tubercle. The screws are placed through the osteotomy fragment and countersunk, and then appropriately sized drill holes are made into the posterior cortex to create lag fixation. In many cases, a small amount of bone may be removed from the medial aspect of the transferred bone fragment if overly prominent.

In patients with instability who have insufficient medial retinacular anatomy, some arthroscopic or open imbrication may be appropriate to reestablish normal length of medial patellofemoral and medial quadriceps femoral restraints. For proper restoration of patellofemoral stability in the presence of lateral patellar tracking, it is important to correct the alignment of the patellofemoral joint by TTT before doing any medial reconstruction.

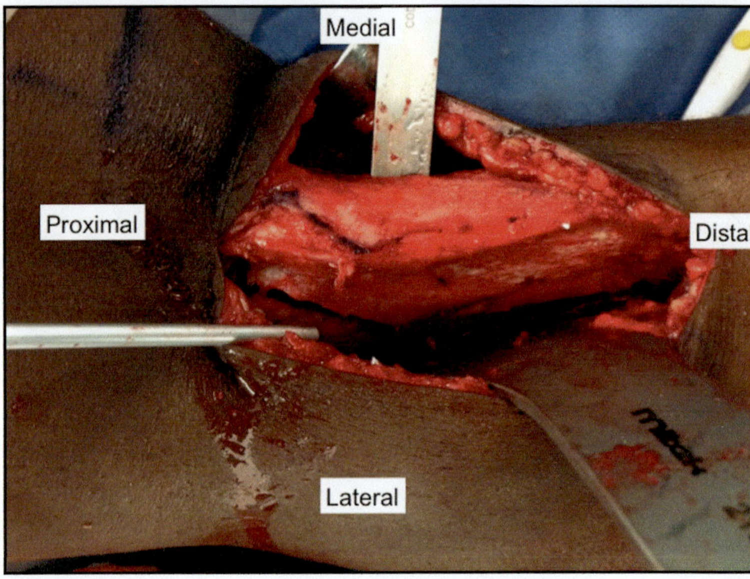

Figure 13-8. Completed lateral connecting osteotomy. Once all osteotomies are complete, the tuberosity is mobilized. (Reprinted with permission from Ganesh Kamath, MD.)

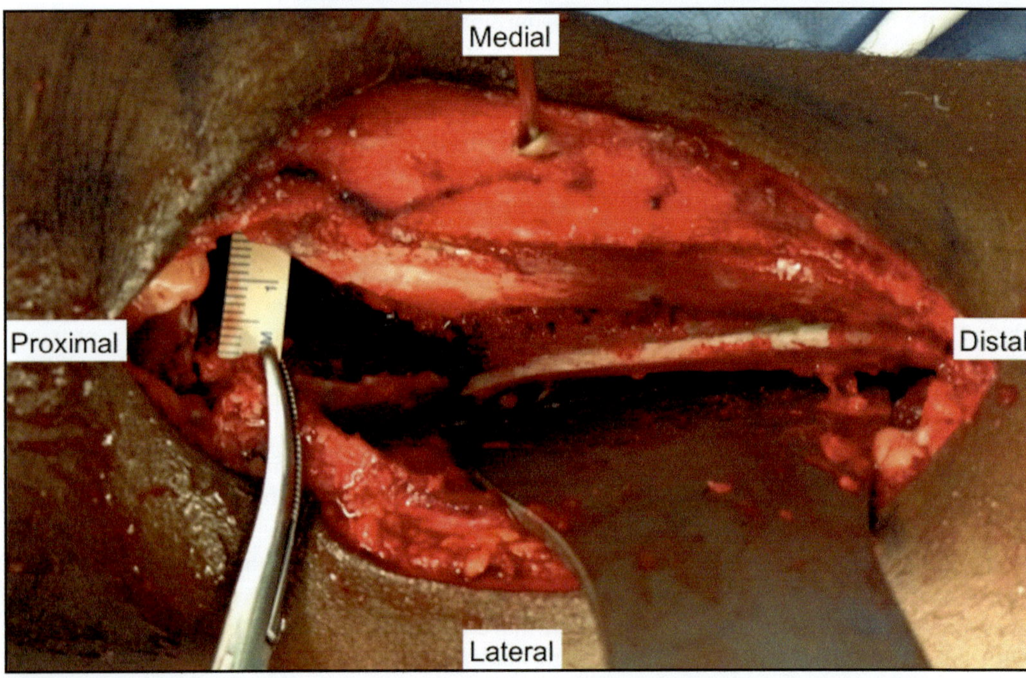

Figure 13-9. K-wire placement into the tibial tuberosity. Measurements can be used to estimate the amount of anteromedialization to be obtained by the tibial tubercle osteotomy. (Reprinted with permission from Ganesh Kamath, MD.)

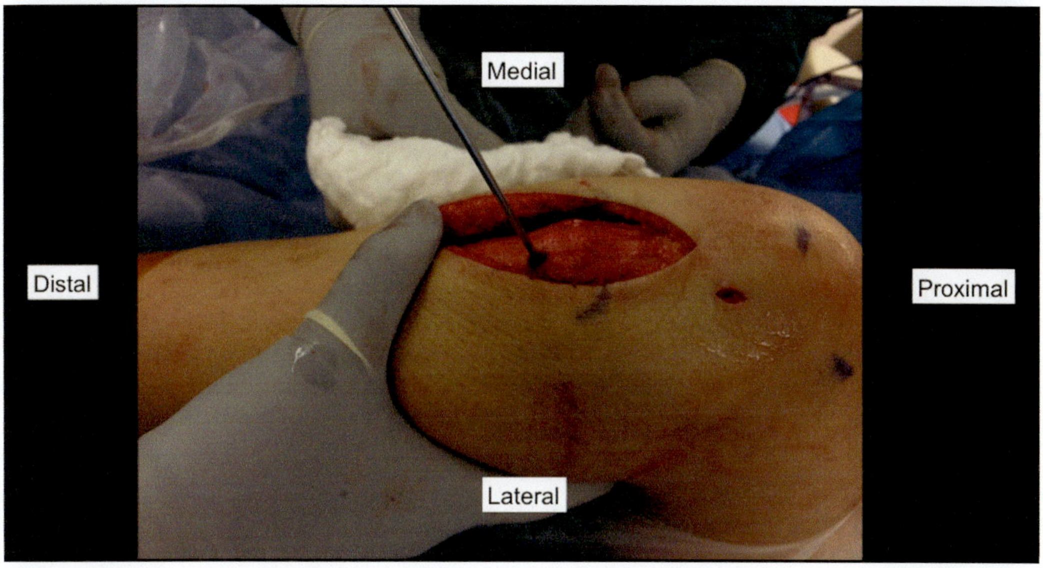

Figure 13-10. K-wire placement into the tibial tuberosity. A K-wire can be placed after the tuberosity is anteromedialized, and arthroscopic evaluation can be used to assess patellar tracking. (Reprinted with permission from Ganesh Kamath, MD.)

Anteromedialization

Exposure is the same as for medial TTT. To perform anteromedial TTT, the entire lateral tibia must be exposed by elevating the tibialis anterior. This becomes particularly important with anteromedial TTT because of the obliquity of the cut, which determines the amount of anteriorization. In order to perform a steep anteromedial TTT, the saw blade is placed immediately adjacent to the medial patellar tendon and then angled posterolaterally such that the saw blade will exit the lateral tibial cortex. Again, the osteotomy is tapered toward the anterior tibial crest distally. In many cases, a 6- to 8-cm longitudinal cut is created. The length is determined by marking the periosteum, starting at the medial patellar tendon insertion and creating a straight line exiting at the anterior tibial crest distally with the desired distance from the proximal tibial tubercle.

When unloading of the distal and lateral patella is of utmost importance, a steeper osteotomy is created. The saw blade must be watched carefully as it exits the lateral tibia cortex, first at the distal aspect and then followed as the cut is brought anteriorly and distally. The saw blade must never exit posteriorly or be out of direct vision of the surgeon. Osteotomes may be used to fine-tune the osteotomy distally to ensure sufficient release while maintaining distal bone continuity.

Distalization

One technique is to bevel the most distal transverse osteotomy so as to lock in the tibial tubercle after the transfer. Finally, the tuberosity is mobilized by making a coronal plane cut and freeing the tibial tubercle fragment with an osteotome. The patellar tendon is dissected in order to allow distal excursion of the tibial tubercle.

Next, the tuberosity is shifted distally and locked into the most distal transverse tibial cut. The tuberosity is then fixed in a lag-time fashion as previously noted.[6,8] Little clinical outcome data exist to support distalization, and some increasing evidence shows that the loads created by altering the Blix curve and retinacular alignment with tubercle distalization can lead to failure of fixation and/or patellofemoral overload and result articular cartilage damage. The best place for tubercle distalization remains to be determined.

Postoperative Protocol

Following TTT, the patient should be anticoagulated. Foot and ankle pumps, ice, elevation, and rest are important for the first 5 days, but the patient may ambulate with crutches for short distances in a protective brace.

After the first few days, the patient should begin daily work on ROM, sitting in a chair, removing the knee immobilizer, and progressing toward a 90-degree bend by 4 weeks postoperatively. Quad sets should be done starting on the first postoperative day. Most patients should be able to bend the knee to 100 to 120 degrees by 6 weeks postoperatively. Physical therapy may start at the discretion of the surgeon, taking care to respect the soft tissue healing of the anterior wound. High-level activity and running should not be performed until at least 6 months postoperatively (Table 13-1). Radiographic evidence of complete healing should be established before any vigorous activities.

Potential Complications

Problems or need for additional surgery after a TTT have been reported to be up to 37% when postoperative hardware removal is considered. The most common complications are listed in Table 13-2.[16]

The prevalence of metaphyseal fractures ranges from 0% to 9.5% in small case series and case reports.[16] Fracture can be prevented by avoiding a notched tibia distally. Careful attention should be made to the thickness of the distal edge of the osteotomy. If it is too large, the fragment will not appropriately hinge during the transfer, and a stress fracture may occur at the level or distal to the osteotomy site. Protected weightbearing postoperatively is also crucial to preventing further propagation of these types of fractures.[17]

Nonunion is a rare complication that may be attributed to heat necrosis from saw use, uneven osteotomy, improper screw placement techniques, and excessive periosteal stripping. Osteotomes may be used to complete the osteotomy so as to avoid necrosis at the cortical edges. A minimalistic approach should also be considered when making the exposure to the anterior tibia, and an attempt to preserve bony blood supply should be paramount.[18]

Hardware irritation has been reported as a common postoperative complaint. Countersinking the traditional 2-by-4.5-mm screws is important to avoid hardware irritation. In biomechanical cadaver studies, 3-by-3.5-mm screws have been proven to withstand similar maximal loads. The lesser prominence of the 3.5-mm screw heads may be a way to avoid hardware irritation.[19]

Vascular injury is a potential catastrophic complication of the tibial tubercle osteotomy. Bifurcation of the popliteal artery has been found to be 8.3 mm from the exit point of the superior screw, and the tibial artery has been found to be 9.0 mm from the inferior screw. Because of the proximity of these large vessels, care should be taken not to plunge past the posterior cortex of the tibia and to always visualize the most posterior saw cut exiting the posterolateral cortex. Tissue protectors should also always be in place to avoid damage to the skin.[20] The lateral tissue protector also must protect the peroneal nerve, which is at risk if the saw or osteotomes are uncontained laterally.

It is important to maintain full-thickness skin flaps during the dissection to prevent wound complications. An appropriate closure of soft tissues may prevent the formation of dead space seromas/hematomas that may lead to secondary infection. Drains may be used at the discretion of the surgeon. Osteomyelitis can occur about 5.8% of the time if there are serious wound complications.

Other rare but important complications include arthrofibrosis, compartment syndrome, and deep venous thrombosis. Arthrofibrosis has a prevalence of about 8.5% but is uncommon by starting early postoperative ROM. Postoperative protocols with use of a hinged knee brace can help allow early ROM and prevent this complication. Compartment syndrome can be prevented

Table 13-1. Postoperative Rehabilitation Protocol

	Weightbearing	Brace	ROM (deg)	Therapeutic Exercises
Phase I 0 to 6 weeks	Nonweight-bearing	0 to 2 weeks Locked in extension for sleep, ambulation, can unlock 0 to 90 degrees 2 to 6 weeks Unlocked	0 to 2 weeks (0 to 30) 2 to 4 weeks (0 to 60) 4 to 6 weeks (0 to 90)	Heel slides, quad/hamstring sets, patellar mobilization in all quadrants, prone hangs, gastroc/soleus stretch,[a] straight leg raising with brace locked in extension, edema control
Phase II 6 to 12 weeks	6 to 8 weeks Advance to weightbearing as tolerated, discontinue crutch use	6 to 8 weeks Unlocked 8 weeks Discontinue use	Maintain full extension and progressive flexion	Progress to normal gait pattern, gastroc/soleus stretch, begin toe raises, closed chain extension, balance exercises, hamstring curls, and stationary bike
Phase III 3 to 5 months	Full, without use of crutches and with a normalized gait pattern	None	Advance to full and pain-free ROM	Advance closed chain strengthening, progress proprioception activities, begin Stairmaster/Nordic Trac and running straight ahead
Phase IV 5+ months	Full	None	Full and pain free	Flexibility/strengthening, progression of function: forward/backward running, cutting, grapevine, initiate plyometric program and sport-specific drills, gradual return to sports participation, maintenance program for strength and endurance

Deg, degrees; ROM, range of motion.

[a]This exercise is to be performed in a nonweightbearing position.

by creating a rent in the tibialis anterior fascia prior to elevating the subperiosteal flap laterally. In addition, the opened anterior-lateral compartment fascia should not be repaired, allowing any potential bleeding a course of egress. Care should be taken to avoid complete anesthetic blocks of the legs (femoral and sciatic combined blocks) as latent compartment syndrome is a recognized (but uncommon) complication associated with lower extremity surgery. In addition, drains may

Table 13-2. Pitfalls and Complications

Pitfalls	*Common Complications*
Failing to unload a distal patellar articular lesion (doing medial tubercle transfer when anteromedial transfer is more appropriate)	Malunion/nonunion
Overmedializing and creating a medial subluxation problem	Vascular injury
Creating an inaccurate osteotomy or notching the tibia	Compartment syndrome
Inadequate fixation	Hardware prominence
Skin injury from the saw blade from inadequate retraction	Pain
Failure to encourage early motion leading to arthrofibrosis	Arthrofibrosis
	Wound complications
	Deep venous thrombosis

be considered when indicated. Thromboembolic prevention should be managed with a thromboembolism-deterrent hose, sequential compression devices, and chemical prophylaxis, including aspirin, enoxaparin, or heparin. Casting is not recommended and may contribute to arthrofibrosis, compartment syndrome, and deep venous thrombosis (see Table 13-2).[16,21]

Top Technical Pearls for the Procedure

1. Allow for full exposure with substantial soft tissue excursion so as to create good tibial cuts and avoid iatrogenic skin injury.
2. Be patient with the tibial cut and establishing a mobile fragment. Inappropriate use of osteotomes and saw blades may create unwanted distal fractures.
3. Perform an adequate post-transfer evaluation, including arthroscopy to evaluate the new tracking pattern between the patella and trochlea.
4. Temporary K-wire fixation allows dynamic evaluation (open and arthroscopic) of patellar alignment after initial tubercle mobilization.
5. Rehabilitation protocols should focus on providing early ROM while protecting the osteotomy site.

References

1. Fulkerson JP, Becker GJ, Meaney JA, Miranda M, Folcik MA. Anteromedial tibial tubercle transfer without bone graft. *Am J Sports Med.* 1990;18(5):490-496.
2. Beck PR, Thomas AL, Farr J, Lewis PB, Cole BJ. Trochlear contact pressures after anteromedialization of the tibial tubercle. *Am J Sports Med.* 2005;33(11):1710-1715.
3. Katchburian MV, Bull AM, Shih YF, Heatley FW, Amis AA. Measurement of patellar tracking: assessment and analysis of the literature. *Clin Orthop Relat Res.* 2003;(412):241-259.
4. Sherman SL, Erickson BJ, Cvetanovich GL, et al. Tibial tuberosity osteotomy: indications, techniques, and outcomes. *Am J Sports Med.* 2013;42(8):2006-2017.

5. Bicos J, Fulkerson JP. Indications and technique of distal tibial tubercle anteromedialization. *Oper Tech Orthop.* 2007;17:223-233.
6. Feller JA. Distal realignment (tibial tuberosity transfer). *Sports Med Arthrosc.* 2012;20(3):152-161.
7. Trinh TQ, Harris JD, Siston RA, Flanigan DC. Improved outcomes with combined autologous chondrocyte implantation and patellofemoral osteotomy versus isolated autologous chondrocyte implantation. *Arthroscopy.* 2013;29(3):566-574.
8. Duchman K, Bollier M. Distal realignment: indications, technique, and results. *Clin Sports Med.* 2014;33(3):517-530.
9. Mihalko WM, Boachie-Adjei Y, Spang JT, Fulkerson JP, Arendt EA, Saleh KJ. Controversies and techniques in the surgical management of patellofemoral arthritis. *Instr Course Lect.* 2008;57:365-380.
10. Crossley K, Bennell K, Green S, Cowan S, McConnell J. Physical therapy for patellofemoral pain: a randomized, double-blinded, placebo-controlled trial. *Am J Sports Med.* 2002;30(6):857-865.
11. Doberstein ST, Romeyn RL, Reineke DM. The diagnostic value of the Clarke sign in assessing chondromalacia patella. *J Athl Train.* 2008;43(2):190-196.
12. Salzmann GM, Weber TS, Spang JT, Imhoff AB, Schöttle PB. Comparison of native axial radiographs with axial MR imaging for determination of the trochlear morphology in patients with trochlear dysplasia. *Arch Orthop Trauma Surg.* 2010;130(3):335-340.
13. Dejour H, Walch G, Nove-Josserand L, Guier C. Factors of patellar instability: an anatomic radiographic study. *Knee Surg Sports Traumatol Arthrosc.* 1994;2(1):19-26.
14. Goutallier D, Bernageau J, Lecudonnec B. The measurement of the tibial tuberosity. Patella groove distanced technique and results (author's transl) [in French]. *Rev Chir Orthop Reparatrice Appar Mot.* 1978;64(5):423-428.
15. Camp CL, Stuart MJ, Krych AJ, et al. CT and MRI measurements of tibial tubercle-trochlear groove distances are not equivalent in patients with patellar instability. *Am J Sports Med.* 2013;41(8):1835-1840.
16. Harrison RK, Magnussen RA, Flanigan DC. Avoiding complications in patellofemoral surgery. *Sports Med Arthrosc.* 2013;21(2):121-128.
17. Luhmann SJ, Fuhrhop S, O'Donnell JC, Gordon JE. Tibial fractures after tibial tubercle osteotomies for patellar instability: a comparison of three osteotomy configurations. *J Child Orthop.* 2011;5(1):19-26.
18. Cosgarea AJ, Freedman JA, McFarland EG. Nonunion of the tibial tubercle shingle following Fulkerson osteotomy. *Am J Knee Surg.* 2001;14(1):51-54.
19. Warner BT, Kamath GV, Spang JT, Weinhold PS, Creighton RA. Comparison of fixation methods after anteromedialization osteotomy of the tibial tubercle for patellar instability. *Arthroscopy.* 2013;29(10):1628-1634.
20. Kline AJ, Gonzales J, Beach WR, Miller MD. Vascular risk associated with bicortical tibial drilling during anteromedial tibial tubercle transfer. *Am J Orthop (Belle Mead NJ).* 2006;35(1):30-32.
21. Tompkins M, Arendt EA. Complications in patellofemoral surgery. *Sports Med Arthrosc.* 2012;20(3):187-193.

Please see videos on the accompanying website at www.routledge.com/9781617119996

SECTION IV

Articular Cartilage

14

Arthroscopic Approach to Knee Osteoarthritis

Timothy M. Bert, MD and Jack M. Bert, MD

Introduction

Osteoarthritis is a common condition treated by a range of nonoperative modalities, including nonsteroidal anti-inflammatory drugs, analgesics, weight loss, activity modification, intra-articular injections of steroids or hyaluronic acid, muscle strengthening, and off-loading the affected compartment with unloader bracing or a heel wedge.[1] When nonoperative measures fail, arthroscopic intervention may be considered. Arthroscopic surgery as a possible intervention to osteoarthritis has been commonly performed to alleviate symptoms and possibly delay future arthroplasty. As the prevalence of arthroscopy has increased, so has the interest in outcomes because there is currently no conclusive evidence that arthroscopy delays or arrests the progression of osteoarthritis.[2]

Conflicting opinions based on the current literature regarding arthroscopic debridement in knee osteoarthritis are explained by the wide range of inclusion criteria, surgical procedures, and outcome measures used in different studies.[3] Arthroscopic debridement comprises a variety of procedures combined into a single operation. Lavage removes the mechanical irritating products and evacuates degradative enzymes potentially contributing to joint degeneration. Partial meniscectomy, articular cartilage shaving, and loose body removal are also commonly performed to improve mechanical symptomatology. On occasion, surgeons also perform a limited synovectomy or osteophyte excision. As a result, the literature has become somewhat confusing and discordant. This controversy has been highlighted in several randomized controlled trials.[4]

Since 2002, there have been 6 randomized controlled trials of arthroscopic management of knee osteoarthritis published, including 2 focusing on the efficacy of arthroscopic debridement and lavage on pain and function[5,6] and 4 on the efficacy of arthroscopic partial meniscectomy in patients with symptomatic meniscal tears and underlying mild to moderate knee osteoarthritis.[7-9]

In a study comparing arthroscopic debridement, arthroscopic lavage, and a placebo group who had skin incisions only, Moseley et al[5] showed no difference at 2-year follow-up between the 3 treatment groups. The conclusion was that the results were similar for the lavage and debridement group compared to the placebo group.[5] Multiple potential biases to this study were

Sgaglione NA, Lubowitz JH, Provencher MT, eds. *The Knee: AANA Advanced Arthroscopic Surgical Techniques* (pp 189-196).

identified. Of the veterans, 44% declined to participate, all procedures were performed by a single surgeon (performance bias), outcomes were self-reported with an invalidated knee score (detection bias), and no patients with positive magnetic resonance imaging (MRI) findings for internal derangement were included in this study.[4,10]

Kirkley et al[6] published a study in 2008 in which patients with moderate to severe osteoarthritis were randomized into the following 2 groups: surgical lavage and arthroscopic debridement with physical and medical therapy vs nonoperative treatment, including physical and medical therapy only. The arthroscopic group had better outcomes at 3 months, but no difference existed at 2 years between the groups.[6] Patients with large symptomatic meniscal tears were excluded from the study. This inclusion bias was the largest flaw in the study because these patients typically benefit from arthroscopic debridement in association with knee osteoarthritis.[4]

Despite Moseley et al's[5] and Kirkley et al's[6] studies, the question of whether surgery is more effective than a standardized nonoperative regimen in patients with symptomatic meniscal tear and concomitant knee osteoarthritis remains unanswered. Four studies have been published in the past several years that begin to address these questions about the role of surgery in patients with meniscal tears and concomitant osteoarthritis.

Herrlin et al[7] evaluated patients with knee pain, meniscal tears on MRI, and radiographic osteoarthritis. They compared 2 groups treated with arthroscopic partial meniscectomy and those treated with exercise alone using multiple functional outcome scores at 6-month and 5-year follow-up. The results were similar at both points of follow-up between patients treated with arthroscopy and those treated with exercise. However, 30% of patients from the nonoperative group did not have satisfactory pain relief and received an arthroscopic partial meniscectomy, noting significant improvement after the procedure.[7]

The Meniscal Tear in Osteoarthritis Research (MeTeOR) Trial shared many design similarities to the study by Herrlin et al[7] but was considerably larger, with 351 subjects from 7 centers. Patients with MRI-documented meniscal tears with radiographic osteoarthritis were randomized to a standardized physical therapy regimen or arthroscopic partial meniscectomy with postoperative physical therapy. Functional outcomes were measured at 6 and 12 months and showed no differences between the groups. Similar to the Herrlin et al[7] study, 30% of the subjects crossed over from nonoperative therapy to surgery.[8]

Yim et al[9] published a randomized controlled trial of arthroscopic partial meniscectomy vs nonoperative regimen focused on strengthening on 102 subjects with symptomatic meniscal tears. They found no significant difference in outcomes at 2-year follow-up. However, unlike Herrlin et al[7] and the MeTeOR trials, only 1 patient crossed over from the nonoperative arm to surgery.[9]

Sihvonen et al[11] reported on a randomized controlled trial of arthroscopic partial meniscectomy vs sham surgery for symptomatic degenerative medial meniscal tear without knee osteoarthritis in 146 patients. Like those of Moseley et al[5] and Kirkley et al,[6] Sihvonen et al's subjects showed no difference in outcomes at 12 months.[11]

Given that the current literature has not been conclusive in showing a clear benefit, arthroscopy continues to be used for patients with arthropathy. Fedorka et al[12] examined the incidence and rates of knee arthroscopy in patients younger than 65 years and the subsequent risk of knee arthroplasty. They found that the conversion rate to arthroplasty was dependent on the age of the patient. Patients in the younger than 65 years age group had a conversion rate of 4.1% within 5 years of arthroscopy for all patients. Patients older than 65 years had a higher conversion rate of 10.2% undergoing arthroplasty within 1 year of arthroscopy. The age of the patient and extent of arthritis play a role in who benefits from an arthroscopy in the presence of arthropathy.[12]

Indications

Regardless of the controversy, arthroscopic surgery is an effective procedure in young and select middle-aged patients with knee osteoarthritis. Patients with severe osteoarthritis do not seem to benefit from arthroscopy.[2] However, some patients with mild to moderate osteoarthritis may have the following:

- Symptomatic meniscus pathology
- Impinging osteophytes
- Loose bodies

Patients with these findings may benefit greatly from arthroscopic treatment. The goal of arthroscopy in this setting is to reduce mechanical irritation and thus reduce symptomatic synovitis. Removal of loose bodies and debridement of unstable cartilage can be performed. The indications for arthroscopic debridement, partial meniscectomy, and/or loose body removal include the discrete chief complaints of the following:

- Acute onset of well-localized joint line pain
- Mechanical symptoms, such as catching or locking[13]

The x-rays should demonstrate normal or near normal alignment, mild to moderate degenerative changes, and a large meniscal tear confirmed by MRI.

Occasionally, an athlete with advanced arthritis may be a candidate for arthroscopy to relieve acute pain and mechanical symptoms. Symptoms typically present as the abrupt onset of a severe, sharp pain in the involved compartment along with catching or locking. The goals of surgery need to be limited to relieve the mechanical symptoms but not the arthritic pain.

Controversial Indications

- Persistent pain with mild to moderate osteoarthritis without specific mechanical symptoms. In at least one study, there appears to some benefit in postponing total knee arthroplasty (TKA) by several years subsequent to arthroscopic debridement.[12]

Pertinent Physical Findings

The primary indication for arthroscopic surgery in a patient presenting with knee osteoarthritis includes the following:

- Distinct presentation of symptoms of well-localized, acute-onset joint line pain
- Mechanical symptoms, such as catching or locking, that have failed nonoperative modalities

Physical examination should include a comprehensive evaluation of the involved knee including the following

- Range of motion (ROM)
- Stability
- Assessing areas of tenderness on palpation
- Presence of an effusion
- Alignment

Particularly, clinical variables that have shown greater improvement after arthroscopic debridement are preoperative joint line tenderness and a positive Steinman test indicative of a torn, unstable meniscus. This has correlated well with the findings of unstable meniscal tissue at the time of surgery.[14] The senior author (JMB) has noted that a positive Steinman test (joint line tenderness at

90 degrees of flexion medially or laterally in internal and external rotation), pain with hyperextension, and effusion almost always confirm a symptomatic torn meniscus. Improved outcomes from arthroscopic debridement are a reduction in pain and mechanical symptoms resulting from loose bodies, displaced articular chondral lesions, and meniscal tears.[2-4]

Pertinent Imaging

Preoperative radiography should consist of the following:

- Standing schuss or Rosenberg view (posteroanterior film of both knees flexed at 30 degrees)
- Lateral view
- Merchant view

Best Test

The schuss view is suggested as the most accurate method for the evaluation of joint-space narrowing in knee osteoarthritis.[15] A standard anteroposterior view may underestimate the amount of osteoarthritis present.

The need for MRI is based on the initial history, examination, x-rays, and response to prior treatment. MRI typically is obtained in patients considered candidates for arthroscopic intervention to assess for loose bodies not visualized on x-rays, meniscal pathology, and potential unstable chondral flaps.[3,4]

Equipment

- Gravity inflow is a common method for infusing the joint. As technology has improved, the fluid pump has gained popularity. It has the advantage of improved hemostasis and higher pressures. Selection of outflow also plays an important role in distention of the joint and providing a clear view. Continuous outflow, whether gravity or suction, will result in greater fluid use; therefore, intermittent outflow controlled by the surgeon or an assistant may be preferable.
- Shavers and occasionally burrs are used during arthroscopy to debride chondral flaps, perform meniscectomies, and shave osteophytes. Shavers are typically available in different sizes and levels of aggressiveness. In general, the smallest and least aggressive shaver should be used.
- The selection and proper use of an arthroscopic camera allows the surgeon to examine all areas of the knee joint efficiently. Most surgeons prefer the 30-degree arthroscope for most procedures. The 70-degree arthroscope is used if a larger view is needed, such as in the posterior aspect of the knee.
- Cannulas are not used frequently in the knee but can be useful for posterior portals. Metal cannulas are useful for posterior portals because shavers can screw into the cannula directly and, with the use of an adapter, the camera can be exchanged between cannulas.
- Other basic working instruments needed for knee arthroscopy include a probe, spinal needle, basket punches (narrow, wide, straight, upbiting, curved, left, right, and back), graspers, cutters, and varying types of shavers, burrs, and cautery. Basket punches are available in various shapes and selection should be based on surgeon preference. More important than the shape, a variety of different angled and curved basket punches should be available so that all areas of the joint can be accessed.

Positioning and Portals

Proper patient positioning is important in terms of patient safety and surgical efficiency. A standard operating room bed is needed. It is the surgeon's responsibility to oversee patient positioning. The use of leg holders is determined by the preoperative diagnosis, surgical plan, and surgeon preference. In most cases, a unilateral leg holder or lateral post is used for the operative leg. Leg holders may include padding, and some others may require you to pad the leg prior to securing it to the leg holder. If you prefer a unilateral holder or lateral post, it will be important to determine how to protect the contralateral leg. The use of a leg holder for the nonoperative leg has been shown to increase the risk of compression to the peroneal nerve.[16] If the foot of the bed is left up for a lateral post, place padding under the nonoperative leg. If the foot is dropped, it is often easiest to place a large pad under the nonoperative thigh to keep the hip flexed.

The advantage of a lateral post is faster setup and positioning, ability to hyperflex the knee, and ease of placing the knee in a figure-4 position. The primary disadvantage is that the leg can slip over the post during valgus stress, which can be prevented by having an assistant push down on the thigh. The major disadvantages associated with a fixed leg holder are the risk of rupturing the medial collateral ligament (MCL) with excess valgus stress and that knee flexion is limited by the lowered portion of the table and inability to move the leg freely.

Step-by-Step Description of the Procedure

A superomedial portal is made using a stab skin incision. A 4.5-cm metal cannula is placed with a dull trochar, and a Christmas tree adaptor is placed (senior author's technique). This serves as the inflow cannula, which allows for rapid large volume inflow into the joint. The arthroscope is placed through a lateral portal, and a drainage tube is placed onto one of the outflow portals. Any loose bodies larger than 3 to 4 mm are grasped with a Schlessinger or a grasping tool through a medial portal and removed (Figure 14-1). Loose debris is removed using motorized shavers connected to suction. If there is a meniscal tear, this should be resected, leaving as much stable rim as possible (Video). More often than not, a 5.5-mm diameter shaver works well to perform the debridement unless the knee is tight medially and requires the use of a shaver with a smaller diameter to avoid injury to the femoral and tibial articular surfaces. Usually, the knee is more lax as a result of degenerative changes in the joint with associated MCL and anterior collateral ligament laxity. A chondroplasty should be performed on all surfaces that have loose fragments adjacent to eburnated bone as well as those with grade III lesions on femoral, tibial, or patellofemoral articular surfaces. After completion of a thorough debridement and chondroplasty in a significantly degenerative knee with grade IV lesions on the femoral and tibial surfaces (Figure 14-2), the instruments are removed, wounds are closed with suture and dressings, and a toe-to-groin ACE wrap is applied. The senior author does not use a tourniquet and injects lidocaine with epinephrine immediately prior to the surgical procedure to afford less bleeding intraoperatively. Usage of a tourniquet has been implicated in an increase in the incidence of phlebitis and pulmonary embolus post arthroscopy.[16]

Postoperative Protocol

The postoperative protocol is based on the specific pathology treated. For loose body removal, chondroplasty, and meniscectomies, rehabilitation may progress aggressively because there is no anatomic structure that requires protection. The protocol should involve 3 phases. Progression to the next phase should be based on clinical criteria and meeting the established goals for each

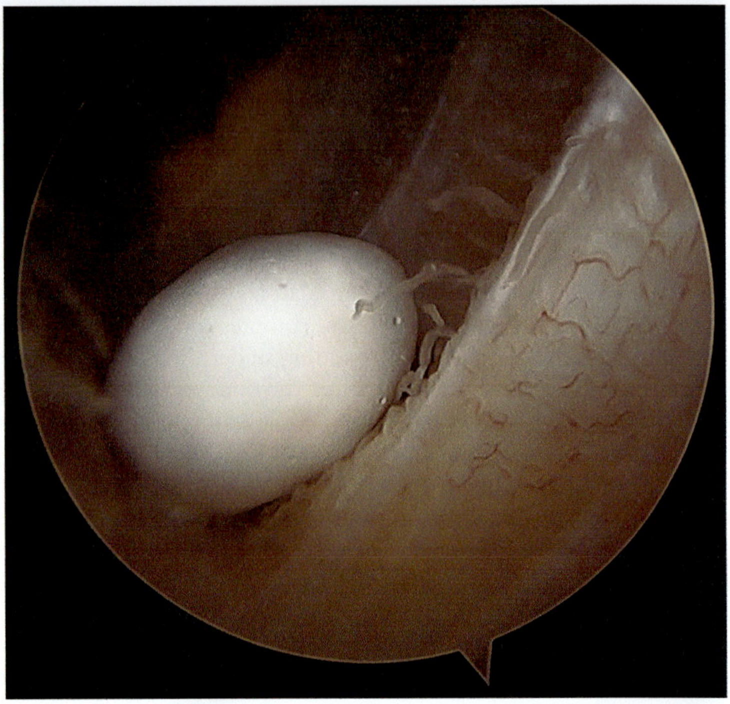

Figure 14-1. Loose body in the medial peripatellar gutter.

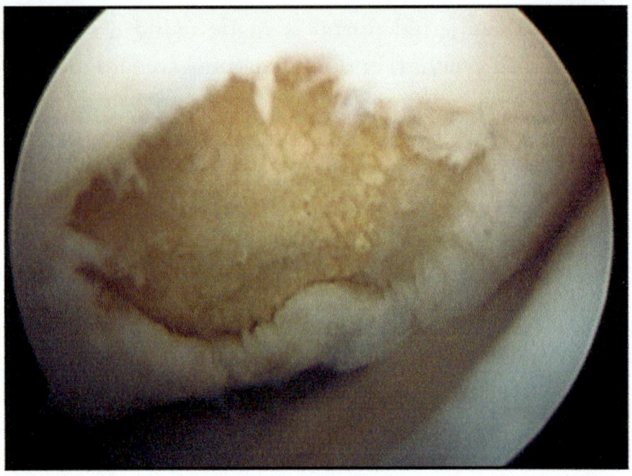

Figure 14-2. Well-contoured bone/cartilage interface of the femoral and tibial surface with grade IV lesions subsequent to debridement.

phase. Phase 1 is the acute phase and consists of diminishing pain and edema, restoring knee ROM, reestablishing quadriceps muscle activity, and educating the patient on weightbearing as tolerated, use of crutches, icing, elevation, and the rehabilitation process. Phase 2 goals are to restore and improve muscle strength and endurance; reestablish full, pain-free ROM; a gradual return to functional activities; restore normal gait without an assistive device; and improve balance and proprioception. Phase 3 goals include enhancing muscular strength and endurance, maintaining full ROM, and returning to sports, functional activities, and work tasks.[2-4]

Potential Complications

Doing knee arthroscopy for any reason results in overall complication rates ranging from 0.8% to 1.8%. Intraoperative complications include further articular cartilage damage (scuffing), instrument breakage, and neurological and vascular injury. The senior author uses a technique of partial release of the MCL with an arthroscopic electrocautery intra-articularly, or a motorized shaver if the joint is tight medially. Creating a Type II MCL tear should have no effect on the patient long term as opposed to an injury to the articular surface, which will cause permanent damage to the articular surface. Capsular herniation can occur when a portion of the capsule is excised near the portal, causing free communication between the joint and subcutaneous tissue. This can be painful and cosmetically displeasing. Postoperative complications can also include thromboembolism, worsening pain, hemarthrosis, infection, effusion and synovitis, complex regional pain syndrome, and infrapatellar contracture.[16-19] It is important to have a thorough medical preoperative assessment, diligent arthroscopic procedure, and careful postoperative management as well.

Conclusion

Arthroscopic debridement can benefit patients with mild to moderate arthritis and mechanical complaints of pain. It can postpone the need for unicompartmental and TKA and is particularly beneficial in younger patients who wish to remain physically active and in patients with significant comorbidities that would make undertaking TKA medically undesirable. The surgeon and the patient must understand that the results of the operation will not completely alleviate the patient's complaints of pain but will afford him or her partial relief and hopefully prevent the necessity of TKA for several years.

Top Technical Pearls for the Procedure

1. Make certain that that all loose bodies and chondral flaps are removed from the joint surface using a motorized shaver and/or grasper.
2. Proceed with medial and/or lateral meniscectomy, removing all unstable meniscal fragments back to a stable rim.
3. Examine the peripatellar gutters, perform a partial synovectomy if there is erythematous redundant synovium, and perform a subpatellar shave for grade II or grade III surface changes.
4. When performing chondroplasty of arthritic joint surfaces, make certain that the edges of grade III lesions are debrided and contoured to avoid sharp edges at the bone-cartilage interface to avoid further detachment of chondral flaps post debridement at the bone-cartilage interface.
5. Do not perform microfracture on the eburnated grade IV joint surfaces subsequent to debridement. There is no evidence that microfracture improves clinical results any better than debridement alone.

References

1. Richmond J, Hunter D, Irrgang J, et al. Treatment of osteoarthritis of the knee (nonarthroplasty). *J Am Acad Orthop Surg.* 2009;17(9):591-600.
2. Dervin GF, Stiell IG, Rody K, Grabowski J. Effect of arthroscopic débridement for osteoarthritis of the knee on health-related quality of life. *J Bone Joint Surg Am.* 2003;85(1):10-19.
3. Bert J. Arthroscopic treatment of degenerative arthritis of the knee. In: Scott WN, Scuderi G, eds. *Insall & Scott Surgery of the Knee.* 5th ed. Philadelphia, PA: Churchill Livingstone; 2012:229-234.
4. Krych AJ, Bert JM, Levy BA. Treatment of OA of the knee in the middle-aged athlete: the role of arthroscopy. *Sports Med Arthrosc.* 2013;21(1):23-30.
5. Moseley JB, O'Malley K, Petersen NJ, et al. A controlled trial of arthroscopic surgery for osteoarthritis of the knee. *N Engl J Med.* 2002;347(2):81-88.
6. Kirkley A, Birmingham TB, Litchfield RB, et al. A randomized trial of arthroscopic surgery for osteoarthritis of the knee. *N Engl J Med.* 2008;359(11):1097-1107.
7. Herrlin S, Hållander M, Wange P, Weidenhielm L, Werner S. Arthroscopic or conservative treatment of degenerative medial meniscal tears: a prospective randomised trial. *Knee Surg Sports Traumatol Arthrosc.* 2007;15(4):393-401.
8. Katz JN, Brophy RH, Chaisson CE, et al. Surgery versus physical therapy for a meniscal tear and osteoarthritis. *N Engl J Med.* 2013;368(18):1675-1684.
9. Yim JH, Seon JK, Song EK, et al. A comparative study of meniscectomy and nonoperative treatment for degenerative horizontal tears of the medial meniscus. *Am J Sports Med.* 2013;41(7):1565-1570.
10. Horng S, Miller FG. Is placebo surgery unethical? *N Engl J Med.* 2002;347(2):137-139.
11. Sihvonen R, Paavola N, Malmivaara A, et al. Arthroscopic partial meniscectomy versus sham surgery for a degenerative meniscal tear. *N Engl J Med.* 2013;369(26):2515-2524.
12. Fedorka CJ, Cerynik DL, Tauberg B, Toossi N, Johanson NA. The relationship between knee arthroscopy and arthroplasty in patients under 65 years of age. *J Arthroplasty.* 2014;29(2):335-338.
13. Marx RG. Arthroscopic surgery for osteoarthritis of the knee? *N Engl J Med.* 2008;359(11):1169-1170.
14. Fond J, Rodin D, Ahmad S, Nirschl RP. Arthroscopic debridement for the treatment of osteoarthritis of the knee: 2 -and 5-year results. *Arthroscopy.* 2002;18(8):829-834.
15. Piperno M, Hellio Le Graverand MP, Conrozier T, Bochu M, Mathieu P, Vignon E. Quantitative evaluation of joint space width in femorotibial osteoarthritis: comparison of three radiographic views. *Osteoarthritis Cartilage.* 1998;6(4):252-259.
16. Bert J, Bert T. Complications of knee arthroscopy. In: *AANA Advanced Arthroscopy: The Knee.* Philadelphia, PA: Saunders Elsevier; 2010:5:37-44.
17. DeLee JC. Complications of arthroscopy and arthroscopic surgery: results of a national survey. *Arthroscopy.* 1985;1:214-220.
18. Small NC. Complications in arthroscopic surgery performed by experienced arthroscopists. *Arthroscopy.* 1998;4:215-221.
19. Rodeo S, Forster R, Weiland A. Current concepts review: neurological complications due to arthroscopy. *J Bone Joint Surg Am.* 1993;75:917-926.

Please see videos on the accompanying website at www.routledge.com/9781617119996

15

Arthroscopic Approaches to Osteochondritis Dissecans

Kevin G. Shea, MD; Nathan L. Grimm, MD; John D. Polousky, MD; Theodore J. Ganley, MD; and Alexandra Styhl, BA

Introduction

Osteochondritis dissecans (OCD) is described as a focal, idiopathic alteration of subchondral bone with risk for instability and disruption of adjacent articular cartilage that may result in premature osteoarthritis.[1] When describing OCD lesions, the parent bone refers to the normal bone structure surrounding the abnormal progeny bone. The cartilage over the progeny bone is part of the OCD lesion, with a well-defined bone margin apparent on imaging.

OCD lesions can be found in the shoulder, elbow, hip, ankle, and foot, but they are most common in the knee. Approximately 60% to 70% occur at the medial femoral condyle and about 20% to 30% at the lateral femoral condyle, with rare cases in the trochlea, patella, and tibial plateau.[2,3] Few higher level of evidence studies have been reported on OCD of the knee, such as randomized clinical trials and prospective cohort studies. Thus, the strength of recommendations for treatment options is limited. The recent 2010 American Academy of Orthopaedic Surgeons Guideline for treatment of OCD of the knee revealed a paucity of high-level research in this area.[4]

In skeletally immature patients, stable OCD lesions (those with intact overlying cartilage) may progress toward healing in the majority of patients, with appropriate activity restrictions, including activity and motion limitations.[5] The specific restrictions and length of nonoperative treatment vary. Different healing rates have been described, with success rates of 60% to 90%[6,7] to less than 60%.[5,8-10] Significant healing may take 6 to 18 months, and prolonged activity restrictions may lead to loss of motion, muscle atrophy, poor treatment compliance, family frustration, and psychosocial impact of prolonged absence from sports participation.[8,11-13]

Sgaglione NA, Lubowitz JH, Provencher MT, eds. *The Knee: AANA Advanced Arthroscopic Surgical Techniques* (pp 197-215).

PART ONE: TREATMENT OF EARLY STAGE, STABLE OSTEOCHONDRITIS DISSECANS LESIONS OF THE KNEE

Indications

- Failure of nonoperative treatment
- Failure of a stable lesion to demonstrate radiographic healing with persistence of clinical symptoms longer than 3 to 6 months[14]
- Arthroscopic demonstration of unstable lesion surface, margins, and fragmentation

Cartilage lesion stability is an important consideration when evaluating OCD lesions. Instability may be assessed by magnetic resonance imaging (MRI) evaluation. Kijowski et al[15] defined criteria for stability in those with open physes based upon the following MRI findings.

Magnetic Resonance Imaging Findings of Instability in Osteochondritis Dissecans With Open Physes

- High T2 signal rim indicates instability only if it is the same signal intensity as the joint fluid, **and**
- The lesion is surrounded by a second, low T2 signal rim **or**
- The lesion demonstrates multiple breaks in the subchondral bone plate
- Cysts suggest instability only if they are large (> 5 mm) or there are multiple

Perhaps the most important determinant of lesion instability is the arthroscopic inspection. In stable lesions, the cartilage surfaces are contiguous and intact. In unstable lesions, the cartilage margins between the surrounding parent bone and involved progeny bone are significantly demarcated or grossly unstable. A recent unpublished classification of OCD lesion of the knee separated these into 2 broad categories, including stable and unstable lesions.[16] Stable lesions are more likely to heal with minimally invasive procedures, whereas unstable lesions may require more complex arthroscopic surgery, internal fixation, arthrotomy, and/or bone grafting. More advanced lesions may not be completely salvageable, requiring more complex procedures, such as osteochondral allografts or autologous bone and cartilage implantation.

Subchondral Bone Drilling/Stimulation for Stable Osteochondritis Dissecans Lesions

This approach includes trans- and retroarticular drilling. Transarticular drilling involves direct drilling (with small K-wires) across the cartilage, into the OCD lesion (or progeny bone), and continuing into the normal (parent) bone. Retroarticular drilling starts in the epiphysis (avoiding the physis) through the parent bone, into the progeny bone, and not drilling through the articular cartilage of the joint (Figure 15-1).

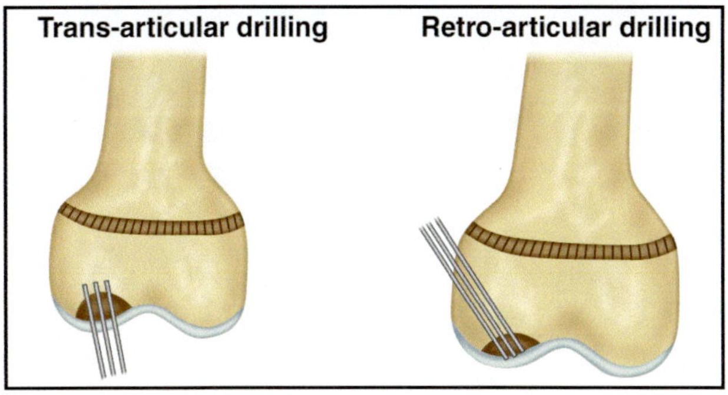

Figure 15-1. Subchondral bone drilling options.

Indications for Subchondral Bone Drilling for Stable Osteochondritis Dissecans Lesions

Trans- and retroarticular of drilling are indicated for skeletally immature patients with stable lesions of the femoral condyles. Studies demonstrate excellent outcomes for both drilling techniques.[12,17-22] Patient selection criteria include the following:

- Diagnosis of OCD
- Lesion located on the medial or lateral femoral condyle
- Lesion considered stable, based on MRI
- Patient deemed skeletally immature based on the following:
  - MRI
  - Bone age film (female younger than 14 years, male younger than 16 years), although results may be better if females are younger than 12, and males younger than 14 by skeletal age
- Completed a 3- to 6-month course of conservative therapy

Patients may be excluded from this protocol for clinical reasons, including the following:

- History of steroid use for other conditions, including autoimmune disease, malignancy, etc
- History of radiation to the affected joint
- Metabolic bone disease
- Sickle cell disease

Trans- vs Retroarticular Subchondral Bone Drilling

Transarticular drilling has been described as retrograde or intra-articular drilling historically. The authors prefer the term *transarticular* because it is a better descriptor for the techniques and avoids confusion with drilling behind the cartilage. Transarticular drilling has the advantage that the technique is straightforward and can be accomplished with minimal drilling orientation challenges, with minimal to no use of the C-arm for imaging (see Figure 15-1). When the lesion can be clearly seen arthroscopically, C-arm use may not be necessary. In some cases with entirely normal-appearing cartilage, the C-arm may be necessary to confirm lesion location. The disadvantage is that the technique crosses the hyaline cartilage, and questions about the long-term impact on cartilage have been raised.[17]

Retro-articular drilling has been described as anterograde or extra-articular, but these latter terms can lead to confusion. Retroarticular drilling has the distinct advantage in that it avoids crossing the hyaline joint cartilage and drills through the normal parent bone of the epiphyseal region into the lesion or progeny bone (see Figure 15-1). The limitations of this technique are longer surgical time, challenges of using the C-arm to obtain ideal images to confirm pin placement,

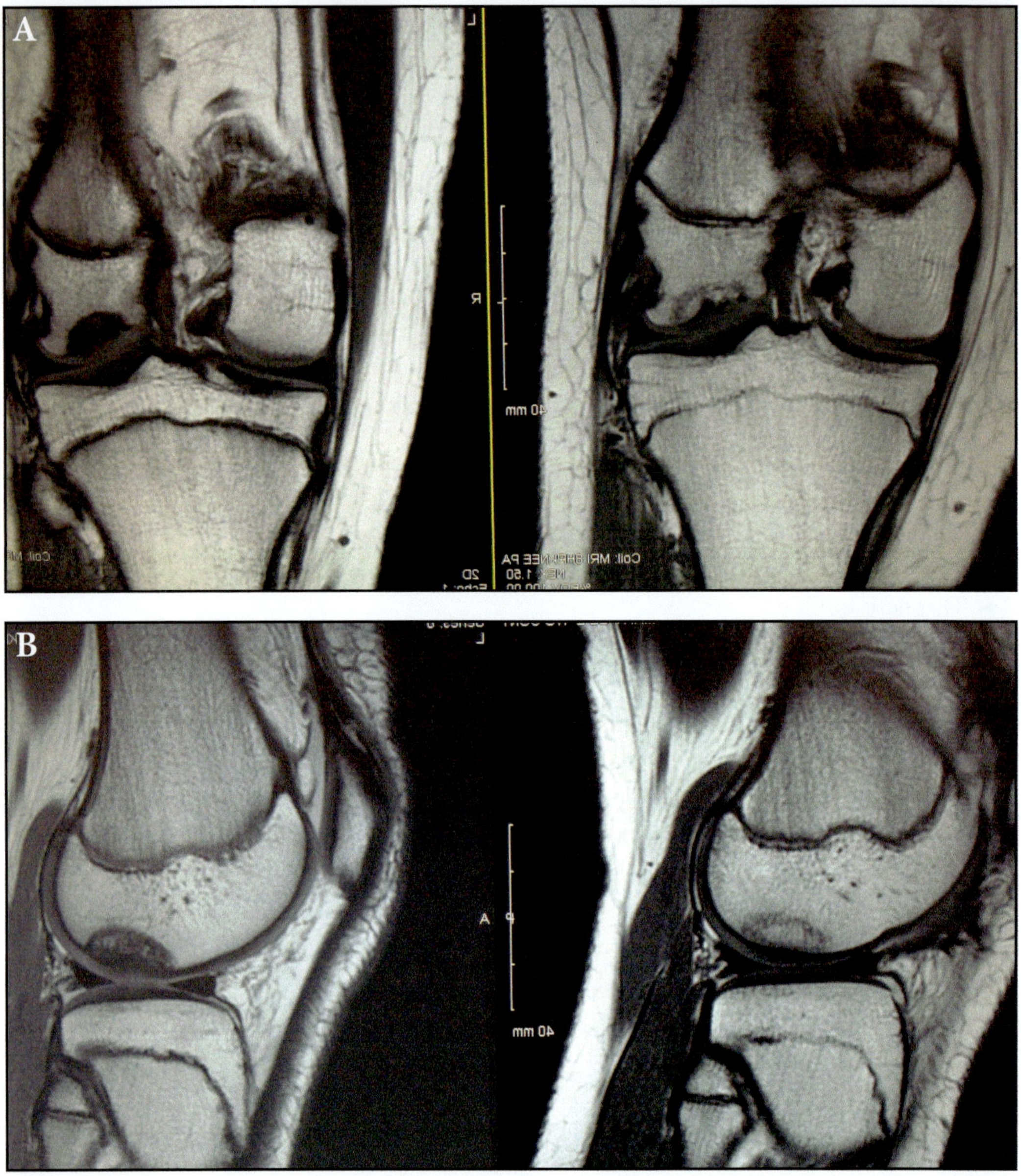

Figure 15-2. MRI findings (A) before and (B) 3 months after drilling in a 13-year-old female soccer player.

and the use of significantly more radiation. The longer radiation exposure has implications for the patient and the operating room team. Surgical technique that consistently produces adequate drilling into the lesion/progeny bone can be challenging; whether this technique can be accurately reproduced in general use is a concern.[18]

Trans- and retroarticular techniques have excellent outcomes at short-term follow-up. Healing rates for transarticular drilling have been reported at 70% to 90% or greater.[12,18,19] Healing rates for retroarticular drilling have been reported at 75% or greater (Figure 15-2).[17,20-22]

Controversial Indications

- OCD lesions with instability should not be treated with isolated subchondral bone drilling. Although this technique may supplement the treatment for more advanced lesions, adjuvant procedures may be required to obtain lesion stability and a healthy subchondral bone environment that promotes healing between the parent and progeny bone.

- Older patients, including those with fusing (closing) or fused (closed) physes, and some larger lesions, are usually not candidates for isolated subchondral bone healing.
- Children with a history of malignancy, autoimmune disease, or other conditions requiring steroid use may develop lesions similar to OCD. These lesions are difficult to treat, and the treatment principles of OCD may not apply.

Pertinent Physical Findings

- Antalgic gait
- Focal localized joint line pain

The best candidates for subchondral bone drilling include those with a history of knee pain, significant growth remaining, and without mechanical symptoms, swelling, or other elements that suggest lesion instability. The Wilson test, which is based upon the principle that the tibial eminence impinges upon the lateral aspect of the medial femoral condyle, is not a consistent finding in these patients and is typically positive in patients with large lesions at the classic lateral aspect medial femoral condyle location.[23,24] Effusion is rarely present, although some patients/families may report a perception of swelling. Mechanical symptoms are rare in stable lesions. In rare cases, patients may have symptomatic plica bands, which can mimic mechanical symptoms in the absence of obvious cartilage breach or fragment instability. The best clinical test for OCD may be having the patient localize the pain over the femoral condyles and eliciting pain with firm palpation in this area. In many cases, these examination findings may be absent, and clinical suspicion is important.

Pertinent Imaging

Four-view series knee x-rays are valuable in the first stage of evaluation. A notch view will frequently reveal lesions that are located more posteriorly on the condyles, making them difficult to visualize on an anteroposterior (AP) view (Figure 15-3). The lateral view should be evaluated closely because the lesions may not be readily apparent without close inspection of the condyles and the trochlea. Merchant and trochlear views will reveal the rare trochlear groove lesions, more commonly seen in the lateral aspect.

In younger patients with smaller and stable lesions, MRI may not be necessary at the first stage of evaluation. Radiographic evaluation may be limited in the ability to detect subtle signs of lesion instability, and MRI is a valuable tool for more comprehensive evaluation of size, location, subchondral changes suggestive of lesion instability, or frank cartilage breach. The authors' usual practice is to obtain an MRI in most patients with an OCD. In addition to the findings described by Kijowski et al,[15] findings on the MRI that suggest instability include the following:

- A clear break/breach in the articular cartilage
- Radially oriented linear markings in the articular cartilage
- Disruption of normal cartilage contour in the progeny region compared with the surrounding bone and cartilage
- Significant T2 sequence signal changes within and/or behind the progeny bone. Signal changes in these regions that mimic the intra-articular fluid are suggestive of a breach in the cartilage surface.[15]

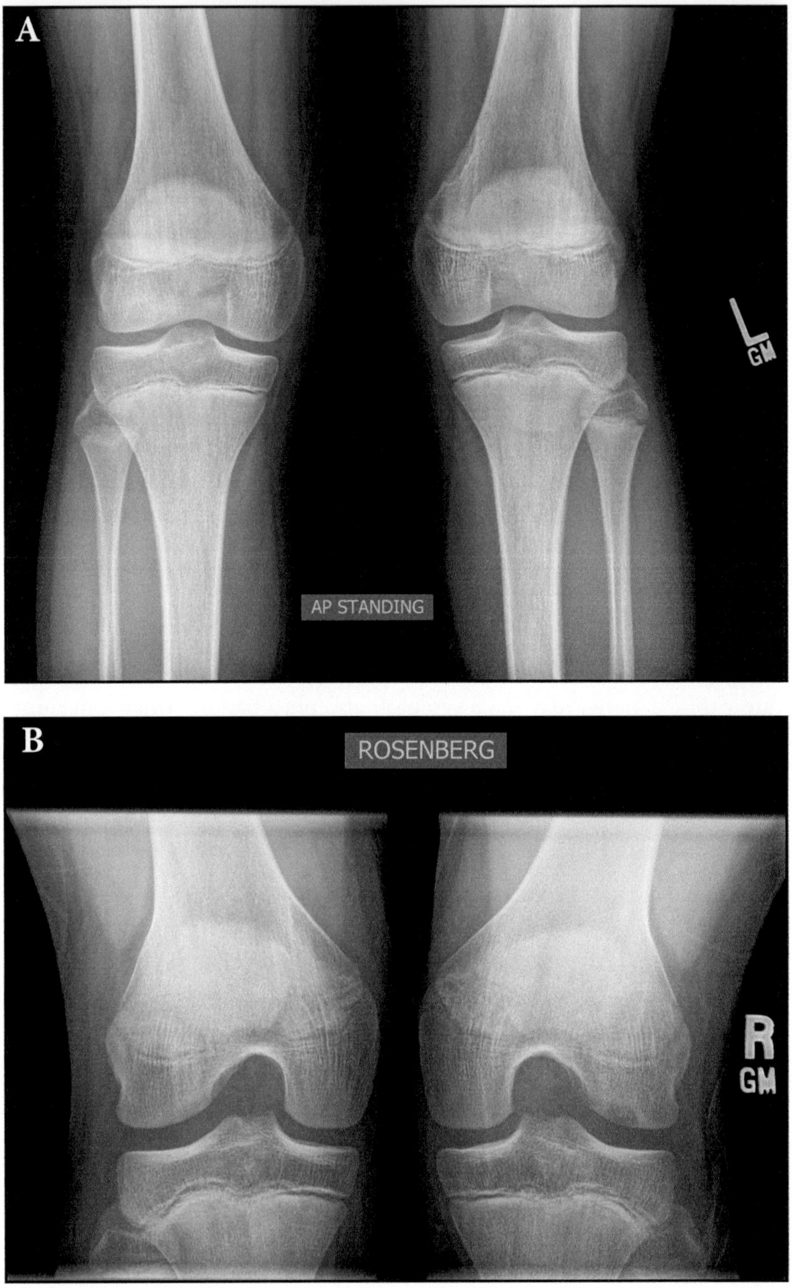

Figure 15-3. (A) AP and (B) notch view with inadequate/adequate visualization of the posterior OCD lesion.

Equipment

The equipment necessary for the procedure includes the following:

- Routine knee arthroscopy equipment
- K-wires of 4 or 9 inches in length. Longer K-wires may be better for retroarticular drilling, but both lengths work well for transarticular drilling.
- K-wire driver. Drivers with an adjustable wire collet are superior to those that use a Jacob's chuck.

- C-arm. The use of a large or small C-arm is appropriate.
  - The large C-arm provides excellent images but may be limited by several factors, including the following:
    - Requirement for extra staff to operate the machine
    - Higher doses of radiation for the patient and operating room staff
  - A relatively new and/or updated small or mini C-arm allows for excellent images in most cases, and the field of view is adequate for seeing the entire knee joint during drilling. This also allows the surgeon to rapidly move the C-arm around the surgical field, and additional operating room staff is not required for operation.
- Heavy-duty needle drivers, such as sternal needle drivers, for K-wire removal in the case of a bent wire
- Parallel pin guide for drilling co-linear pins. These are available in many small fragment screw sets.

Positioning and Portals

Different patient positioning options exist for the surgeon. The use of an operating room table with the knee hanging off the edge of the table is a consistent arthroscopic positioning used by many surgeons. The use of a knee holder may make C-arm visualization more challenging, and the surgeon may consider forgoing the use of a thigh holder for this reason. This allows for more flexibility of the thigh, knee, and leg position, to obtain the ideal orientation for the C-arm.

Another patient position is to use a fully extended and radiolucent operating room table in which the knee may be fully extended and supported by the end of the table (Figure 15-4). The knee may be flexed and the thigh internally/externally to allow for optimal C-arm positioning and visualization of the OCD lesion during drilling. The thigh may be positioned such that it rotates off the side of the table, allowing the C-arm to easily image the knee joint off the side of the table (Figure 15-5).

Step-by-Step Description of the Procedure

- Availability of images: Review all previous MRIs and x-rays at the start of the case, and have these available during the case to guide drilling. A close inspection of these images just before and during the case can help plan the guide pin orientation. The preoperative planning will greatly increase the efficiency of the drilling and improve the surgeon's confidence in the accuracy of the drilling.
- Position the C-arm and monitor such that the surgeon will be able to see the knee x-ray without looking away from the operative field. The surgeon should avoid looking over his or her shoulder or away from the surgical field because this may impact drilling accuracy. The hand holding the K-wire driver may change position if the surgeon's head is moved away from the surgical field to look at the monitor.
- Tourniquet use is at the discretion of the surgeon, although in the authors' experience, these cases can be performed with excellent visualization without the use of a tourniquet.

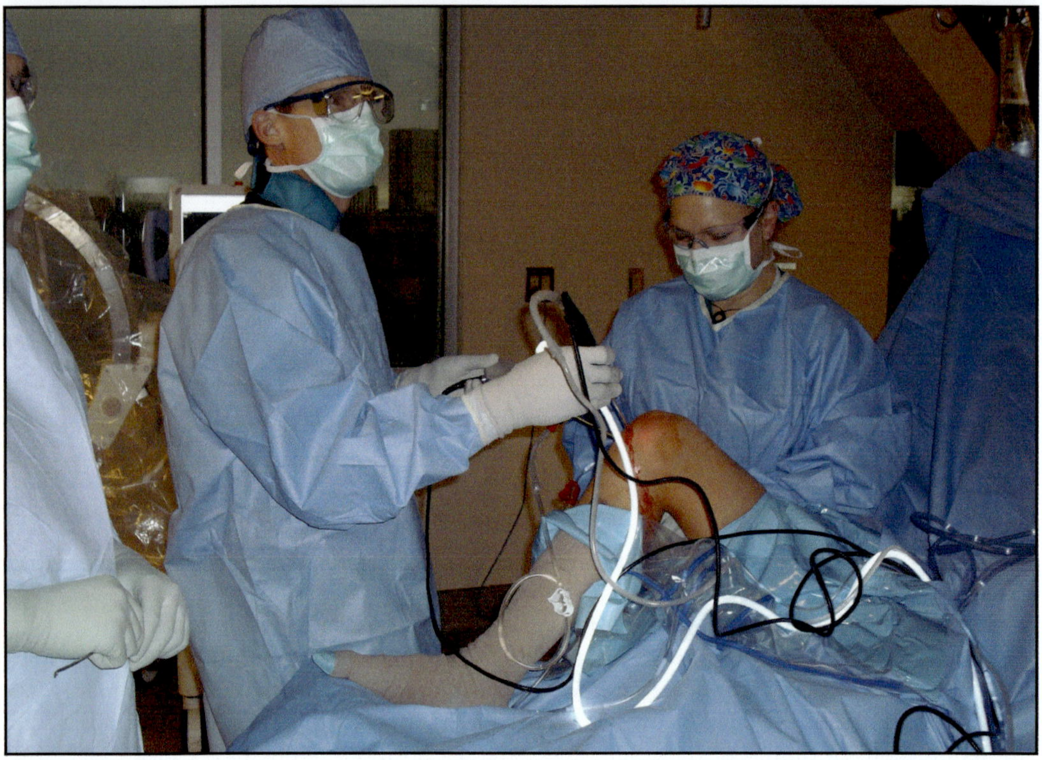

Figure 15-4. Leg position with the end of the table in full extension.

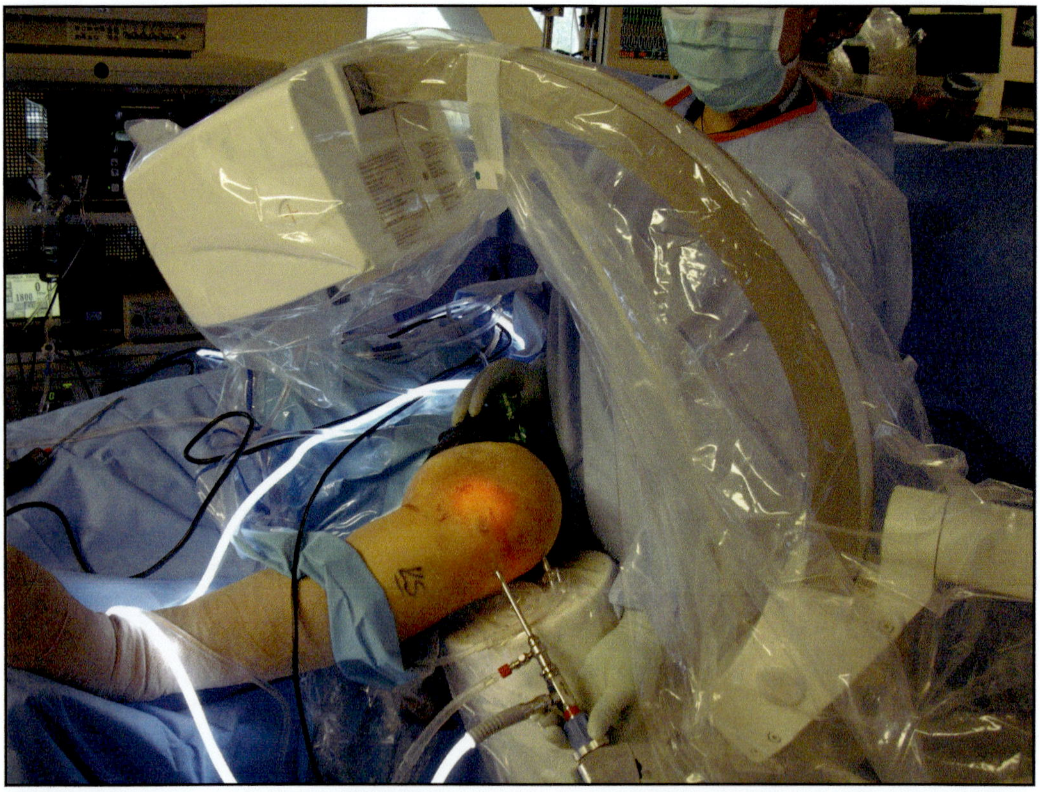

Figure 15-5. Thigh position with mini C-arm use. The thigh can be flexed and externally rotated to allow for visualization of the OCD lesion and K-wire drilling.

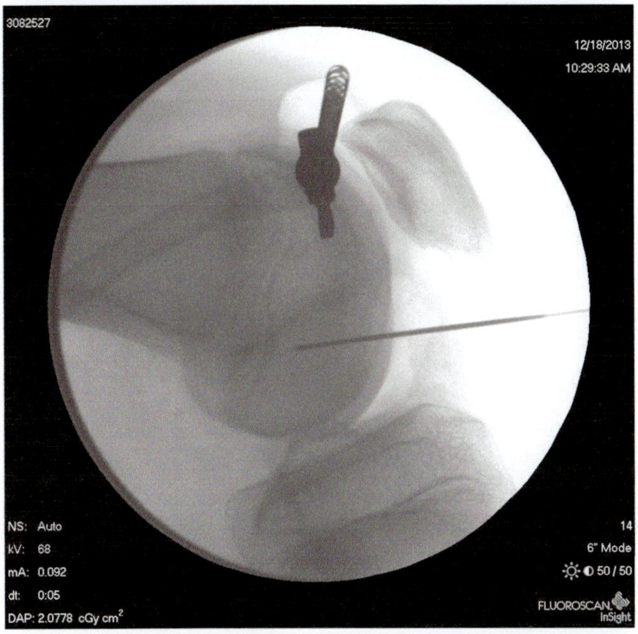

Figure 15-6. Lateral C-arm view showing the depth of the penetration of OCD drilling.

- Perform a routine diagnostic arthroscopy to confirm the absence of other joint pathology, including chondral free bodies, significant plica bands, etc. Routine anterolateral and anteromedial portals are used. In some cases, the OCD lesion may be better seen by using the light source on a lower setting to reduce the reflected light form the hyaline cartilage surfaces. This can be especially helpful if the overlying cartilage is completely normal.
- The K-wires should be positioned as perpendicular as possible to the lesion. Changing the degree of knee flexion/extension can help with wire placement. K-wire drilling may be done through the portals or directly through the skin.
- Avoid bending the wires during placement. If this occurs, it is safer to remove the wires without the K-wire driver. If the driver is used on a bent pin, the pin may shear off at the bend due to the relatively high torque applied to the pin. A stout needle driver can be used to gently remove a bent pin and avoid breaking the pin off in the bone or at the cartilage surface.
- Carefully monitor the depth of K-wire penetration. For transarticular drilling, penetration into the parent bone beyond a few centimeters may not be necessary (Figure 15-6). Place the K-wire on the surface of the cartilage and then grasp the collet driver away from the skin surface. The distance from the skin surface and the collet driver should equal the desired depth of penetration. The K-wire is advanced until the collet tip contacts that skin, ensuring an appropriate depth of drilling into the lesion and normal bone.
- In most cases, the K-wire orientation will be perpendicular to the cartilage and/or the lesion/progeny bone. In some cases, orientation may be less than perpendicular due to lesion location.

Transarticular Drilling

- K-wire selection: Historically, 0.0625-in wires have been used in previous publications. To minimize the trauma to the articular hyaline cartilage, the use of 0.045- or 0.054-in wires may be selected. These wires have sufficient stiffness for transarticular drilling.
- Drill hole density: Typically, 4 to 5 drill holes are passed per square centimeter.

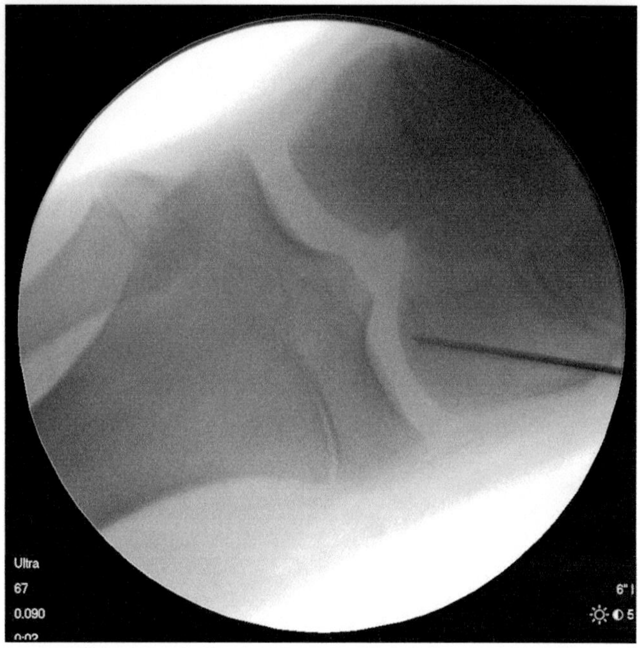

Figure 15-7. This image demonstrates retroarticular drilling, which is behind the cartilage, but avoids the physis of the medial femoral condyle.

- Drill hole depth: The use of imaging can help guide this. Ideally, the drill holes will cross the progeny bone and enter the parent bone by about a 1 to 2 cm or slightly more. The K-wire can be grasped outside of the knee with a gap between the tip of the driver and the patient's skin surface. This gap can approximate the depth of penetration desires, and when the tip of the driver contacts the skin, no further advancement of the wire is necessary. In all cases, be aware of the potential for injury to neurovascular structures about the knee. It is also important to be aware of the physis because drilling should not penetrate the physis.
- When the surface cartilage is entirely normal, use of the C-arm may be necessary to identify the appropriate drilling location. The use of AP, lateral, and oblique imaging may be advantageous in this situation.

Retroarticular Drilling

- Drilling must be performed under AP and lateral fluoroscopic guidance, as described by Edmonds et al,[17] Kocher et al,[18] and Boughanem et al.[20]
- The entrance point of the K-wires is distal to the femoral physis, traversing the epiphysis, directed toward the OCD progeny bone. Review of x-ray and MRI sequences can help determine the optimal starting point for drilling. C-arm images should be used to ensure that these pins are not crossing the physis (Figure 15-7).
- The larger-diameter K-wire of 0.0625 in may be a better choice than the 0.054- or 0.045-in K-wire. This larger diameter wire is stiffer and may be easier to orient the K-wire in the optimal drilling position for drilling. Remember, this K-wire will traverse a longer region of bone prior to entering the progeny bone of the OCD lesion.
- The first K-wire should aim to enter the more central region of the OCD lesion. After drilling is complete with this wire, this can act as a guide for secondary drilling. The use of a small drill guide with multiple drill hole options can help with secondary drilling. Place the drill guide over the K-wire that is in a near central location of the OCD lesion. This drill guide can now rotate around this centrally placed wire to facilitate the placement of appropriately spaced but nearly parallel drill holes (Figure 15-8).

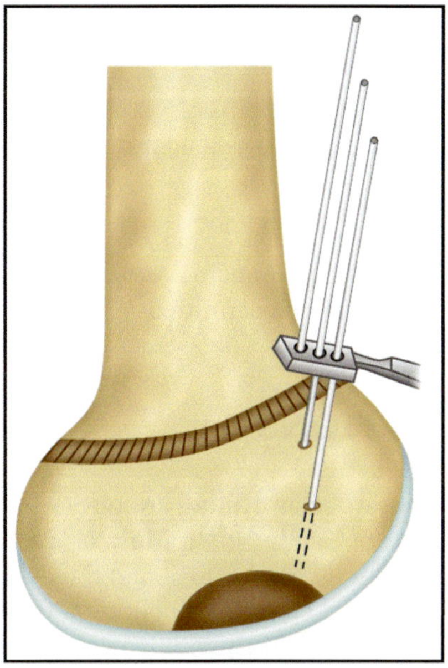

Figure 15-8. Retroarticular drilling with use of a parallel drill guide.

- To provide the patient with a less noticeable scar, a small incision about 5 to 8 mm can be used. This incision is centered around the first pin, and subsequent K-wire passes can performed through the incision. This single incision may cause less of a scar compared to multiple K-wire marks through the skin.
- Perform a minimum of 4 to 8 wire passes per square centimeter (to ensure adequate disruption of sclerotic bone margin of the OCD lesion). Additional wire passes may be advantageous (because additional wire passes are theorized to not be disruptive to the health of the articular cartilage) as described in published techniques.[18,20]

Avoid crossing the progeny bone into the hyaline articular cartilage. If the K-wire is advanced slowly, you may see the vibration and movement of the cartilage above the progeny bone without penetrating the articular cartilage and entering the joint.

Intercondylar Notch Drilling

Kawasaki et al[22] described a form of retroarticular drilling through the intercondylar notch that can be used for medial and lateral femoral condyle drilling. With this technique, the K-wire is drilled at an oblique angle through the intercondylar notch and traversing the progeny and parent bone. This technique has the advantage of avoiding transarticular drilling, and it may require less radiation and C-arm use than previously described for retroarticular drilling techniques. This technique may be limited for cases in which the subchondral lesion/progeny bone is shallow, and thus, the K-wire may not adequately traverse the involved bone (Video of Notch Drilling Retroarticular).

Postoperative Protocol

All patients will be prescribed formal outpatient physical therapy, beginning within 1 week of surgery, to include the following features:

- Weeks 0 to 6: Nonweightbearing with crutches
- After 6 weeks: Weightbearing as tolerated
- Continuous passive motion machines are not used routinely due to variation in insurance coverage, family, and institutional resources.

- Prescribed aquatic therapy is not used routinely due to insurance coverage limitations.
- During the nonweightbearing phase, patients will be allowed the following:
  - Full range of motion of the affected knee
  - Strength training will be allowed within the weightbearing guidelines, including isometric thigh and leg activity
  - Stationary bike with zero or minimal resistance
- Recreational swimming following confirmation of wound healing (minimum 2 weeks postoperatively) will be allowed, but breaststroke and whip kicks will not be permitted.

Potential Complications

Fortunately, acute surgical complications for retro- and transarticular drilling are rare. Most studies have reported no or rare perioperative complications.[12,17-19,21,23,25-31] Most of these studies lacked significant follow-up beyond the phase of subchondral bone healing, and thus, the long-term impact on joint health and articular cartilage is unknown. The main complication from this surgery may be failure to obtain adequate healing. This may be more likely with larger lesions, lesions in older patients, or lateral femoral condyle lesions. Counseling the patient and family about the possibility of incomplete healing, as well as the need for future surgery, is important.

Pins may break off during drilling, and the techniques to avoid this, or to avoid shearing off the pins in the joint, are described in the surgical technique.

Top Technical Pearls for the Procedure

1. Evidence of lesion instability: Review the MRI sequences thoroughly before the case to confirm the absence of obvious signs of lesion instability. Evidence of lesion stability may require different preoperative planning and additional instrumentation.
2. Use of preoperative images: These images will guide your drilling and complement your C-arm views. Visualize the orientation and depth of penetration on these images prior to starting the case. The images should be readily available during the case to guide the location, orientation, and depth of drilling.
3. Avoid bending K-wires: If these become bent during insertion, use caution with removal. Use of a needle driver to remove these pins is ideal because it can prevent the K-wire from shearing at the bend. The torque of the K-wire driver is sufficient to shear the K-wires at the bend.
4. C-arm position: Position the C-arm carefully to allow easy image visualization that does not require the surgeon to look away from the surgical field. The large and small C-arm can be used for these cases, although the small C-arm results in a fraction of the radiation exposure to the operating room staff and patient. Prior to draping the patient, the C-arm should be brought into the field to ensure that adequate images can be obtained to see the location and depth of drilling. The positioning for retroarticular drilling can be more difficult than transarticular drilling.
5. For retroarticular drilling, starting the K-wire just below the physis can help with pin orientation. Use of a parallel drill guide can help with K-wire placement (see Figures 15-7 and 15-8).

PART TWO: ADJUVANT SCREW FIXATION AND SUBCHONDRAL BONE DRILLING IN ASSOCIATION WITH EARLY STAGE OSTEOCHONDRITIS DISSECANS UNSTABLE LESIONS

Indications

When the lesion has some instability, the placement of arthroscopic fixation may be indicated. If the instability is minimal and the cartilage surface is predominantly intact, arthroscopic screw or pin fixation may be used for lesion stabilization, in combination with subchondral bone drilling. Fixation options include metallic screws and/or bioabsorbable screws or pins.

Controversial Indications

- In cases of significant instability, such as trap door lesions or those with significant or complete detachment (trap door lesion or completely detached fragment), more advanced arthroscopic or mini open procedures may be necessary. These lesions are more common in skeletally mature patients but can be seen in skeletally immature patients. In addition to drilling and fixation, debridement of necrotic bone from the lesion/progeny bone and abnormal subchondral bone may be necessary, along with supplemental autogenous bone grafting.
- In some cases, cartilage salvage of the progeny fragment may not be possible; in these cases, a cartilage implantation technique may be necessary. These techniques are beyond the scope of this chapter.

Pertinent Physical Findings

These findings may be similar to the previously described stable lesions. In many cases, the symptoms will be more significant, including the presence of mechanical symptoms and effusion.

Pertinent Imaging

MRI is indicated for preoperative evaluation and planning for these patients. Signs of instability on MRI have been described previously.

Equipment

- The equipment used for this procedure is similar to that described for subchondral bone drilling. The choice of fixation devices will be at the discretion of the surgeon.

Figure 15-9. Cartilage lesion thickness and screw fixation.

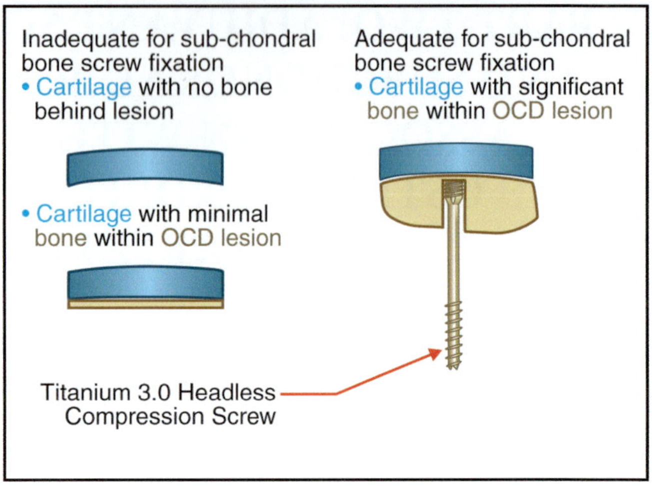

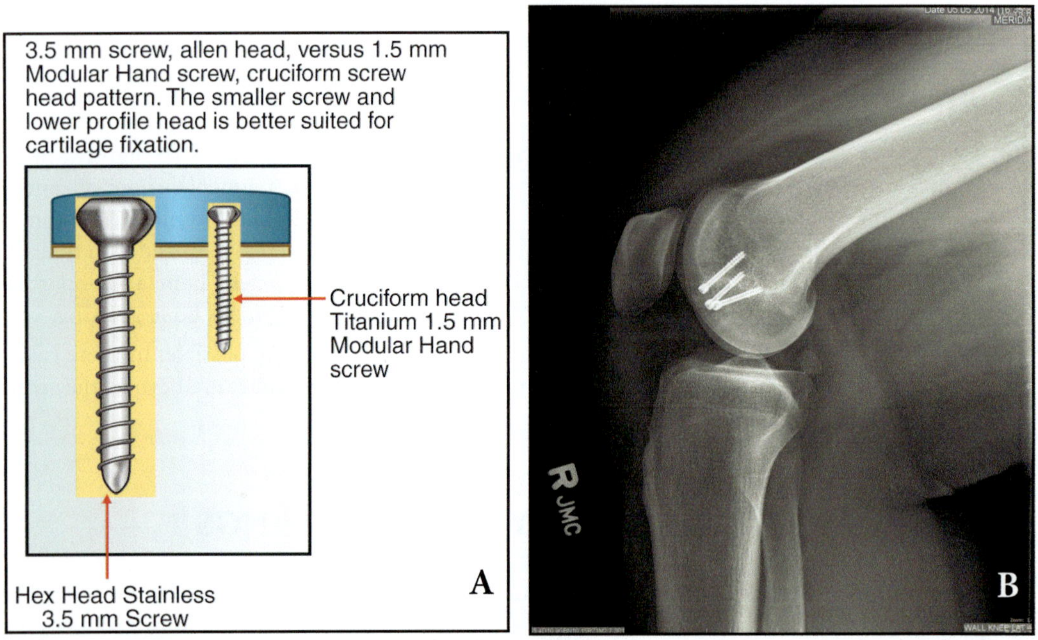

Figure 15-10. (A, B) Countersunk screws within the cartilage.

- Screw options will require some form of countersinking.
  - When the lesion (progeny) bone is of adequate size, the screws can be recessed completely below the cartilage within the subchondral bone (Figure 15-9). Countersink options include 3.0 Headless compression screws (Synthes), Acutrak 2 Headless Compression screws (Acumed), and Arthrex variable pitch small diameter screws. These screws may not need to be removed. Screw designs with variable pitch threads may produce improved compression of the lesion/progeny bone into the parent bone. Close follow-up is important to ensure the screws do not start to back out of the subchondral bone and penetrate into the joint.
  - When the lesion (progeny) bone is of inadequate size for countersinking into the subchondral bone of the lesion, fixation within the cartilage alone is an option. This screw choice should have a low profile head that allows it to be countersunk below the surface of the cartilage 1 to 2 mm, such as 1.5-mm modular hand screws (Synthes; Figure 15-10).

- In all cases, screw backout or prominence are concerns because this can cause damage to the opposite cartilage surfaces. In some cases, second-look arthroscopy and early screw removal may be necessary to avoid these types of complications. In all cases in which screws are not fully recessed in the subchondral bone, the authors routinely remove these about 4 to 6 weeks after placement.

- Bioabsorbable screw and pin options include the following.
  - Pins: These can be placed with relative ease. The ability to obtain compression with these devices is limited. In some cases, the portion of the pin within the articular cartilage may not dissolve adequately. This lack of absorption can lead to problems with the following:
    - Scoring of the articular cartilage on the opposite joint surface
    - A portion of the pin becomes a free body in the joint, leading to some symptoms.
    - In some cases, the pins may start to back out of the bone.
    - In the authors' experience, there is a tendency for the surgeon to leave the pins too proud within the cartilage. These pins should be countersunk in the cartilage to avoid backout and damage to other cartilage surfaces.
  - Screws: The size of the bioabsorbable screw head may be larger than comparable shaft diameter metallic screws. Although these may work well in lesions with adequate bone for subchondral bone fixation, the size of the screw head may leave a larger cartilage entry track than metallic screws. The heads of these screws may not adequately absorb and can become free bodies within the joint. In lesions with inadequate subchondral bone substance, these screws may be limited in the ability to obtain adequate cartilage purchase or may cut through the cartilage. These screws may also form expanding cysts around the screws, during screw absorption.
- Cannulated screw options may be placed arthroscopically, but noncannulated options may require a small arthrotomy in some cases. Titanium screw options also exist for recessed and superficial fixation and may allow for better MRI evaluation postoperatively when compared with stainless screw options (see Figure 15-9).

Positioning and Portals

This is identical to the options discussed for subchondral bone drilling.

Step-by-Step Description of the Procedure

- Lesion/progeny stability is evaluated. If the lesion is stable or has minimal signs of instability, routine subchondral drilling may be performed.
- If the patient is a candidate for adjuvant fixation, ensure that the lesion does not have significant instability. In cases with significant instability or concerns about the condition of the progeny bone, autogenous bone grafting may be necessary via an arthrotomy.
- Study the MRI sequences in detail to determine if the progeny bone lesion is adequate for subchondral bone fixation, or if surface cartilage fixation is appropriate.
- Cannulated systems are easily placed arthroscopically. Place the guide wires perpendicular to the OCD surface. In some cases, slight deviation from the perpendicular may be necessary. Accessory portals can be used for this, including small, vertically oriented portals through the patella tendon.

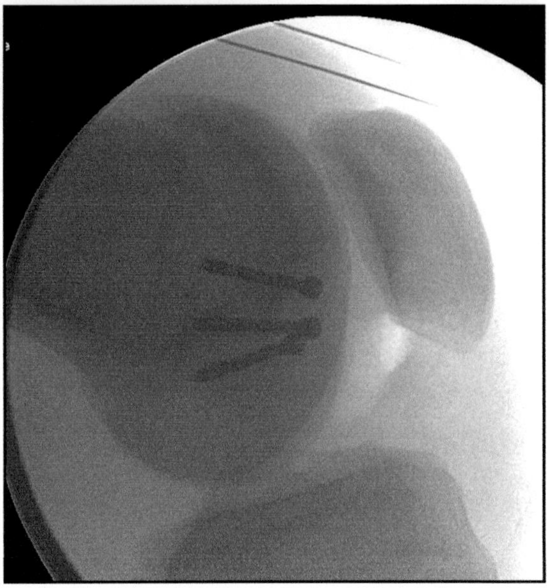

Figure 15-11. C-arm image showing the screw within the subchondral bone of the OCD lesion.

- If adequate subchondral lesion/progeny bone exists for fixation, a screw option with a low profile, fully recessed device may be selected. This screw will be placed below the level of the cartilage, with all fixations depending upon the surrounding bone of the lesion (see Figure 15-9). The depth of penetration can be verified in the following 2 ways.
  - After the screw is placed, look down the screw hole through the layer of cartilage and bone. The head of the screw should be fully recessed in the bone, not within the articular cartilage.
  - The C-arm can be used, and multiple oblique angles may be necessary to ensure that the screw head is completely recessed in the bone (Figure 15-11).
- If the subchondral bone is inadequate for recessed screw fixation in the bone, a device that obtains fixation in the cartilage may be used. This includes bioabsorbable pins and some screw options. Screw options with a very low profile screw head are probably ideal for this, to avoid screw prominence and contact with the opposite joint surface, and loss of fixation if the device descends too far into the cartilage substance. Screws that are not fully recessed into the subchondral bone will need to be removed early.

Postoperative Protocol

During clinical follow-up visits, x-rays are used to confirm that the fixation is still in place and not migrating or backing out. These films can be compared with the intraoperative C-arm images. The rehabilitation protocol is similar to the protocol for subchondral bone drilling. In cases in which surface fixation is used, the authors routinely perform a second-look arthroscopy and perform implant removal. The time for removal varies but typically occurs between 4 and 8 weeks. In cases in which the screw heads are not fully recessed into the subchondral bone, the authors limit impact activities until the hardware has been removed. Early full knee range of motion is encouraged in most cases.

Potential Complications

Routine complications described previously with subchondral bone drilling are applicable here. Failure of fixation, which leads to pins and/or screws backing out, are of concern, and this needs to be monitored closely by imaging and patient evaluation. Fracture of a portion of the bioabsorbable fixation devices can occur and lead to development of symptoms. In rare cases, reactions to the biocomposite material can also produce synovitis and cystic lesions in the subchondral bone.

Top Technical Pearls for the Procedure

1. Evidence of lesion instability: Review the MRI sequences thoroughly before the case to confirm the absence of obvious signs of lesion instability. Evidence of lesion stability may require different preoperative planning and need for additional instrumentation or fixation devices.
2. Use of preoperative images: These images will guide your guide wire drilling and complement your C-arm views. Visualize the orientation and depth of penetration on these images prior to starting the case. The images should be readily available during the case to guide the location, orientation, and depth of drilling.
3. Careful selection of implants for stabilization and avoiding complications with implants is important.
4. For metallic implants, the use of the C-arm to take multiple tangential views at the cartilage surface will help confirm the subchondral bone placement of the screws.
5. When surface fixation is used, a second-look arthroscopy and implant removal are indicated. That typically is scheduled between 4 and 8 weeks postoperatively. When the screw heads are not fully recessed into the subchondral bone, impact activities are limited until the hardware has been removed.

Conclusion

Treating young patients with OCD can be some of the most satisfying work, and OCD lesions are also some of the most challenging cartilage conditions that are treated by sports/arthroscopy surgeons. The prognosis for younger patients is overall good, but older patients are less likely to heal with observation or minimally invasive procedures. Future multicenter research on this condition will be necessary to determine optimum treatment protocols.

Acknowledgments

The authors would like to thank Benton Heyworth, MD, and Jake Jacobs for their feedback on this chapter.

References

1. Edmonds EW, Shea KG. Osteochondritis dissecans: editorial comment. *Clin Orthop Relat Res.* 2013;47(14):1105-1106.
2. Kessler JI, Nikizad H, Shea KG, Jacobs JC Jr, Bebchuk JD, Weiss JM. The demographics and epidemiology of osteochondritis dissecans of the knee in children and adolescents. *Am J Sports Med.* 2014;42(2):320-326.
3. Kocher MS, Tucker R, Ganley TJ, Flynn JM. Management of osteochondritis dissecans of the knee: current concepts review. *Am J Sports Med.* 2006;34(7):1181-1191.
4. Chambers HG, Shea KG, Anderson AF, et al. Diagnosis and treatment of osteochondritis dissecans. *J Am Acad Orthop Surg.* 2011;19(5):297-306.
5. Wall E, Von Stein D. Juvenile osteochondritis dissecans. *Orthop Clin North Am.* 2003;34(3):341-353.
6. Linden B. Osteochondritis dissecans of the femoral condyles: a long-term follow-up study. *J Bone Joint Surg Am.* 1977;59(6):769-776.
7. Sales de Gauzy J, Mansat C, Darodes PH, Cahuzac JP. Natural course of osteochondritis dissecans in children. *J Pediatr Orthop B.* 1999;8(1):26-28.
8. Cahill BR, Phillips MR, Navarro R. The results of conservative management of juvenile osteochondritis dissecans using joint scintigraphy: a prospective study. *Am J Sports Med.* 1989;17(5):601-606.
9. Cepero S, Ullot R, Sastre S. Osteochondritis of the femoral condyles in children and adolescents: our experience over the last 28 years. *J Pediatr Orthop.* 2005;14(1):24-29.
10. Pill SG, Ganley TJ, Milam RA, Lou JE, Meyer JS, Flynn JM. Role of magnetic resonance imaging and clinical criteria in predicting successful nonoperative treatment of osteochondritis dissecans in children. *J Pediatr Orthop.* 2003;23(1):102-108.
11. Hughston JC, Hergenroeder PT, Courtenay BG. Osteochondritis dissecans of the femoral condyles. *J Bone Joint Surg Am.* 1984;66(9):1340-1348.
12. Aglietti P, Buzzi R, Bassi PB, Fioriti M. Arthroscopic drilling in juvenile osteochondritis dissecans of the medial femoral condyle. *Arthroscopy.* 1994;10(3):286-291.
13. Hefti F, Beguiristain J, Krauspe R, et al. Osteochondritis dissecans: a multicenter study of the European Pediatric Orthopedic Society. *J Pediatr Orthop.* 1999;8(4):231-245.
14. Flynn JM, Kocher MS, Ganley TJ. Osteochondritis dissecans of the knee. *J Pediatr Orthop.* 2004;24(4):434-443.
15. Kijowski R, Blankenbaker DG, Shinki K, Fine JP, Graf BK, De Smet AA. Juvenile versus adult osteochondritis dissecans of the knee: appropriate MR imaging criteria for instability. *Radiology.* 2008;248(2):571-578.
16. Carey JL, Wall EJ, Shea KG, et al. *Reliability of the ROCK Osteochondritis Dissecans Knee Arthroscopy Classification System—multi-center validation study.* Paper presented at: AOSSM Annual Meeting; September 2013.
17. Edmonds EW, Albright J, Bastrom T, Chambers HG. Outcomes of extra-articular, intra-epiphyseal drilling for osteochondritis. *J Pediatr Orthop.* 2010;30(8):870-878.
18. Kocher MS, Micheli LJ, Yaniv M, Zurakowski D, Ames A, Adrignolo AA. Functional and radiographic outcome of juvenile osteochondritis dissecans of the knee treated with transarticular arthroscopic drilling. *Am J Sports Med.* 2001;29(5):562-566.
19. Bradley J, Dandy DJ. Results of drilling osteochondritis dissecans before skeletal maturity. *J Bone Joint Surg Br.* 1989;71(4):642-644.
20. Boughanem J, Riaz R, Patel RM, Sarwark JF. Functional and radiographic outcomes of juvenile osteochondritis dissecans of the knee treated with extra-articular retrograde drilling. *Am J Sports Med.* 2011;39(10):2212-2217.
21. Adachi N, Deie M, Nakamae A, Ishikawa M, Motoyama M, Ochi M. Functional and radiographic outcome of stable juvenile osteochondritis dissecans of the knee treated with retroarticular drilling without bone grafting. *Arthroscopy.* 2009;25(2):145-152.
22. Kawasaki K, Uchio Y, Adachi N, Iwasa J, Ochi M. Drilling from the intercondylar area for treatment of osteochondritis dissecans of the knee joint. *Knee.* 2003;10(3):257-263.
23. Conrad JM, Stanitski CL. Osteochondritis dissecans: Wilson's sign revisited. *Am J Sports Med.* 2003;31(5):777-778.

24. Wilson JN. A diagnostic sign in osteochondritis dissecans of the knee. *J Bone Joint Surg Am.* 1967;49(3):477-480.
25. Anderson AF, Richards DB, Pagnani MJ, Hovis WD. Antegrade drilling for osteochondritis dissecans of the knee. *Arthroscopy.* 1997;13(3):319-324.
26. Donaldson LD, Wojtys EM. Extraarticular drilling for stable osteochondritis dissecans in the skeletally immature knee. *J Pediatr Orthop.* 2008;28(8):831-835.
27. Hayan R, Phillipe G, Ludovic S, Claude K, Jean-Michel C. Juvenile osteochondritis of femoral condyles: treatment with transchondral drilling. Analysis of 40 cases. *J Child Orthop.* 2010;4(1):39-44.
28. Ojala R, Kerimaa P, Lakovaara M, et al. MRI-guided percutaneous retrograde drilling of osteochondritis dissecans of the knee. *Skeletal Radiol.* 2011;40(6):765-770.
29. Guhl JF. Arthroscopic treatment of osteochondritis dissecans: preliminary report. *Orthop Clin North Am.* 1979;10(3):671-683.
30. Lee CK, Mercurio C. Operative treatment of osteochondritis dissecans in situ by retrograde drilling and cancellous bone graft: a preliminary report. *Clin Orthop Relat Res.* 1981;(158):129-136.
31. Louisia S, Beaufils P, Katabi M, Robert H; French Society of Arthroscopy. Transchondral drilling for osteochondritis dissecans of the medial condyle of the knee. *Knee Surg Sports Traumatol Arthrosc.* 2003;11(1):33-39.

Please see videos on the accompanying website at www.routledge.com/9781617119996

16

Arthroscopic Marrow Stimulation Including Microfracture, Nanofracture, and Marrow Augmentation Scaffold Stimulation Techniques

Ethan Kellum, MD, MS; Darius Lin, MD; and Kai Mithoefer, MD

Introduction

Articular cartilage injuries affect an estimated 900,000 individuals in the United States every year and result in considerable morbidity and disability for affected individuals, with a substantial associated burden on the health care system.[1] It has been well established that injury to the chondral surface does not readily repair itself. However, previous experience has shown that this limited spontaneous repair capacity of articular cartilage can be overcome if there is access to the mesenchymal stem cells (MSCs) in the subchondral bone marrow, which can be achieved with different so-called marrow stimulation techniques. Penetration of the subchondral bone plate leads to outflow of growth factors, cytokines, and bone marrow-derived MSCs from the subchondral bone marrow, with formation of a pluripotent clot in the chondral defect that stimulates the formation of fibrohyaline repair cartilage.

Evolution of Marrow Stimulation Techniques

Kenneth Pridie, an English athlete and orthopedic surgeon, described the first marrow stimulation technique known as Pridie drilling in 1959.[2] This technique involved penetrating the subchondral bone with multiple drill holes. However, there was concern of thermal necrosis created in the subchondral bone by the drilling process.[3] In the early 1980s, Insall et al[4] and Johnson[5] independently reported on arthroscopic abrasion arthroplasty. This method used a motorized burr to remove the top 1 to 3 mm of subchondral bone in the cartilage defect, creating bleeding and access to the subchondral bone marrow. The pitfall with this procedure was the potential for compromise of the subchondral bone plate. Popularized by Steadman et al[6] in the 1980s, microfracture has become a widely used marrow stimulation procedure that is generally regarded as safe and cost effective. The microfracture technique involves debridement of the chondral defect, with exposure of the subchondral bone and subsequent removal of the calcified cartilage layer.[7] Specifically designed arthroscopic awls are then used to create small holes (ie, microfractures) in the subchondral bone plate throughout the defect to avoid thermal necrosis. The holes are approximately 4 mm deep and 3 to 4 mm apart to maintain subchondral bone plate biomechanics. The microfracture

Sgaglione NA, Lubowitz JH, Provencher MT, eds. *The Knee: AANA Advanced Arthroscopic Surgical Techniques* (pp 217-229).

holes allow bone marrow contents, including MSCs, to flow out into the defect and form a super clot that promotes development of fibrohyaline cartilage repair tissue.[8-10] Experimental studies by Chen et al[11-13] reported that the use of the conical microfracture awls can lead to compaction of the subchondral bone with subchondral fracture and osteocyte necrosis. Moreover, they found that the microfracture may result in a sealing effect from the subchondral bone marrow. In contrast in their rabbit model, they found that cooled drilling allowed better egress of marrow content than microfracture and potential for improved repair cartilage tissue volume and quality. These findings have stimulated a renaissance of subchondral drilling and have led to the development of a modified drilling technique (Powerpick, Arthrex) that limits the risk of thermal necrosis and the reported adverse subchondral bone effects of microfracture. Another approach to reducing the reported deleterious effect of microfracture on the subchondral bone and to optimize bone marrow access has been described by Benthien and Behrens.[14] This so-called nanofracture technique (Arthrosurface) involves the use of a cannulated aiming device with a 1-mm diameter needle that is penetrated 9 mm deep into the subchondral marrow. It has been proposed that this technique generates a "smaller, deeper, better" solution with more hyaline character of the repair cartilage compared to traditional microfracture technique. However, prospective studies have not yet demonstrated the clinical superiority of modified drilling techniques and nanofracture compared to the original awl microfracture technique.

Clinical Application of Marrow Stimulation

Although no validated treatment algorithm exists for treating articular cartilage lesions in the knee, the arthroscopic microfracture technique is commonly used as a first-line option and frequently serves as the standard technique against which other cartilage repair procedures are compared.[15-17] In addition, second-generation microfracture augmentation and scaffold stimulation (MASS) technologies have been developed and are described briefly in this chapter. Therefore, this chapter primarily focuses on the indications, contraindications, surgical technique, and clinical outcomes of the microfracture and MASS techniques (ie, autologous matrix-induced chondrogenesis [AMIC], BioCartilage [Arthrex], and BST-CarGel [Piramal Healthcare]). Based on current recommendations, indications and contraindications for modified drilling and nanofracture are equal to those established for microfracture, making the following descriptions applicable also for these novel technologies.

Indications

Microfracture, MASS, drilling, or nanofracture are indicated for symptomatic, high-grade (grade III to IV) chondral defects of the knee in active patients who are physiologically too young for arthroplasty. This technique is most successfully used as a first-line treatment of isolated lesions up to 4 cm^2 involving the femoral condyles, trochlea, and patella. Prerequisites for successful microfracture include adequate range of motion (ROM), appropriate axial alignment or patellar tracking, ligamentous stability, and the ability to comply with the postoperative rehabilitation. Adjuvant procedures may be performed simultaneously to address coexisting pathology without negative effects of the complex procedures on the postoperative functional outcome and activity level. Detailed indications and contraindications for microfracture are as follows:

- Symptomatic cartilage lesions of the femur, patella, or tibia (including incidental defects)
- Defect size smaller than 4 cm^2
- Short preoperative duration of symptoms (optimally < 12 months)
- Patient age (optimally < 45 years)

Contraindications

- Generalized degenerative joint changes
- Limited patient compliance
- Uncontained chondral lesions
- Severe axial malalignment greater than 5 degrees for femoral condyle lesions (surgical realignment required)
- Patellar maltracking or instability for patellofemoral lesions
- High-grade ligamentous instability (surgical stabilization required for translation > 10 mm)
- Tumor
- Infection
- Inflammatory arthropathy
- Systemic cartilage disorder

Controversial Indications

- Preoperative duration of symptoms greater than 12 months
- Body mass index (BMI) greater than 30 kg/m^2
- Meniscal deficiency
- Moderate to advanced chondropenia
- Defect size greater than 4 cm^2
- Patient age older than 60 years

Patient History

Obtaining a thorough history in patients with knee cartilage defects is a critical first step in selecting appropriate candidates for microfracture. Symptoms from cartilage defects are usually nonspecific and can mimic other knee pathology, such as meniscal tears. Pain with weightbearing is often present with impact activities. Catching and locking sensation can occur from cartilage flaps of larger defects. Joint effusion is frequently reported, particularly after demanding impact activities. Defects of the femoral condyles often produce focal tenderness over the condyle rather than the joint line. Patellar or trochlear lesions usually lead to pain when ambulating stairs, driving a car, getting out of a chair, or in a squatting position. Symptoms of patellar instability may be reported. Articular cartilage defects may present acutely (eg, joint trauma, such as knee ligament tears) or chronically. Any history of previous knee surgeries should be noted because marrow stimulation techniques are most effective as a first-line treatment.

Pertinent Physical Findings

Physical examination includes evaluation of gait pattern as well as hip, knee, and ankle ROM. The knee should be routinely evaluated for ligamentous instability, patellar maltracking or instability, or lower-extremity malalignment. Any joint effusion should be noted. Depending on the defect's location and size, mechanical symptoms may or may not be present and may overlap with meniscal tests. The patient's BMI should be assessed using height and weight for standardized calculation because it has been shown to correlate with functional outcome after microfracture.[9,18,19] The best test usually is precise focal point tenderness over the chondral lesion with potential painful catching and/or crepitus.

Pertinent Imaging

Plain x-rays, including weightbearing anteroposterior, lateral, Rosenberg, long-leg, and Merchant views, can help identify osteochondral lesions, joint space narrowing, patellar maltracking, or lower-extremity malalignment. Cartilage-sensitive magnetic resonance imaging (MRI) presents a sensitive, specific, and accurate tool for noninvasive diagnosis of articular cartilage injury.[18] It provides useful information about meniscal and ligamentous status, subchondral bone, lesion size, and depth. Due to the pathologic changes in the surrounding cartilage, the final size of the defect usually is larger than the defect size measured on preoperative MRI.[1]

Equipment

- 30-degree arthroscope
- Graspers
- Small (3.5-mm) arthroscopic shaver
- Sharp ring curette
- Microfracture awls (30 to 90 degrees)
- Nanofracture guide (15 degrees)
- Nanofracture needles
- Powerpick system (30- or 45-degree tips with a top length of 4 mm [regular] and 6 mm [Powerpick Extend; Arthrex])

Positioning and Portals

Positioning of the extremity must allow knee motion without limitation. A tourniquet is placed on the proximal thigh but is not routinely inflated. Portals are positioned according to the location of the cartilage lesion to provide optimal access to the articular cartilage defect. Standard anterolateral and anteromedial portals can be used for lesions of the central femoral condyles. For defects of the posterior condyles, portals should be placed lower to facilitate access and visualization of the defects. Far medial or lateral portals can be added if necessary. Superolateral portals can be helpful for patellar and trochlear lesions. A thorough diagnostic arthroscopy is performed to identify any additional intra-articular pathology, such as meniscal tears, ligamentous disruption, patellar maltracking, or multiple cartilage defects. Surgical treatment of meniscal pathology is addressed before microfracture, whereas ligamentous reconstruction is performed after microfracture to allow for better visualization. Simultaneous treatment of concomitant pathology avoids repetitive operative morbidity and associated prolonged rehabilitation.

Step-by-Step Description of the Procedure

Step 1

The cartilage defect is identified, and existing cartilage flaps are debrided back to a stable and healthy peripheral margin using an arthroscopic shaver or ring curette (Figure 16-1). The size of the articular lesion is measured with a calibrated probe and recorded. If debridement reveals that the lesion is not contained by an intact cartilage margin, microfracture or MASS techniques

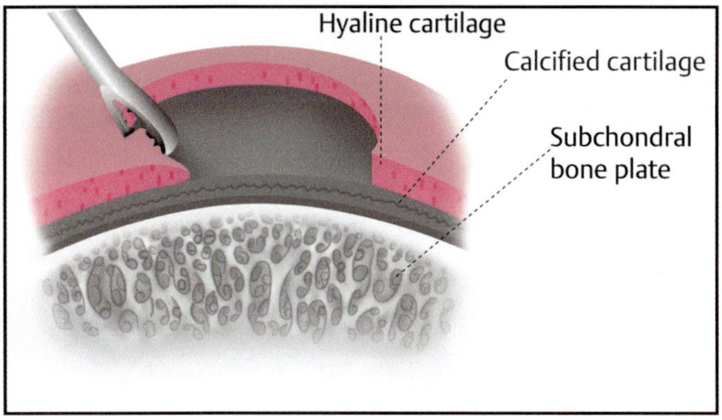

Figure 16-1. Schematic drawing demonstrating debridement of the loose cartilage flaps to create a stable peripheral cartilage margin using an arthroscopic shaver. (Adapted from Mithoefer K, Williams RJ 3rd, Warren RF, et al. Chondral resurfacing of articular cartilage defects in the knee with the microfracture technique. Surgical technique. *J Bone Joint Surg Am.* 2006;88[Suppl 1][Pt 2]:294-304.)

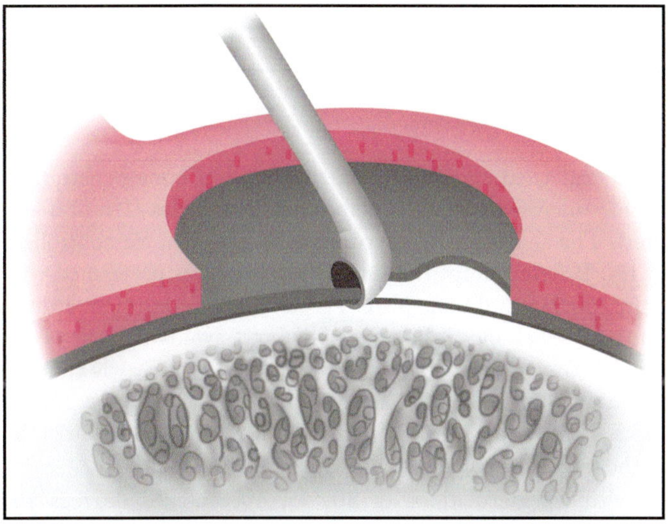

Figure 16-2. Drawing showing the gentle intraoperative debridement of the calcified cartilage using a curette for manual feedback control. (Adapted from Mithoefer K, Williams RJ 3rd, Warren RF, et al. Chondral resurfacing of articular cartilage defects in the knee with the microfracture technique. Surgical technique. *J Bone Joint Surg Am.* 2006;88[Suppl 1][Pt 2]:294-304.)

cannot be used because sufficient pooling of the marrow clot cannot be achieved. The ROM in which the lesion articulates with the opposing joint surface is carefully recorded. Knowledge of this range of contact has important implications for postoperative rehabilitation.

Step 2

A curette is used to carefully remove the calcified cartilage layer from the base of the lesion (Figure 16-2). The calcified cartilage layer is a thin layer between the deep zone of the cartilage and subchondral bone and can increase in thickness with age. Removal of the calcified cartilage has been shown to improve bonding of the repair tissue to the subchondral bone after microfracture.[20] The calcified cartilage can be difficult to differentiate visually but can be distinguished more easily from the hard underlying subchondral bone plate by tactile feedback. Use of a curette provides better manual feedback than use of an arthroscopic shaver and avoids excessive debridement with thinning of the subchondral bone. Excessive removal of the subchondral bone may stimulate subchondral bone overgrowth and should be avoided. This phenomenon is observed in 25% to 49% of patients after microfracture and leads to relative thinning of the overlying repair cartilage layer with resultant biologic and biomechanical implications for the repair tissue quality.

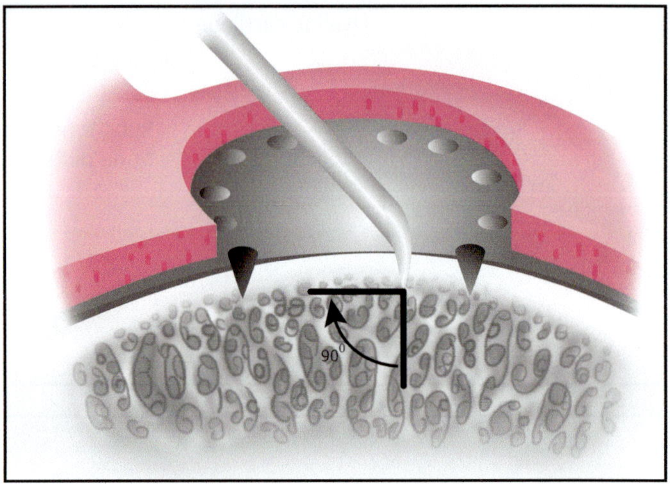

Figure 16-3. Drawing illustrating the subchondral penetrations with perpendicular alignment of the instrument for optimal penetration of the subchondral bone plate. (Adapted from Mithoefer K, Williams RJ 3rd, Warren RF, et al. Chondral resurfacing of articular cartilage defects in the knee with the microfracture technique. Surgical technique. *J Bone Joint Surg Am.* 2006;88[Suppl 1][Pt 2]:294-304.)

Step 3

Following appropriate removal of the calcified cartilage layer, subchondral bone penetrations are created using commercially available microfracture awls, nanofracture needles (1-mm diameter), or microdrills (1.5-mm diameter). The shape of the instruments is designed for controlled-depth penetration of the instrument tip. Penetration of the subchondral bone is performed with the instrument tip perpendicular to the subchondral bone plate. Perpendicular alignment ensures appropriate depth of penetration into the subchondral bone marrow and avoids skiving of the microfracture awl tip during impact with the mallet. Skiving of the microfracture awls can create large longitudinal disruptions of the subchondral bone plate and may affect its biomechanical integrity. Skiving can also be avoided by gently toeing in the tip of the instrument. The risk for skiving is reduced significantly with the nanofracture and microdrilling techniques.

Microfracture awls are available with tip angulations of 30, 45, 60, and 90 degrees and facilitate access to cartilage lesions in all areas of the knee joint. For femoral condyle or trochlear lesions, the 30- or 45-degree awls readily provide perpendicular alignment of the instrumentation (Figure 16-3). Knee motion can also help to optimize instrument positioning. The 90-degree awl is frequently used for patellar defects. Perpendicular penetration of the 90-degree awl through the patellar subchondral bone plate is facilitated by impacting the grip of the instrument rather than its end. This technique in combination with manual stabilization and counterpressure on the patella will help to prevent skiving of the instrument (Figure 16-4). Nanofracture guides (Arthrosurface) are available at a 15-degree angle, and microdrills (Powerpick) are available with 30- and 45-degree tip angles allowing for depth of penetration from 4 to 6 mm. Nanofracture and microdrilling allow for technically easier penetration of the subchondral bone plate.

Subchondral bone penetrations are created on the periphery of the defect first and are then continued toward the center of the lesion using a systematic spiral pattern (Figure 16-5). This systematic approach provides homogeneous distribution of the holes throughout the entire cartilage defect and maximizes adherence of the mesenchymal clot at the base (Figure 16-6). Three- to 4-mm-wide bone bridges are carefully maintained between the individual holes to preserve subchondral bone plate integrity and function. Release of fatty droplets from the subchondral bone holes indicates adequate depth of the penetration. Once the entire defect has been treated, any bony debris on the rim of the holes is removed by curettage or arthroscopic shaver. Adequate release of blood and marrow fat droplets from the holes can also be confirmed by eliminating arthroscopic pump pressure. Once adequate access to the subchondral bone marrow has been ensured, the arthroscope is removed from the joint. No drains are used to avoid removal of the pluripotent mesenchymal clot from the cartilage defect by suction or direct abrasion by the drain

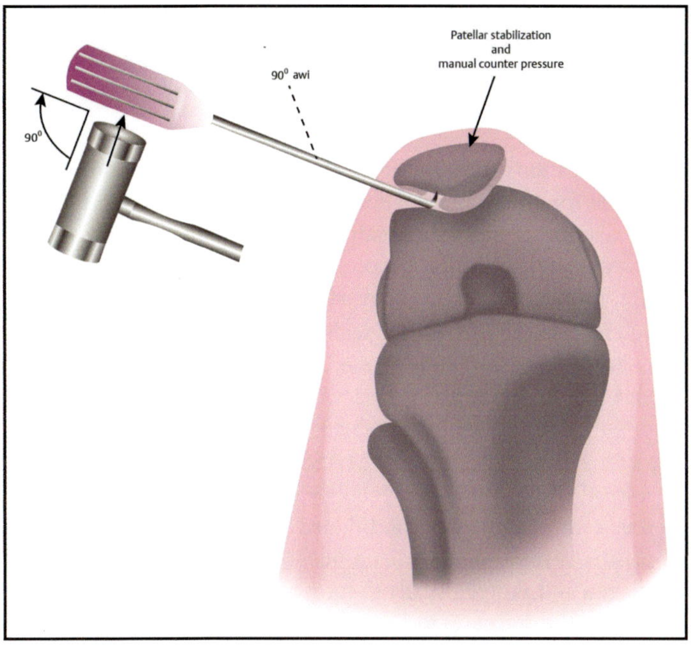

Figure 16-4. Drawing illustrating the technique for microfracture of patellar lesions. (Adapted from Mithoefer K, Williams RJ 3rd, Warren RF, et al. Chondral resurfacing of articular cartilage defects in the knee with the microfracture technique. Surgical technique. *J Bone Joint Surg Am.* 2006;88[Suppl 1][Pt 2]:294-304.)

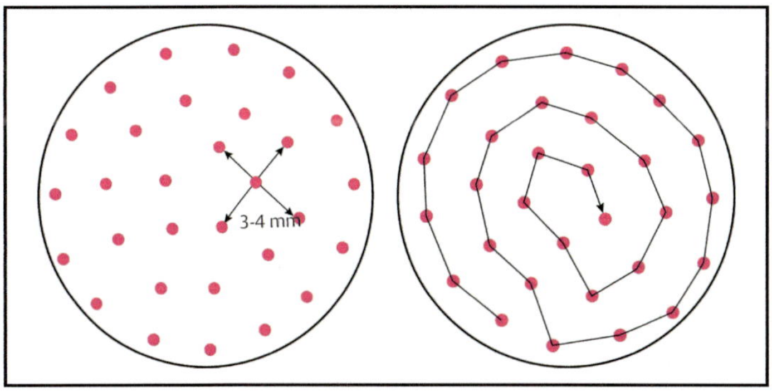

Figure 16-5. Illustration of the systematic spiral pattern to ensure homogeneous distribution of the subchondral penetrations while maintaining sufficient subchondral bone bridges between individual penetrations. (Adapted from Mithoefer K, Williams RJ 3rd, Warren RF, et al. Chondral resurfacing of articular cartilage defects in the knee with the microfracture technique. Surgical technique. *J Bone Joint Surg Am.* 2006;88[Suppl 1][Pt 2]:294-304.)

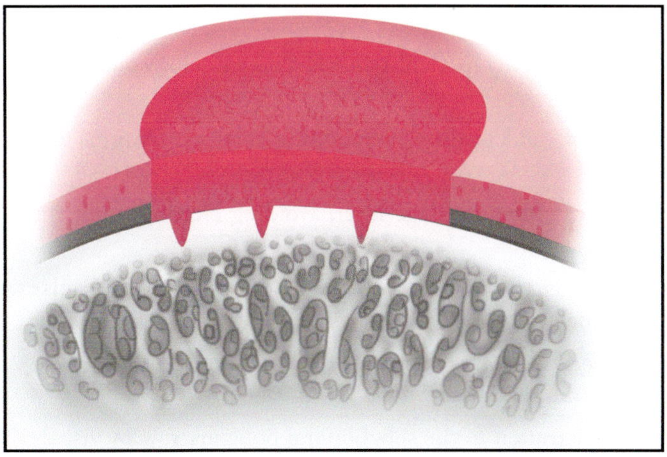

Figure 16-6. Schematic drawing showing the pooling of the mesenchymal clot in the treated cartilage defect and the anchoring effect of the microfracture penetrations. (Adapted from Mithoefer K, Williams RJ 3rd, Warren RF, et al. Chondral resurfacing of articular cartilage defects in the knee with the microfracture technique. Surgical technique. *J Bone Joint Surg Am.* 2006;88[Suppl 1][Pt 2]:294-304.)

during postoperative joint mobilization. A compression dressing is placed, and cryotherapy is used routinely for control of postoperative swelling.

MASS

MASS techniques have the same indications/contraindications as microfracture-alone techniques. Lesion preparation is identical as for microfracture techniques; care should be taken to remove the calcified cartilage without disrupting the subchondral bone and create stable vertical walls of the lesion. Each technique has nuances to the procedure, but each mainly includes lesion preparation, microfracture/nanofracture, product mixture, and product delivery.

Following lesion preparation and microfracture, the AMIC technique (Geistlich) uses a slightly undersized porcine collagen membrane (type I or III) that is formed by a template (aluminum). The membrane is placed into the lesion and secured with a fibrin clot created from the patient's own blood after undergoing centrifuging or with commercially available fibrin glue.[21]

The BioCartilage technique provides a 1-step, off-the-shelf, MASS technology that can be used with microfracture, nanofracture, or microdrilling (Powerpick). Following preparation of the defect, the patient's blood is drawn and prepared into autologous conditioned plasma by defined centrifugation. The autologous conditioned plasma is then mixed with a micronized extracellular allograft cartilage matrix containing type II collagen and proteoglycans to form a thick but fluid paste that is then injected into the cartilage defect, filling the defect up to 1 mm below the level of the surrounding native articular cartilage. Fibrin glue is then applied over the implanted BioCartilage paste to seal the lesion flush with the surrounding cartilage and is allowed to cure for 5 to 10 minutes.[22] The technique is traditionally done with mini-arthrotomy but can also be performed arthroscopically (Figure 16-7).

The BST-CarGel technique is also designed to promote hyaline cartilage regeneration in conjunction with bone marrow stimulation technique for the repair of articular cartilage. BST-CarGel uses an off-the-shelf, minimally invasive, 1-step procedure. BST-CarGel uses a scaffold augmentation with chitosan, a natural glucosamine polysaccharide derived from the exoskeleton of crustaceans with proven biocompatibility, biodegradability, and natural adhesiveness. Following the marrow stimulation of the cartilage defect, BST-CarGel is mixed with whole blood drawn from the patient, and the liquid gel is then applied into the defect, filling it flush with the surrounding cartilage. Depending on the lesion location, patient positioning should be designed to allow for gravity to optimize lesion fill with the gel. The mixture is allowed to set in the lesion for approximately 15 minutes.[23]

Specific Steps

1. Perform a complete arthroscopic joint survey to identify associated pathology and assess joint cartilage status.
2. Debride the chondral defect to stable and healthy surrounding cartilage margins and determine the final defect size.
3. Gently but thoroughly remove the calcified cartilage layer, avoiding bleeding from the subchondral bone.
4. Start subchondral bone penetrations in the periphery of the defect with perpendicular access of the instrument tip to the defect base.
5. Systematically penetrate the subchondral bone plate using a spiral pattern, leaving 3 to 4 mm between individual subchondral bone holes.
6. Ensure appropriate depth of the penetration to the subchondral bone marrow by visualization of fat droplets or bleeding from the individual subchondral bone holes.
7. Close the portal incisions tightly and avoid drain placement.

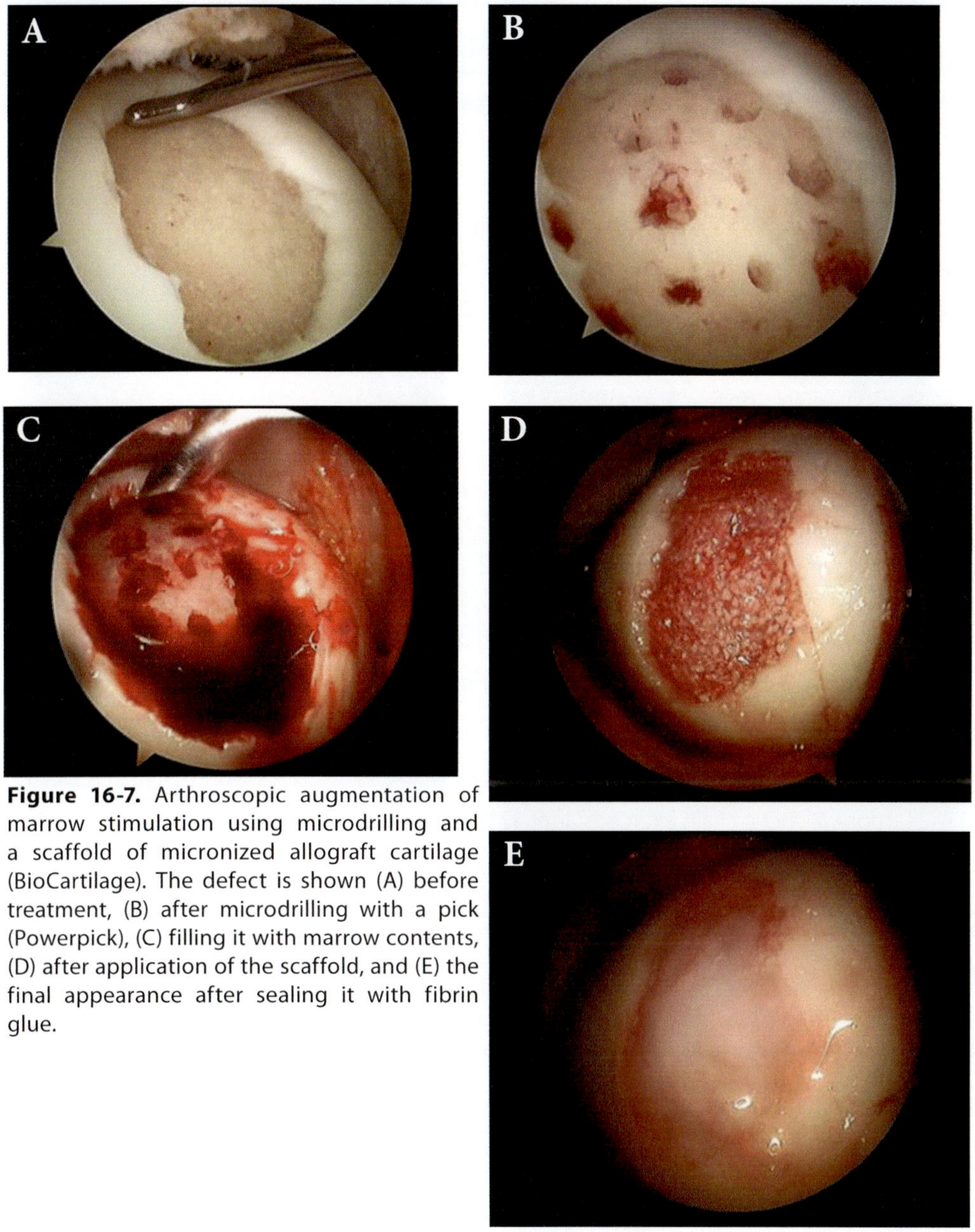

Figure 16-7. Arthroscopic augmentation of marrow stimulation using microdrilling and a scaffold of micronized allograft cartilage (BioCartilage). The defect is shown (A) before treatment, (B) after microdrilling with a pick (Powerpick), (C) filling it with marrow contents, (D) after application of the scaffold, and (E) the final appearance after sealing it with fibrin glue.

Postoperative Protocol

Appropriate rehabilitation following treatment of articular cartilage defects of the knee with marrow stimulation helps MSC differentiation in the clot while avoiding detrimental compression and shear forces on the developing repair cartilage tissue. Rehabilitation presents a critical component for successful treatment outcome and follows different guidelines for femorotibial lesions and patellofemoral defects (Table 16-1). Although general timelines can be useful, progression through rehabilitation should be done individually based on the lesion characteristics, surgical details, and patient symptoms. Concomitant procedures, such as ligament reconstruction, meniscal surgery, or osteotomy, may alter the postoperative rehabilitation protocol.

Table 16-1. Microfracture/Nanofracture/Microdrilling Rehabilitation Timeline*

Femoral Defects

- Touchdown weightbearing for 2 weeks then progress 25% per week
- Continuous passive motion 6 to 8 hours/day for 6 weeks
- Closed kinetic chain exercises (biking) without resistance at 2 weeks
- Start limited-arc open kinetic chain exercises at 6 to 8 weeks
- Initiate impact exercises (jogging) at 4 months if no pain/effusion
- Start plyometric drills at 5 months
- Return to cutting, jumping activities at 5 to 6 months
- Sport-specific skill program and functional progression at 6 months
- Gradual return to high-impact athletics by 6 to 8 months

Patellar/Trochlear Defects

- Weightbearing as tolerated for 8 weeks with brace locked at 0 to 20 degrees
- Continuous passive motion 6 hours/day for 6 to 8 weeks at 0 to 45 degrees
- Start closed kinetic chain exercises without resistance at 2 to 4 weeks
- Limited-arc range of motion exercises until 12 weeks
- Start open kinetic chain exercises after 12 to 16 weeks
- Initiate impact activities at 6 to 7 months
- Return to high-impact athletics at 8 to 12 months

*Individualized progression is recommended based on patient's lesion characteristics and symptoms rather than fixed timelines.

Potential Complications

- Insufficient debridement to a stable peripheral cartilage margin and failure to remove the calcified cartilage layer can limit attachment of the repair tissue to the subchondral bone and surrounding intact cartilage.
- Compromise of subchondral bone plate integrity from limited distance between subchondral holes, skiving of instruments, or excessive calcified cartilage debridement
- Insufficient depth penetration of the subchondral bone and the low density of the penetrations may reduce the quality and quantity of the repair cartilage tissue.
- Premature weightbearing can lead to clot displacement or limit attachment to the surrounding cartilage or base.
- Aggressive removal of the calcified cartilage layer can promote subchondral bone overgrowth.

Results

Over the past 2 decades, many studies have shown good short-term follow-up results after microfracture.[24-28] Several factors were identified that affected the clinical outcome after microfracture and included age (better results with age older than < 40 years), lesion location, duration of symptoms (< 12 months), lesion size (< 4 cm^2), preoperative activity level (Tegner score > 4), BMI (< 30 kg/m^2), and competitive level for athletes (better return to sport in competitive athletes).[1,18,19,24,25,29] Microfracture effectively improved knee function in many studies during the first 24 months postoperatively, but the reports on durability of the initial functional improvement conflicted with several studies that reported decreases from the initial improvement and higher failure rates after 2 years.[18,19,30] Two studies in professional athletes document the decline in performance in the short term.[30,31] Eighty-three percent of National Basketball Association players returned to sport, although they had fewer games played, points per game, and steals per game.[32] Long-term follow-up has demonstrated that gradual functional decline can occur after the initial functional improvement observed in the first 2 years after microfracture. Systematic review of 6 long and 9 short-term studies suggested functional results may be limited beyond 5 years after microfracture. However, average functional improvement after microfracture remained higher than preoperative levels even beyond 10 years after microfracture, and similar gradual functional decrease has been observed for other cartilage repair techniques over time, demonstrating the common need for further scientific and technical advances to optimize the outcome from articular cartilage repair despite the promising results from first-generation technologies.[8,10,18,19,27,29,31,33] New technologies, such as nanofracture and microdrilling, may help to overcome some of the technical and outcome limitations associated with microfracture, but more scientific studies are needed to systematically evaluate the clinical efficacy of these promising new techniques.

Most recently, the outcome of MASS techniques has been studied. The data are currently limited to short-/medium-term data, and long-term studies need to be completed. Gille et al[34] showed a significant improvement in Lysholm and visual analog scale scores of 57 patients at 2 years undergoing AMIC. When compared to microfracture alone, AMIC shows no significant improvement of clinical scores or MRI defect filling at 1 and 2 years.[35] Although BST-CarGel treatment compared to microfracture alone showed a significantly greater defect filling and more hyaline cartilage-like T2 values, it did not show a greater clinical benefit.[23]

Top Technical Pearls for the Procedure

1. Careful preoperative patient counseling and close cooperation with well-trained physical therapists improves postoperative rehabilitation.
2. Gentle but thorough removal of calcified cartilage improves repair tissue volume and adherence.
3. Systematic placement of subchondral bone holes optimizes clot adherence, MSC distribution, and reduces the risk of subchondral bone collapse and bony overgrowth.
4. Use criteria-based progression during postoperative rehabilitation that avoids activity-related pain and swelling.
5. Modified drilling or nanofracture can reduce the risk of skiving associated with microfracture awls and allows for well-controlled penetration of the subchondral bone even in difficult-to-reach areas, such as the patella.

References

1. Mithoefer K, McAdams T, Williams RJ, Kreuz PC, Mandelbaum BR. Clinical efficacy of the microfracture technique for articular cartilage repair in the knee: an evidence-based systematic analysis. *Am J Sports Med.* 2009;37(10):2053-2063.
2. Pridie KH. A method of resurfacing osteoarthritic knee joints. *J Bone Joint Surg Br.* 1959;41(3):618-619.
3. Bert JM, Maschka K. The arthroscopic treatment of unicompartmental gonarthrosis: a five-year follow-up study of abrasion arthroplasty plus arthroscopic debridement and arthroscopic debridement alone. *Arthroscopy.* 1989;5(1):25-32.
4. Insall JN, Hood RW, Flawn LB, Sullivan DJ. The total condylar knee prosthesis in gonarthrosis. A five to nine-year follow-up of the first one hundred consecutive replacements. *J Bone Joint Surg Am.* 1983;65(5):619-628.
5. Johnson LL. Arthroscopic abrasion arthroplasty historical and pathologic perspective: present status. *Arthroscopy.* 1986;2(1):54-69.
6. Steadman JR, Rodkey WG, Singleton SB, Briggs KK. Microfracture technique for full-thickness chondral defects: technique and clinical results. *Oper Tech Orthop.* 1997;7(4):300-304.
7. Hunt SA, Jazrawi LM, Sherman OH. Arthroscopic management of osteoarthritis of the knee. *J Am Acad Orthop Surg.* 2002;10(5):356-363.
8. Steadman JR, Miller BS, Karas SG, Schlegel TF, Briggs KK, Hawkins RJ. The microfracture technique in the treatment of full-thickness chondral lesions of the knee in National Football League players. *J Knee Surg.* 2003;16(2):83-86.
9. Mithoefer K, Williams RJ III, Warren RF, et al. Chondral resurfacing of articular cartilage defects in the knee with the microfracture technique. Surgical technique. *J Bone Joint Surg Am.* 2006;88(suppl 1, pt 2):294-304.
10. Steadman JR, Briggs KK, Rodrigo JJ, Kocher MS, Gill TJ, Rodkey WG. Outcomes of microfracture for traumatic chondral defects of the knee: average 11-year follow-up. *Arthroscopy.* 2003;19(5):477-484.
11. Chen H, Hoemann CD, Sun J, et al. Depth of subchondral perforation influences the outcome of bone marrow stimulation cartilage repair. *J Orthop Res.* 2011;29(8):1178-1184.
12. Chen H, Sun J, Hoemann CD, et al. Drilling and microfracture lead to different bone structure and necrosis during bone-marrow stimulation for cartilage repair. *J Orthop Res.* 2009;27(11):1432-1438.
13. Chen H, Chevrier A, Hoemann CD, Sun J, Ouyang W, Buschmann MD. Characterization of subchondral bone repair for marrow-stimulated chondral defects and its relationship to articular cartilage resurfacing. *Am J Sports Med.* 2011;39(8):1731-1740.
14. Benthien JP, Behrens P. Reviewing subchondral cartilage surgery: considerations for standardized and outcome predictable cartilage remodeling. *Int Orthop.* 2013;37(11):2139-2145.
15. Gudas R, Gudaitė A, Pocius A, et al. Ten-year follow-up of a prospective, randomized clinical study of mosaic osteochondral autologous transplantation versus microfracture for the treatment of osteochondral defects in the knee joint of athletes. *Am J Sports Med.* 2012;40(11):2499-2508.
16. Knutsen G, Drogset JO, Engebertson L, et al. A randomized trial comparing autologous chondrocyte implantation with microfracture. Findings at five years. *J Bone Joint Surg Am.* 2007;89(10):2105-2112.
17. Saris DB, Vanlauwe J, Victor J, et al. Treatment of symptomatic cartilage defects of the knee: characterized chondrocyte implantation results in better clinical outcome at 36 months in a randomized trial compared to microfracture. *Am J Sports Med.* 2009;37(suppl 1):10S-19S.
18. Mithoefer K, Williams RJ III, Warren RF, et al. The microfracture technique for the treatment of articular cartilage lesions in the knee. A prospective cohort study. *J Bone Joint Surg Am.* 2005;87(9):1911-1920.
19. Mithoefer K, Williams RJ III, Warren RF, et al. High-impact athletics after knee articular cartilage repair: a prospective evaluation of the microfracture technique. *Am J Sports Med.* 2006;34(9):1413-1418.
20. Frisbie DD, Morisset S, Rodkey WG, Steadman JR, McIlwraith CW. Effects of calcified cartilage on healing of chondral defects treated with microfracture in horses. *Am J Sports Med.* 2006;34(11):1824-1831.
21. Benthien JP, Behrens P. The treatment of chondral and osteochondral defects of the knee with autologous matrix-induced chondrogenesis (AMIC): method description and recent developments. *Knee Surg Sports Traumatol Arthrosc.* 2011;19(8):1316-1319.
22. Abrams GD, Mall NA, Fortier LA, Roller BL, Cole BJ. BioCartilage: background and operative technique. *Oper Tech Sports Med.* 2013;21(2):116-124.

23. Stanish WD, McCormack R, Forriol F, et al. Novel scaffold-based BST-CarGel treatment results in superior cartilage repair compared with microfracture in a randomized controlled trial. *J Bone Joint Surg Am.* 2013;95(18):1640-1650.
24. Kreuz PC, Erggelet C, Steinwachs MR, et al. Is microfracture of chondral defects in the knee associated with different results in patients aged 40 years or younger? *Arthroscopy.* 2006;22(11):1180-1186.
25. Kreuz PC, Steinwachs MR, Erggelet C, et al. Results after microfracture of full-thickness chondral defects in different compartments in the knee. *Osteoarthritis Cartilage.* 2006;14(11):1119-1125.
26. Miller BS, Steadman JR, Briggs KK, Rodrigo JJ, Rodkey WG. Patient satisfaction and outcome after microfracture of the degenerative knee. *J Knee Surg.* 2004;17(1):13-17.
27. Miller BS, Briggs KK, Downie B, et al. Clinical outcomes following the microfracture procedure for chondral defects in the knee: a longitudinal data analysis. *Cartilage.* 2010;1:108-112.
28. Salzmann GM, Sah B, Südkamp NP, Niemyer P. Clinical outcome following the first line, single lesion microfracture at the knee joint. *Arch Orthop Trauma Surg.* 2013;133(3):303-310.
29. Blevins FT, Steadman JR, Rodrigo JJ, Silliman J. Treatment of articular cartilage defects in athletes: an analysis of functional outcome and lesion appearance. *Orthopedics.* 1998;21(7):761-768.
30. Gobbi A, Nunag P, Malinowski K. Treatment of chondral lesions of the knee with microfracture in a group of athletes. *Knee Surg Sports Traumatol Arthrosc.* 2005;13(3):213-221.
31. Gobbi A, Karnatzikos G, Kumar A. Long-term results after microfracture treatment for full-thickness knee chondral lesions in athletes. *Knee Surg Sports Traumatol Arthrosc.* 2014;22(9):1986-1996.
32. Harris JD, Walton DM, Erickson, BJ, et al. Return to sport and performance after microfracture in the knees of National Basketball Association players. *Orthop J Sports Med.* 2013;1(6):1-7.
33. Goyal D, Keyhani S, Lee EH, Hui JH. Evidence-based status of microfracture technique: a systematic review of level I and II studies. *Arthroscopy.* 2013;29(9):1579-1588.
34. Gille J, Behrens P, Volpi P, et al. Outcome of autologous matrix induced chondrogenesis (AMIC) in cartilage knee surgery: data of the AMIC Registry. *Arch Orthop Trauma Surg.* 2013;133(1):87-93.
35. Anders S, Volz M, Frick H, Gellissen J. A randomized, controlled trial comparing autologous matrix-induced chondrogenesis (AMIC®) to microfracture: analysis of 1- and 2-year follow-up data of 2 centers. *Open Orthop J.* 2013;7:133-143.

Please see videos on the accompanying website at www.routledge.com/9781617119996

17

Autogenous Osteochondral Transplantation

Ryan Michels, MD and Nicholas A. Sgaglione, MD

Introduction

Symptomatic focal advanced grade III/IV osteochondral defects in the knee present a unique treatment dilemma for clinicians. It is well known that damaged cartilage lacks the ability to heal with restorative type II hyaline tissue. Autogenous osteochondral transplantation (AOT) is a viable treatment option in the properly selected patient. D'Aubigné first described AOT in 1945 as a pedunculated patellar graft. Campanacci used a similar procedure for patients with osteo-articular defects from giant cell tumor resections.[1] Later press-fit technology was pioneered by Outerbridge and reported in 1995. This technique resulted in improved knee scores and demonstrated well-fixed integrated grafts on second-look arthroscopy.[2] In an effort to eliminate the need for an invasive arthrotomy, all-arthroscopic techniques have been described, with optimal results.

The main advantage of AOT over other articular cartilage biological resurfacing methodologies (ie microfracture) is the predictable restoration of viable hyaline cartilage and bone-to-bone autogenous graft healing. A histologic analysis of 7 patients after AOT showed viability of hyaline cartilage structure and healing of subchondral bone at 2 to 12 months.[3] This restoration is thought to be the key to the success of AOT procedures. Gudas et al[4,5] published a randomized trial of 60 young athletes demonstrating the success of AOT over microfracture. They reported higher return to sport and higher knee scores at 3- to 10-year follow-up. More recently, Krych et al[6] reported higher activity levels following AOT compared to microfracture procedures. Marcacci reported[7] 76.7% good or excellent results at 7-year follow-up with an all-arthroscopic approach in a prospective study of 30 patients. Barber et al[8] reported an improvement of Lysholm score from 44 preoperatively to 84 at 2-year follow-up.

The term *mosaicplasty,* originally described by Hangody et al,[9] refers to the use of smaller, 3- to 5-mm-diameter autologous grafts. This allows for less potential donor site morbidity and more available graft tissue in the native knee. It is possible to fill one large defect with several small plugs to restore the native contour of the condyle.[9] The advantage of using multiple smaller grafts is greater potential to restore complex surface topography of certain lesions. The disadvantages include less potential hyaline and more intergraft clefting. Treatment results confirming

Sgaglione NA, Lubowitz JH, Provencher MT, eds. *The Knee: AANA Advanced Arthroscopic Surgical Techniques* (pp 231-242).

the advantages of smaller grafts have been reported by Filardo et al,[10] who found a significant number of patients complaining of pain attributed to donor site morbidity in a study of 31 patients after femoral condyle AOT. In a large multicenter trial including 383 patients with 2- to 17-year follow-ups, Hangody et al[11] demonstrated 91% good to excellent results with femoral AOT and 74% good to excellent results with patellofemoral AOT. More recently, in a prospective study of 33 patients, Astur et al[12] reported significant improvement of knee scores and osseous integration on magnetic resonance imaging (MRI) after patellofemoral AOT.

Advantages[13]

- Arthroscopic outpatient procedure/minimally invasive techniques
- Single point of service index cost-effective procedure
- Hyaline cartilage and subchondral bone full tissue restoration
- Long-term outcome data results at 7 to 10 years demonstrate success

Disadvantages[13]

- Donor site morbidity
- Limited donor site availability
- Technically challenging procedure
- Areas of intergraft fibrocartilage due to incongruent geometric configuration of grafts

Indications

- Symptomatic and active patient with focal osteochondral pathology
- Focal articular cartilage lesions on the medial or lateral femoral condyles, patella, and central trochlea
- Defect size of 10 to 25 mm in diameter or 15 to 250 mm^2 in area
- Patient age younger than 50 years
- Rehabilitation compliant
- Ligamentous stability
- Lack of significant degenerative changes
- Lack of significant varus/valgus deformity
- Lack of significant patellofemoral joint deformity
- Lack of rheumatoid disease or crystal arthropathy

Controversial Indications

- Lesions smaller than 10 mm
- Lesions larger than 400 mm^2
- History of patellofemoral pain syndrome

Pertinent Physical Findings

Although no test has 100% sensitivity or specificity, there are physical examination findings that can suggest an osteochondral defect. Patients may have the following:

- Antalgia
- Effusion
- Soft tissue swelling
- Diminished range of motion (ROM)
- Abnormal patellofemoral tracking
- Crepitus may be palpated with ROM testing

Best test: Palpable focal point tenderness with demonstrable clunk or mechanical catching over the site of the symptomatic lesion is considered the best and most clinically correlative physical examination test.

- Wilson's test may be useful to identify an osteochondritis dissecans lesion on the medial condyle.
  - When performing Wilson's test, the patient is examined in a seated position with the tibia internally rotated, with the legs dangling off of the examination table. Have the patient extend the knee to approximately 30 degrees. A positive test is noted if the maneuver elicits pain. Next, external rotation of the tibia, with unloading of the medial compartment, results in reduction of the pain.

Pertinent Imaging

- Anteroposterior and 45-degree posteroanterior standing x-rays, including lateral, notch, and sunrise/Merchant views
- Full-length hip-to-ankle standing x-rays to calculate the lower-extremity mechanical axis
- High-resolution MRI improves the accuracy of assessment of the cartilaginous defect, including width, length, and depth and which can also be used to measure tibial tuberosity to trochlear groove distance
- Computed tomography arthrogram if MRI is contraindicated (can also measure tibial tuberosity to trochlear groove distance)

Equipment

- Standard arthroscopy equipment
  - Fluid pump
  - Radiofrequency ablation tool
  - Oscillating shaver
  - Calibrated defect measuring probe/ruler
- Sharp ring curettes
- Proprietary disposable harvesting/trephine system, including the following:
  - Donor site harvester trephine/tubed cutter device

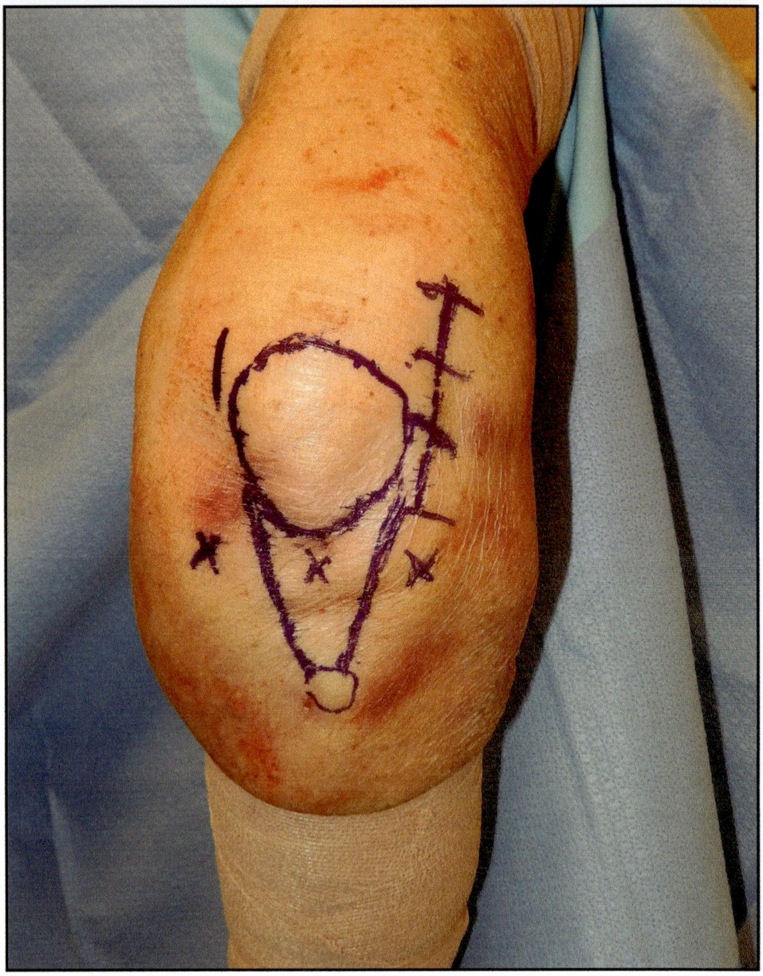

Figure 17-1. The operative knee with portals marked.

- ▹ Defect recipient site preparation harvester trephine/tubed cutter device (with 1-mm offset smaller diameter than donor harvester to ensure press-fit)
- ▹ Calibrated alignment rod
- ▹ Insertion tamp

Positioning and Portals

Proper portal placement and knee position is key to the harvest and implantation of plugs (Figure 17-1). The patient is placed supine on the operating room table, and a lateral post or leg holder is applied. Typically, an extended knee position is used for autograft harvesting, whereas a flexed position is used for graft plug implantation. Proprietary knee positioning devices can be used that sterilely affix to the operating room table and facilitate precise maintenance of the knee flexion angle using Velcro material fastening surfaces (Figure 17-2). These devices firmly position the knee and minimize motion that can alter graft plug harvest or insertion.

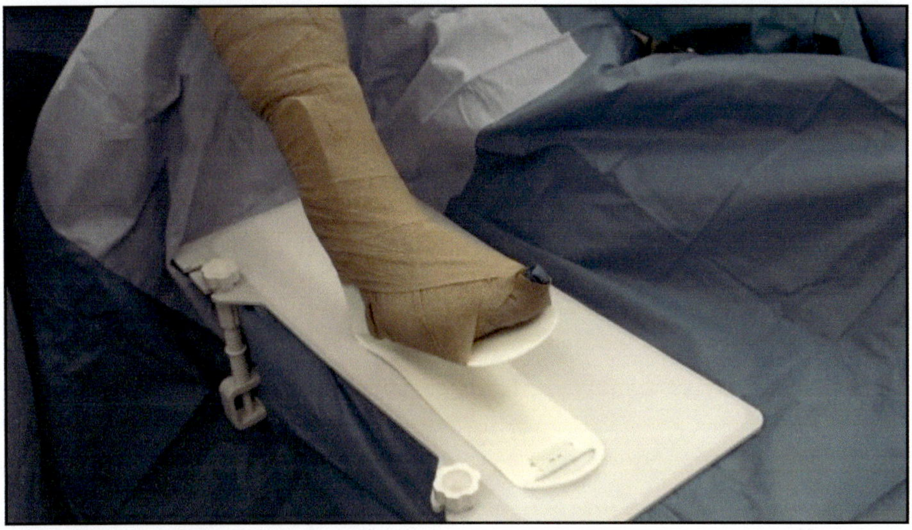

Figure 17-2. Proprietary knee positioner that uses Velcro to maintain the knee flexion angle to ensure perpendicular harvesting and grafting.

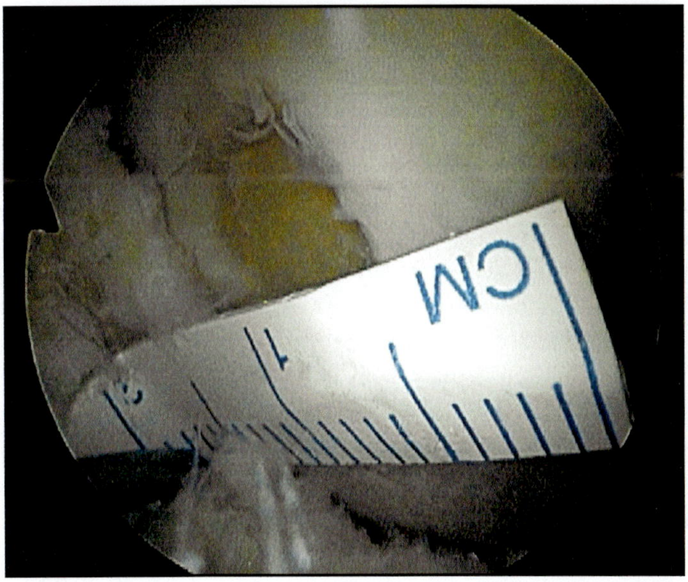

Figure 17-3. Defining the lesion and measuring its dimensions.

Step-by-Step Description of the Procedure

Assessment of the Recipient Lesion Site

Arthroscopic assessment of the defect site is performed along with arthroscopic diagnostic evaluation for concomitant pathology. The recipient site width, length, and depth are measured and templated (Figure 17-3). Sizing cylinder tubes facilitate calculation of how many grafts are needed and what size required to resurface the defect. Templating of the defect is best performed and planned by centering the apex sentinel graft plug and then layering out the perimeter. Arthroscopic visualization of the site from multiple portals along with insertion vector analysis using 18-gauge spinal needles is required to best assess the optimal angle of perpendicular graft insertion.

Figure 17-4. Available harvest sites. The preferred harvest site is the superolateral flare.

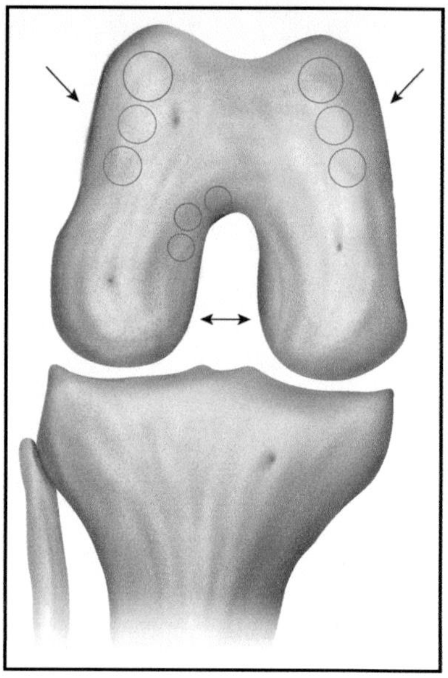

Harvest Site Choices

There are 3 accepted harvest sites for osteochondral graft selection. These are the far medial and lateral superior surfaces of the trochlear flare superior to the sulcus terminalis (of lateral femoral condyle) and the intercondylar notch, particularly in the area where a notchplasty would be performed during anterior cruciate ligament reconstruction surgery (Figure 17-4). These areas of the knee joint are subject to lower contact pressures during knee joint loading, thereby representing the potentially safest harvest sites. Most authors recommend harvesting grafts from the medial and lateral condyles to maintain a perpendicular articular surface for implantation to avoid incongruency at the implantation site. The donor sites typically heal with fibrocartilage.[14-16]

Harvest Technique

Debridement of the fat pad is helpful and necessary for appropriate visualization. Standard medial and lateral peripatellar tendon portals are made. It is important to position the portals close to and adjacent to the patellar tendon.

Once the area of harvest has been selected, it is useful to create a satellite portal such that the donor harvester device can be applied perpendicular to the chondral surface (Figure 17-5). These portals should be vertically oriented and extensile. Extending the portal sites for harvesting can facilitate harvesting an osteochondral graft with a perpendicular cartilage surface (Figure 17-6). An extended portal incision may require closure to maintain fluid pressure in the knee for the remaining steps of the procedure. If necessary, a transpatellar tendon portal can be used for harvesting trochlear cartilage. The standard graft plug diameter used is typically 4 to 10 mm.[17] The donor site harvester is placed against the surface of the cartilage and is gently impacted with a mallet to a depth of 13 to 15 mm.[13] Once the donor harvester is inserted to the appropriate depth, rotation is performed to cut and disengage the graft from the subchondral bone. Special care must be taken to avoid levering and/or toggling of the harvester devices as this will decrease the stability of the press-fit.[18]

The same portal can be used for adjacent harvesting if acceptable perpendicularity is achieved. Separation of each harvest site by 2 mm of bone is important, as is care taken to address the underlying curvature of the harvest site to avoid convergence of the graft harvest site base, which

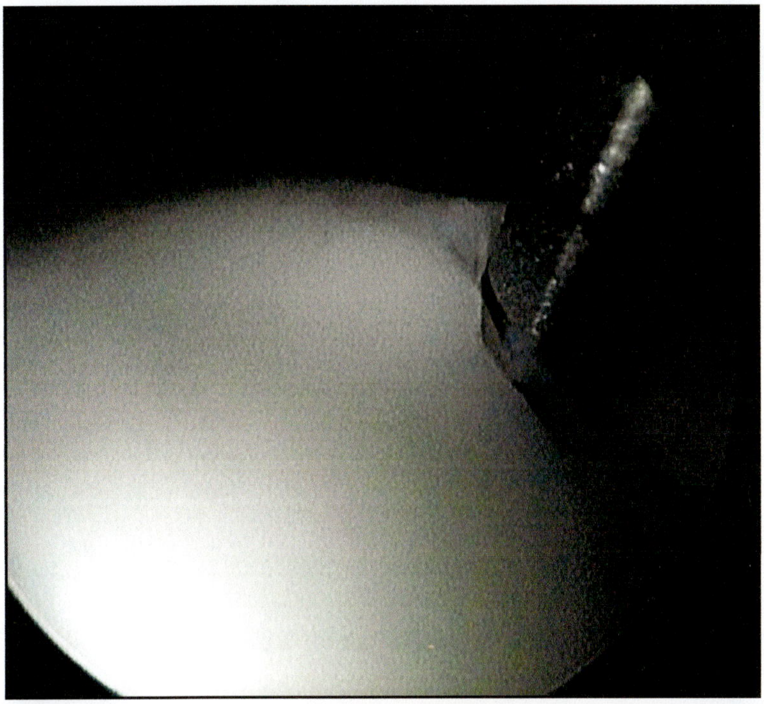

Figure 17-5. Mini-arthrotomy can be used for open harvest. Arthrotomy can be closed with suture to maintain fluid pressure for the remainder of the case.

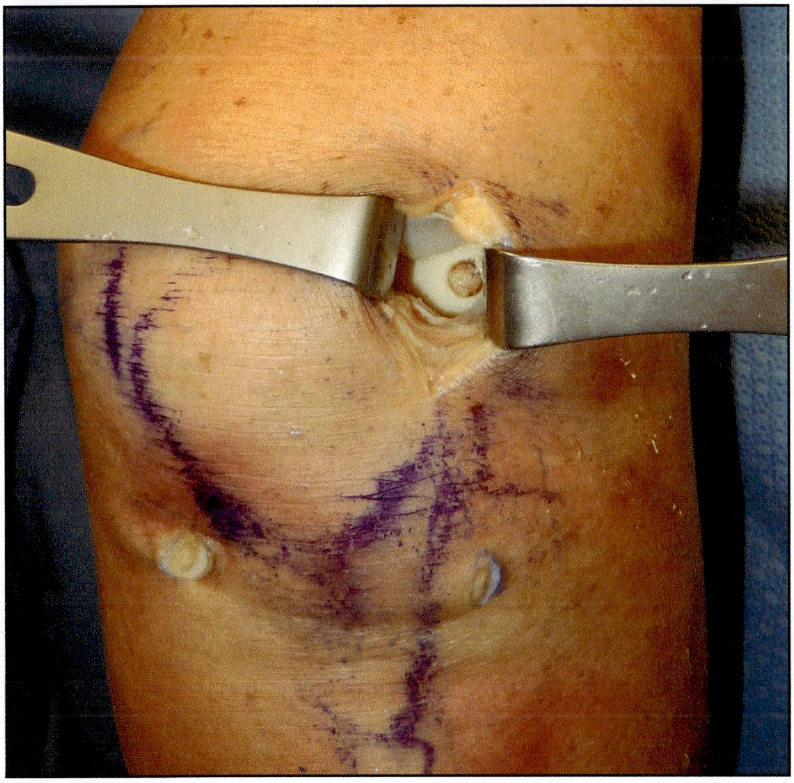

Figure 17-6. Perpendicular harvesting on the superolateral flare.

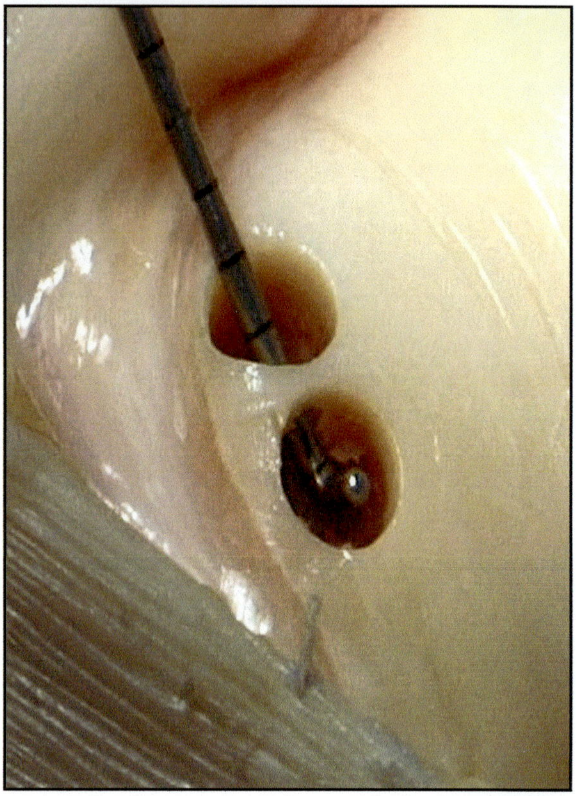

Figure 17-7. Convergence when performing multiple harvests due to the curvature of the femoral condyle.

can result in iatrogenic fracture (Figure 17-7). Small adjustments in the flexion of the knee can aid in this. Once removed, the donor graft plug must be inspected for its integrity, size, and chondral cap thickness.

Lesion/Recipient Site Preparation

The lesion recipient site must be prepared such that it will accept a graft/plug and create a congruous surface with the surrounding cartilage. The lesion should be curetted of fibrous tissue to define the true pathologic extent of the defect. The surrounding perimeter of the defect should be prepared, creating perpendicular walls. Commercially available systems have a recipient site harvester used to cut the recipient site to the bone in order to seat the osteochondral autografts. Of note, the harvesting device is 1 mm larger in diameter compared to the recipient cite trephine. For example, the 8-mm donor harvester trephine outer diameter is 9 mm, whereas the recipient site harvester trephine is exactly 8 mm in diameter to perfectly accept the graft and create a press-fit flush perpendicular surface. The underlying bone socket cut should be several millimeters less than the graft plug length. When a 15-mm plug is obtained, the lesion recipient site should be cut to a depth of 13 mm.

Graft Insertion

Graft position is critical to the success of plug implantation. The cartilaginous surface of the graft must be flush with the surrounding native cartilage. A height mismatch can cause early failure of the graft. Countersunk grafts lead to cartilage thickening, fibrous overgrowth, or even cartilage necrosis. Proud grafts also lead to failure via surface shear and toggling, which can result in graft fissuring and underlying clefting. Combination of small and large graft plugs can lead

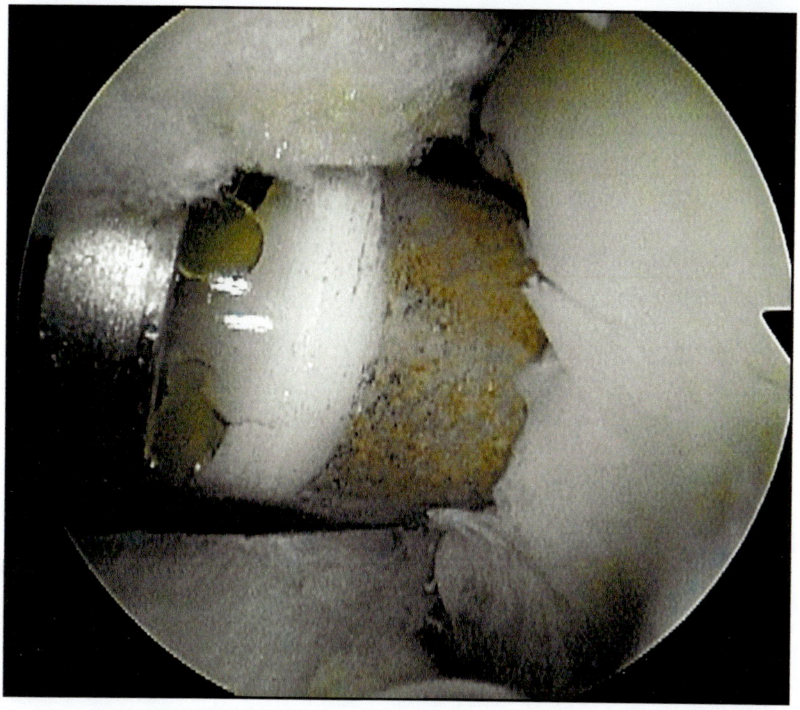

Figure 17-8. Perpendicular insertion of the graft. The graft is visualized through the clear insertion tube.

to near 100% defect coverage with congruent a surface.[9,19,20] The graft should be gently manually impacted (Figure 17-8). Use of a mallet can result in graft chondrocyte injury or fissuring of the plug.[13] Once all plugs have been placed, carefully assess the congruency of the surface (Figure 17-9). Proud plugs will be subject to compression fissuring and potential breakdown with weightbearing, and incongruent plugs significantly alter the biomechanics of the cartilaginous surface.[19,21]

Postoperative Protocol

Limiting weightbearing until bone-to-bone graft healing occurs is important to avoid graft subsidence. Early ROM to avoid stiffness is important.[9] Protocols typically commence with immediate motion and nonweightbearing limitations for 1 to 3 weeks. Progressive weightbearing begins at 2 to 6 weeks and full weightbearing at 6 weeks. Patients are typically withheld from sports for 3 to 6 months.[9,13]

Potential Complications

Chondrocyte viability in graft plugs is a concern for AOT procedures. Huntley et al[22] demonstrated chondrocyte death in human tissue from arthroplasty resections at the periphery or the graft plugs that had been harvested with standard techniques. The zone of death of chondrocytes they describe suggests that the border of the plugs will heal to fibrocartilage rather than a hyaline structure, although this has not been shown in vivo. The plugs can fracture during harvest, decreasing the number of available plugs. The necessity for perpendicular articular surface leads to converging plug bases. This can alter the depth of the plug.

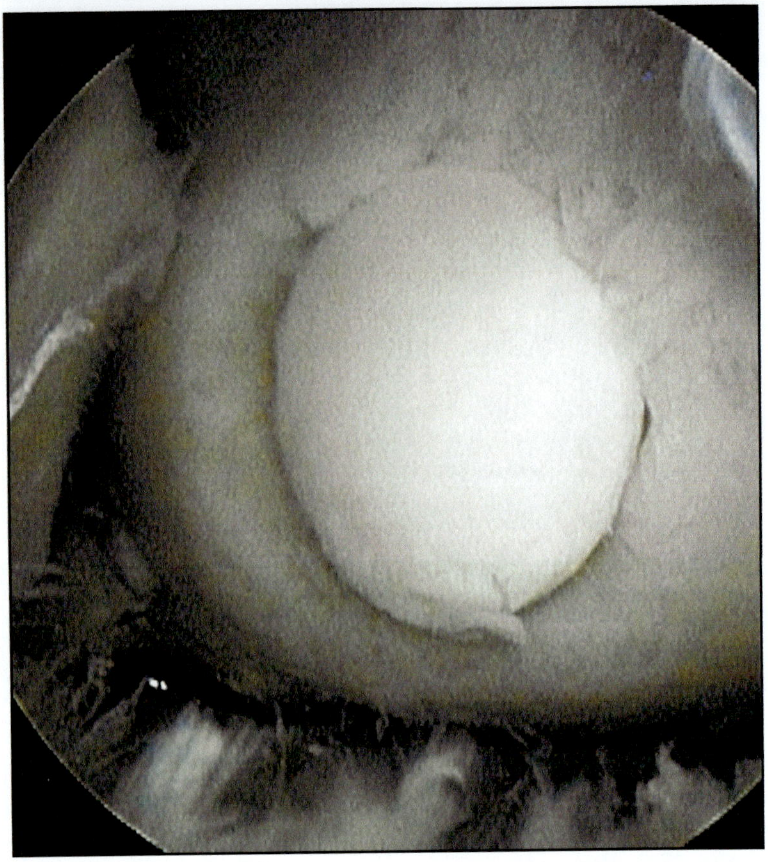

Figure 17-9. The defect site after restoration.

Immediate perioperative complications can include painful hemarthrosis, infection, and venous thromboembolism. Complications that may require a revision procedure include harvest site fracture, arthrofibrosis, patellofemoral pain, clefting, cavitation, and subchondral cyst formation.[6] Clinical outcomes include subjective, objective, functional, radiologic, and histologic parameters. Tetta et al[23] described MRI evaluation of postoperative AOT patients. They reported that clinical results are correlated to postoperative imaging.[23]

Top Technical Pearls for the Procedure

1. A 13- to 15-mm plug depth allows for bony healing at the plug base.
2. Place larger plugs in the center and then work toward resurfacing the perimeter.
3. Preserve bony recipient site walls to optimize press-fit configuration and bone-to-bone healing.
4. Low-impact harvesting and manual plug insertion avoids graft injury.
5. Use recipient site bone plugs to graft the harvest site by reversing the bone plugs.

References

1. Chen E, Sgaglione NA. Osteochondral autograft plug transfer. In: Scott WN, ed. *Insall & Scott Surgery of the Knee.* 5th ed. Philadelphia, PA: Churchill Livingstone; 2012:178-194.
2. Outerbridge HK, Outerbridge AR, Outerbridge RE. The use of a lateral patellar autologous graft for the repair of a large osteochondral defect in the knee. *J Bone Joint Surg Am.* 1995;77(1):65-72.
3. Barber FA, Chow JC. Arthroscopic osteochondral transplantation: histologic results. *Arthroscopy.* 2001;17(8):832-835.
4. Gudas R, Gudaitė A, Pocius A, et al. Ten-year follow-up of a prospective, randomized clinical study of mosaic osteochondral autologous transplantation versus microfracture for the treatment of osteochondral defects in the knee joint of athletes. *Am J Sports Med.* 2012;40(11):2499-2508.
5. Gudas R, Gudaitė A, Mickevičius T, et al. Comparison of osteochondral autologous transplantation, microfracture, or debridement techniques in articular cartilage lesions associated with anterior cruciate ligament injury: a prospective study with a 3-year follow-up. *Arthroscopy.* 2013;29(1):89-97.
6. Krych AJ, Harnly HW, Rodeo SA, Williams RJ III. Activity levels are higher after osteochondral autograft transfer mosaicplasty than after microfracture for articular cartilage defects of the knee: a retrospective comparative study. *J Bone Joint Surg Am.* 2012;94(11):971-978.
7. Marcacci M, Kon E, Delcogliano M, Filardo G, Busacca M, Zaffagnini S. Arthroscopic autologous osteochondral grafting for cartilage defects of the knee: prospective study results at a minimum 7-year follow-up. *Am J Sports Med.* 2007;35(12):2014-2021.
8. Barber FA, Chow JC. Arthroscopic chondral osseous autograft transplantation (COR procedure) for femoral defects. *Arthroscopy.* 2006;22(1):10-16.
9. Hangody L, Vásárhelyi G, Hangody LR, et al. Autologous osteochondral grafting—technique and long-term results. *Injury.* 2008;39(suppl 1):S32-S39.
10. Filardo G, Kon E, Perdisa F, Balboni F, Marcacci M. Autologous osteochondral transplantation for the treatment of knee lesions: results and limitations at two years' follow-up. *Int Orthop.* 2014;38(9):1905-1912.
11. Hangody L, Dobos J, Baló E, Pánics G, Hangody LR, Berkes I. Clinical experiences with autologous osteochondral mosaicplasty in an athletic population: a 17-year prospective multicenter study. *Am J Sports Med.* 2010;38(6):1125-1133.
12. Astur DC, Arliani GG, Binz M, et al. Autologous osteochondral transplantation for treating patellar chondral injuries: evaluation, treatment, and outcomes of a two-year follow-up study. *J Bone Joint Surg Am.* 2014;96(10):816-823.
13. Sgaglione NA, Chen E, Bert JM, Amendola A, Bugbee WD. Current strategies for nonsurgical, arthroscopic, and minimally invasive surgical treatment of knee cartilage pathology. *Instr Course Lect.* 2010;59:157-180.
14. Ahmad CS, Cohen ZA, Levine WN, Ateshian GA, Mow VC. Biomechanical and topographic considerations for autologous osteochondral grafting in the knee. *Am J Sports Med.* 2001;29(2):201-206.
15. Garretson RB III, Katolik LI, Verma N, Beck PR, Bach BR, Cole BJ. Contact pressure at osteochondral donor sites in the patellofemoral joint. *Am J Sports Med.* 2004;32(4):967-974.
16. Bartz RL, Kamaric E, Noble PC, Lintner D, Bocell J. Topographic matching of selected donor and recipient sites for osteochondral autografting of the articular surface of the femoral condyles. *Am J Sports Med.* 2001;29(2):207-212.
17. Keeling JJ, Gwinn DE, McGuigan FX. A comparison of open versus arthroscopic harvesting of osteochondral autografts. *Knee.* 2009;16(6):458-462.
18. Duchow J, Hess T, Kohn D. Primary stability of press-fit-implanted osteochondral grafts. Influence of graft size, repeated insertion, and harvesting technique. *Am J Sports Med.* 2000;28(1):24-27.
19. Pearce SG, Hurtig MB, Clarnette R, Kalra M, Cowan B, Miniaci A. An investigation of 2 techniques for optimizing joint surface congruency using multiple cylindrical osteochondral autografts. *Arthroscopy.* 2001;17(1):50-55.
20. Huang FS, Simonian PT, Norman AG, Clark JM. Effects of small incongruities in a sheep model of osteochondral autografting. *Am J Sports Med.* 2004;32(8):1842-1848.
21. Koh JL, Wirsing K, Lautenschlager E, Zhang LO. The effect of graft height mismatch on contact pressure following osteochondral grafting: a biomechanical study. *Am J Sports Med.* 2004;32(2):317-320.

22. Huntley JS, Bush PG, McBirnie JM, Simpson AH, Hall AC. Chondrocyte death associated with human femoral osteochondral harvest as performed for mosaicplasty. *J Bone Joint Surg Am.* 2005;87(2):351-360.
23. Tetta C, Busacca M, Moio A, et al. Knee osteochondral autologous transplantation: long-term MR findings and clinical correlations. *Eur J Radiol.* 2010;76(1):117-123.

Please see videos on the accompanying website at www.routledge.com/9781617119996

18

Osteochondral Allograft Transplantation

V. Franklin Sechriest II, MD; David B. Merkow, BA;
Brian J. Cole, MD, MBA; and William Bugbee, MD

Introduction

Patients with symptomatic chondral and osteochondral defects of the knee are commonly encountered in orthopedic practice. Left untreated, cartilage lesions may contribute to chronic joint irritation and inflammation resulting in early progression of osteoarthritis.[1] This increasingly common clinical problem has led surgeons and scientists to pursue and refine biologic solutions for joint restoration.[2] Fresh osteochondral allograft (OCA) transplantation is a technique that has been successfully used for primary treatment of a wide spectrum of articular injuries and joint diseases as well as for the salvage of failed cartilage repair. For the surgeon, use of fresh OCA provides an opportunity to achieve durable biological joint restoration. For the patient, this procedure provides predictable symptomatic relief and lasting functional improvement with the possibility of delaying or eliminating the need for arthroplasty.[3]

Indications

- Diagnosis
  - In general, conditions of the knee indicated for treatment with fresh OCA include large chondral and osteochondral lesions secondary to the following:
    - Osteochondritis dissecans (Figure 18-1)
    - Focal avascular necrosis
    - Other conditions involving cartilage disease or absence of subchondral bone (ie, fracture malunion)
    - Failed cartilage repair procedures (ie, microfracture, osteochondral autologous transfer, autologous chondrocyte implantation)
    - Degenerative knee conditions (select cases) in which arthroplasty is relatively contraindicated[4]

Sgaglione NA, Lubowitz JH, Provencher MT, eds. *The Knee: AANA Advanced Arthroscopic Surgical Techniques* (pp 243-255).

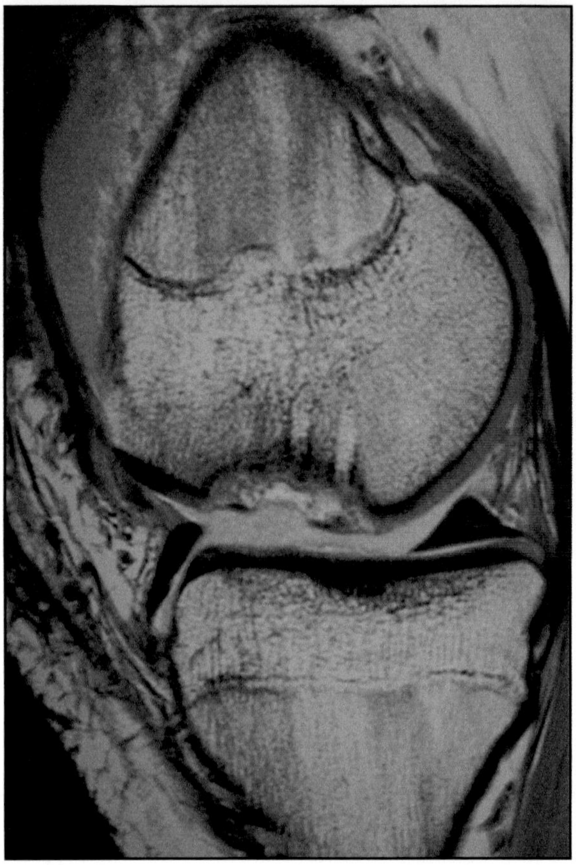

Figure 18-1. The most common indication for osteochondral allografting is osteochondritis dissecans with an unsalvageable fragment, as shown in this MRI.

- Lesion size and location
  - Primary management of chondral or osteochondral defects (≤2 cm^2)
  - Larger/deeper lesions of the femoral condyles (>2 cm^2 to ≤10, 6 to 10 mm deep) for which other techniques may be less effective, contraindicated, and/or limited by availability of donor tissue
  - Tibial chondral defects
    - Entire tibial and meniscal surface may be transplanted
  - Bipolar (ie, "kissing") lesions of the femur and tibia
    - Relatively indicated when secondary changes occur on the nontraumatized side of the lesion
    - Less successful than treatment of unipolar cartilage defects
- Salvage
  - Management of clinical failure of primary OCA transplantation
  - Success rates comparable to primary allografting[5]

Relative Contraindications

- Age
  - No absolute age limitations
  - Inferior outcomes have been reported in older patients (ie, age >40 years)[6]

- Comorbid conditions
    - Uncorrected joint malalignment and/or ligamentous instability
    - Meniscal insufficiency
    - Inflammatory arthropathy
    - Diffuse degenerative arthrosis
    - Morbid obesity, body mass index (BMI) > 30 kg/m^2

Pertinent Physical Findings

- Historical points
    - Focus on the location, duration, and onset of knee symptoms, including the following predictors of significant intra-articular pathology:
        - Knee swelling
        - Mechanical symptoms
        - Joint instability
    - Review all prior conservative and/or surgical treatments.
    - Screen for risk factors of osteonecrosis and any contraindications to OCA transplantation.
    - Patient age, sex, BMI, activity level, and expectations should influence patient selection.
- Physical examination findings
- Evaluation of the entire affected extremity is required, with attention to the following:
    - Limb malalignment and/or rotational deformity, diffuse hyperlaxity, and/or ipsilateral hip/ankle disorders
    - A focused examination of the knee joint should assess the following:
        - Joint alignment, range of motion (ROM), ligamentous stability, and function during gait
        - Presence of swelling/effusion, muscular atrophy, and tenderness to palpation at the site of the lesion
            - ◊ Best test: Correlation of chondral lesion locations with the patient's symptomatic complaints or site of tenderness is the best test to predict the outcome of osteochondral allografting
        - A dynamic strength assessment, particularly of the quadriceps[7]

Pertinent Imaging

- X-rays
    - Standing anteroposterior view with the knee in full extension (weightbearing) to assess anterior joint space narrowing and to allow tissue banks to size-match allografts
        - Use a marker to correct for magnification[8]
            - ◊ Femoral lesions: Width of the affected condyle is measured, with an acceptable match considered as allograft condyle within ± 2 mm[9]
            - ◊ Tibial lesions: Width of the affected tibial plateau is measured from the medial to lateral cortex just distal to the articular surface.

  - Standing posteroanterior view with the knee flexed 45 degrees (weightbearing) to assess posterior joint space narrowing
  - Lateral view to assess patellofemoral relationship (ie, alta or baja)
  - Patellar view to assess the presence of trochlear or patellar dysplasia, patellar tilt, and/or maltracking
  - Standing bilateral long-leg alignment view to measure the mechanical axis through the knee
- Magnetic resonance imaging (MRI)
  - To assess cartilage integrity and bone quality of/adjacent to articular lesion as well as concomitant ligamentous and/or meniscal pathology
  - The true size of the articular lesion may be underestimated.[10]
- Conventional computed tomography (CT)
  - To quantify the extent of bone involvement, bone quality, and/or evaluate patellofemoral relationship (ie, tibial tubercle to trochlear groove distance)
- Single-photon emission CT
  - A hybrid imaging technique that combines bone scintigraphy with high-resolution CT images is useful in patients for whom MRI is contraindicated and/or when image quality is impaired by retained metallic implants.[11]
- Arthroscopic images
  - Photographic images recorded during previous surgical procedures provide insight into defect dimensions, degree of containment, and associated pathology.
  - They may obviate the need for another diagnostic knee arthroscopy.

Equipment

The equipment required depends on the surface to be grafted and the surgical technique used. For most contained defects of the femoral condyles, a press-fit technique can be performed using commercially available systems (Arthrex) that simplifies site preparation, donor harvesting, and graft insertion (Figure 18-2).[12] However, if the size or location of the lesion does not permit use of a dowel-type press-fit system, the surgeon should be prepared to perform the shell graft technique. Because shell grafts require measured resection and sculpting of bone and cartilage, additional surgical equipment on hand should include calipers, depth-gauge, high-speed burr, reciprocating and oscillating saws, bone files, and/or rasps. In addition, use of fluoroscopy is critical for the treatment of certain large knee defects (ie, tibial plateau) and may enhance accuracy when treating other anatomic locations as well. For either technique, the allograft is opened and inspected prior to surgical incision to ensure it is acceptable for implantation. Although most grafts can be press-fit without fixation, multiple options for graft fixation should be available, including bioabsorbable pins and/or low-profile interfragmentary screws 3 mm in diameter or less.

Positioning and Portals

The patient is positioned supine with a proximal thigh tourniquet. A leg or foot holder helps to position and maintain the knee in flexion between 70 and 110 degrees (Figure 18-3). Prophylactic antibiotics are administered at the induction of anesthesia. The operative extremity is prepared and draped to permit an anterior approach to the knee. Old incision sites are marked. If an

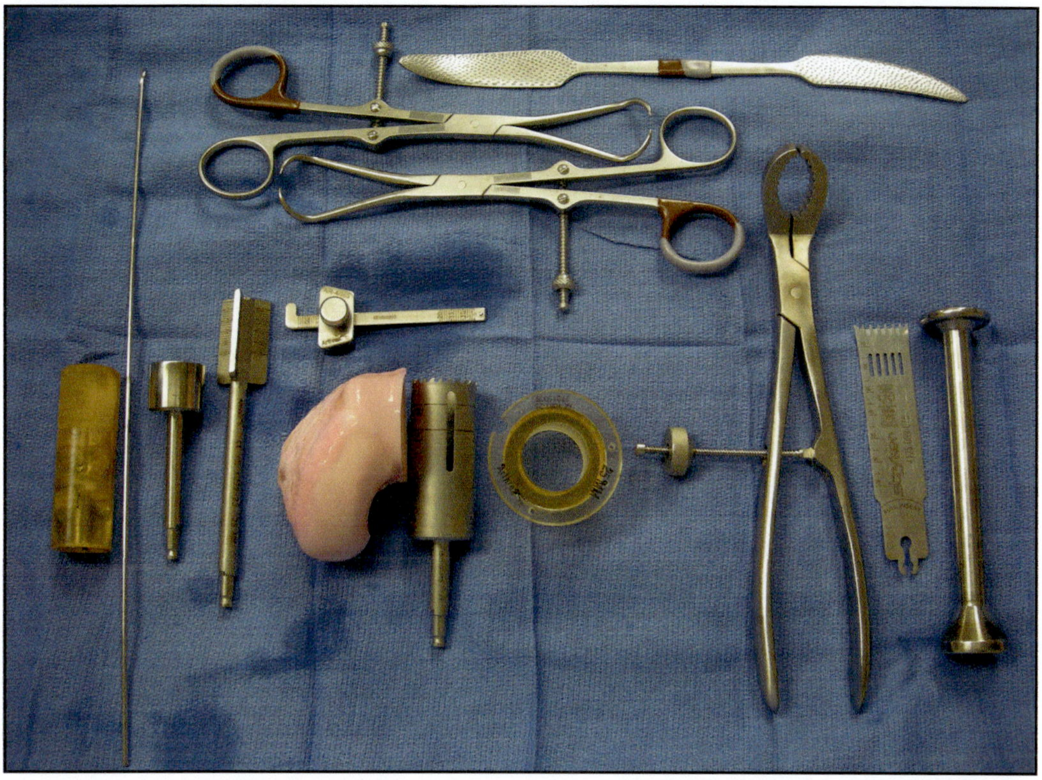

Figure 18-2. Typical instruments used to prepare and insert a plug-type allograft.

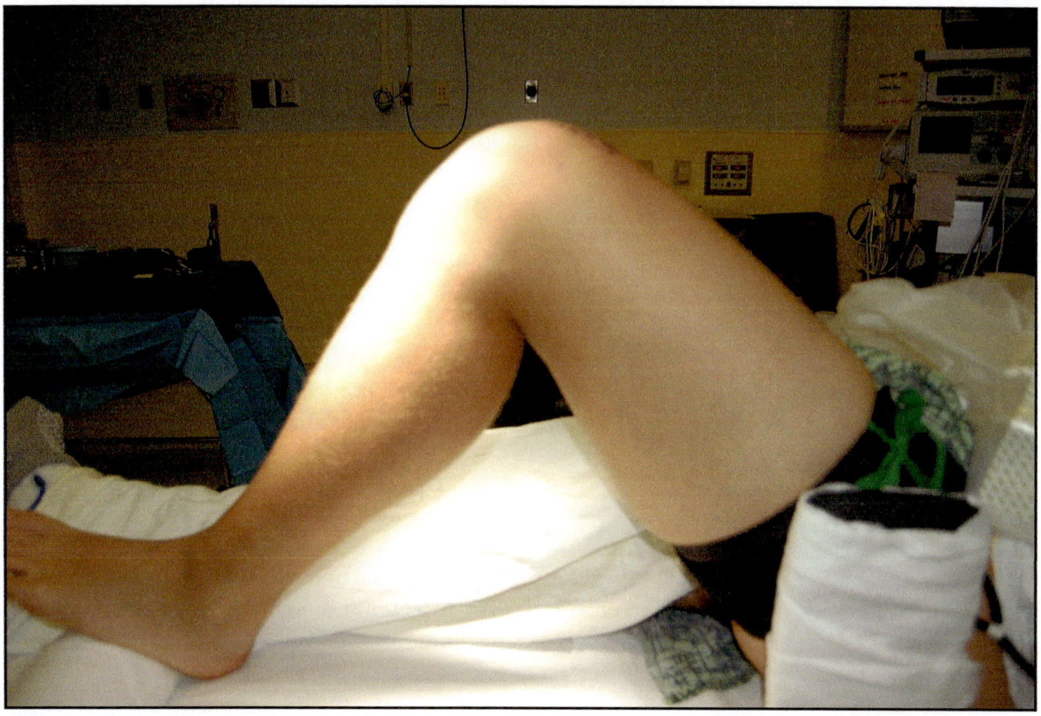

Figure 18-3. Stable limb positioning that allows for various degrees of knee flexion facilitates exposure of the lesion.

osteotomy is planned, it may be advantageous to have access to the ipsilateral anterior superior iliac spine as a source of autograft bone and as a reference to evaluate alignment. A diagnostic arthroscopy may be performed before the OCA transplantation to confirm lesion size and/or to treat coexisting pathology.

Step-by-Step Description of the Procedure

Management of Concomitant Pathology

For cartilage defects of the knee, if malalignment is present, realignment osteotomy is required to decrease the load on the graft. In general, opening wedge high tibial osteotomy is used to correct varus malalignment, and opening wedge lateral distal femoral osteotomy is used to correct valgus deformity.[13] For the patellofemoral joint, optimization of patellofemoral biomechanics may result in better outcomes, although this has not been proven in the context of osteochondral allografting. Therefore, in the setting of a patellofemoral lesion, tibial tubercle anteriorization or anteromedialization may be performed to transfer load and/or correct maltracking.[14] Management of ligament and meniscal deficiency is critical to normalization of compartment contact stresses and shear forces. Ligament reconstruction and/or meniscal allograft transplantation may be performed concomitantly with osteochondral transplantation to optimize graft survival and improve clinical outcome.[15]

Surgical Exposure

A standard midline incision is made. Depending on lesion location, a medial or lateral arthrotomy may be used. Once the joint capsule has been incised and the retractors have been placed, the knee is brought into the degree of flexion that presents the lesion into the arthrotomy site. In some cases, when the lesion is posterior, detachment and reflection of the meniscus may aid exposure. Angled retractors are placed medially and laterally to expose the condyle. A carefully placed retractor into the notch is useful to aid in patellar retraction (Figure 18-4). Extension of the deep incision proximally and distally aids in patellar mobilization.

Lesion Inspection and Preparation

The articular lesion is inspected to define the margins. Surrounding damaged cartilage and bone is debrided to facilitate accurate sizing of the lesion. The lesion is assessed to determine the allograft shape that will best match the defect. The 2 techniques for OCA preparation include the press-fit circular plug technique and the shell graft technique. Whenever possible, the press-fit technique is preferred based on the relative ease in achieving a precise graft fit and the low likelihood for need of supplemental internal fixation. If the lesion is not amenable to a press-fit OCA, a shell graft may be used.

Dowel or Plug Technique (Video)

The size of the OCA is estimated using the commercially available cannulated, cylindrical sizing guides. Each guide is positioned to encompass the defect and thereby determine the optimal plug diameter. The guide must sit flush with the surrounding normal cartilage to properly restore the geometry of the articular surface. If the lesion is between 2 sizes, begin with the smaller size. Once a size has been determined, ensure that the available graft can accommodate the harvesting of this size graft as anatomic differences can occur that may change the surgical plan (ie, the surgeon may choose to place two 20-mm grafts rather than one 30-mm graft if the allograft condyle

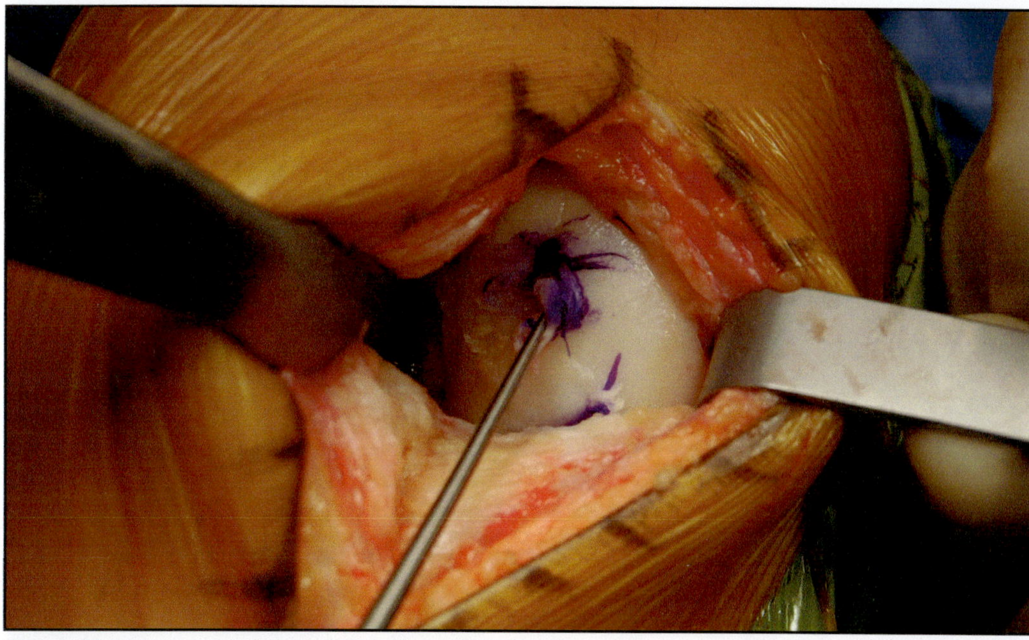

Figure 18-4. Exposure of the lesion with small arthrotomy and retractor placement. This patient has a failed microfracture of the medial femoral condyle.

is too narrow to harvest a 30-mm diameter graft). Recipient site preparation begins with placement of a guide wire through the cylindrical sizing guide into the center of the lesion, perpendicular to the articular surface. The cartilage surface is scored, and a cannulated counter bore reamer is used to remove the articular cartilage and 3 to 4 mm of subchondral bone. In deeper lesions, the pathologic bone is removed until there is healthy, bleeding bone. Generally, for treatment of chondral defects, depth does not exceed 6 to 8 mm (Figure 18-5). For treatment of osteochondral lesions, depth may reach up to 10 mm. The authors rarely find it necessary or appropriate to ream more than 8 mm total depth. The reamings are collected and may be used to graft osseous defects (cysts) or to optimize the position of the graft. At this point, the guide pin can be removed. If necessary, multiple perforations can be made in the base of the defect using a K-wire to promote vascular inflow. A skin marker is used to mark the 12 o'clock position for reference, and depth measurements are made and recorded in the 4 quadrants of the recipient site. A ruler or depth gauge is used to measure and record the socket depth at the 3, 6, 9, and 12 o'clock positions. The recipient socket is now complete and ready for the press-fit OCA.

The corresponding anatomic location of the recipient site is identified on the donor allograft. The allograft is then secured to the allograft workstation platform or held with clamps and positioned such that the appropriate diameter bushing may be positioned perpendicular to the articular surface, matching the orientation used to create the recipient site. The cylindrical sizing tube is used to confirm that the selected angle will match the contour of the defect, and the 12 o'clock position is marked with a surgical marker. The appropriate size-coring reamer is passed through the bushing and advanced through the entire depth. Once harvested from the donor condyle, the graft is removed as a long cylindrical plug. An oscillating saw can be used to release the graft from the donor condyle. The depths for the 4 quadrants of the recipient site are transferred to the graft, and the allograft plug thickness is customized using a microsagittal saw to trim excess bone to the thickness matching the recipient site. Just before insertion, it is beneficial to bevel the edges of the osseous portion with a small rongeur or rasp to facilitate the initial press-fit into the recipient socket. The donor graft should be irrigated copiously with a pulsatile lavage to remove blood and marrow cells to decrease the risk of a host immune response.[16] The donor graft is positioned by

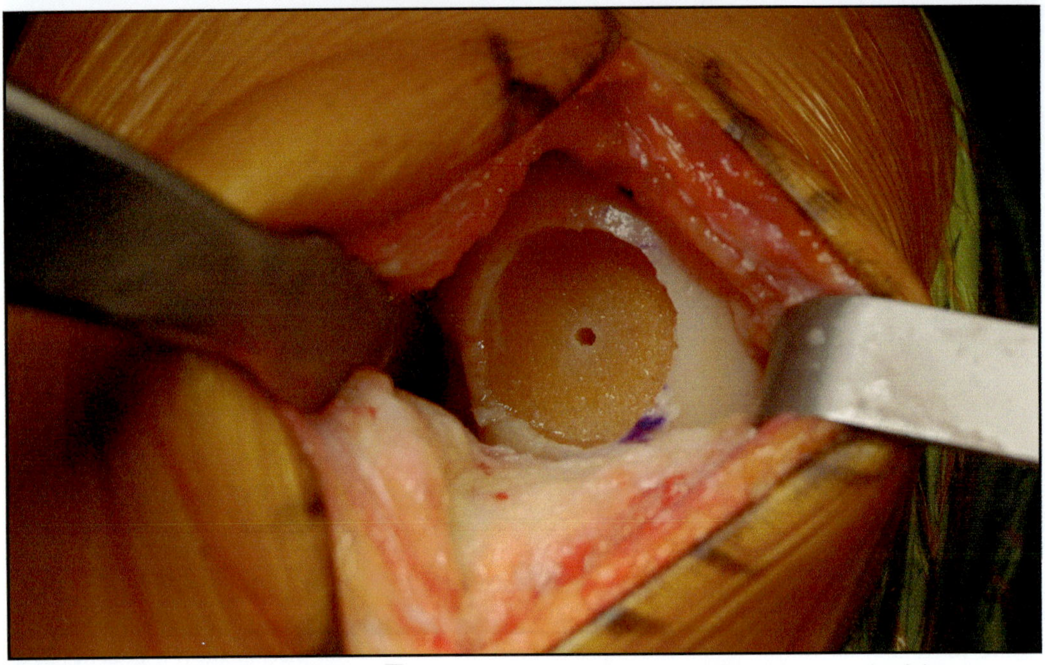

Figure 18-5. Preparation of the defect site is complete. Note the relatively shallow depth of the site.

aligning the markings and is pressed into place by hand. The authors prefer to use passive knee ROM to initially seat the graft, and then gentle tamping can be performed to fully seat the graft, but excessive impact loading with a mallet during allograft insertion may damage the extracellular matrix and/or result in chondrocyte death. If the graft does not fit, dilating the recipient site with a slightly oversized tamp or reinserting the guide wire and reaming deeper may be considered or the graft can be further trimmed or beveled. The final resting position of the graft should be flush relative to the surrounding articular surface, although the authors accept stepoffs of less than 1 mm (Figure 18-6).[17] If the graft is unstable or has an exposed edge, absorbable pins or biocompression screws are used. For large femoral defects, more than 1 press-fit OCA plug may be required. The "snowman technique" facilitates coverage of a greater condylar area using a second press-fit plug (Figure 18-7). In this technique, the first graft is secured with a small K-wire or, if necessary, definitively fixed with biocompression screws to prevent dislodgement during preparation of the second overlapping site. Care is taken to minimize space between multiple grafts as this may lead to formation of biomechanically inferior fibrocartilage and/or lack of articular congruity (ie, cobble stoning) which may alter biomechanics and negatively affect clinical outcome.

Shell Technique

For uncontained or asymmetric lesions or for lesions in locations that are difficult to access on the femur, a free-hand technique is required to match donor tissue to the recipient defect. A skin marker is used to outline the shape of the defect, and a 15-blade scalpel is used to incise the remaining cartilage, which is then removed using sharp curettes. A high-speed burr is then used to remove the underlying pathologic bone to expose healthy bleeding bone. Creation of a simple recipient site geometry (ie, rectangle or trapezoid) simplifies subsequent freehand sizing of the OCA. After the recipient site is prepared, the donor graft is roughly fashioned with a microsagittal saw. It is best to make the initial cuts slightly wider than measured to oversize the donor graft. A series of trial fittings and repeated measurement guide sculpting of the donor tissue to achieve a precise fit.

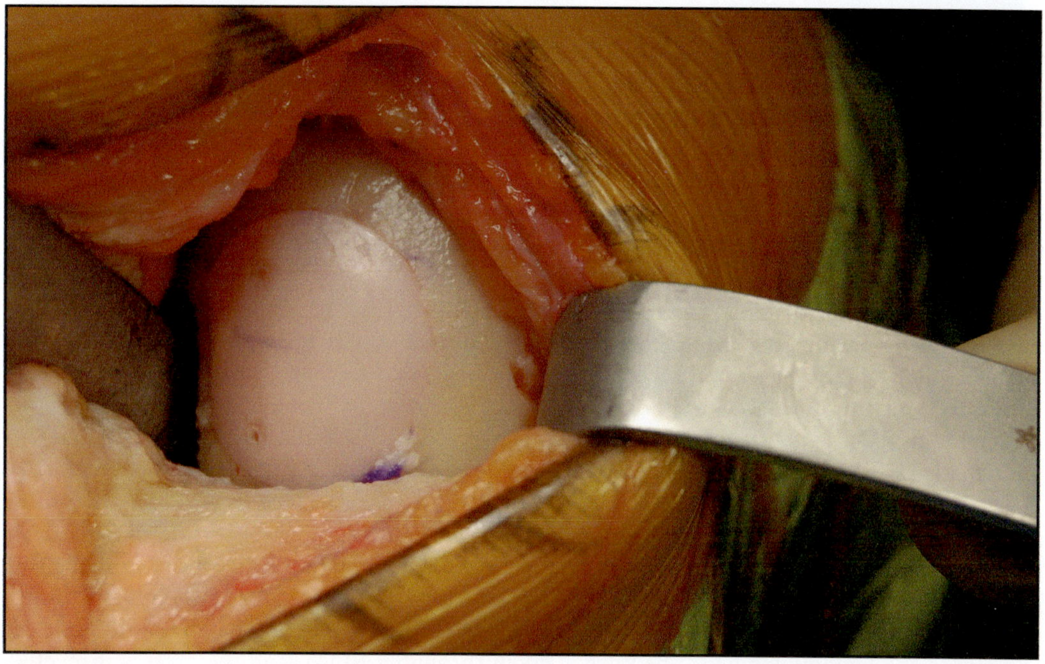

Figure 18-6. The graft has been inserted in appropriate orientation, and a flush press-fit has been obtained.

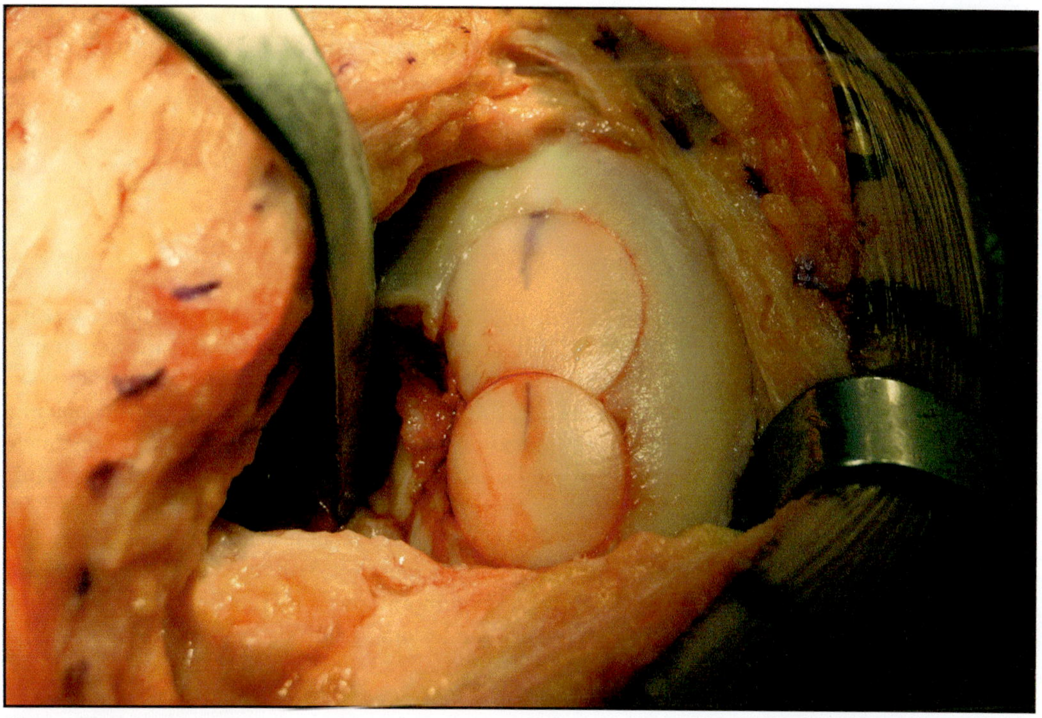

Figure 18-7. In this patient, 2 overlapping grafts have been used in the "snowman" configuration.

For the patella, although smaller lesions may be successfully managed with press-fit circular grafts, larger lesions are managed with a technique similar to that used in total knee arthroplasty. Patellar thickness is measured with calipers and resection of the articular surface is performed, maintaining at least 12 mm of residual bone. The donor graft is then resected in a similar fashion. The allograft is then lavaged and seated in the appropriate position. The graft is then secured with interfragmentary screw fixation from the anterior surface of the patella into the subchondral bone beneath the median ridge of the graft. Afterward, an assessment of patellar tracking will determine the need for any additional soft tissue or bony realignment procedures.

Large post-traumatic tibial plateau lesions are managed with a technique similar to that used in unicompartmental knee arthroplasty. Under fluoroscopic guidance, en bloc resection of the meniscotibial unit with an "L-cut" is performed. Two freehand cuts are made to resect a minimal amount of subchondral bone. K-wires or arthroplasty jigs may be used to assist the surgeon with these cuts. Measurements of the length and width of the resected surface and the joint space gap allow estimation of the required allograft dimensions. Next, the donor graft is secured in the graft holder, and the desired dimensions are marked. Ideally, tibial plateau grafts are 8 to 12 mm thick, which is typical for restoring plateau height after fracture malunion. A reciprocating saw is used to make the vertical cut, and an oscillating saw is used to make the horizontal cut referencing off the marks placed on the graft margins. Once sculpted to the optimal size and shape, the graft is lavaged and carefully inserted in the anatomic position adjacent to the femoral condyle. The knee is taken through a ROM, and the graft is inspected visually and under fluoroscopy to assess graft position and restoration of the joint line and tibial slope. Revisions are made as necessary to optimize graft fit and position as well as overall joint alignment and mechanics. The graft is then fixed with 2 interfragmentary screws placed from the submeniscal articular margin at the midcoronal and anterior positions. After fixation of the bone, the meniscus is repaired in the standard fashion.

Postoperative Protocol

Phase I: 0 to 4 Weeks

In the first phase of rehabilitation, patient goals are to control pain and swelling, restore muscle control, improve knee ROM, and protect the allograft. Patients are allowed unrestricted early nonweightbearing motion unless a concurrent procedure dictates otherwise. Weightbearing status varies based on lesion location, but the general goal is to avoid placing stress on the transplanted area. Patients with tibial or femoral grafts are restricted to toe-touch weightbearing for 6 weeks. Patients with patellofemoral grafts are permitted weightbearing as tolerated in extension but are limited to between 30 and 45 degrees of active flexion. In addition to passive- and active-assisted knee ROM, exercises include stretching and isometric strengthening of the quadriceps, hamstrings, and gluteus muscles. Although knee braces are not required, they may be useful for patients with patellofemoral grafts by limiting knee flexion to less than 45 degrees.[18] For patients with bipolar knee lesions, an unloader brace may be useful as they progress to full weightbearing.

Phase II: 4 to 12 Weeks

In the second phase, patient goals are to regain full ROM, a normalized gait, and the ability to perform functional activities of daily life. Stretching and isometric strengthening exercises are continued as weightbearing is progressed. Typically, once the patient has adequate quadriceps control and can perform a straight leg raise without an extension lag, initiation of a stationary cycle is appropriate. Gait training and closed chain exercises are introduced. For focal lesion treated with a single plug graft, full weightbearing is generally allowed by 6 to 8 weeks. Patients with large or complex grafts are restricted to partial weightbearing for 8 to 12 weeks.

Phase III: 12 to 18 Weeks

The final phase of rehabilitation varies based on the goals and expectations of the patient. For the patient with a goal of performing activities of daily living, a transition is made to a maintenance home exercise program. Recreational sports are not reintroduced until joint rehabilitation is complete and radiographic healing has been demonstrated, which generally occurs no earlier than 4 to 6 months postoperatively. In athletes, this phase focuses on advanced strengthening, core stabilization, proprioception, and gradual return to sport-specific training. At a minimum, athletes should demonstrate full knee ROM, no effusion, joint stability, excellent dynamic strength, and have clinical and radiographic evidence of complete graft incorporation before returning to the highest level of activity. Ideally, high-loading activities should be avoided until at least 6 to 12 months postoperatively.[19]

Potential Complications

Early Complications

Use of a limited arthrotomy and emphasis on early motion is advised to avoid arthrofibrosis. Superficial and deep surgical site infections may occur and must be distinguished based on laboratory markers, physical examination, and joint aspiration. The risk of surgical site infection is low as long as the graft is processed and handled properly and graft lavage and appropriate perioperative antibiotics are used. Allograft-related complications, such as disease transmission, infection, and immunogenic reaction, are rare but may arise.[20-23] Occasionally, patients may develop recurrent sterile effusions related to overuse or an immune-mediated synovitis. These symptoms typically resolve with symptomatic management (ie, aspiration, rest, ice, compression) without requiring graft removal. Graft failure with fragmentation and collapse may occur. Delayed or nonunion of the allograft is extremely rare but may occur with use of larger allografts or in patients with compromised subchondral bone.[24]

Late Complications

Late graft failure may be characterized by fracture of the graft, incomplete remodeling of the graft-bone interface, and/or resorption of allograft tissue. Graft fragmentation and collapse may result from incomplete healing with host bone due to limited revascularization.[25] Progression of the underlying disease process (ie, additional chondral lesions, osteoarthritis, avascular necrosis) may result in recurrent or persistent symptoms independent of graft status.

Top Technical Pearls for the Procedure

1. Prior to surgical incision, ensure the OCA is for the correct patient, the correct knee, and the correct anatomic location. Inspect the allograft tissue to confirm adequacy of the size-match and overall quality.
2. When using the press-fit technique, during preparation of the recipient site, ensure the cylinder-sizing guide is placed perpendicular to the joint surface to ensure a uniform socket for the donor plug.
3. During preparation of the recipient site articular surface, limit the depth of the recipient socket (eg, 5 to 8 mm) to reduce the amount of allograft bone that must ultimately heal/incorporate. Save subchondral bone from reaming to fill defects or adjust height of the OCA.
4. Pulse lavage of the OCA prior to insertion will decrease marrow elements and immunogenicity of allograft bone.
5. After implantation, if the OCA is not secure, fix with a bioabsorbable compression screw that is advanced to a level just below the articular surface and just beneath the subchondral plate.

References

1. Heir S, Nerhus TK, Røtterud JH, et al. Focal cartilage defects in the knee impair quality of life as much as severe osteoarthritis: a comparison of knee injury and osteoarthritis outcome score in 4 patient categories scheduled for knee surgery. *Am J Sports Med.* 2010;38(2):231-237.
2. Moran CJ, Pascual-Garrido C, Chubinskaya S, et al. Restoration of articular cartilage. *J Bone Joint Surg Am.* 2014;96(4):336-344.
3. Raz G, Safir OA, Backstein DJ, Lee PT, Gross AE. Distal femoral fresh osteochondral allografts: follow-up at a mean of twenty-two years. *J Bone Joint Surg Am.* 2014;96(13):1101-1107.
4. Yu J, Bugbee WD. Osteochondral allograft transplantation. In: Williams RJ III, ed. *Cartilage Repair Strategies.* Totowa, NJ: Humana Press Inc; 2007:167-191.
5. Horton MT, Pulido PA, McCauley JC, Bugbee WD. Revision osteochondral allograft transplantations: do they work? *Am J Sports Med.* 2013;41(11):2507-2511.
6. Behery O, Siston RA, Harris JD, Flanigan DC. Treatment of cartilage defects of the knee: expanding on the existing algorithm. *Clin J Sport Med.* 2014;24(1):21-30.
7. Sharma L, Dunlop DD, Cahue S, Song J, Hayes KW. Quadriceps strength and osteoarthritis progression in malaligned and lax knees. *Ann Intern Med.* 2003;138(8):613-619.
8. Highgenboten CL, Jackson A, Aschliman M, Meske NB. The estimation of femoral condyle size. An important component in osteochondral allografts. *Clin Orthop Relat Res.* 1989;(246):225-233.
9. Latterman C, Romine SE. Osteochondral allografts: state of the art. *Clin Sports Med.* 2009;28(2):281-301.
10. Campbell AB, Knopp MV, Kolovich GP, et al. Preoperative MRI underestimates articular cartilage defect size compared with findings at arthroscopic knee surgery. *Am J Sports Med.* 2013;41(3):590-595.
11. Mucha A, Dordevic M, Hirschmann A, et al. Effect of high tibial osteotomy on joint loading in symptomatic patients with varus aligned knees: a study using SPECT/CT [published online ahead of print May 11, 2014]. *Knee Surg Sports Traumatol Arthrosc.*
12. Arthrex. Allograft OATS (Osteochondral Autograft Transfer System) Surgical Technique. Available at: http://jrfortho.org/images/prod-files/Allograft_OATS%C2%AE_(Osteochondral_Autograft_Transfer_System).pdf. Accessed on July 30, 2015.
13. Minzlaff P, Feucht MJ, Saier T, et al. Osteochondral autologous transfer combined with valgus high tibial osteotomy: long-term results and survivorship analysis. *Am J Sports Med.* 2013;41(10):2325-2332.

14. Pascual-Garrido C, Slabaugh MA, L'Heureux DR, Friel NA, Cole BJ. Recommendations and treatment outcomes for patellofemoral articular cartilage defects with autologous chondrocyte implantation: prospective evaluation at average 4-year follow-up. *Am J Sports Med.* 2009;37(suppl 1):33S-41S.
15. Harris JD, Cavo M, Brophy R, Siston R, Flanigan D. Biological knee reconstruction: a systematic review of combined meniscal allograft transplantation and cartilage repair or restoration. *Arthroscopy.* 2011;27(3):409-418.
16. Hunt HE, Sadr K, Deyoung AJ, Gortz S, Bugbee WD. The role of immunologic response in fresh osteochondral allografting of the knee. *Am J Sports Med.* 2014;42(4):886-891.
17. Koh JL, Wirsing K, Lautenschlager E, Zhang LO. The effect of graft height mismatch on contact pressure following osteochondral grafting: a biomechanical study. *Am J Sports Med.* 2004;32(2):317-320.
18. Cole BJ, Pascual-Garrido C, Grumet RC. Surgical management of articular cartilage defects in the knee. *Instr Course Lect.* 2010;59:181-204.
19. Krych AJ, Robertson CM, Williams RJ III; Cartilage Study Group. Return to athletic activity after osteochondral allograft transplantation in the knee. *Am J Sports Med.* 2012;40(5):1053-1059.
20. Kainer MA, Linden JV, Whaley DN, et al. Clostridium infections associated with musculoskeletal-tissue allografts. *N Engl J Med.* 2004;350(25):2564-2571.
21. American Association of Tissue Banks. Standards for tissue banking. Available at: http://www.aatb.org/. Accessed July 16, 2014.
22. Centers for Disease Control and Prevention (CDC). Update: allograft-associated bacterial infections—United States, 2002. *MMWR Morb Mortal Wkly Rep.* 2002;51(10):207-210.
23. Tugwell BD, Patel PR, Williams IT, et al. Transmission of hepatitis C virus to several organ and tissue recipients from an antibody-negative donor. *Ann Intern Med.* 2005;143(9):648-654.
24. Ball ST, Amiel D, Williams SK, et al. The effects of storage on fresh human osteochondral allografts. *Clin Orthop Relat Res.* 2004;(418):246-252.
25. Oakeshott RD, Farine I, Pritzker KP, Langer F, Gross AE. A clinical and histologic analysis of failed fresh osteochondral allografts. *Clin Orthop Relat Res.* 1988;(233):283-294.

Please see videos on the accompanying website at www.routledge.com/9781617119996

19

Approach to Chondral Damage in the Patellofemoral Joint

Randy Mascarenhas, MD, FRCSC; Shane J. Nho, MD, MS; and Jack Farr, MD

Introduction

Chondral defects of the patellofemoral joint can be caused by overuse, traumatic injury, and pathoanatomy. As such, the patellofemoral joint remains the most common location for articular cartilage defects of the knee.[1] Most of these lesions are asymptomatic and found incidentally at the time of knee arthroscopy, but some may be symptomatic. The key to proper management is to sort through the multiple potential etiologies of the patient's patellofemoral pain and assign a component to the cartilage defect. This is a diagnosis by exclusion because the aneural chondral defect contributes to the pain through its effect on the sensory nerves in the bone, capsule, and synovium. For patients with chondral lesions that have been assigned as a contributing component to the overall patellofemoral pain, a spectrum of treatment may be indicated based on the size and location of the defect in addition to patient-related and anatomic factors. These treatments include arthroscopic and open procedures and combinations of both. This chapter focuses on providing a framework for the surgical management of symptomatic chondral defects of the patellofemoral joint via an algorithmic approach.

Indications

- Failed thorough comprehensive nonoperative management
- Pain is directly attributed to the documented chondrosis by imaging and/or arthroscopy (no atypical or global pain)
- Chondral lesion is grade III or IV modified Outerbridge (International Cartilage Repair Society grades IIIA, IIIB, IIIC, IIID, IVA, or IVB, noting the environment is optimized for patellofemoral force/contact area, tracking, and stability
- Lesion size appropriate for considered treatment (< 3 cm^2 in diameter osteochondral autograft transfer; > 3 cm^2 in diameter osteochondral allograft transplant or cell therapy)[2]

Sgaglione NA, Lubowitz JH, Provencher MT, eds. *The Knee: AANA Advanced Arthroscopic Surgical Techniques* (pp 257-268).

Controversial Indications

- Bipolar lesions
- Marrow stimulation of patellar lesions[3]
- Autologous chondrocyte implantation (ACI) after prior microfracture/marrow stimulation[4,5]
- When age and lesion size would allow consideration of patellofemoral arthroplasty
- Worker's compensation cases[6]
- Open growth plates
- Elevated body mass index (BMI; > 35 kg/m^2 or > 40 kg/m^2)[6]
- Cell therapy alone in the presence of marked bone marrow lesion(s)

Contraindications

- Atypical pain (complex regional pain syndrome)
- Pain not directly attributable to the chondrosis
- Patient not willing to follow the rehabilitation program and/or future activity modification

Pertinent Physical Findings

Patients with symptomatic lesions generally describe anterior knee pain deep to the patella or in the distribution of the infrapatellar fat pad. Activities with impact or those that require increased knee flexion may exacerbate symptoms. These patellofemoral loading activities include ascension and descension of stairs, prolonged sitting, running, jumping, kneeling, and squatting.[7] Patients may complain of crepitus or clicking with range of motion (ROM) and also may describe the presence of effusions. Details should be ascertained regarding the presence of any preceding traumatic inciting event, history of patellar instability, and previous surgeries. Having the patient use a knee pain diagram may also be helpful.[8]

- Assessment gait and standing coronal plane alignment
- Patient sitting: Patellar tracking (central, lateral, J sign frank subluxation or dislocation) and the presence of crepitus
- Supine position: Standard knee examination assessing ligament laxity, areas of focal pain (with emphasis on point tenderness of the medial and lateral facets of the patellar), presence of an effusion, and provocative testing. Assess pelvic flexibility and hamstring flexibility.
- Supine position: Patellar-specific evaluation involves patellar mobility medial and lateral displacement, proximal and distal glide, and tilt. Apprehension is noted medially and laterally, especially in those with prior lateral release. The involved limb muscle bulk and strength is compared to the asymptomatic limb.
- Lateral position: Ober testing for iliotibial band flexibility
- Prone position: Test quadriceps flexibility, internal and external rotation of the hips, and foot progression angle
- Functional testing: Double- and single-leg squats and/or stepping up forward and backward on a small step to assess weakness of the hip abductors and gluteal muscles resulting in pelvic tilt and dropping of the opposite limb causing functional internal rotation and valgus positioning. (These tests may elicit more pain and crepitus than the manual examination.)

Nonoperative Management

Initial nonoperative management is to educate the patient on why he or she is having pain. For example, is the primary problem structural, inadequate muscle/soft tissue balance, or overuse? Patients need to understand their personal "envelope of function" and that all patients are unique and must stay within their own body limits. Physical therapy is key and should include a comprehensive "core to floor" program that is similar in some aspects to an anterior cruciate ligament prevention program. Attention is focused on quadriceps, core, abductor, and gluteal strengthening in addition to flexibility, patellar mobilizations, and physiotaping. Anti-inflammatory drugs and/or cortisone injections may aid in symptom control while the patient undergoes physical therapy. A patellar stabilizing brace may be useful if the patient has a history of patellar instability. This aggressive nonsurgical regimen should continue for a minimum of 6 weeks and should be pursued until muscle strength and flexibility defects are improved, which can require up to 6 months in some patients. Surgery should be considered in the patient who remains symptomatic despite regaining near full ROM and near normal strength. Such patients should also have a chondral defect that is logically contributing to the majority of their symptoms.

Pertinent Imagining

X-Rays

- Standing anteroposterior, posteroanterior, flexion weightbearing and hip-to-ankle alignment view if coronal plane malalignment is suspected
- True lateral x-ray to evaluate trochlear dysplasia and patellar tilt.[9] Patellar height is most commonly reported as a ratio using the Caton-Deschamps or Blackburne-Peel method.
- Low flexion angle axial view, such as the Merchant view, to assess patellar position in relation to the trochlea and for identifying the subluxation. (In most patients, this view assesses the distal aspect of the trochlea and will underestimate patellofemoral chondral wear that occurs in the mid aspect.)

Magnetic Resonance Imaging

- Magnetic resonance imaging (MRI) allows articular cartilage defect visualization.[10,11]
- Axial and sagittal cuts are most useful for evaluating the patellofemoral compartment.
- T1- and T2-weighted images can be used to assess the chondral surfaces of the patella and trochlea; T2 fat-suppressed imaging should be used to identify underlying subchondral bone marrow lesions.
- The presence of trochlear dysplasia can be confirmed directly in 2-dimensional and further enhanced with 3-dimensional reconstructions.
- Effusions and loose bodies are noted.
- Tibial tubercle to trochlear groove (TT-TG) distance and tibial tuberosity to posterior cruciate ligament distance (TT-posterior cruciate ligament) are measured on axial MRI cuts. (More than 50% of patients with symptomatic patellofemoral disease will have a TT-TG distance greater than 20 mm compared to 5% of asymptomatic knees.[12]) Computed tomography (CT) and MRI TT-TG measurements are not in strict agreement.[13]

Computed Tomography

- Allows for quad active view of alignment and patellar positioning through ROM
- Alternative measurement for tuberosity distances
- Assesses bone quality, especially if there are regions of deficiency

Computed Tomography or Magnetic Resonance Arthrogram

- Thin sectioning may allow more detailed measurement of the defect.
- Assessing delamination or unstable osteochondral lesions

Equipment

- Arthroscopic debridement
  - 3.5- or 4.5-mm high-speed shaver
  - Curved shaver
- Marrow stimulation: Microfracture awls with a variety of curves
  - K-wires
  - Power drill
  - Ring curettes
  - Arthroscopic scalpel
- Osteochondral autograft
  - Osteochondral plug harvest set from company of surgeon's choice
  - Donor plug harvester
  - Cannulated reamer or tubular chisel
  - Calibrated ruler
  - Donor plug inserter or bone tamp
- Osteochondral allograft
  - Allograft set from a company of the surgeon's choice
  - Cannulated circular reamers
  - Calibrated ruler
  - Coring reamer
  - Pulsatile lavage
  - Oversized bone tamp
- ACI
  - Harvesting awl for initial biopsy
  - Ring curettes
  - 6-0 suture
  - Periosteal patch or collagen membrane
  - Fibrin glue
  - Small angiocatheter and syringe
  - Sterile saline
  - Autologous chondrocytes in vials

- Particulated juvenile allograft cartilage (PJAC) transplantation
  - Ring curettes
  - 6-0 suture
  - Periosteal patch or collagen membrane
  - Fibrin glue
  - Small angiocatheter and syringe
  - Sterile saline
  - PJAC

Positioning and Portals

Patients should be placed supine on the operating table with a bump under the ipsilateral hip of the affected knee. A tourniquet may be used during the approach and then deflated. A radiolucent operative table should be used to facilitate intraoperative fluoroscopy if the surgeon feels fluoroscopy may aid the scheduled procedure.

Step-by-Step Description of the Procedure

Arthroscopic Debridement

Arthroscopy may be performed using standard inferomedial and inferolateral portals with an optional outflow portal. Portals may need to be moved distal to facilitate access to the undersurface of the patella. Unstable articular cartilage flaps should be debrided mechanically with a small-radius, high-speed shaver.[14] Use of electrocautery or radiofrequency devices for chondral debridement is generally discouraged due to the potential for damage to the adjacent cartilage secondary to heat production.[15,16] The noncutting portion of the shaver can be placed at the base of the articular cartilage to allow for amputation of any fibrillated fronds. A curved shaver may be useful to reach some lesions. For smaller lesions, marrow stimulation or osteochondral autograft transplantation can be performed following debridement. However, larger lesions will require a second procedure for osteochondral allograft transplantation or cell-based treatment, such as ACI or PJAC. Patients indicated for ACI require cartilage biopsy at the time of staging the arthroscopy to provide a medium for cell expansion. Generally, 200 to 300 g of full-thickness articular cartilage from the intercondylar notch is required and can be harvested with the use of a curved scoop.

Marrow Stimulation

Microfracture of patellar defects generally leads to less promising results than those obtained when the procedure is performed for symptomatic defects on the femoral condyles.[17] Microfracture may be performed via open or arthroscopic means. If open access is required, a laterally based arthrotomy allows avoidance of the vastus medialis obliquus. The incision extends from the superior pole of the patella to the patellar tendon and may be extended further distally to expose the entire tibial crest if a tibial tubercle osteotomy is being performed concomitantly with the patellofemoral cartilage procedure. Lesions are debrided down to sharp margins with stable, vertical walls of healthy articular cartilage surrounding the defect. A curette or arthroscopic scalpel removes the calcified cartilage layer from the defect without penetrating the subchondral bone. Multiple perforations are then made 2 to 3 mm apart in the subchondral bone by starting at the periphery and moving toward the center of the defect (Figure 19-1). This can be done with a

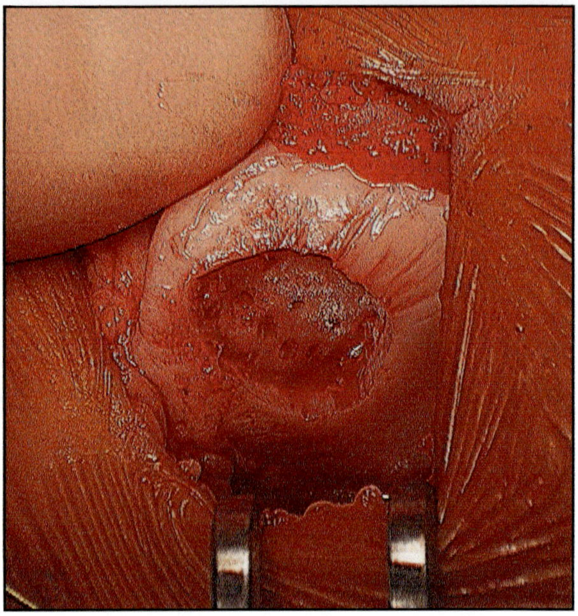

Figure 19-1. Microfracture of a trochlear defect is performed through a parapatellar arthrotomy and the creation of stable vertical walls. The calcified cartilage layer is removed and multiple perforations are made 2 to 3 mm apart to encourage marrow stimulation.

microfracture awl, K-wire, or drill with care taken to not fracture the subchondral bone between perforations. Drilling with saline irrigation may be specifically useful on the patella where the subchondral bone is thicker because awls with a 90-degree curve may still skive.

Osteochondral Autograft

Osteochondral autograft plug harvest and implantation may be performed via arthroscopic or open means. If performed arthroscopically, accessory portals may be required to achieve perpendicular access to the donor and recipient sites and should be confirmed with spinal needle localization. Once the lesion has been debrided to a stable base, a sizing tool is placed arthroscopically through the appropriate portal or through a mini-arthrotomy to determine the size of the defect and the number of donor plugs required to fill the lesion. Graft harvest is then performed from the intercondylar notch, the trochlea, or just proximal to the sulcus terminalis. Using a plug harvester placed directly perpendicular to the donor site, an osteochondral plug of 6 to 11 mm in diameter and 8 to 12 mm long is taken from a location of the surgeon's choice. Multiple plugs may be harvested if needed and should be inspected for length and slope after removal. The recipient site is then prepared with a tubular chisel placed perpendicular to the defect or by placing a guide pin into the center of the defect and reaming over it with a cannulated circular reamer. A calibrated measuring device is used to measure the recipient socket at the 3, 6, 9, and 12 o'clock positions to ensure that the donor graft(s) can be oriented in the correct position to match slope before implantation in a press-fit fashion. It is imperative that articular congruency be maintained, but it is preferable to have the graft slightly recessed rather than proud if congruency cannot be achieved.[18]

Osteochondral Allograft

A standard parapatellar arthrotomy is performed, and the patella is everted to expose the chondral defect. A cylindrical guide is placed over the defect to perform appropriate sizing, and the 12 o'clock position is marked. A guide pin is placed through the center of the guide to a depth of 2 cm, and the guide is removed. A cannulated reamer is placed over the guide pin, and the defect is reamed to a depth of 6 to 8 mm. The depth of the recipient site is then measured at the 3, 6, 9, and 12 o'clock positions with a small ruler to allow precise allograft preparation and to minimize the chances of the

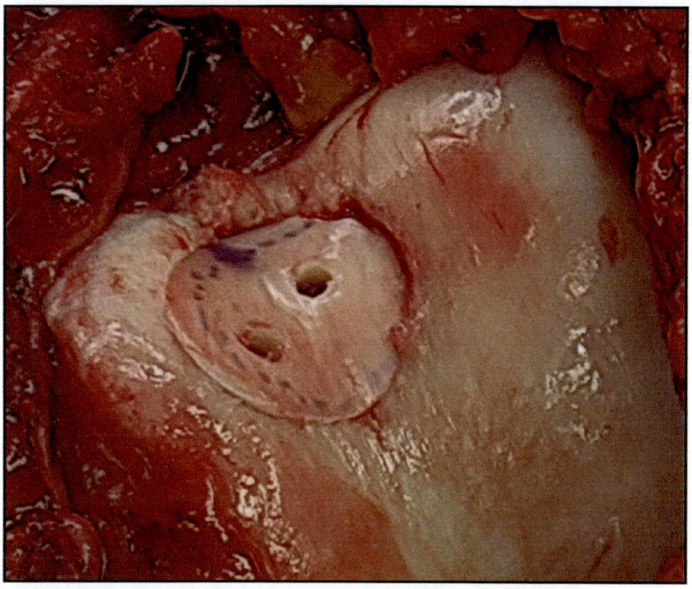

Figure 19-2. Trochlear osteochondral allograft fixed with biocompression screws.

graft being proud or recessed. The donor graft is prepared using a coring reamer of appropriate size with adjustments being made to the depth based on the recipient site measurements. The donor plug is irrigated using pulsatile lavage to wash out marrow elements and is inserted into the recipient site in a press-fit manner with gentle use of an oversized tamp (Figure 19-2).

Autologous Chondrocyte Implantation

As previously mentioned, ACI requires a staged procedure in which cartilage biopsy is performed during the initial staged arthroscopy to facilitate chondrocyte cell expansion, which can take 6 to 12 weeks. When the cells are ready, ACI is performed through a standard parapatellar arthrotomy with the patella everted to expose the defect (Figure 19-3). Similar to the microfracture procedure, the patellar or trochlear defect is then prepared with vertical peripheral walls, and the calcified cartilage layer is removed (Figure 19-4). A periosteal patch or collagen membrane in the same shape as the defect can be used to cover the lesion, and cells may be placed on the patch/membrane prior to suturing to allow for chondrocyte adherence. The patch/membrane is then sewn to the periphery of the defect using 6-0 suture with interrupted stitches spaced 3 to 4 mm apart evenly around the periphery (Figure 19-5). The suture needle should pass from patch to cartilage, with the knots placed on the patch surface. Fibrin glue is then placed around the periphery while leaving a small opening in the superior aspect of the patch. A leak test may be performed if the patch was not seeded with cells by using a small angiocatheter to inject sterile saline through the opening in the construct while monitoring for leaks. Fibrin glue or sutures are used to correct any deficiencies in the integrity of the patch, and then the angiocatheter is used to inject the remaining cells in the defect through the superior opening. The opening is then closed with sutures and fibrin glue. This step is omitted for the seeded patch technique, and the cells are injected after suturing and gluing.

Particulated Juvenile Allograft Cartilage

PJAC transplantation may be formed in a similar fashion to ACI for large, contained grade III/IV defects of the patellofemoral joint with intact subchondral bone. The defect is prepared in the same fashion as required for ACI, and the particulated cartilage tissue is then mixed with fibrin glue and placed into the defect (Figure 19-6). The particulated tissue should be left slightly

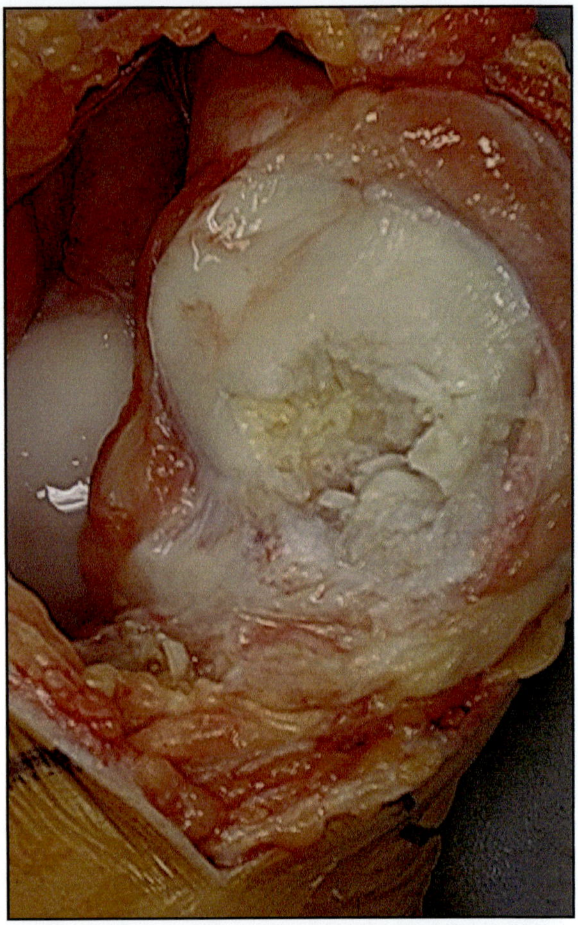

Figure 19-3. A lateral parapatellar arthrotomy is used to evert the patella and access the patellar defect.

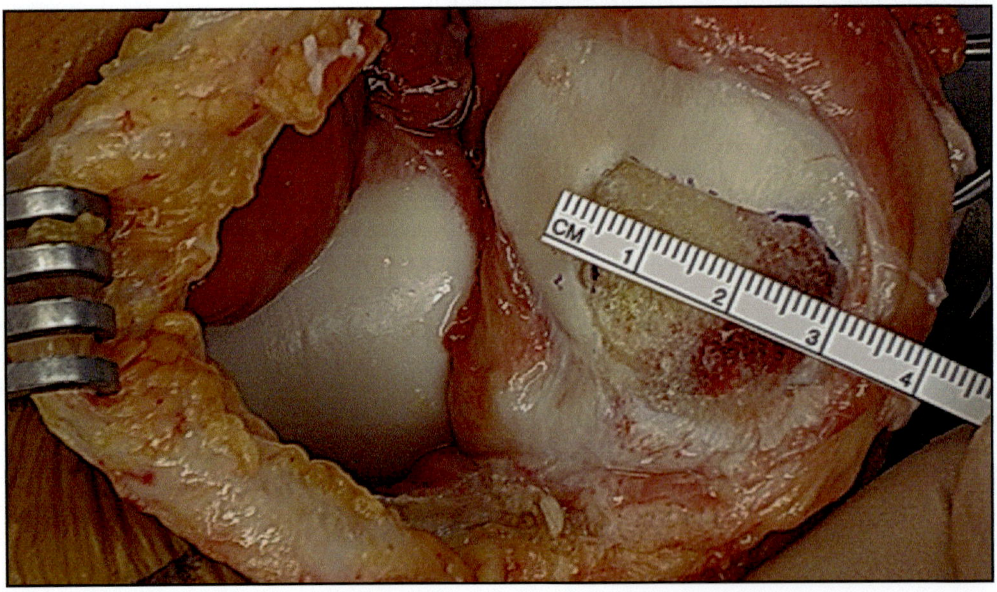

Figure 19-4. The margins of the defect are sharply debrided, and the calcified cartilage is removed.

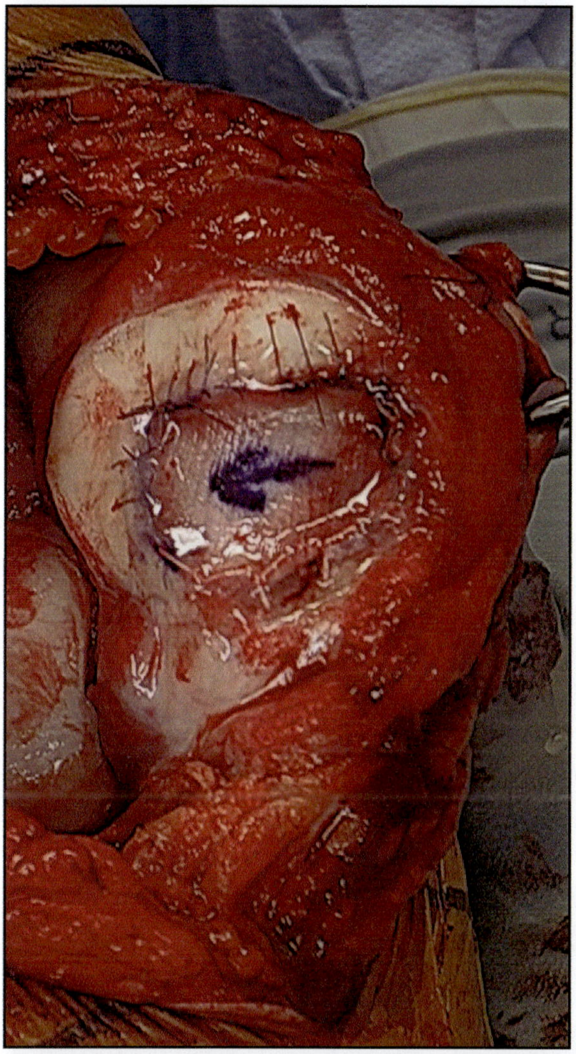

Figure 19-5. A periosteal patch or collagen membrane is sewn over the lesion to allow for infusion of chondrocytes into the defect.

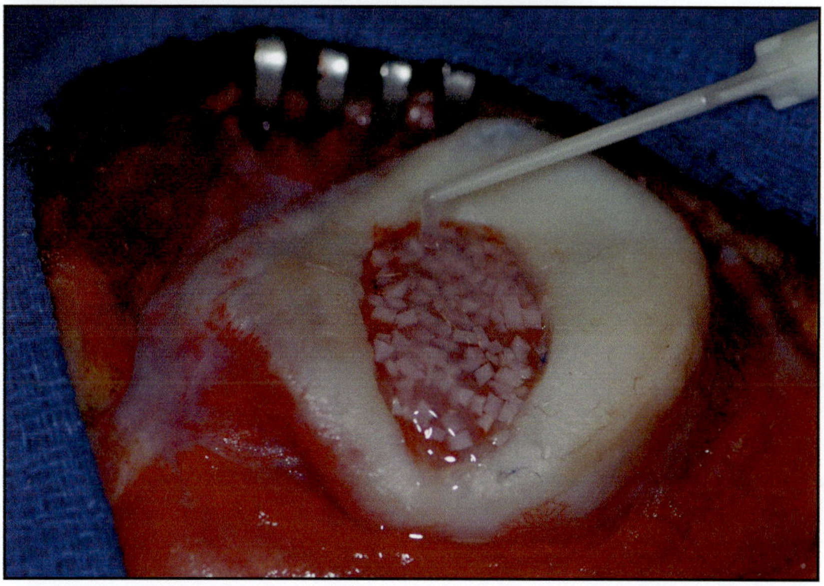

Figure 19-6. PJAC is mixed with fibrin glue and placed into the trochlear defect.

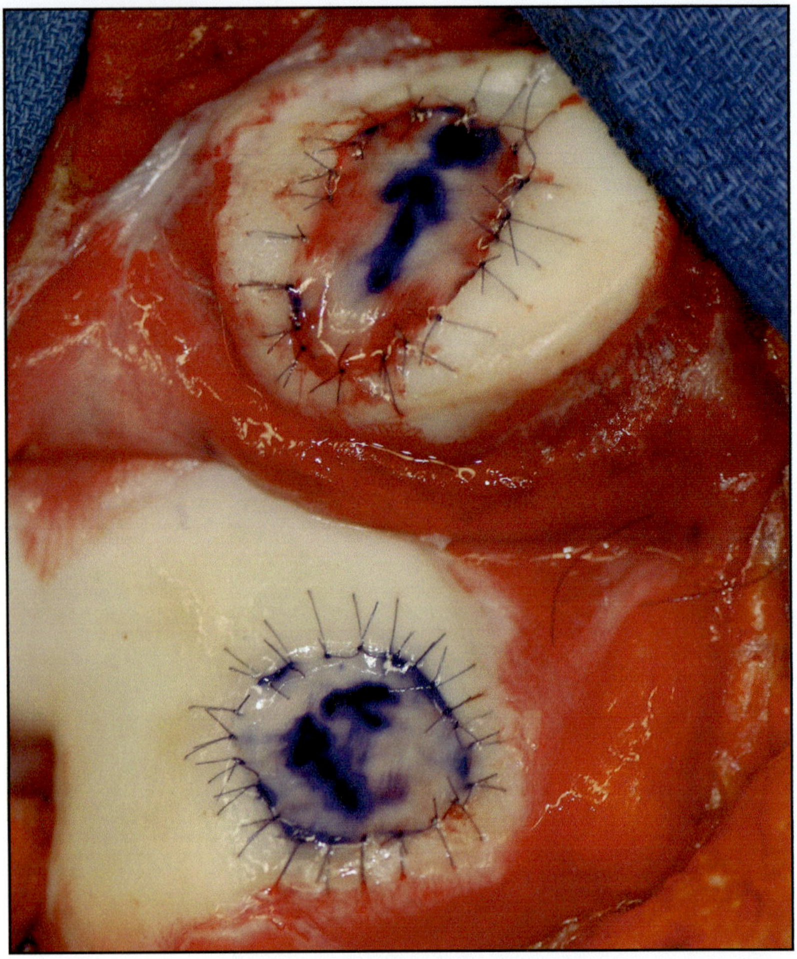

Figure 19-7. A collagen membrane may be sewn over a patellar and/or trochlear defect after insertion of the mixture of DeNovo NT and fibrin glue into the defect.

recessed because there is a tendency for the cells to grow upward and outward. The mixture should be allowed to set before closure and may be sealed with a fibrin glue seal around the margins of the defect or sewing a collagen membrane in place (Figure 19-7).

Postoperative Protocol

If arthroscopic debridement alone is performed, patients are allowed full weightbearing and full knee ROM. However, weightbearing is only allowed in extension for 4 to 6 weeks if microfracture, cartilage transplantation, or ACI is performed so as to not unduly load the patellofemoral joint with flexion weightbearing. In addition, weightbearing is protected for 6 weeks if a tibial tubercle osteotomy is performed in conjunction with the patellofemoral cartilage. Continuous passive motion is started immediately postoperatively and is typically used for 6 to 8 hours per day. ROM is set from 0 to 30 degrees and is increased by 5 to 10 degrees daily so that patients have nearly full flexion by 6 to 8 weeks postoperatively. A brace is worn locked in extension for the first week postoperatively but can be removed for continuous passive motion and exercises. The brace is then gradually opened in 20-degree increments per week and can be discontinued when active quadriceps control is achieved to the extent that a straight leg raise can be performed with extensor lag. Microfracture patients generally may be ready to return to strenuous activities by 6 months postoperatively, whereas patients undergoing cartilage transplantation or ACI may require as long as 12 months to return to impact activities and as long as 18 months to reach maximum medical improvement.

Potential Complications

Standard postoperative complications, such as infection, wound complications, complex regional pain syndrome, and deep venous thrombosis, may be encountered with all procedures. Patients undergoing microfracture may undergo intralesional osseous overgrowth within the treated defect, and research is currently ongoing to confirm whether microfracture may reduce the potential efficacy of any future cell-based therapies for the treated lesion. Patch overgrowth may occur in patients treated with cell-based therapies, such as ACI and PJAC, and osteochondral allograft treatment carries with it risks of disease transmission and graft resorption along with the potential to delaminate or collapse. Osteochondral autografts may lead to development of postoperative pain due to donor site morbidity and cyst formation.

Top Technical Pearls for the Procedure

1. Use a small-radius, high-speed shaver for mechanical debridement of symptomatic cartilage flaps rather than radiofrequency or electrocautery devices. This reduces the risk to the surrounding healthy cartilage.
2. Ensure that the symptomatic patellofemoral defect is debrided to stable vertical walls with sharp margins and that the calcified cartilage layer is removed before microfracturing the subchondral bone.
3. Ensure that instruments approach the donor and recipient sites in a perpendicular fashion to enable proper graft harvest and implantation when performing osteochondral autograft implantation.
4. Avoid dog-ears and multiple suture passes when securing the periosteal patch or collagen membrane with 6-0 suture when performing ACI.
5. If open exposure to a patellofemoral defect is required, use a lateral parapatellar arthrotomy to minimize violation of the quadriceps.

References

1. Curl WW, Krome J, Gordon ES, Rushing J, Smith BP, Poehling GG. Cartilage injuries: a review of 31,516 knee arthroscopies. *Arthroscopy.* 1997;13(4):456-460.
2. Hangody L, Füles P. Autologous osteochondral mosaicplasty for the treatment of full-thickness defects of weight-bearing joints: ten years of experimental and clinical experience. *J Bone Joint Surg Am.* 2003;85(suppl 2):25-32.
3. Kreuz PC, Steinwachs MR, Erggelet C, et al. Results after microfracture of full-thickness chondral defects in different compartments in the knee. *Osteoarthritis Cartilage.* 2006;14(11):1119-1125.
4. Minas T, Von Keudell A, Bryant T, Gomoll AH. The John Insall Award: a minimum 10-year outcome study of autologous chondrocyte implantation. *Clin Orthop Relat Res.* 2014;472(1):41-51.

5. Pestka JM, Bode G, Salzmann G, Südkamp NP, Niemeyer P. Clinical outcome of autologous chondrocyte implantation for failed microfracture treatment of full-thickness cartilage defects of the knee joint. *Am J Sports Med.* 2012;40(2):325-331.
6. Ding C, Cicuttini F, Scott F, Cooley H, Boon C, Jones G. Natural history of knee cartilage defects and factors affecting change. *Arch Intern Med.* 2006;166(6):651-658.
7. Crossley KM, Cowan SM, Bennell KL, McConnell J. Knee flexion during stair ambulation is altered in individuals with patellofemoral pain. *J Orthop Res.* 2004;22(2):267-274.
8. Post WR, Fulkerson J. Knee pain diagrams: correlation with physical examination findings in patients with anterior knee pain. *Arthroscopy.* 1994;10(6):618-623.
9. Malghem J, Maldague B. Depth insufficiency of the proximal trochlear groove on lateral radiographs of the knee: relation to patellar dislocation. *Radiology.* 1989;170(2):507-510.
10. Potter HG, Linklater JM, Allen AA, Hannafin JA, Haas SB. Magnetic resonance imaging of articular cartilage in the knee. An evaluation with use of fast-spin-echo imaging. *J Bone Joint Surg Am.* 1998;80(9):1276-1284.
11. Shindle MK, Foo LF, Kelly BT, et al. Magnetic resonance imaging of cartilage in the athlete: current techniques and spectrum of disease. *J Bone Joint Surg Am.* 2006;88(suppl 4):27-46.
12. Dejour H, Walch G, Nove-Josserand L, Guier C. Factors of patellar instability: an anatomic radiographic study. *Knee Surg Sports Traumatol Arthrosc.* 1994;2(1):19-26.
13. Camp CL, Stuart MJ, Krych AJ, et al. CT and MRI measurements of tibial tubercle-trochlear groove distances are not equivalent in patients with patellar instability. *Am J Sports Med.* 2013;41(8):1835-1840.
14. Federico DJ, Reider B. Results of isolated patellar debridement for patellofemoral pain in patients with normal patellar alignment. *Am J Sports Med.* 1997;25(5):663-669.
15. Edwards RB III, Lu Y, Uthamanthil RK, et al. Comparison of mechanical debridement and radiofrequency energy for chondroplasty in an in vivo equine model of partial thickness cartilage injury. *Osteoarthritis Cartilage.* 2007;15(2):169-178.
16. Ryan A, Bertone AL, Kaeding CC, Backstrom KC, Weisbrode SE. The effects of radiofrequency energy treatment on chondrocytes and matrix of fibrillated articular cartilage. *Am J Sports Med.* 2003;31(3):386-391.
17. Mithoefer K, Williams RJ III, Warren RF, et al. The microfracture technique for the treatment of articular cartilage lesions in the knee. A prospective cohort study. *J Bone Joint Surg Am.* 2005;87(9):1911-1920.
18. Koh JL, Wirsing K, Lautenschlager E, Zhang LO. The effect of graft height mismatch on contact pressure following osteochondral grafting: a biomechanical study. *Am J Sports Med.* 2004;32(2):317-320.

Please see videos on the accompanying website at www.routledge.com/9781617119996

20

Articular Cartilage Transplantation

Kenneth R. Zaslav, MD

Introduction

Articular cartilage implantation or transplant, first described by Brittberg et al[1] in 1994, has been performed in the United States since 1996. The literature is now replete with a plethora of reports, including more than 15- to 20-year follow-up for the treatment of focal chondral defects in the knee.[2-6] Its first and current Food and Drug Administration (FDA)-approved use is as a second-line treatment for previous failed chondral debridement, microfracture, or osteoarticular autograft treatment of a focal articular cartilage defect in the medial, lateral, or trochlear femoral condyle. Recent experience has shown it to be effective in knees with deep osteochondral defects, osteochondritis dissecans,[7] primary treatment of large chondral defects up to 7 cm^2, and in multiple lesions.[8] Patellofemoral lesions have also been successfully treated when effectively combined with patellar realignment.[9] Despite these excellent medium- and long-term peer-reviewed reports, its widespread use in the United States remains limited, and the procedure is most often performed in specialty centers. Most recent data estimate that approximately 11,000 implants are performed worldwide annually, mostly in the United States and Europe, with a small number in Asia. Relative contraindications include kissing lesions, presence of uncorrected malalignment, meniscal deficiency, and ligament instability. Presence of infection or synovial inflammatory disease is also a contraindication.

Over the past decade, several technical improvements have been published regarding the technique and have been put into popular use as off-label uses of this technology. In addition, rehabilitation protocols have progressed to allow earlier load bearing while protecting the nascent cartilage. Lastly, newer cellular technologies with collagen matrix and hyaluronan seeding, plus collagen gel and atelocollagen-based cell transport vehicles, have been reported in other countries and approved for use.

Sgaglione NA, Lubowitz JH, Provencher MT, eds. *The Knee: AANA Advanced Arthroscopic Surgical Techniques* (pp 269-282).

Indications

- Focal chondral post-traumatic defects of the medial, lateral, and trochlear femoral condyles. Although well-contained lesions are preferable, partially uncontained lesions can be addressed with specific techniques
- Age range 15 to 55 years
- Osteochondritis dissecans
- Knee must have or the surgeon must provide adequate ligament stability, limb alignment, and adequate meniscal function.

Controversial Indications

- Multiple lesions in the same knee, including kissing lesions of the opposite condyle
- Patellar lesions with or without concomitant instability or malalignment. Issues of malalignment or instability must be addressed at the time of implantation for good results.
- Lesions in patients with concomitant varus or valgus malalignment and degenerative lesions. Must address alignment with high tibial or distal femoral osteotomy as well.
- Chronologically older active patients with focal defects and younger teenagers prior to physeal closure

Pertinent Physical Findings

As with all orthopedic surgical procedures, accurate patient selection is critical to the success of this procedure. A complete history and physical examination is the first critical step in this process. Patients with chondral defects usually report symptoms similar to many knee pathologies, including swelling, pain, and mid-range instability and mechanical symptoms, including catching or locking sensations. Symptoms may come on insidiously over time or may begin immediately after a sudden shearing or compression-type injury. Physical examination usually does not rely on a single diagnostic examination test but will often be a diagnosis of exclusion once simple ligament or meniscal tests are not clearly positive but joint line pain and tenderness or effusions are present. The final diagnostic evaluation will always be the arthroscopic examination performed at the time of biopsy. This evaluation will confirm the presence or absence of kissing lesions and the amount of functional meniscus remaining. Lastly, this examination will determine if there is generalized chondropenia or thick, healthy cartilage surrounding the lesion.

Common physical findings include the following:

- Crepitance
- Effusion
- Joint line tenderness

Pertinent Imaging

- Weightbearing anteroposterior, lateral, Rosenberg, and patellofemoral x-rays
- Long-leg alignment scanogram from hip to ankle to evaluate alignment and the need for concomitant osteotomy

- Magnetic resonance imaging (MRI): Standard 1.5 or 3 T scanner. Delayed gadolinium-enhanced MRI of cartilage or T2 mapping may be helpful but is often not necessary to evaluate articular lesions.
- Possible computed tomography to evaluate patella alta, trochlear dysplasia, and tibial tubercle to trochlear groove (TT-TG) distance to evaluate patellofemoral alignment and stability.[10]

Patient Counseling

These procedures are significant undertakings for patients, their families, and the surgeon. The cost and postoperative requirements are considerable; therefore, it is essential that the surgeon offer a comprehensive teaching and counseling program and effectively help these patients make a truly informed consent about these complex surgical choices. Often, these decisions may occur over more than one visit. Patients should be made aware not only of the existing research and potential success rates, along with the typical discussion of surgical risks, but should also be instructed in the considerable postoperative precautions and rehabilitation needed to truly make this procedure a success. Educating patients about the maturation phases of cartilage is important for them to understand the protective weightbearing phases postoperatively and restrictions from work and daily activities that will be important to ensure success. In addition, a discussion of the patient's expectations at 1 and 2 years postoperatively from a work and athletic perspective is essential. The physician should discuss what actual change in lifestyle and sports participation is possible. It is also essential to stress that these are salvage procedures and often may be performed with multiple concomitant procedures. Therefore, the patient should expect some secondary small procedures to maximize results, which may include lysis of adhesions, excision of a thickened fat pad or plica, or partial patch detachment and/or hardware removal if applicable. These secondary surgical procedures are not failures but should be considered essential to returning the patient to the best function possible for the longest period of time. If these issues are discussed upfront, patients are cooperative and sanguine about their progress. If these complications occur postoperatively but they were not effectively discussed prior to primary surgery, it may have a negative effect on the surgeon-patient relationship later on and lead to poorer prognosis.

Arthroscopic Diagnosis/ Final Decision Making and Cell Harvest

Once the patient has decided to move forward with the evaluation, a first-stage, outpatient arthroscopic procedure is scheduled. Simple diagnostic arthroscopy is performed and minimal concomitant pathology may be addressed simultaneously with partial meniscectomy, plica resection, or chondral debridement of partial-thickness defects. The meniscal volume and ligament integrity can be confirmed and any kissing lesions noted. The joint is also evaluated in regard to the character of the lesion (ie, single, multiple, or well contained or not). In addition, the thickness or health of the surrounding cartilage can help determine if this patient is not presenting with a traumatic chondral injury but perhaps a knee that is heading for arthritis and happened to have a traumatic event prior to presentation. The latter patients with diffuse disease are poorer candidates for joint restoration procedures and may be better candidates for metallic joint resurfacing or osteotomy.

If the patient meets the final criteria for cartilage transplant, the cell harvest is performed at this time. Approximately 300 to 400 mg of normal cartilage is required. This amount is estimated as 3 Tic Tac–sized biopsies of full-thickness cartilage from a nonweightbearing area, including a small amount of subchondral bone. The author's preferred safe location is the intercondylar notch near where notchplasty was performed in the earlier days of anterior cruciate ligament reconstruction. Medial trochlear areas away from the articulating patellofemoral joint are also available as in osteochondral autograft transfer system procedures; however, some mechanical symptoms may occur from fibrous infill here. An angled or ring curette is used to harvest the full-thickness biopsy. The cells closest to the lamina splendens may be the best for growth, so it is important to get to the basal area of cartilage by the bone interface. Cells are then placed in the provided commercial medium and sent for culture. The cell company will isolate and culture chondrocytes and can return between and 4 and 12 million chondrocytes for transplant on the day of surgery within 3 to 4 weeks.

Treating the Entire Organ: Addressing Concomitant Pathology

Several authors have reminded us that aiming for a smooth, white surface but not addressing the rest of the joint usually yields poor results in joint resurfacing.[11,12] The knee has several important structures, and all must be addressed for success in cartilage reconstruction. Ligament and meniscal integrity is important to protect the newly transplanted cells. Transplanting them into the same hostile milieu in which they were damaged will be a waste of time and expense. Meniscal tears, if repairable, should be repaired; however, small partial meniscectomy, less than one-third of the meniscus, may be tolerated. However, larger loss of volume of the meniscus or any loss of the outer peripheral ring integrity, losing effective hoop stress, will have to be addressed by concomitant or prior meniscal transplant to achieve successful restoration of function. The anterior or posterior cruciate ligaments, if not intact, need to be reconstructed, and all malalignment has to be addressed. The most common malalignment encountered is medialization of the weightbearing line or mild varus. Through osteotomy, one should aim to bring weightbearing to neutral or slightly lateral just a few millimeters off the midline for optimum success. For these varus knees, concomitant opening-wedge high tibial valgus osteotomy has been successful. For valgus knees, distal femoral osteotomy may be preferred. Osteotomy techniques are covered elsewhere in this volume.

More recently, other structures in this complex joint organ have been recognized as equally important to the long-term success of cartilage repair procedures. First, the subchondral bone integrity and flexibility needs to be maintained. Many authors believe one of the etiologies for poor long-term results post standard microfracture may be internal osteophytes from the microfractures that act to stiffen the subchondral plate.[13] Minas et al[14] reported poorer results with articular cartilage implantation after failed microfracture in the presence of these osteophytes. As far back as the 1970s, Pugh et al[15] postulated that loss of normal flexibility and increased stiffness in subchondral bone may be the primary change in osteoarthritis that causes thinning of the overlying articular cartilage. Therefore, addressing bony abnormalities and restoring normal subchondral architecture may be equally important to the long-term success of these procedures as regenerating hyaline cartilage.[16] The final aspect of normal joint homeostasis and cartilage health is the synovial milieu. The pH and viscoelasticity of the normal joint fluid are an important part of cartilage health and are important in nurturing articular cartilage repair. In the future, use of chemical manipulation with better defined platelet-rich plasma, hyaluronic acid, or bone morphogenic proteins may prove to be important in healthy cartilage reconstitution; however, large prospective studies on the effects of these adjuncts have not yet been completed or reported.

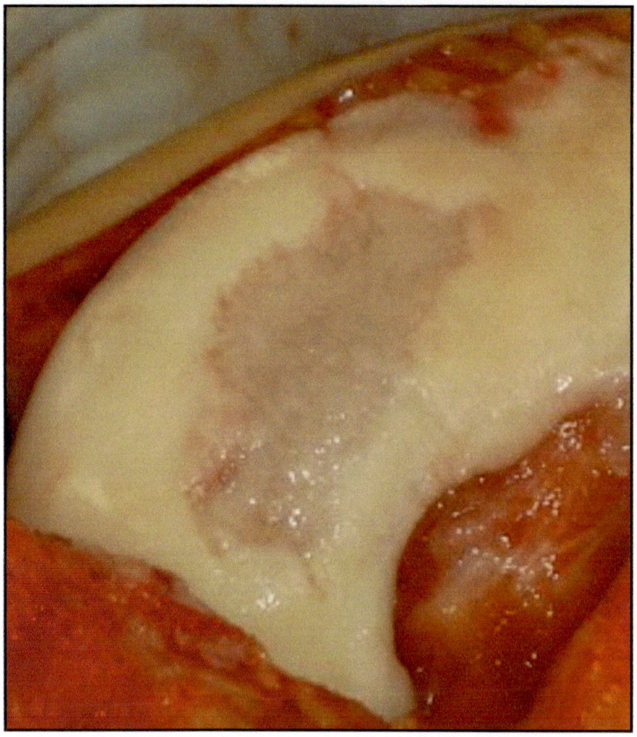

Figure 20-1. Large medial femoral chondral grade III lesion. Note the well-contained borders and good surrounding cartilage. There is no significant bony defect.

Standard FDA-Approved Technique

The original articular cartilage implantation technique was first described by Lars Peterson and has remained successful over time.[1] The knee is entered for a medial condyle lesion through a standard medial parapatellar arthrotomy. Central weightbearing lesions may be approached through minimal incisions, sparing the extensor mechanism, but multiple lesions, and larger lesions especially with posterior extension, will necessitate using more extensile exposures as one would do for total knee arthroplasty. Eversion of the patella yields excellent access to most of the condyle and trochlea. For patellar lesions, one would consider performing a distal tibial tubercle osteotomy to realign concomitant malalignment and provide more adequate exposure to the articular surface of the patella. Lateral condyle lesions may be approached through medial parapatellar arthrotomy with patellar eversion, or smaller central lesions can be approached directly through a limited lateral arthrotomy with possible extension proximally through a lateral subvastus approach. Posterolateral lesions often necessitate taking down the anterior horn of the lateral meniscus and removing a periosteal sleeve of the lateral capsule, along with internal rotation of the foot.

Once the lesion is located, one must assess the surrounding cartilage (Figure 20-1). The lesion then needs to be debrided to provide a good stable rim for attachment. Although this may necessitate enlarging the original confines of the lesion seen arthroscopically, experience has shown that debridement to stable perpendicular walls, if possible, is important to creating a stable long-term repair. Early failures were reported with minimal debridement and sutures through less-than-optimum cartilage. Gel-soaked thrombin sponges and/or small sponges soaked in epinephrine are helpful to achieve hemostasis in the defect. To avoid fibrocartilaginous repair, one aims for a dry bed with little to no bleeding in the defect to avoid contamination of the cells by marrow constituents. Although the calcified cartilage layer should be removed to allow proper cell attachment as with proper preparation for microfracture, the subchondral plate should not be damaged. If there are stiff central osteophytes in the lesion from previous treatment or bone injury, one

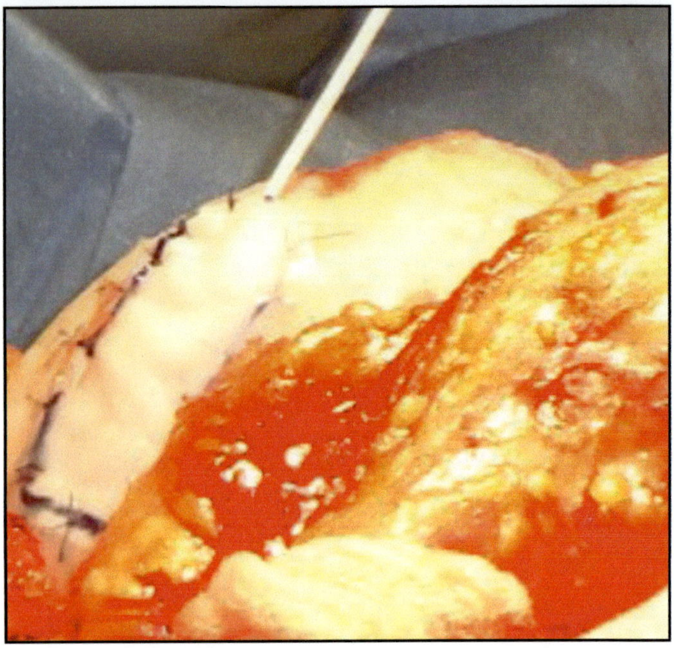

Figure 20-2. Cells being placed under the patch from a tuberculin syringe after suturing and fibrin glue placement.

should flatten these with a burr. These central osteophytes usually do not bleed because they are quite sclerotic. Minas et al[14] showed that placing cells and patches over these may often lead to cell transplant failure if not addressed.

Once debridement and preparation are complete, the lesion is measured, and a patch will be taken to fit the exact size. In the standard FDA-approved protocol, a patch is taken from the proximal tibial or distal femoral periosteum. Distal femoral periosteum is usually reserved for older patients with thin to nonexistent tibial periosteum because it is often too thick in younger subjects. The tibial periosteum is harvested from just distal to the pes anserine bursa to a size 2 mm larger in diameter than the lesion to be covered because the periosteum often shrinks during harvest. Care to remove the full depth of the periosteum down to the bone is important because the layer closest to the bone has some progenitor cells, which may aid in the repair. The cambium layer side of the periosteum is then placed down toward the lesion and sewn into place with 6-0 or 5-0 Vicryl suture.

The repair is then checked to see if it is water tight with the application of 0.3 cc of saline delivered by a tuberculin syringe under the patch via the superior corner where the final suture is left unplaced. Once placed, if there is no leak, the saline is removed with the tuberculin syringe so as not to dilute the ultimate chondrocyte suspension. Fibrin glue (Tisseal; Baxter) is then added to the periphery of the repair, and the final superior stitch remains open. The cultured chondrocytes are then drawn up using appropriate Carticel (Vericel Inc) technique and delivered under the patch by a similar tuberculin syringe after which the final stitch is placed and followed by fibrin glue (Figure 20-2).

Equipment

- Standard open knee tray with at least 2 "Z" retractors
- Small pads soaked in 1% epinephrine and thrombin to decrease intralesional bleeding and gel-soaked thrombin pads
- Narrow sharp periosteal elevator
- 5-0 and 6-0 Vicryl suture (preferably dyed purple)

Positioning and Portals

The patient is positioned in the supine position with a tourniquet on thigh and the leg draped free. Positioning is similar to a total knee procedure allowing the knee to be flat or flexed to 45 or 95 degrees as needed during the procedure.

Enhanced Techniques for Articular Cartilage Implantation

Although first-generation articular cartilage implantation remains the only FDA-approved cartilage transplant procedure in the United States, surgeons have worked to improve the procedure to allow for quicker surgery and lower risk of secondary surgical procedures. The first enhancement came with the use of a collagen patch with a technique known as CACI (collagen-covered autologous chondrocyte implantation). A type I to III porcine collagen membrane, approved for dental use in the United States (Bioguide; Geistlich), can be used instead of the periosteal patch as an off-label use. This decreases early postoperative discomfort from the periosteal harvest and its longer incision, and more importantly has been shown to decrease the complication of patch hypertrophy and detachment, leading to a significant decrease in secondary arthroscopic procedures to address these issues.[17,18] The patch is measured and cut similar to the periosteal patch; however, it can be cut closer to the true size of the defect because no shrinkage occurs. It will then be sewn on using the same approved Carticel technique with 5-0 or 6-0 Vicryl suture.

A more recent technical development first described by Neimeyer et al[19] uses the collagen membrane as a cell carrier instead of as a barrier. This technique, referred to as cell-seeded CACI, allows the surgeon to perform an in-theater-prepared matrix-associated articular cartilage implantation.[19] In this case, the surgeon places cells onto the collagen membrane prior to sewing on the membrane. The defect and patch are prepared in the usual fashion; however, prior to sewing on the patch, the cells are placed on the rough side of the collagen patch and allowed to sit for 10 minutes to attach to the collagen matrix (Figure 20-3). A thin layer of fibrin glue is applied to the base of the chondral defect, and then the cells and patch are placed upon it with the rough side down and are then attached with several sutures (5-0 or 6-0 Vicryl) followed by application of fibrin glue to the periphery as in the usual technique. This will potentially give a better distribution of cells along the entire patch and avoid any efflux of cell-containing liquid suspension out the sides. Although this procedure has been reported to have equal success rates as standard articular cartilage implantation, longer-term study is needed to see if there are any long-term clinical or graft survival benefits to these modifications. These modifications of the original procedure are considered off-label use of the cultured chondrocytes, and patients should be made aware of these enhancements.

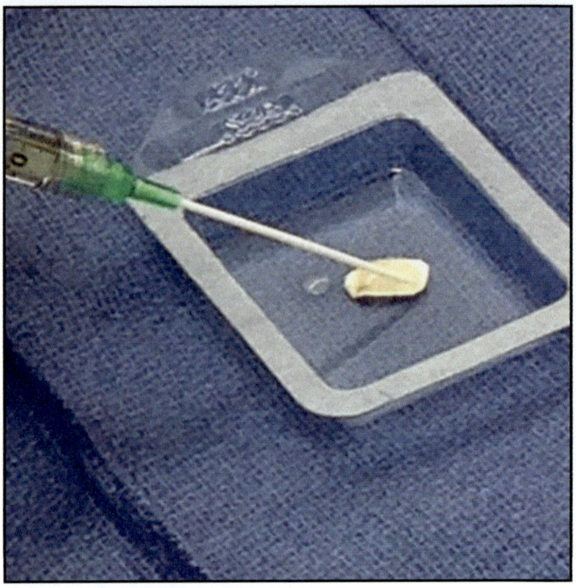

Figure 20-3. Placing cells on collagen type I/III matrix to perform cell-seeded collagen articular cartilage implantation.

Second-Generation Articular Cartilage Implantation: Membrane-Associated Articular Cartilage Implantation

Three companies (Vericel, Aesculap, and Histogenics) have taken the same isolated and cultured chondrocytes and grown them in the laboratory on a membrane for more secure attachment. The cells are grown in 2- or 3-dimensional cultures, are seeded on the membrane, and are then shipped in a sterile container rather than a liquid cell suspension. These have been placed using open and arthroscopic procedures in multiple European centers with good success rates.[20,21] These implants are not yet available for general use in the United States, although multicenter Good Clinical Practice Level I studies comparing these techniques with microfracture are underway now in the United States by all 3 companies.

Technique for Deep Bony Defects and Osteochondral Dissecans

This technique can be effective not only with chondral defects but with osteochondral defects. The cells and membrane alone can fill a defect of bone up to 7 to 8 mm, but once the defect reaches depths of 1 cm or more, a bony procedure is also needed. The surgeon can perform a 2-stage procedure with burring and bone graft first and return later for CACI or, more commonly, perform a sandwich technique as described by Peterson et al.[22] Deep osteochondral dissecans lesions often have dead bone, even beneath the level of the bone visualized on the lesion arthroscopically; therefore, preoperative MRI evaluation to judge the depth of bone involvement is essential (Figure 20-4). A flexible subchondral architecture is essential to long-term success of these implants. Therefore, one should first debride the lesion of loose dead fragments, use a high-speed burr to get to good bleeding bone, and then drill into the bone below to the level of cyst formation seen on MRI to stimulate healthy bone reconstitution. Next, the author recommends taking cancellous bone from the proximal tibia. A cortical window is cut just below the tibial tubercle, and the osteochondral autograft transfer system harvester (Arthrex) can be used to harvest multiple plugs

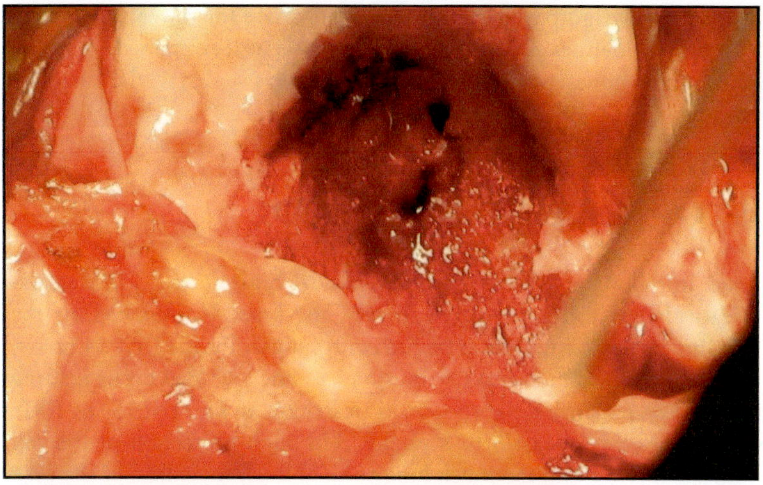

Figure 20-4. Large lateral femoral condyle deep grade IV osteochondral defect after failure of open reduction and internal fixation of the fragment 2 years prior in a 17-year-old athletic male.

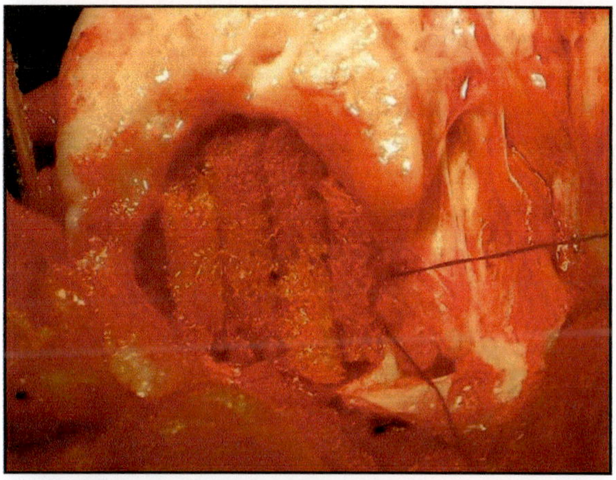

Figure 20-5. Defect prepared and filled with cancellous bone plugs from the tibia as part 1 of the sandwich technique. Note the suture anchor placed for patch attachment peripherally in area of poor cartilage containment.

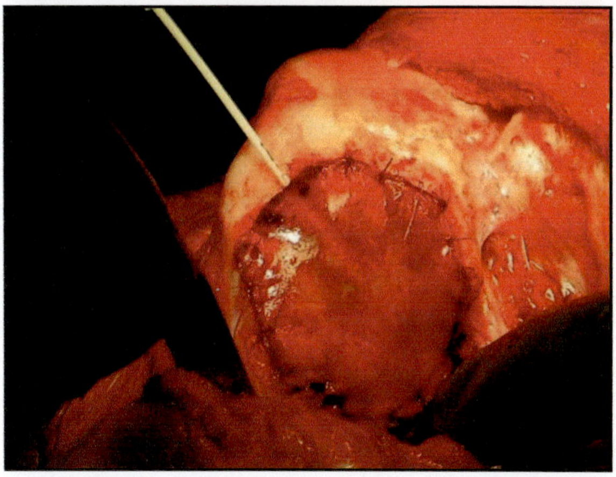

Figure 20-6. Final stage of Peterson's sandwich technique method. Cultured chondrocytes are placed between the 2 patch layers.

of cancellous bone to place in to fill the defect to the normal anatomic subchondral bone plate level (Figure 20-5). A collagen or periosteal patch is then sewn with a rough or cambium layer face up over the bone graft to prevent blood infusion into the chondrocyte implant. A second collagen patch is then sewn on top with the rough side facing down as usual, and the cells can be placed between the 2 membranes using the usual proper Carticel technique (Figure 20-6). If these lesions are poorly contained, strict nonweightbearing might be appropriate for 4 weeks and then progress along the original Carticel guidelines. However, if the lesion is well contained, minimal partial weightbearing may be begun postoperatively with foot flat as with usual articular cartilage implantation.

Postoperative Protocol

Patients are placed in a knee immobilizer or off-the-shelf T-ROM brace locked in extension for the first 6 hours postoperatively. At 6 hours postoperatively, the brace is unlocked, or the immobilizer removed, and continuous passive motion is begun continuously for the first 24 hours. After that, many surgeons recommend continuous passive motion or some low-load cyclic loading 6 hours per day for the first week. The patient's weightbearing is restricted to foot flat 15- to 20-lb partial weightbearing with 2 crutches for at least 6 to 8 weeks. Although protection of the cell transplant is important to avoid shear stress and too much longitudinal load, some load at the cell-bone interface and cyclic motion is useful for stimulating chondrocyte growth and maturation. For poorly contained lesions, nonweightbearing may be needed for a few weeks, but most patients may begin partial weightbearing immediately. The amount of weightbearing also varies based on the location of the lesion. If the lesion is in the central weightbearing area of medial or lateral femoral condyle, the load is more slowly applied; however, trochlear lesions and lesions more posterior in the condyle can accept more rapid partial weightbearing as tolerated because they are not loaded in the normal gait cycle. Immediate weightbearing for patellofemoral lesions is appropriate once quadriceps recovery allows, but active open chain extension must be avoided for the first month in these patients to avoid the shear stresses in this area that would most likely affect the implant in this region.

Cyclic loading is appropriate once ROM allows, and early pool exercises, once the incision is effectively sealed, can allow earlier low-load functional activity.

Protocols have been previously published for the appropriate progression to full weightbearing and progressive resistance exercises,[23] and in recent years, surgeons and therapists have begun to accelerate the full weightbearing process from an average of 10 to 12 weeks to 6 to 8 weeks. No untoward effects have been noted in early studies to date of these accelerated rehabilitation programs; however, it is important for sports medicine surgeons to note that these accelerated programs allow for stress protection early up to 6 weeks and are not as aggressive as usual ligament reconstruction protocols.[24]

Concomitant meniscal transplant or ligament reconstruction will also affect rehabilitation protocols; however, osteotomy, which used to delay weightbearing when open-wedge osteotomy was performed with weaker implants, can now tolerate rapid weightbearing if larger, stronger implants or newer weightbearing bone or bone substitute wedges are used.

Potential Complications

The most common complications reported with open articular cartilage implantation include patch hypertrophy, partial patch detachment, and adhesions. These complications most often show up in the first 4 to 6 months postoperatively and may need to be addressed with arthroscopic evaluation and surgery. In the early prospective studies of the use of articular cartilage implantation for second-line treatment, these complications were reported as commonly as 30% to 49% but once addressed had no effect on the ultimate success rate.[3] Since the use of CACI and cell seeded–articular cartilage implantation, these complications rates have significantly decreased to less than 5% to 10%.[18] Therefore, the need for secondary surgical procedures has significantly

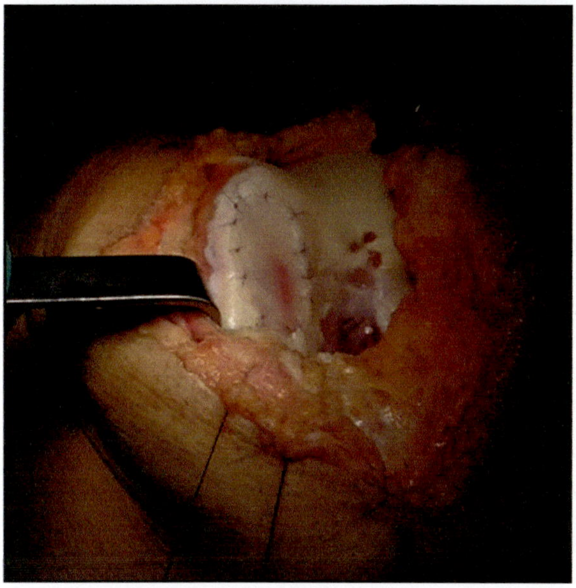

Figure 20-7. Matrix-associated chondrocyte transplant (6 cm^2) in the medial femoral condyle using the Novocart 3D implant (Aesculap). This implant has cloned chondrocytes distributed throughout the 3D matrix.

decreased. Rarer complications include infection and deep venous thrombosis, which are both less than 1% to 2% but have been reported, as with most limb surgeries.[3]

Although these are complex surgeries with long postoperative recuperative periods, significant serious adverse events are rare if good surgical and postoperative protocols are followed.

New Techniques on the Horizon

Although the FDA's rigorous demands for Level I prospective randomized studies on large populations for new Biologic License Applications has made it difficult to bring new cellular cartilage products to market in the United States, newer cellular transplant technologies have been reported throughout the world with good results and potential clinical benefits. Currently, 2 Good Clinical Practice FDA-approved clinical trials are ongoing for new chondrocyte products in the United States, including one for the Novocart 3D matrix-associated cell product by Aesculap and a second for Neocart by Histogenics. In addition, the data from a recent 4-year prospective randomized Good Clinical Practice trial of matrix-associated products by Genzyme (MACI), now owned by Vericel Inc, have been completed in Europe and published with good results and may soon be under consideration by the FDA.[20] A study of a single-stage autologous minced cartilage technique by Johnson and Johnson (Cartilage Autograft Implantation System [CAIS]) was halted, as was a study on the use of cultured allogeneic children's chondrocytes due to the difficulty of enrolling patients with pure cartilage lesions that had no concomitant pathology, such as malalignment, meniscal, or ligament insufficiency that needed to be addressed.

In Europe and Asia, several technologies have achieved regulatory approval and are in common use. The Novocart 3D MACI product has been used safely for more than 10 years in Germany and central Europe and has made the application of these cells already grown in a 3D matrix easy to place surgically.[21] In addition, many surgeons have also performed these matrix-associated articular cartilage implantation procedures arthroscopically.[25] Several other matrix-associated products have been used and reported, but due to new stringent laboratory regulatory licensing requirements recently initiated in the European Union, the production of these products has been discontinued except in exempted university settings in specific countries where centers may make their own cultured cell product for their own use only (Figure 20-7). Although Vericel Inc

(Carticel) is the sole provider of cultured chondrocytes in the United States, throughout most of Europe, the only product available is Chondroselect (formerly Tigenix), which is now marketed exclusively by Sobi.

In England, Shetty reported on a collagen gel–based articular cartilage implantation, originally described with Kim in Korea, that can be performed arthroscopically or open and distributes the chondrocytes evenly within a collagen gel with thrombin and fibrinogen. After standard defect preparation as previously described in this chapter, this gel product can be easily applied to fill these defects arthroscopically under gas insufflation. For this purpose, he uses the same double injector the authors use for fibrin glue in the standard procedure.[26,27] In Japan, authors have similarly worked to decrease the variability in the fluid injection of cells under membrane by suspending cells in a matrix of atelocollagen, with good to excellent results in prospective studies.[27,28] Although these newer techniques have many potential technical and biologic benefits to creating a stable cartilage repair, longer-term studies are needed to see if these new constructs yield a more durable repair than existing techniques.

Top Technical Pearls for the Procedure

1. Preoperative evaluation with x-rays, including scanograms and adequate patellofemoral views, and MRI is necessary to properly plan operative treatment and select patients for successful treatment.
2. Address all concomitant pathology with prior surgery or at the time of definitive cell transplant. Address all parts of the knee organ.
3. Debride all loose and undermined cartilage edges to stable shoulders surrounding the lesion before measuring and preparing the patch.
4. Avoid subchondral penetration and efflux of marrow contents. Stop any significant hemorrhage into the lesion with thrombin- and epinephrine-prepared sponges prior to attaching the cells or patch.
5. Sew from the patch side to the cartilage side so knots are on the patch. Have a scrub technician place mineral oil on all sutures just before use.

References

1. Brittberg M, Lindahl A, Nilsson A, Ohlsson C, Isaksson O, Peterson L. Treatment of deep cartilage defects in the knee with autologous chondrocyte transplantation. *N Engl J Med.* 1994;331(14):889-895.
2. Mandelbaum BR, Browne JE, Fu F, et al. Articular cartilage lesions of the knee. *Am J Sports Med.* 2000;26(6):853-861.
3. Zaslav K, Cole B, Brewster R, et al. A prospective study of autologous chondrocyte transplantation in patients with failed prior treatment for articular cartilage defect of the knee: results of the Study of Articular Repair (STAR) clinical trial. *Am J Sports Med.* 2009;37(1):42-55.
4. Peterson L, Brittberg M, Kiviranta I, Akerlund EL, Lindahl A. Autologous chondrocyte transplantation. Biomechanics and long-term durability. *Am J Sports Med.* 2002;30(1):2-12
5. Peterson L, Vasiliadis HS, Brittberg M, Lindahl A. Autologous chondrocyte implantation: a long-term follow-up. *Am J Sports Med.* 2010;38(6):1117-1124.

6. Biant LC, Bentley G, Vijayan S, Skinner JA, Carrngton RW. Long-term results of autologous chondrocyte implantation in the knee for chronic chondral and osteochondral defects. *Am J Sports Med.* 2014;42(9):7-11.
7. Cole BJ, DeBerardino T, Brewster R, et al. Outcomes of autologous chondrocyte implantation in Study of the Treatment of Articular Repair (STAR) patients with osteochondritis dissecans. *Am J Sports Med.* 2012;40(9):2015-2022.
8. Minas T, Gomoll AH, Solhpour S, Rosenberger R, Probst C, Bryant T. Auotologous chondrocyte implantation for joint preservation in early osteoarthritis. *Clin Orthop Related Res.* 2010;468(1):147-157.
9. Gillogly SD, Arnold RM. Autologous chondrocyte implantation and anteromedialization for isolated patellar cartilage lesions: 5- to 11-year follow-up. *Am J Sports Med.* 2014;42(4):912-920.
10. Farr J. Specific considerations for patellofemoral chondral disease. In: Cole BJ, Gomoll AH, eds. *Biologic Joint Reconstruction.* Thorofare, NJ: SLACK Incorporated; 2009:187-201.
11. Minas T. *A Primer in Cartilage Repair and Joint Preservation of the Knee.* Philadelphia, PA: Elsevier; 2011.
12. Buckwalter JA. Evaluating methods of restoring cartilaginous articular surfaces. *Clin Orthop Rel Res.* 1999;(367 suppl):S224-S238.
13. Mithoefer K, McAdams T, Williams RJ, Kreuz PC, Mandelbaum BR. Clinical efficacy of the microfracture technique for articular cartilage repair in the knee: an evidence-based systematic analysis. *Am J Sports Med.* 2009;37(10):2053-2063.
14. Minas T, Gomoll AH, Rosenberger R, Royce RO, Bryant T. Increased failure rate of autologous chondrocyte implantation after previous treatment with marrow stimulation techniques. *Am J Sports Med.* 2009;37(5):902-908.
15. Pugh JW, Radin EL, Rose RM. Quantitative studies of subchondral cancellous bone. Its relationship to the state of its overlying cartilage. *J Bone Joint Surg Am.* 1974;56(2):313-321.
16. Richardson JB. Sub-chondral bone: current concepts. In: Brittberg M, Imhoff A, Madry H, Mandelbaum B, eds. *Cartilage Repair: Current Concepts.* Surrey, UK: DJO Publications; 2010.
17. Gooding CR, Bartlett W, Bentley G, Skinner JA, Carrington R, Flanagan A. A prospective, randomized study comparing two techniques of autologous chondrocyte implantation for osteochondral defects of the knee: periosteum covered versus type I/III collagen covered. *Knee.* 2006;13(3):203-210.
18. Gomoll AH, Probst C, Farr J, Cole BJ, Minas T. Use of a type I/III collagen membrane decreases reoperation rates for symptomatic hypertrophy after autologous chondrocyte implantation. *Am J Sports Med.* 2009;37(suppl 1):20S-23S.
19. Neimeyer P, Lenz P, Kreuz PC, et al. Chondrocyte-seeded type I/III collagen membrane for autologous chondrocyte transplantation: prospective 2-year results in patients with cartilage defects of the knee. *Arthroscopy.* 2010;26(8):1074-1082.
20. Saris D, Price A, Widuchowski W, et al. Matrix-applied characterized autologous cultured chondrocytes versus microfracture: two-year follow-up of a prospective randomized trial. *Am J Sports Med.* 2014;42(6):1384-1394.
21. Zak L, Albrecht C, Wondrasch B, et al. Results 2 years after matrix-associated autologous chondrocyte transplantation using the Novocart 3D scaffold: an analysis of clinical and radiological data. *Am J Sports Med.* 2014;42(7):1618-1627.
22. Peterson L, Minas T, Brittberg M, Lindahl A. Treatment of osteochondritis dissecans of the knee with autologous chondrocyte transplantation: results at two to ten years. *J Bone Joint Surg Am.* 2003;85(suppl 2);17-24.
23. Hambly K, Bobic V, Wondrasch B, Van Assche D, Marlovits S. Autologous chondrocyte implantation postoperative care and rehabilitation: science and practice. *Am J Sports Med.* 2006;34(6):1020-1038.
24. Edwards PK, Ackland TR, Ebert JR. Accelerated weightbearing rehabilitation after matrix-induced articular chondrocyte implantation in the tibiofemoral joint: early clinical and radiological outcomes. *Am J Sports Med.* 2014;41(10):2314-2324.
25. Kon E, Gobbi A, Filardo G, Delcogliano M, Zaffagnini S, Maracci M. Arthroscopic second-generation autologous chondrocyte implantation compared with microfracture for chondral lesions of the knee: prospective nonrandomized study at 5 years. *Am J Sports Med.* 2009;37(1):33-41.
26. Choi NY, Kim BW, Yeo WJ, et al. Gel-type autologous chondrocyte implantation (Chondron) implantation for treatment of articular cartilage defects of the knee. *BMC Musculoskelet Disord.* 2010;11:103.

27. Gomoll AH, Kamei G, Ochi M, Shetty AA, Zaslav K. Technical enhancements and update on chondrocyte implantation. *Oper Tech Orthop.* 2014;24:35-47.
28. Katsube K, Ochi M, Uchio Y, et al. Repair of articular defects with cultured chondrocytes in Atellocollagen gel. Comparison with cultured chondrocytes in suspension. *Arch Orthop Trauma Surg.* 2000;120(3-4):121-127.

Please see videos on the accompanying website at www.routledge.com/9781617119996

21

Novel Techniques in Articular Cartilage Restoration

Adam B. Yanke, MD; David B. Merkow, BA;
Annemarie K. Tilton, BS; and Brian J. Cole, MD, MBA

PART ONE: DENOVO NT

Introduction

DeNovo NT (Zimmer) is minced (1-mm cubes) juvenile allograft cartilage delivered with fibrin glue indicated for the treatment of chondral defects with minimal to no bone loss. One benefit of DeNovo NT is the use of juvenile tissue, which has been shown to have a considerably greater ability to produce proteoglycans and stimulate matrix production compared to adult sources of chondrocytes.[1,2] An additional feature is that juvenile cells are less immunogenic than their adult counterparts.[1] Because DeNovo NT supplies viable cells, it has a shelf-life of 44 days from the date it was harvested and typically needs to be ordered prior to surgery, similar to an osteochondral allograft. The technique can be applied in an open or arthroscopic fashion; however, the arthroscopic method is significantly more demanding.

Outcomes for DeNovo NT have only recently been reported. Tompkins et al[3] reported on patellar defects (2.4 ± 1.2 cm^2) at 28 months using a density of 1 unit per 1.3 cm^2. This is twice the density recommended by the manufacturer. In this setting, there was an 89% mean defect fill on magnetic resonance imaging (MRI), and 2 of 15 patients required a debridement for hypertrophy. Farr et al[4] reported on a similar patient population and reported no reoperations at 2 years in 25 patients; the study also demonstrated statistically significant improvements over baseline levels for multiple measures of pain, symptoms, activities of daily living, and sports and recreation.

Indications

- In general, the indications for DeNovo NT mirror that of autologous chondrocyte implantation (ACI).

Sgaglione NA, Lubowitz JH, Provencher MT, eds. *The Knee: AANA Advanced Arthroscopic Surgical Techniques* (pp 283-296).

- International Cartilage Repair Society grade III cartilage lesion (cartilage defect > 50% cartilage depth but with minimal bone loss, possibly extending down to but not through the subchondral bone)
- Lesion size > 2 cm^2 after debridement
- Minimal to no bone loss
  - Can possibly be performed in conjunction with bone grafting as described in ACI, although there are no data to support this technique
- Preferentially used in the patellofemoral joint
- Body mass index less than 30 to 34 kg/m^2

Relative Contraindications

- Bipolar lesion
- Significant subchondral bone edema
- > 5 mm of untreated bone loss (osteochondritis dissecans)
- Unaddressed meniscectomy or malalignment
- Potentially decreased outcomes in the setting of prior microfracture based on ACI data[5,6]

Pertinent Physical Findings

- Effusions are probably the most important examination finding demonstrating significant intra-articular pathology
- Patellofemoral defects
  - One-finger sign in which a patient points to the front of the patella and describes the pain being deep to this location
  - Patellar grind test, placing downward force on the patella during flexion and extension
- Associated pathology
  - Varus/valgus alignment
  - Patellar instability/apprehension

Pertinent Imaging

- X-rays
  - Anteroposterior standing: Anterior tibiofemoral arthritis
  - Posteroanterior flexion weightbearing: Posterior tibiofemoral arthritis
  - Lateral: Patellar alta/baja
  - Merchant: Patellofemoral joint space narrowing, tilt, and tracking
- MRI (necessary for all patients to evaluate the following)
  - Cartilage integrity
  - Cartilage quality (delayed gadolinium-enhanced MRI of cartilage, fast-spin echo, or other cartilage-specific sequences)
  - Subchondral bone edema

- ▹ Associated pathology
  - Meniscus status
  - Ligament status
  - Tibial tubercle to trochlear groove (TT-TG) distance
- Computed tomography (CT)
  - ▹ Considered for patients with significant bone loss, cystic change, or as an alternative to measure the TT-TG distance in the setting of concomitant planned tibial tubercle osteotomy

Equipment

- DeNovo NT needs to be requested prior to surgery because it is viable tissue that is not generally made available as an on-the-shelf option.
- The manufacturer recommends 1 package per 2.5-cm^2 defect.
- Arthroscopy setup is based on surgeon preference.
- Small curettes and ring curette if available

Positioning and Portals

- Supine with the leg of the bed extended
- Lateral post
- Tourniquet

Step-by-Step Description of the Procedure

Diagnostic Arthroscopy

- The procedure should begin with standard diagnostic arthroscopy (inferolateral viewing portal and inferomedial working portal with optional outflow).
- Evaluate the entire knee and the lesion to determine the lack of unexpected contraindications or concomitant pathology, even in the setting of a relatively recent index arthroscopy indicating a patient for DeNovo NT.

Arthrotomy

- The authors prefer performing an arthrotomy to access the cartilage defect. The location of the incision depends on the location of the defect, with a lateral arthrotomy preferred for a patellofemoral or lateral femoral condyle defect and a medial vastus sparing approach for other defects.

Defect Preparation

- Similar to any cartilage procedure, the defect should be debrided to stable healthy walls that are vertical in nature.

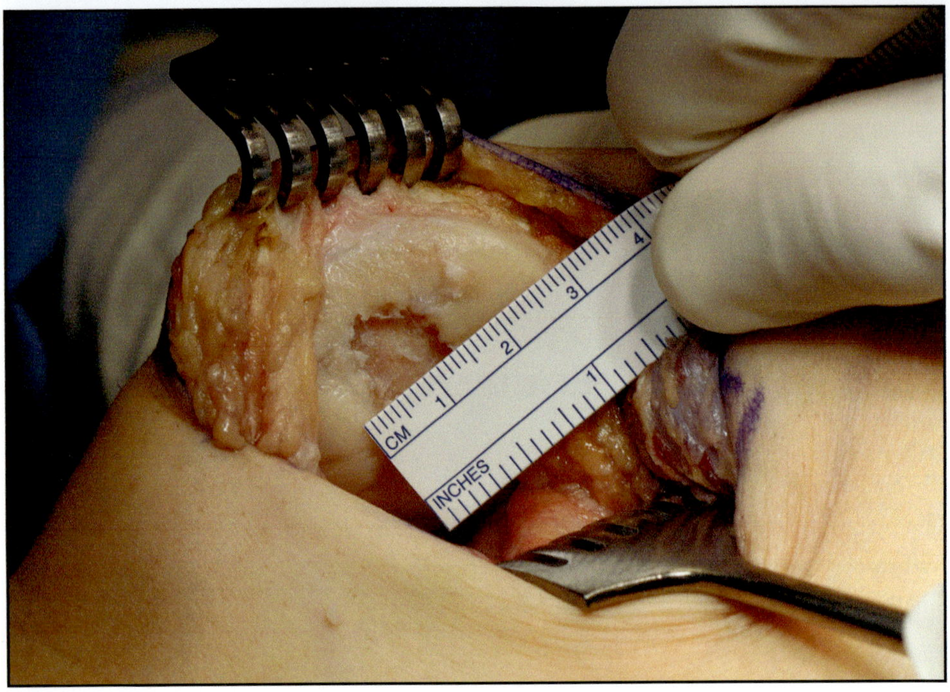

Figure 21-1. Sizing of a patellar defect through an arthrotomy after debridement.

- The bed of the defect should be free of any diseased tissue, and care should be taken to attempt removal of the calcified cartilage layer without gaining access to the subchondral bone elements.
- Measure the defect to ensure the size is as expected (Figure 21-1).

DeNovo NT Application Directly Into the Defect

- Although there are several methods to apply DeNovo NT, the authors' preferred method is preparing the implant directly into the defect.
- To begin, the remaining media from the DeNovo NT package should be aspirated (Figure 21-2).
- The minced cartilage can then be placed directly into the defect site, which is immediately covered with fibrin glue.
- Care should be taken to avoid the fibrin being proud to the bordering healthy chondral surface to avoid displacement.
- After the fibrin has set, gently range the knee to ensure construct stability.

Extra-Articular DeNovo NT Preparation and Placement

- Alternatively, the DeNovo NT implant can be prepared on the back table.
- A piece of sterile foil can be pressed into the defect to form a negative mold (Figure 21-3).
- This is then filled with the DeNovo NT and fibrin glue (Figure 21-4).
- As this sets, place fibrin glue in the base of the defect and press in digitally to decrease bleeding from the defect bed (Figure 21-5).

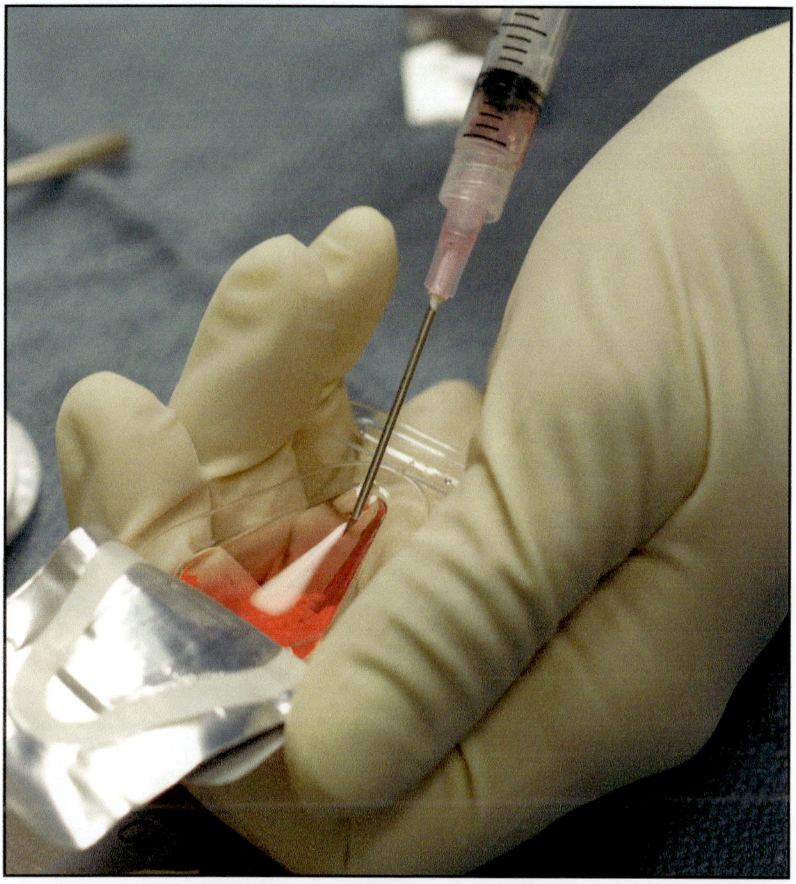

Figure 21-2. Removing the media from the DeNovo NT implant on the back table.

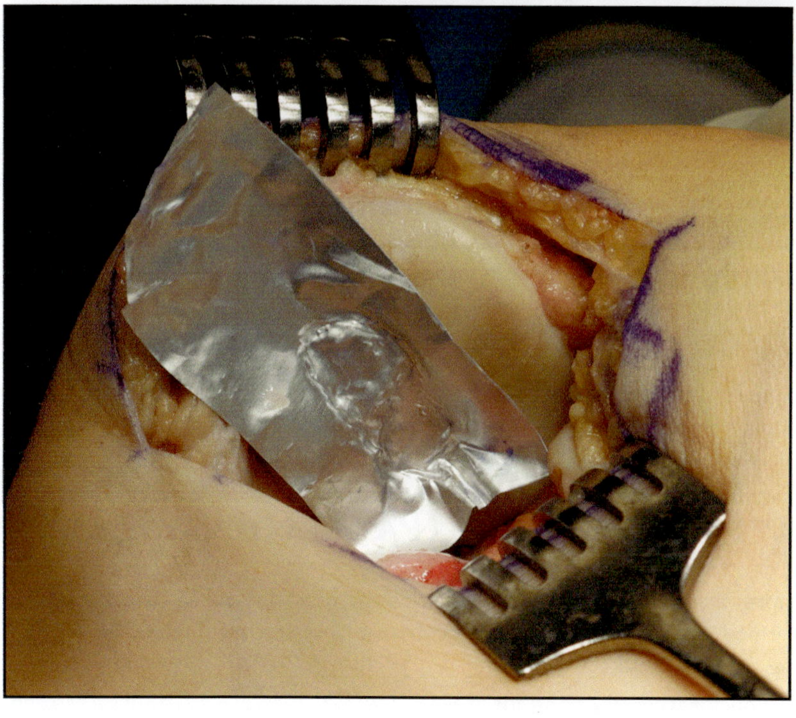

Figure 21-3. Foil placed in a patellar defect to create a negative mold for DeNovo NT placement.

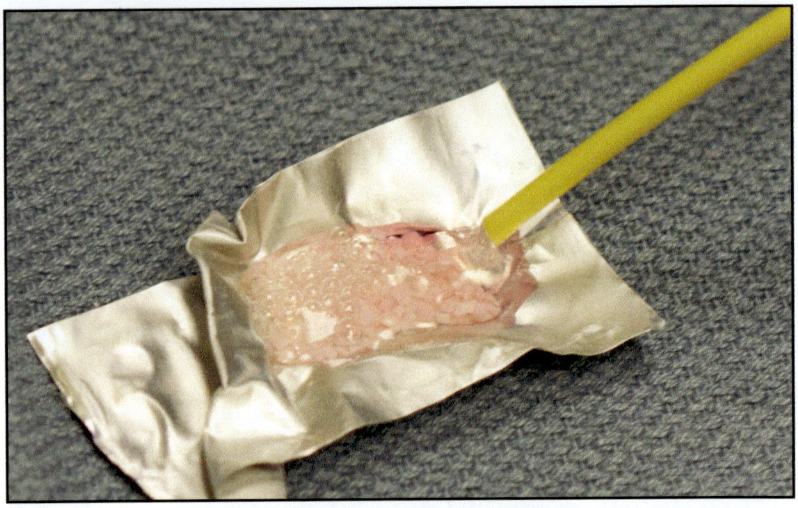

Figure 21-4. Fibrin being added to the DeNovo NT placed in the negative mold.

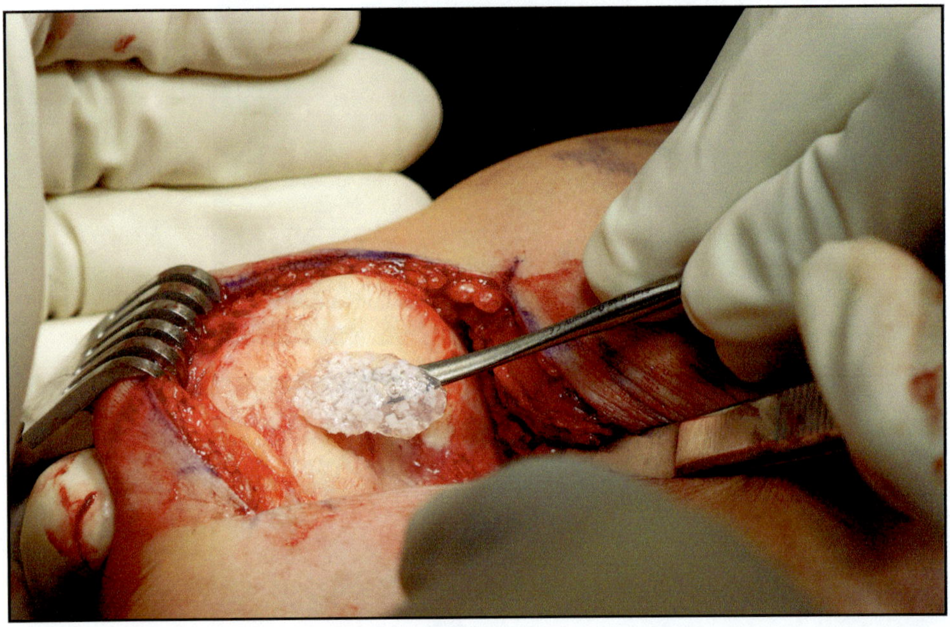

Figure 21-5. The implant is lifted from the foil using an elevator and is placed into the defect after fibrin has been placed in the base of the defect.

- Finally, set the pre-prepared DeNovo implant into the defect bed and ensure stability with knee range of motion (ROM) (Figure 21-6).

Postoperative Protocol (Patellofemoral)

- Weightbearing: Perform weightbearing as tolerated with the brace locked in extension if no osteotomy was performed. Limit weightbearing to nonweightbearing from 0 to 2 weeks and partial weightbearing at 2 to 4 weeks if osteotomy was performed.
- Brace: Lock in extension for weightbearing for at least 2 weeks, increase by 20 degrees each week until full, and then discontinue.

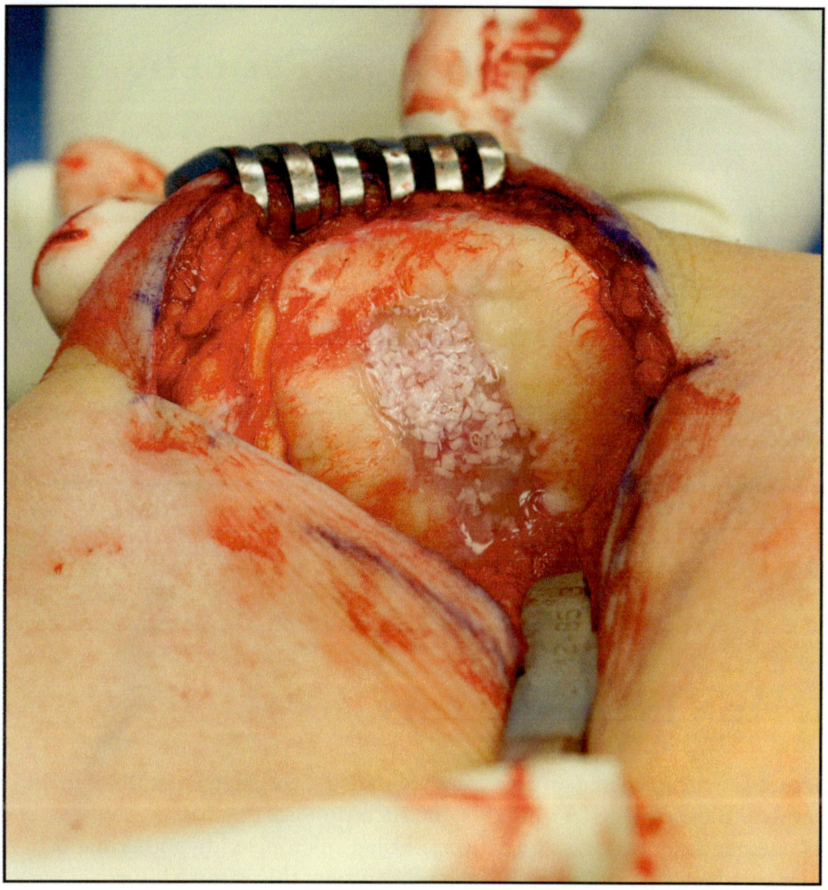

Figure 21-6. The final DeNovo NT implant placed in the patellar defect with fibrin placed over the implant after placement.

- ROM: Continuous passive motion (CPM) is performed out of the brace for 6 hours per day from 0 to 45 degrees for 3 weeks and is then increased by 5 to 10 degrees per day until it reaches 90 degrees by 6 weeks. Discontinue it thereafter.
- Exercises: At weeks 1 to 4, perform quadriceps sets and straight leg raises with hamstring isometrics. At weeks 4 to 10, perform isometric closed chain exercises with balance and bike at 8 weeks. At 6 to 8 months, perform fast walking on a treadmill and light plyometric activity. High-impact activities thereafter are limited and advanced as tolerated as long as symptoms do not recur.

Potential Complications

- Lack of integration/graft displacement
- Graft hypertrophy
- Risk of infection/allograft transmission
- Chondrocytes have not been shown to stimulate proliferation of allogeneic or xenogeneic lymphocytes or promote graft rejection immune responses

Top Technical Pearls for the Procedure

1. Ensure adequate defect sizing if performing a staged procedure in order to place the appropriate amount of DeNovo NT.
2. Do not perform arthroscopically unless you feel you can get the same result as when performing an arthrotomy.
3. Correct associated pathology to optimize the results (eg, osteotomy, meniscal allograft transplantation, medial patellofemoral ligament reconstruction, etc).
4. Ensure that the fibrin glue is not proud relative to the surrounding cartilage.
5. Do not take shortcuts on the rehabilitation; there is no quick fix for cartilage damage and the time required to promote integration and tissue stability.

PART TWO: BIOCARTILAGE

Introduction

Although microfracture is not considered an emerging technology, the augmentation of microfracture continues to evolve. BioCartilage (Arthrex) is one such product that acts as a clot stabilizer that also involves autogenous growth factor delivery. Using micronized hypothermic dehydrated allograft articular cartilage that is 100 to 300 microns in size, this is mixed in equal parts of an autologous blood solution, such as platelet-rich plasma (PRP). This mixture can be delivered arthroscopically or through an open technique. After placement, fibrin glue is used to maintain the graft in the defect site. BioCartilage does not contain a viable cell source and has a shelf-life of 5 years. Although comparing it to microfracture is favorable in clinical use and basic science in vivo large animal models, no clinical outcomes regarding BioCartilage have been reported.

Indications[7,8]

- In general, the indications for BioCartilage mirror that of microfracture alone.
- Grade III/IV cartilage lesion
- Lesion size <2 to 4 cm^2 after debridement
- No bone loss
- Preferentially used on the femoral condyle, trochlea, tibia, and hard-to-reach locations
- Body mass index <30 to 34 kg/m^2
- No prior cartilage repair surgery
- Better outcomes if Tegner score is >4 and symptoms last for <12 months

Relative Contraindications

- Bipolar lesion
- Significant subchondral bone edema

- Unaddressed meniscectomy or malalignment
- Larger (> 4 cm^2) shallow defect with primary microfracture may decrease the potential outcomes of future interventions, such as ACI

Pertinent Physical Findings

- Effusions are probably the most important examination finding demonstrating significant intra-articular pathology.
- Femoral defects
  - Tenderness directly over the femoral condyle. (If it is a distal femoral lesion, it is easiest to palpate directly with the knee in flexion.)
- Associated pathology
  - Varus/valgus alignment
  - Joint line tenderness and prior meniscectomy

Pertinent Imaging

X-rays

- Anteroposterior standing: Anterior tibiofemoral arthritis
- Posteroanterior flexion weightbearing: Posterior tibiofemoral arthritis
- Lateral: Patellar alta/baja
- Merchant: Patellofemoral joint space narrowing, tilt, and tracking

MRI (necessary for all patients to evaluate the following)

- Cartilage integrity
- Cartilage quality (delayed gadolinium-enhanced MRI of cartilage, fast-spin echo, or other cartilage-specific sequences)
- Subchondral bone edema
- Associated pathology
  - Meniscus status
  - Ligament status
  - TT-TG distance

CT

- A consideration for patients with significant bone loss, cystic change, or as an alternative to measure the TT-TG distance in the setting of concomitant planned tibial tubercle osteotomy

Equipment

- Arthroscopy setup based on surgeon preference
- Small curettes and ring curette if available
- Microfracture awls and/or powered device to create subchondral access
- BioCartilage comes in 1-cc packages that are to be mixed with 1 cc of PRP or less; this typically is enough volume to cover any indicated lesion.

- BioCartilage Mixing and Delivery System
- PRP system of choice

Positioning and Portals

- Supine with the leg of the bed extended
- Lateral post
- Tourniquet

Step-by-Step Description of the Procedure

- Diagnostic arthroscopy: Standard diagnostic arthroscopy (inferolateral viewing portal and inferomedial working portal with optional outflow)
- Evaluate the entire knee and the lesion to determine the lack of unexpected contraindications or concomitant pathology, even in the setting of a relatively recent index arthroscopy indicating a patient for BioCartilage arthrotomy.
  - The authors prefer performing an arthrotomy to access the cartilage defect. The location of the incision depends on the location of the defect, with a lateral arthrotomy preferred for a patellofemoral or lateral femoral condyle defect and a medial vastus-sparing approach for other defects.
- Defect preparation
  - Similar to any cartilage procedure, the defect should be debrided to stable healthy walls that are vertical in nature.
  - The bed of the defect should be free of any diseased tissue, and care should be taken to attempt removal of the calcified cartilage layer without gaining access to the subchondral bone elements.
- Perform microfracture
  - The bed of the defect should then be microfractured, which is described elsewhere (Figure 21-7).
- BioCartilage preparation
  - Open the BioCartilage vial and prepare equal parts of PRP (Figure 21-8).
  - The mixture should be workable and viscous. Start by adding part of the PRP until you can mold the mixture. This may not require the entire PRP volume (Figure 21-9).
- BioCartilage application
  - After BioCartilage preparation, the defect can be approached by arthrotomy or arthroscopy.
  - If applying via arthroscopy, Touhy needles can be used.
  - Applying through an arthrotomy can be performed with a freer elevator and digital pressure.
  - This is then covered with a layer of fibrin glue, making sure that this is not overly proud compared to the surrounding cartilage (Figure 21-10).
  - The final construct should be stable after putting the knee through a ROM (Figure 21-11).

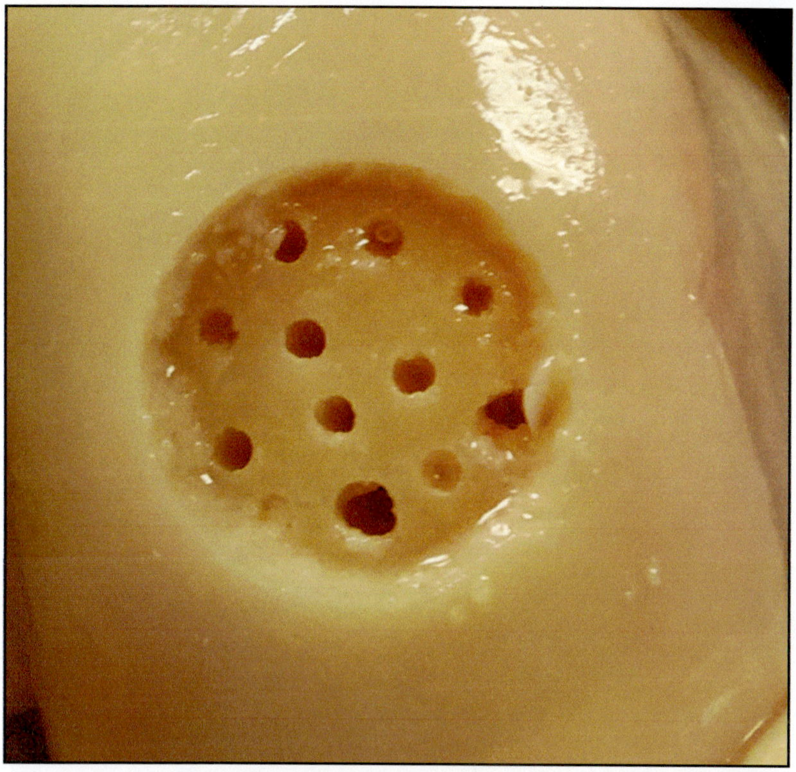

Figure 21-7. Cadaveric example of a prepared cartilage defect with microfracture performed.

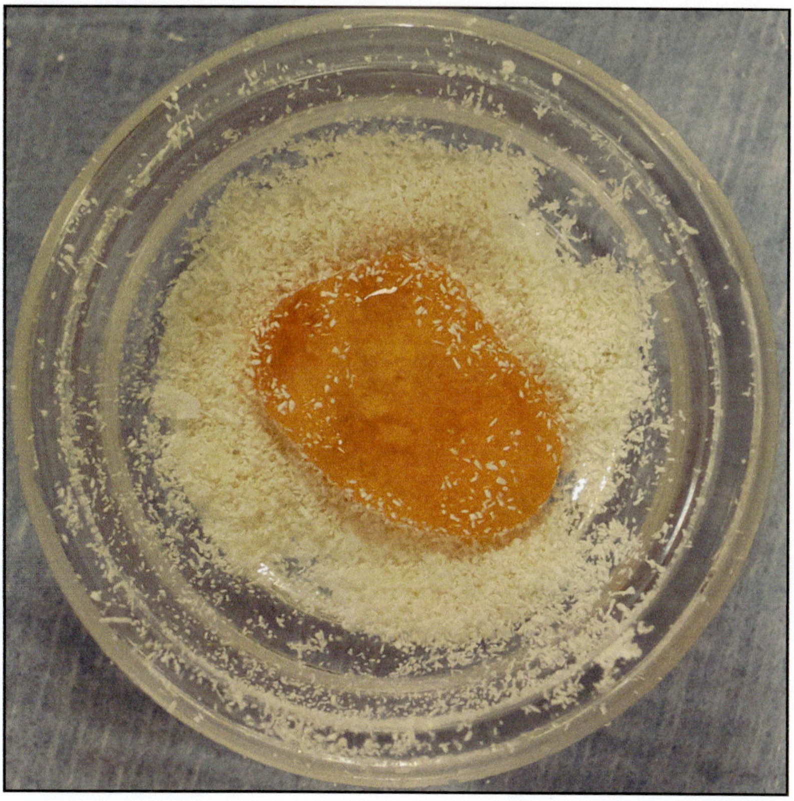

Figure 21-8. BioCartilage added to equal parts of PRP.

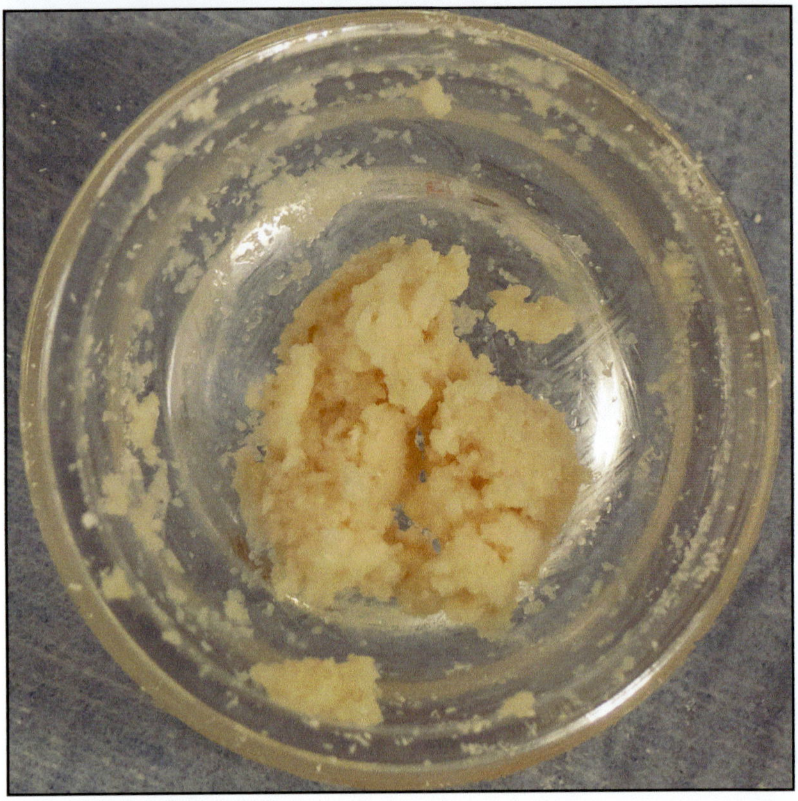

Figure 21-9. The BioCartilage and PRP mixture prepared for placement into the defect. Note the viscosity and workable texture.

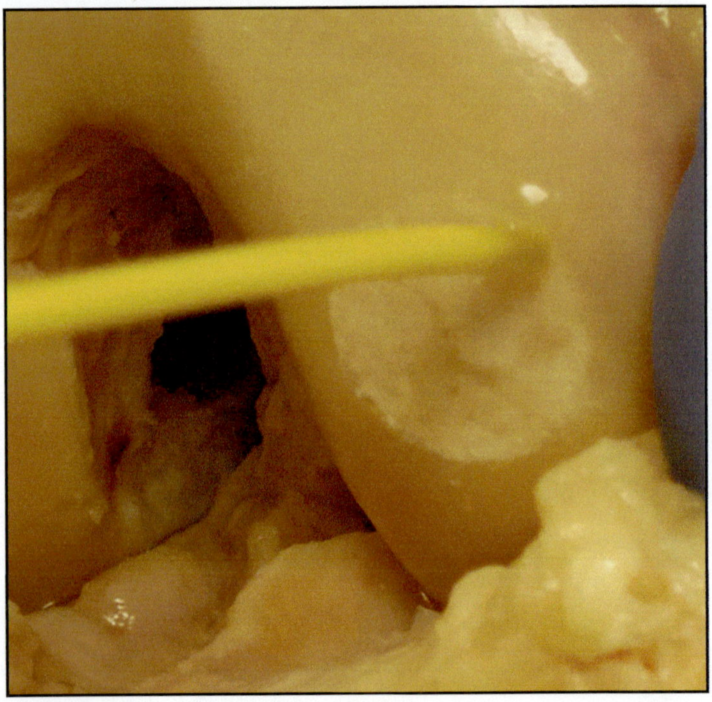

Figure 21-10. The BioCartilage implant has been placed into the femoral condyle defect, and fibrin glue is placed over this to improve stability.

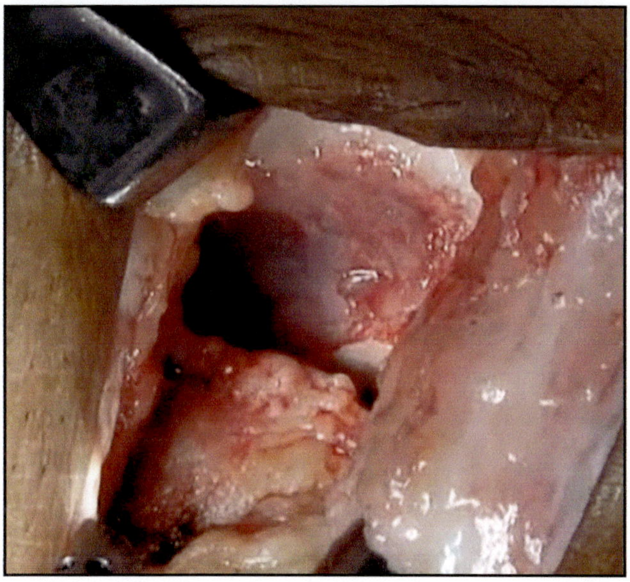

Figure 21-11. A clinical example of the BioCartilage implant after placement in a femoral condyle defect.

Postoperative Protocol (Femoral Condyle)

- Weightbearing: Weeks 0 to 2: Nonweightbearing. Weeks 2 to 6: Foot flat weightbearing (30 to 40 lb with use of 1 crutch). Weeks 6 to 12: Progress to full weightbearing and normal gait.
- Brace: Weeks 0 to 2: Locked in full extension (removed for CPM or manually cycle leg and exercise). Weeks 2 to 4: Gradual brace unlocking as lower-extremity control returns.
- ROM: Weeks 0 to 4: CPM for 6 to 8 hours/day (may be broken up into 2-hour increments) at 1 cycle/minute or manually cycle the leg. Begin at 0 to 30 degrees and increase 5 to 10 degrees daily per patient comfort. The patient should gain at least 90 degrees by week 4 and 120 to 130 degrees by week 6 or manually cycle the leg. Full active ROM is allowed thereafter.
- Exercises: Weeks 0 to 2: Quadriceps sets, straight leg raises, hamstring isometrics (complete exercises in the brace if quadriceps control is inadequate). Weeks 2 to 6: Begin progressive closed chain exercises. Open chain exercises with emphasis on quadriceps and core muscles (customized to the site of the lesion). Weeks 10 to 12: Progress closed chain exercises using resistance less than patient's body weight, progress to unilateral closed chain exercises, begin balance activities, and perform biking with progressive load 30 minutes per day as possible. Months 3 to 6: Advance bilateral and unilateral closed chain exercises, with emphasis on concentric/eccentric control; continue with biking, StairMaster, and treadmill; and progress balance activities.
  - Respect the chondrocyte graft with closed chain activities (if anterior, avoid loading in full extension; if posterior, avoid loading in flexion greater than 45 degrees).
  - All phases are to include an emphasis on terminal extension and patellar mobility.
  - If pain or swelling occurs with any activities, they must be modified to decrease symptoms.

Potential Complications

- Microfracture site pain
- Osseous overgrowth at the site of microfracture
- Subchondral cyst formation

Top Technical Pearls for the Procedure

1. Do not short-change the microfracture part of the procedure; ensure proper technique with calcified cartilage layer removal and adequate marrow access confirmed visually.
2. Do not perform the procedure arthroscopically unless you feel you can get the same result as achieved with an arthrotomy.
3. Do not add excessive PRP to the BioCartilage; keep it viscous for placement.
4. Ensure that the fibrin glue is not proud relative to the surrounding cartilage.
5. Check knee ROM after finishing to ensure the BioCartilage is retained within the defect.

References

1. Adkisson HD, Gillis MP, Davis EC, Maloney W, Hruska KA. In vitro generation of scaffold independent neocartilage. *Clin Orthop Relat Res.* 2001;(391 suppl):S280-S294.
2. Bonasia DE, Martin JA, Marmotti A, et al. Cocultures of adult and juvenile chondrocytes compared with adult and juvenile chondral fragments: in vitro matrix production. *Am J Sports Med.* 2011;39(11):2355-2361.
3. Tompkins M, Hamann JC, Diduch DR, et al. Preliminary results of a novel single-stage cartilage restoration technique: particulated juvenile articular cartilage allograft for chondral defects of the patella. *Arthroscopy.* 2013;29(10):1661-1670.
4. Farr J, Tabet SK, Margerrison E, Cole BJ. Clinical, radiographic, and histological outcomes after cartilage repair with particulated juvenile articular cartilage: a 2-year prospective study. *Am J Sports Med.* 2014;42(6):1417-1425.
5. Minas T, Gomoll AH, Rosenberger R, Royce RO, Bryant T. Increased failure rate of autologous chondrocyte implantation after previous treatment with marrow stimulation techniques. *Am J Sports Med.* 2009;37(5):902-908.
6. Pestka JM, Bode G, Salzmann G, Südkamp NP, Niemeyer P. Clinical outcome of autologous chondrocyte implantation for failed microfracture treatment of full-thickness cartilage defects of the knee joint. *Am J Sports Med.* 2012;40(2):325-331.
7. Mithoefer K, McAdams T, Williams RJ, Kreuz PC, Mandelbaum BR. Clinical efficacy of the microfracture technique for articular cartilage repair in the knee: an evidence-based systematic analysis. *Am J Sports Med.* 2009;37(10):2053-2063.
8. Kreuz PC, Steinwachs MR, Erggelet C, et al. Results after microfracture of full-thickness chondral defects in different compartments in the knee. *Osteoarthritis Cartilage.* 2006;14(11):1119-1125.

Please see videos on the accompanying website at www.routledge.com/9781617119996

22

Proximal Tibial and Distal Femoral Osteotomy

Robert Litchfield, MD, FRCSC and Annunziato Amendola, MD

Introduction

High tibial osteotomy (HTO) for the treatment of varus gonarthrosis isolated to the medial compartment of the knee was first described by Jackson et al in 1958[1] and popularized by Coventry.[2] Valgus-producing HTO for medial joint gonarthrosis has evolved from a lateral closing wedge to a medial opening wedge, and both techniques are recognized as joint-preserving alternatives to unicompartmental and total knee arthroplasty, specifically in younger patients.[3,4] Many studies have shown good patient-reported outcomes and survivorship following limb realignment with an HTO for medial joint gonarthrosis.[5,6] A varus-producing distal femoral osteotomy (DFO) can be performed to unload the lateral compartment with valgus malalignment, which also provides good results.[7]

The use of HTO and DFO for the treatment of gonarthrosis follows the theory of limb realignment in the coronal plane in order to unload the affected knee compartment and transfer the weightbearing forces through the healthy knee compartment.[5,8] Valgus-producing osteotomies to unload the medial compartment are typically performed with an HTO (medial opening wedge or lateral closing wedge), whereas varus producing-osteotomies to unload the lateral compartment are performed with a DFO (medial opening wedge or lateral closing wedge) or lateral opening wedge HTO.

Osteotomies can also be used in the treatment of ligamentous instability in the setting of malalignment. Coronal plane realignment can be used to protect ligamentous reconstructions.[9-12] In addition, altering the tibial slope on the sagittal plane can be performed to treat posterior (PCL) or anterior cruciate ligament (ACL) insufficiency.[13,14] Corrections to the tibial slope can be performed with a direct anterior wedge osteotomy or through a medial or lateral wedge biplanar osteotomy (to address coronal and sagittal alignment).[13]

Multiple HTO and DFO techniques have been described in the literature for a variety of conditions, both gonarthrosis and ligamentous instability. This chapter describes the authors' technique of a medial opening wedge HTO for medial gonarthrosis and medial closing wedge DFO for lateral gonarthrosis.

Sgaglione NA, Lubowitz JH, Provencher MT, eds. *The Knee: AANA Advanced Arthroscopic Surgical Techniques* (pp 297-311).

Indications

High Tibial Osteotomy (Medial Opening Wedge)

- Gonarthrosis isolated to the medial compartment with varus malalignment
- Age younger than 60 years
- Good range of motion (ROM)
- Ligamentous knee stability[5] (but it is indicated in some ACL-/PCL-deficient patients)
- Associated with meniscal or osteochondral transplantation

Controversial Indications

- Knee with significant motion loss
- Inflammatory arthritis
- Associated patellofemoral or low-grade contralateral compartment arthritis (compartment that the mechanical axis is shifting to needs to be relatively well preserved)
- Advanced age[5,6,15]
- Obesity[5]
- Relative contraindications include smoking and diabetes mellitus given the increased rate of complications in these patient populations.

Distal Femoral Osteotomy (Medial Closing Wedge)

- Gonarthrosis isolated to the lateral compartment and valgus malalignment[7]
- Primary femoral deformity
- Large correction (ie, > 12 degrees of valgus deformity)[16,17]
- Lateral opening wedge HTO can be considered for small corrections, with the advantage of correcting the deformity in extension and flexion; DFO only corrects the deformity in extension.[16]

Contraindications

- Contraindications for a DFO include advanced age, stiffness, tricompartmental disease, and inflammatory arthritis.[7,18,19]

Pertinent Physical Findings

- Gait assessment: Any varus thrust observed during the patient's gait cycle should be noted because this can indicate a double or triple varus knee.[10]
- Alignment can be observed clinically by having the patient stand with his or her heels together and knees pointing forward and facing the examiner.
- Peripheral vascular: Assess peripheral pulses, skin, venous disease, and presence of hair.
- ROM: The knee should be brought through a ROM and compared to the contralateral knee (note recurvatum and loss of flexion or extension).
- Ligamentous knee examination should be performed to rule out any injury to the ACL, PCL, lateral collateral ligament, medial collateral ligament (MCL), or posteromedial corner (PMC). It is common to find pseudolaxity if there is increased wear of one of the compartments.

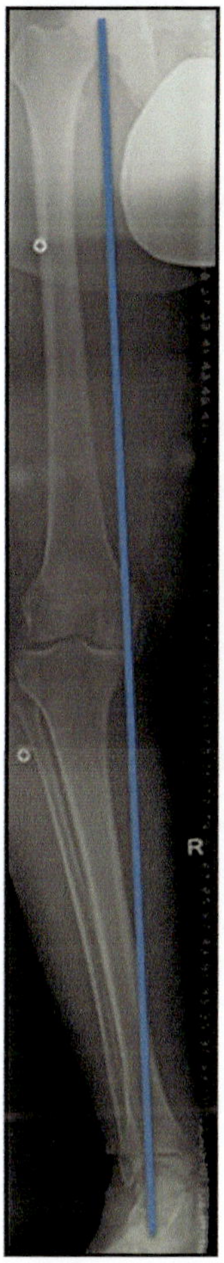

Figure 22-1. Draw the mechanical axis of the leg from the center of the hip to the center of the ankle.

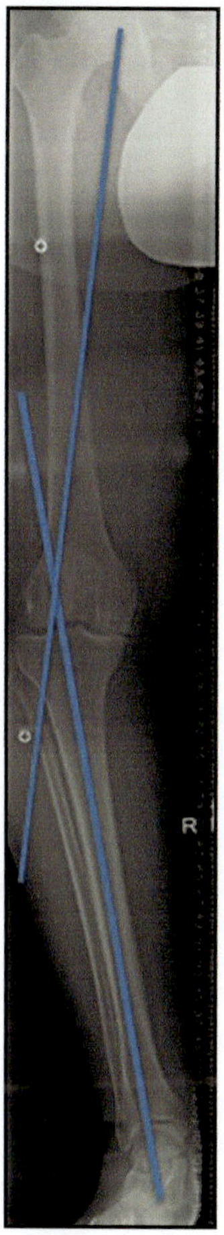

Figure 22-2. From the center of the hip, draw a line to the desired correction point in the lateral compartment and a line to that point from the center of the ankle.

Pertinent Imaging

- Bilateral weightbearing
- Anteroposterior (AP) in full extension
- Rosenberg or tunnel view (AP in 30 to 45 degrees of flexion)
- Lateral
- Skyline views
- Weightbearing hips-to-ankles AP x-ray to assess weightbearing axis and calculate correction[20]

When unloading the medial compartment with a valgus-producing osteotomy, most authors aim to correct the weightbearing line to intersect in the lateral compartment at Fujisawa's point, 62.5% along the medial to lateral width of the tibia.[15,21] However, correction to Fujisawa's point is largely arbitrary, as this has never been validated.[22] The authors believe that correction to the midpoint of the lateral tibial spine downslope is sufficient. Studies in the authors' gait analysis laboratory suggest that this reduces the adduction moment during the gait cycle by 50% on average (unpublished data). The method for calculating the degree of correction in a medial opening wedge HTO is shown in Figures 22-1 through 22-3. Calculations for the varus-producing osteotomy are similar; however, when performing a varus-producing osteotomy, it is largely accepted to correct the alignment to neutral.[7]

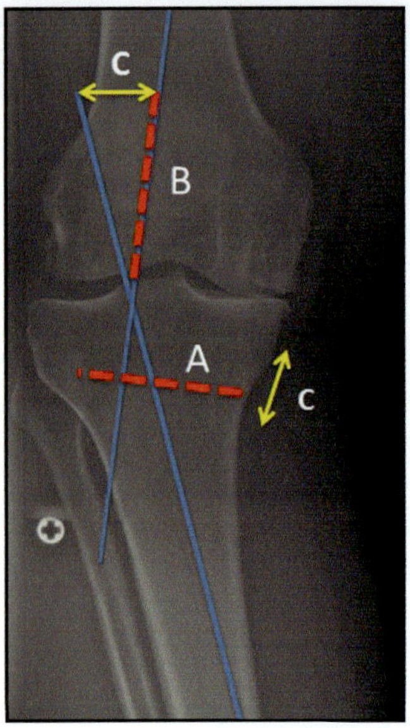

Figure 22-3. Draw line A, which represents the osteotomy; this line stops 7 to 10 mm inside the lateral cortex of the tibia. Draw line B, which is identical in length to line A. Distance C represents the amount the osteotomy will need to be opened for the desired mechanical axis to be achieved.

Equipment

- Fluoroscopy
- Radiolucent operating room table
- Positioning bundle
- Large curved blunt Hohmann retractor (Figure 22-4) for posterior retraction
- Narrow curved retractor (see Figure 22-4) for anterior retraction
- Calibrated pin (or break-away pins)
- Oscillating saw
- Wide and narrow flexible osteotomes (Figure 22-5)
- Opening wedge (Figure 22-6A)
- Laminar spreader (optional) (Figure 22-6B)
- Plate fixation (TomoFix, Puddu plate, Contourlock, iBalance)
- Bone graft, synthetic or allograft (optional)

Positioning and Portals

The patient should be positioned supine on a radiolucent operating table. A tourniquet is applied to the thigh for intraoperative hemostasis. A sterile positioning bundle can be placed underneath the knee and leg during the osteotomy for optimum positioning during fluoroscopy. The same sterile positioning bundle can be placed under the heel to obtain knee extension prior to fixation. If knee arthroscopy is indicated, an arthroscopy setup can easily be added to the osteotomy setup.

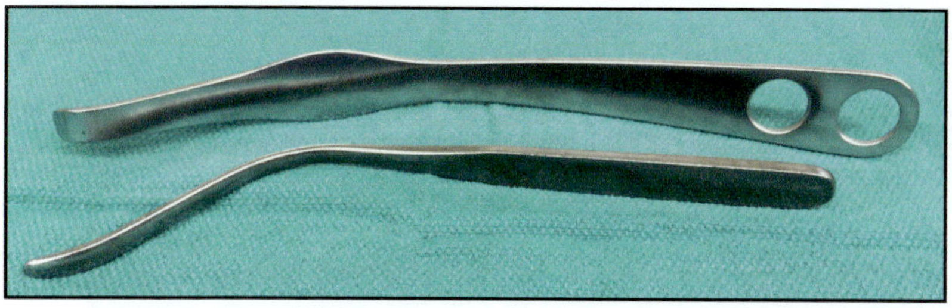

Figure 22-4. A blunt-tipped Hohmann retractor is useful along the posterior tibial cortex. A bent Lane retractor is useful above the tibial tubercle to retract the patellar tendon laterally.

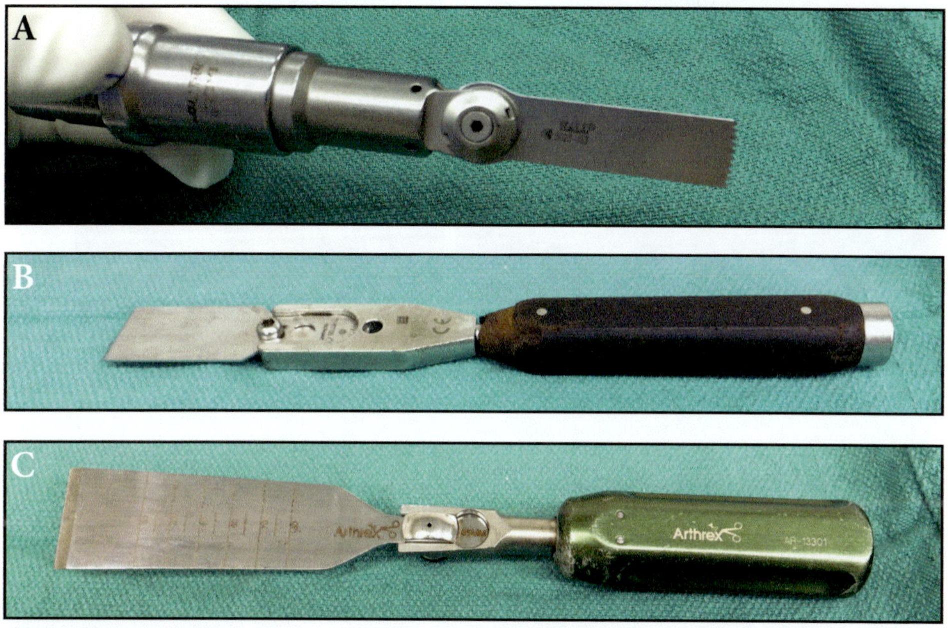

Figure 22-5. (A-C) Thin, sharp osteotomes are useful following a limited saw cut followed by a calibrated osteotome to ensure the lateral hinge is maintained.

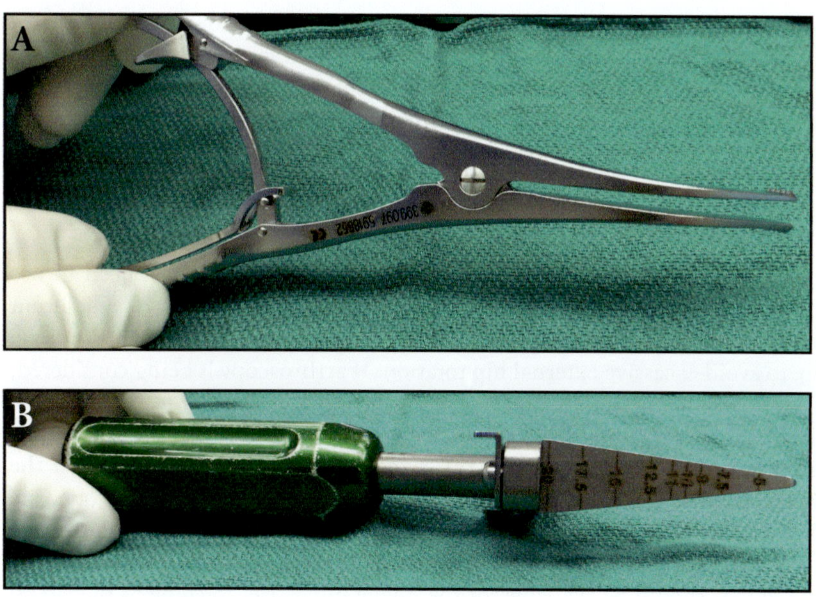

Figure 22-6. (A, B) A laminar spreader or a calibrated wedge is helpful to maintain the osteotomy open.

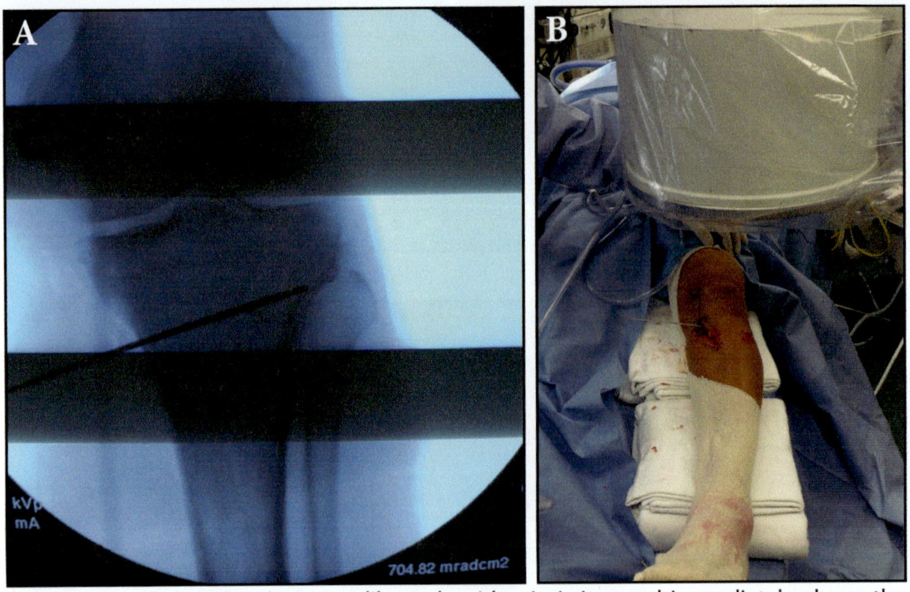

Figure 22-7. (A, B) A break-away calibrated guide pin is inserted immediately above the proposed plane of the osteotomy under fluoroscopic guidance. It is best to bring the C-arm from the operative side and perform the surgery from the medial position.

Step-by-Step Description of the Procedure

Surgery starts with a well thought out preoperative plan, including calculating the desired correction in the coronal and sagittal planes as mentioned previously (see Figures 22-1 through 22-3).

Anesthetic Considerations

The standard at the authors' institution is a general anesthetic with or without a supplementary regional block at the discretion of the anesthetic team. The exception to this is when a tibial tubercle osteotomy or biplanar cut is anticipated, which would violate the anterior compartment of the lower leg; it is best to avoid a regional block for fear of masking a potential compartment syndrome. This is not an issue with standard medial opening tibial wedge HTO (MOWHTO) or DFO.

Positioning

Fluoroscopic guidance is essential to perform an osteotomy; therefore, one will need to use a radiolucent operating table. The author uses a trauma table or, more frequently, a radiolucent extension on a standard operating table. One may consider a small bolster, such as a 3-L saline bag, under the operative hip, to avoid excessive external hip rotation. If arthroscopy is being considered, lateral posts can be easily added to the setup. A pneumatic tourniquet is applied to the proximal thigh and can be inflated at the surgeon's discretion; once a surgeon is experienced, tourniquet times are routinely less than an hour. Plan to have a full-sized C-arm fluoroscopy unit enter the surgical field from the same side as the operative leg with the surgeon operating from the opposite side (Figure 22-7). The C-arm will move in and out as needed by having it move from a proximal position over the hip to a more distal position over the knee when required. The C-arm should be draped, and appropriate drapes should be available for the image intensifier to come to the lateral position. After standard draping with an extremity drape or U-drapes (for distal femoral access),

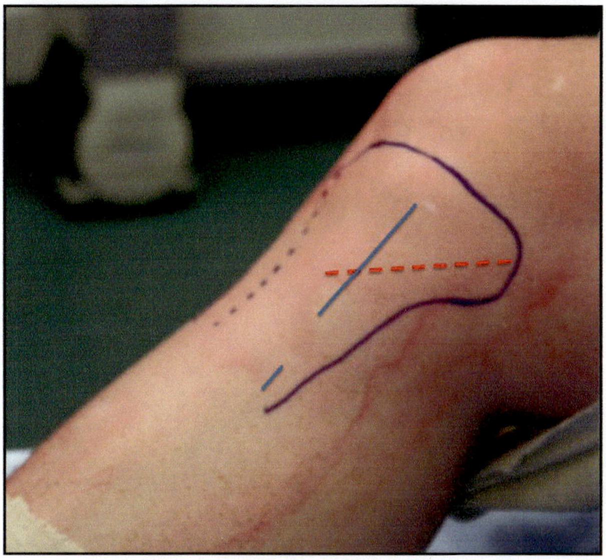

Figure 22-8. A 6- to 7-cm incision is made starting 1 cm below the joint line, a second stab incision is useful for filling the distal holes in the plate. The red dotted line represents an alternate incision.

the operative side can be elevated above the nonoperative side using a positioning pack (sterile sheets or towels); this places the knee in slight flexion and makes it easier to retract and to get a lateral x-ray when needed.

Medial Opening Tibial Wedge High Tibial Osteotomy

The surgical approach for a proximal MOWHTO should respect future surgical approaches; for this reason, the authors favor a medial longitudinal incision based midway between the tibial tubercle and the posteromedial border of the tibia (Figure 22-8). After dissection through skin and subcutaneous tissue, the first layer of fascia can be exposed using blunt dissection with a surgical sponge. The sartorius fascia is then incised just above and inline with the gracilis tendon and the pes anserine is released 1 cm off the tibial attachment (Figure 22-9). The surgeon will now have an excellent look at the MCL tibial attachment. Using cautery, the PMC of the fascial attachment (popliteus) is elevated off the metaphyseal flare of the tibia posterior to the MCL for a length of 3 to 5 cm. Using a Cobb or a periosteal elevator, the soft tissue on the posterior aspect of the tibia can be gently elevated. During this step, be sure to direct the instrument toward the posterior cortex of the tibia. Next, a blunt-tipped Hohmann retractor is placed across the tibia, feeling bone on the tip of the instrument as it is inserted (Figure 22-10). This instrument will be in direct line with the proposed osteotomy. The tibial tubercle is then identified, as is the medial border of the patellar tendon in the proximal aspect of the wound. Open the fascia longitudinally medial to the tendon to facilitate insertion of a blunt retractor (bent Lane or Hohmann) beneath the tendon. A small release of 5 mm or so of the medial aspect of the tendon insertion on the tubercle will enhance the view. The C-arm is then brought into the surgical field to guide insertion of a break-away pin at the upper margin of where the surgeon plans to cut the tibia. At this stage, the tibial width is measured using the calibrated pin. The authors prefer a fairly horizontal plan to the osteotomy, with the lateral target being the metaphyseal flare of the tibia, not the fibular head. Use a wide osteotome to plan the plane of the cut to pass just on the top of the tibial tubercle. In the sagittal plane, the cut can follow the tibial slope; therefore, angling back 10 degrees or so will give the surgeon more proximal bone for subsequent screw fixation. Once the plane of the cut is chosen, use the osteotome as a cutting guide and mark the cut line with electrocautery (Figure 22-11). The MCL is not elevated but is cut through horizontally in the line of the osteotomy (authors' preference); if the surgeon prefers, the MCL can be elevated and

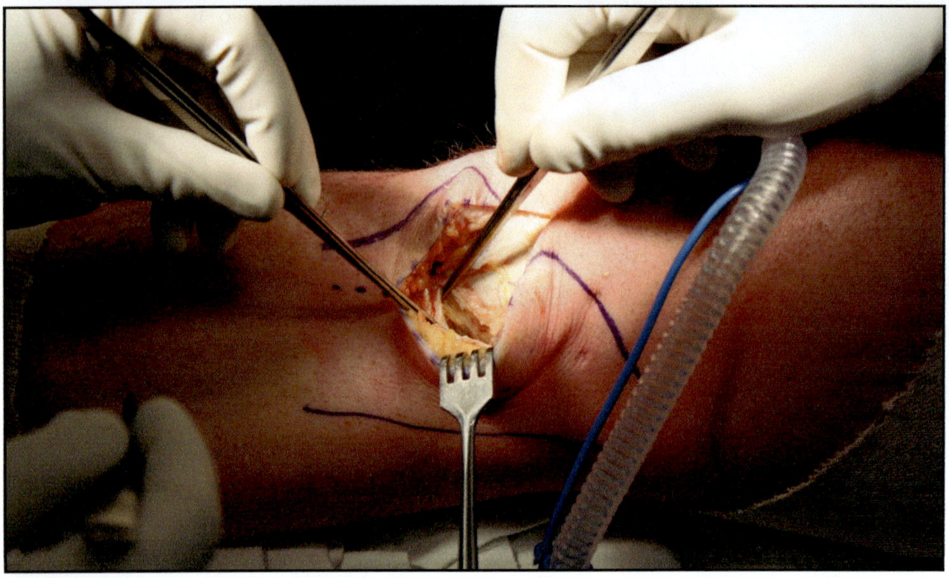

Figure 22-9. Following dissection through the skin and subcutaneous tissue, the sartorius fascia is opened just above the gracilis tendon and the pes anserinus is released off the tibia for 1 cm distally.

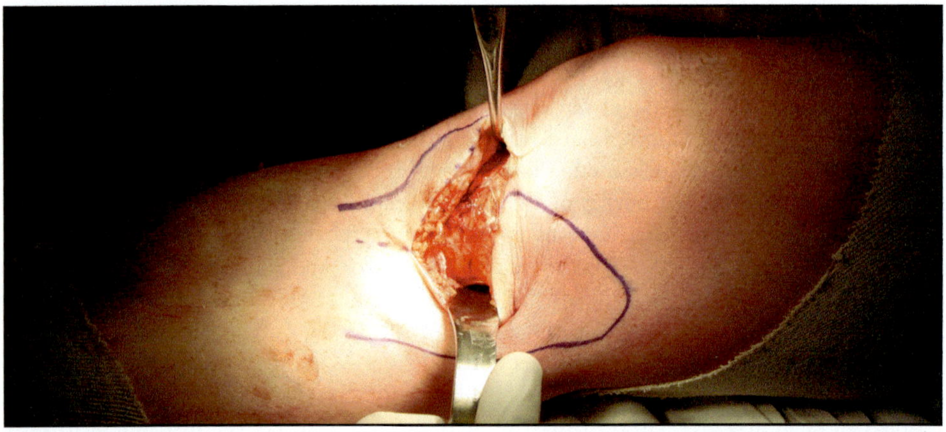

Figure 22-10. The pes anserinus tendons are retracted distally, the posteromedial edge of the tibia is identified, and the attachment of the popliteus muscle is elevated off the flare of the tibia. A Cobb elevator can be gently inserted directly on the posterior tibial cortex and a blunt Hohmann retractor slid across the posterior tibia. This is a key step in protecting neurovascular structures posteriorly.

allowed to fall back over the osteotomy at the end of the procedure. A small oscillating saw blade is chosen (45 mm long), and the cut is made staying perfectly inline and below the guide pin. Commit to the plane of the cut, especially anterior to the pin, so that the surgeon does not wander more proximally toward the joint than desired. Once the initial cut is made with the saw, thin osteotomes can be used. Keep a 10-mm bridge of bone on the lateral side and use the C-arm to follow each step. During cutting, the retractors should remain in the same plane as the saw or osteotome for safety. Once the surgeon feels he or she has completed the desired cut, a wide, firm osteotome can be inserted, and mobility of the osteotomy can be assessed by gently levering on this instrument. Usually, if minimal movement is noted, the posterior cortex needs to be cut a little further. To open the osteotomy, you can use stacked osteotomes or wedges to open to the desired amount. The authors like to use the equipment from the original Puddu set along with laminar

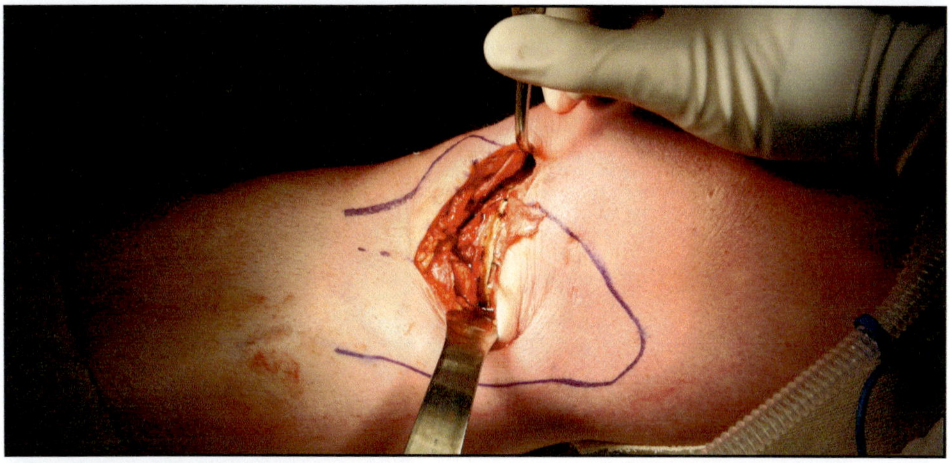

Figure 22-11. The osteotomy is planned out from a point anteriorly just at the patellar tendon attachment on the tibial tubercle to a point angling posteriorly and distally. The superficial MCL can be elevated up or cut directly in line with the proposed osteotomy. This does not destabilize the medial side of the knee.

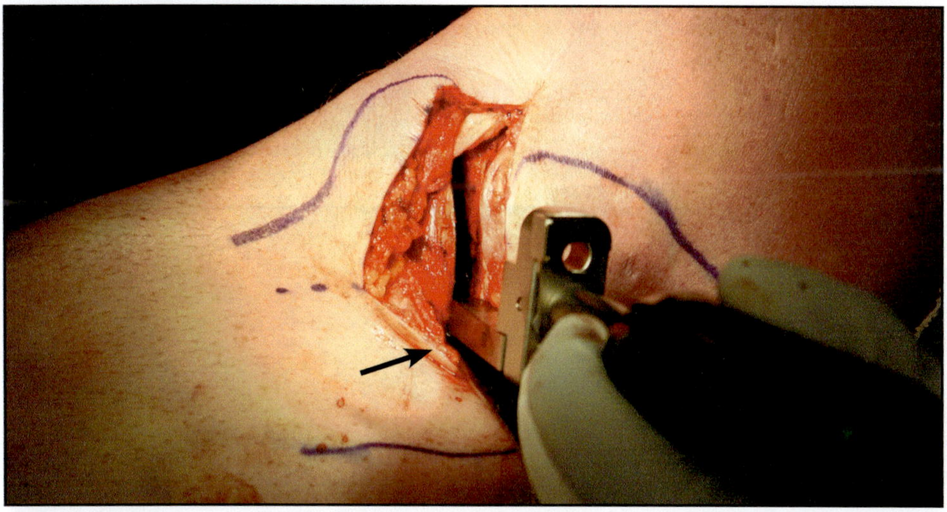

Figure 22-12. Upon completion of the osteotomy, a calibrated wedge or laminar spreader is used to open the osteotomy. Be sure to keep the wedge to the very posterior aspect to avoid increasing tibial slope and also to stay out of the way of plate positioning.

spreaders as needed. Gauge the amount of opening off the posteromedial aspect of the osteotomy; to keep the slope neutral, do not use a wedge more anteriorly because this will open the front and increase the slope (this can be desirable in cases of PCL insufficiency but not in cases of ACL insufficiency or medial arthrosis; Figure 22-12). It is important to try to maintain the integrity of the lateral column of bone to prevent translation and maintain stability. The tip of the osteotomy on the lateral side should always be closer to the lateral cortex than to the lateral joint line; this will avoid intra-articular fractures (Figure 22-13).

Once the osteotomy is complete and is held open with a wedge or laminar spreader to the desired amount, one can then apply hardware to maintain the correction. The authors prefer a locking plate to maintain axial and rotational stability during the consolidation period. The plate is placed on top of the fascial layer using spacer screws to hold the plate slightly off the bone (Figure 22-14). While

Figure 22-13. Intra-articular fractures can be avoided by creating a more horizontal cut and targeting the tibial metaphyseal flare rather than the tip of the fibula. The dotted line represents a safer trajectory.

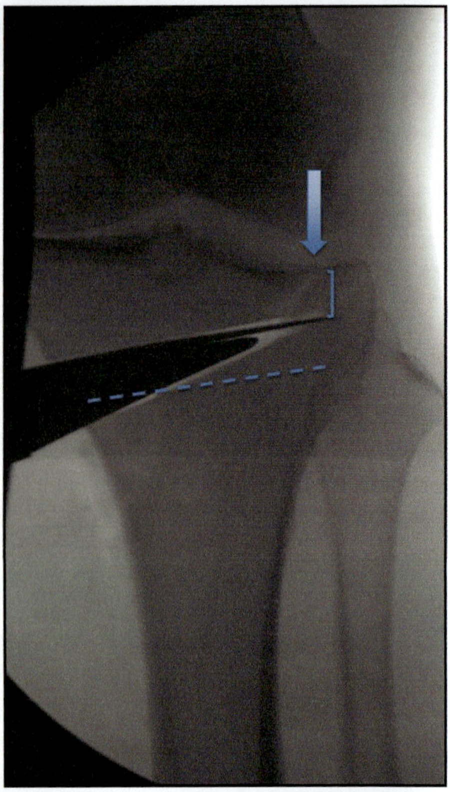

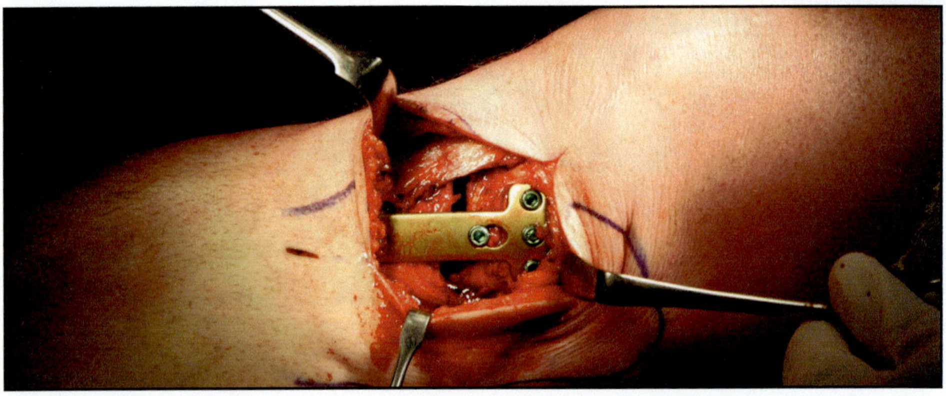

Figure 22-14. A locking plate is then inserted subcutaneously superficial to the pes anserinus, minimizing any periosteal stripping. Spacer screws can help hold the plate from compressing the soft tissues as it is fixed. A small stab wound facilitates distal fixation. Grafting the defect can be performed with autograft, allograft, or bone graft substitutes.

inserting screws using the C-arm to confirm safe positioning, one can usually place 4 locking screws proximal and distal to the osteotomy with proper plate position. Check the lateral fluoroscopic view to ensure that screws are not extending beyond the posterior cortex. After one is satisfied with the fixation, one may consider filling the defect with bone graft or a bone graft substitute (Figure 22-15). The authors prefer allograft cancellous chips combined with 1 g of vancomycin for corrections of greater than 8 mm; no graft is used for smaller corrections. The wound is closed over a one-eighth-in suction drain that is removed the following day. One may chose an icing sleeve and/or a hinged knee brace for added comfort.

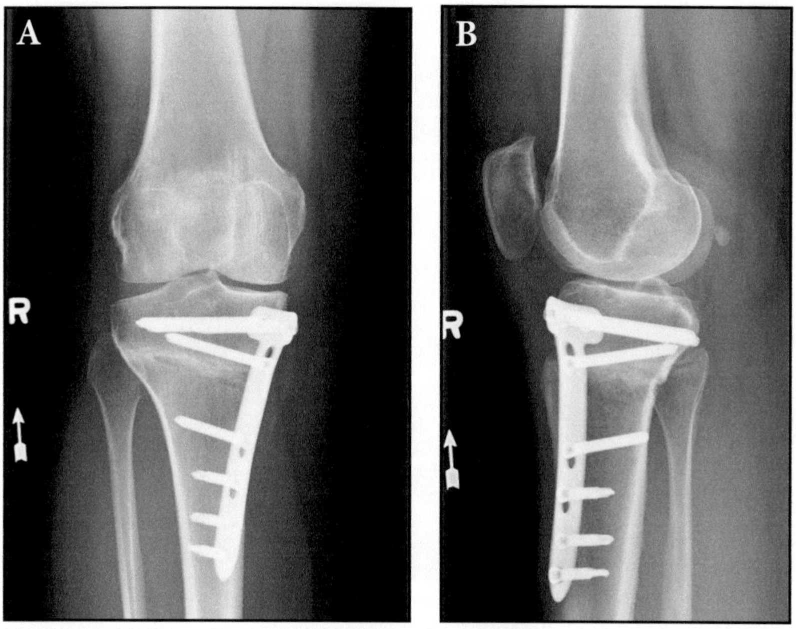

Figure 22-15. AP and lateral radiographs of a completed MOWHTO with locking plate.

Medial Closing Wedge Distal Femoral Osteotomy

Patients with valgus alignment with the weightbearing axis extending through a diseased lateral compartment are candidates for a varus-producing procedure. For small corrections less than 10 mm, the authors prefer to correct below the knee with a lateral opening tibial osteotomy.[16] The indications for varus-producing osteotomies include isolated lateral compartment arthrosis with the medial and patellofemoral compartments having Outerbridge changes of grade II or less. The patient should be physiologically young, preferably with a healthy body mass index, and a nonsmoker, with more than 90 degrees knee flexion.

This section focuses on patients requiring larger corrections, including those with primarily femoral-sided valgus deformity. On the femoral side, a lateral opening or medial closing procedure can achieve the desired correction; the advantages of medial closing are that the hardware is less prominent medially, the closing wedge technique is stable, and union occurs quickly.

The setup for medial closing wedge DFO is the same as for MOWHTO with a radiolucent table that allows visualization from the hip to the ankle using a C-arm. The image intensifier is brought in from the affected side, and the surgeon works from the opposite (medial) side. A tourniquet is used as desired, and preoperative antibiotics are given routinely. The incision is medial to the midline and longitudinal to facilitate any future reconstructions. The incision extends from the distal pole of the patella proximally for 15 cm. After dissection through the skin and subcutaneous tissue, the lower border of the vastus medialis is identified; in order to mobilize the vastus, the medial patellofemoral ligament is incised and later repaired. The vastus medialis is mobilized off the intermuscular septum, taking care to cauterize any perforating vessels. The distal two-fifths of the medial femur can be safely exposed before encountering the adductor canal and the femoral artery. A blunt retractor (Hohmann, Bennett, or curved knee) is placed beneath the vastus to retract it anteriorly. The intermuscular septum is carefully elevated off the PMC of the femur at the supracondylar level at the proposed osteotomy site, and a blunt Hohmann retractor is placed across the posterior femur directly on the bone to prevent neurovascular injury during the osteotomy. The periosteum is left intact to maintain vascularity. The hardware can then be trialed

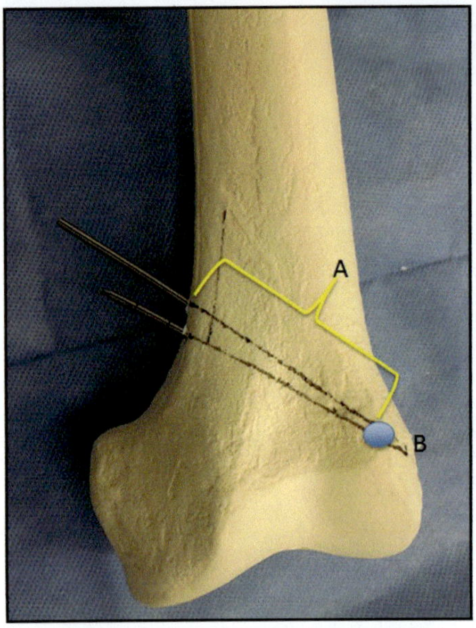

Figure 22-16. Medial femoral closing wedge osteotomy to correct valgus deformity. Two pins are inserted equal distance A, converging upon point B, which is just above the trochlea and 10 mm medial to the cortex.

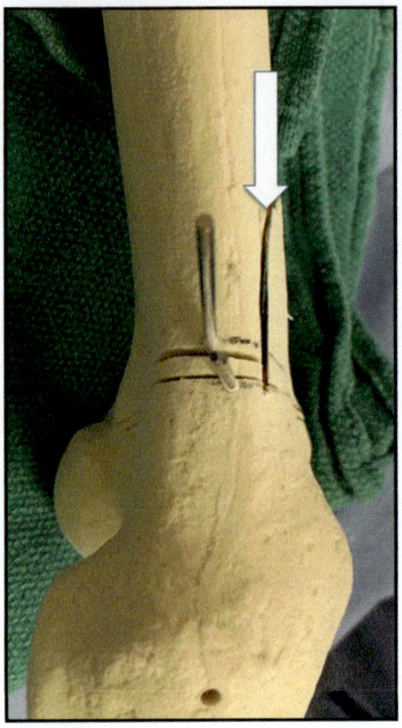

Figure 22-17. On the lateral view, an optional biplane cut is demonstrated (arrow).

on the medial femur with fluoroscopic guidance. The authors prefer to use the Medial TomoFix Plate (DePuy Synthes). The plate is lined up with the anterior aspect of the plate flush with the anterior cortex of the femur. There is room for 4 screws above and below the osteotomy. The lower cut of the osteotomy should be approximately 10 mm above the superior extent of the trochlea; a small arthrotomy may be necessary to palpate this landmark. The proposed osteotomy is then marked using electrocautery on the medial cortex perpendicular to the long axis of the femur. To make the osteotomy close with cortical contact, one should have both limbs of the osteotomy of equal length with the apex 10 mm medial to the lateral cortex (Figure 22-16). The apex should be below the level of the medial epicondyle because the MCL will provide additional restraint to translation of the osteotomy (Figure 22-16, blue dot). K-wires can be used as cutting guides, being sure to account for the thickness of the saw blade when planning the wedge. While using the saw, use plenty of irrigation to avoid heat build-up on the blade. The posterior Hohmann retractor should be right in line with the saw at all times. A series of osteotomes can be used to complete the cuts as needed. The bone wedge is then removed. A biplanar cut can be performed as an option to increase the stability and surface area of the osteotomy (Figure 22-17). Fixation is then achieved using standard fracture fixation techniques to achieve compression across the osteotomy site (Figures 22-18 through 22-20).

Postoperative Protocol

Patients are kept overnight in most situations, although with healthy younger patients with good perioperative pain management, one can consider outpatient surgery. Prophylactic antibiotics and anticoagulation can be given per the surgeon's preference. The brace is locked at 0 degrees overnight then unlocked after a dressing change and drain removal the following morning. The brace is set at 0 to 90 degrees. During the first 2 weeks, the patient is on crutches and is

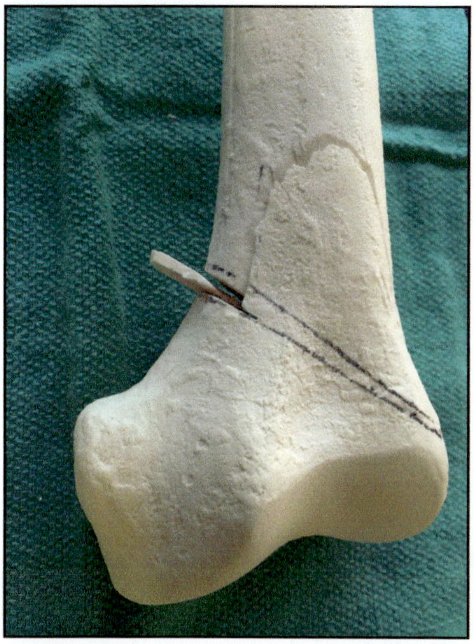

Figure 22-18. The medial wedge of bone is removed.

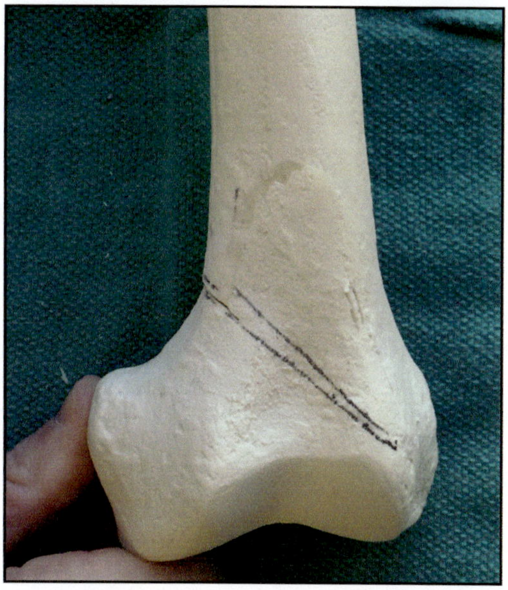

Figure 22-19. The osteotomy is closed with a varus load to the leg.

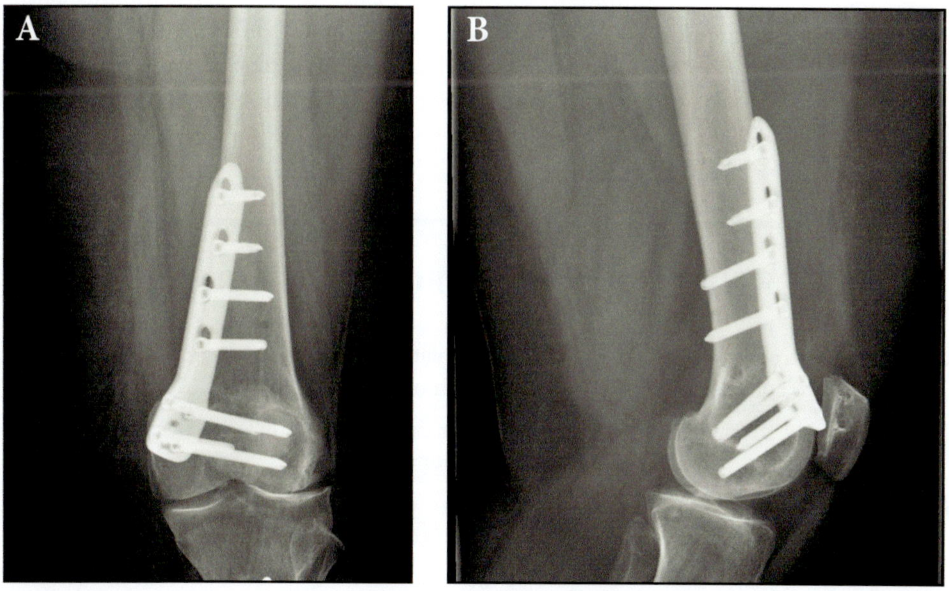

Figure 22-20. (A, B) A medial closing wedge femoral osteotomy is secured with a locking plate. If performed as described, this is a very stable construct that will tolerate early weightbearing and motion.

feather-touch weightbearing. The patient is reassessed for wound healing at this stage and is then allowed to put as much weight as tolerated through the operative leg so long as no complications with the fixation are noted on x-rays. In general, it takes another 3 or 4 weeks of crutch usage before patients can walk without aids. The brace is removed for therapy, and full ROM and isometric quadriceps and hamstring exercises are encouraged. The use of a stationary bike without resistance and water therapy are allowed when the wound is well healed. After 6 weeks, the brace is discontinued, and progressive closed chain strengthening is used. Patients are followed routinely at 2, 6, 12, 26, and 52 weeks. It is not uncommon for the osteotomy to take a full 6 months to unite and 1 year to remodel.

Potential Complications

Complications can be looked at in 3 classes. Class 1 includes complications considered minor that do not require treatment and do not affect outcome. Class 2 complications require nonoperative medical treatment. Class 3 complications are more severe and required surgical management and/or long-term medical treatment. A review of complications on 323 osteotomies performed in the authors' center was performed.[23] The incidence of complications is multifactorial and is influenced by the following factors: body mass index, systemic illness (diabetes mellitus), size of the correction, hardware system used, and how and when one defines delayed union.

Class 1 complications included undisplaced lateral cortex breach (20%), displaced lateral cortical breach 2 mm or greater (6%), delayed wound healing (6%), undisplaced tibial plateau fracture (3%), hematoma (3%), and increased tibial slope (1%). Class 2 complications included delayed union after 3 months that resolved by 6 months (12%), cellulitis (10%), limited hardware failure (broken screw; 4%), stiffness (1%), deep vein thrombosis (1%), and chronic regional pain syndrome (1%). Class 3 complications included aseptic nonunion (3%), deep infection (2%), chronic regional pain syndrome (1%), gross hardware failure and correction loss (1%), and additional surgery (3%).

These complications can be minimized by careful patient selection (avoid insulin-dependent diabetics) and meticulous technique (avoid penetrating the lateral cortex or cutting proximally toward the plateau), including wound closure. Use a locking plate system to minimize mechanical failure during bone healing. If these issues are avoided, the important class 3 complication rate is low (3% reoperation rate). One additional issue is the need for hardware removal; in the authors' experience, this is necessary 30% to 40% of the time.

Top Technical Pearls for the Procedure

1. Measure twice, cut once! Be precise in templating the correction and use the C-arm frequently to confirm the direction and length of the osteotomy.
2. Minimize the amount of soft tissue stripping during your approach because this likely leads to increased pain and bleeding and slower union.
3. Do not work through undersized wounds because this limits the view and safe retraction and can lead to wound edge necrosis and delayed wound healing or infection.
4. Use a locking plate. This takes some of the issues relating to lateral cortex integrity out of play and allows the patient to bear weight safely.
5. Do not rush to equalize the patient's leg lengths with shoe lifts because most will accommodate within the first 6 months.

References

1. Jackson JP, Waugh W, Green JP. High tibial osteotomy for osteoarthritis of the knee. *J Bone Joint Surg Br.* 1969;51(1):88-94.
2. Coventry MB. Osteotomy of the upper portion of the tibia for degenerative arthritis of the knee. A preliminary report. *J Bone Joint Surg Am.* 1965;47:984-990.
3. Smith TO, Sexton D, Mitchell P, Hing CB. Opening- or closing-wedged high tibial osteotomy: a meta-analysis of clinical and radiological outcomes. *Knee.* 2011;18(6):361-368.
4. Hoell S, Suttmoeller J, Stoll V, Fuchs S, Gosheger G. The high tibial osteotomy, open versus closed wedge, a comparison of methods in 108 patients. *Arch Orthop Trauma Surg.* 2005;125(9):638-643.
5. Amendola A, Bonasia DE. Results of high tibial osteotomy: review of the literature. *Int Orthop.* 2010;34(2):155-160.
6. Floerkemeier S, Staubli AE, Schroeter S, Goldhahn S, Lobenhoffer P. Outcome after high tibial open-wedge osteotomy: a retrospective evaluation of 533 patients. *Knee Surg Sports Traumatol Arthrosc.* 2013;21(1):170-180.
7. Puddu G, Cipolla M, Cerullo G, Franco V, Gianni E. Osteotomies: the surgical treatment of the valgus knee. *Sports Med Arthrosc.* 2007;15(1):15-22.
8. Saithna A, Kundra R, Modi CS, Getgood A, Spalding T. Distal femoral varus osteotomy for lateral compartment osteoarthritis in the valgus knee. A systematic review of the literature. *Open Orthop J.* 2012;6:313-319.
9. Noyes FR, Barber SD, Simon R. High tibial osteotomy and ligament reconstruction in varus angulated, anterior cruciate ligament-deficient knees. A two- to seven-year follow-up study. *Am J Sports Med.* 1993;21(1):2-12.
10. Noyes FR, Barber-Westin SD, Hewett TE. High tibial osteotomy and ligament reconstruction for varus angulated anterior cruciate ligament-deficient knees. *Am J Sports Med.* 2000;28(3):282-296.
11. Dejour H, Neyret P, Boileau P, Donell ST. Anterior cruciate reconstruction combined with valgus tibial osteotomy. *Clin Orthop Relat Res.* 1994;(299):220-228.
12. Trojani C, Elhor H, Carles M, Boileau P. Anterior cruciate ligament reconstruction combined with valgus high tibial osteotomy allows return to sports. *Orthop Traumatol Surg Res.* 2014;100(2):209-212.
13. Giffin JR, Shannon FJ. The role of the high tibial osteotomy in the unstable knee. *Sports Med Arthrosc.* 2007;15(1):23-31.
14. McNamara I, Birmingham TB, Fowler PJ, Giffin JR. High tibial osteotomy: evolution of research and clinical applications—a Canadian experience. *Knee Surg Sports Traumatol Arthrosc.* 2013;21(1):23-31.
15. Rossi R, Bonasia DE, Amendola A. The role of high tibial osteotomy in the varus knee. *J Am Acad Orthop Surg.* 2011;19(10):590-599.
16. Collins B, Getgood A, Alomar AZ, et al. A case series of lateral opening wedge high tibial osteotomy for valgus malalignment. *Knee Surg Sports Traumatol Arthrosc.* 2013;21(1):152-160.
17. Healy WL, Anglen JO, Wasilewski SA, Krackow KA. Distal femoral varus osteotomy. *J Bone Joint Surg Am.* 1988;70(1):102-109.
18. Stahelin T, Hardegger F, Ward JC. Supracondylar osteotomy of the femur with use of compression. Osteosynthesis with a malleable implant. *J Bone Joint Surg Am.* 2000;82(5):712-722.
19. Wang JW, Hsu CC. Distal femoral varus osteotomy for osteoarthritis of the knee. Surgical technique. *J Bone Joint Surg Am.* 2006;88(suppl 1 pt 1):100-108.
20. Dugdale TW, Noyes FR, Styer D. Preoperative planning for high tibial osteotomy. The effect of lateral tibiofemoral separation and tibiofemoral length. *Clin Orthop Relat Res.* 1992;(274):248-264.
21. Fujisawa Y, Masuhara K, Shiomi S. The effect of high tibial osteotomy on osteoarthritis of the knee. An arthroscopic study of 54 knee joints. *Orthop Clin North Am.* 1979;10(3):585-608.
22. Amis AA. Biomechanics of high tibial osteotomy. *Knee Surg Sports Traumatol Arthrosc.* 2013;21(1):197-205.
23. Martin R, Birmingham TB, Willits K, Litchfield R, Lebel ME, Giffin JR. Adverse event rates and classifications in medial opening wedge high tibial osteotomy. *Am J Sports Med.* 2014;42(5):1118-1126.

Please see videos on the accompanying website at www.routledge.com/9781617119996

SECTION V

Ligaments

23

Arthroscopic Anterior Cruciate Ligament Repair

Walter Shelton, MD and Taylor Mathis, MD

Introduction

The anatomy of the cruciate ligaments has been described as far back as the Egyptians in 3000 BC. Around 170 AD, Galen first described the anterior cruciate ligament (ACL) as a supportive structure of the knee that prevented abnormal knee motion.[1,2] Through the 1800s, the understanding of the ACL evolved, and near the turn of the 20th century, the first case reports of repair of the ACL emerged.[3,4] An estimated 175,000 ACL reconstructions are performed each year, with revision rates reported from 1.5% to 20%.[5-8] In the 1970s, reports of primary ACL repair with or without augmentation were successful in approximately 70% of cases with higher success in proximal tears. This overall 20% to 30% failure rate led to the abandonment of ACL repair in most cases.[9-14] The trouble with interpretation of early studies was that these studies included many midsubstance tears, which have clearly shown a lesser potential for healing. However, Marshall et al[12] reported a series of ACL repairs, including 56 of 70 patients with midsubstance, mop-end tears. Using a multiple-looped, varying-depth suture repair, the group overall achieved a 90% return to sports with 68% at preinjury level of function.[12] Higgins and Steadman[15] reported a series of elite downhill skiers who underwent primary ACL repair with iliotibial band tenodesis. They had an average return to competitive skiing at 9.1 months in all but 3 skiers, pain-free function in 78%, and a normal pivot shift in 85% of patients.[15] The belief that the ACL lacked the potential to heal was widely held,[16,17] despite several studies showing definite healing of a torn ACL.[18-20] Arthroscopic reconstruction techniques improved, and a rapid shift to ligament reconstruction took place.

Recent advances in orthobiologics have demonstrated promising results of primary ACL repair in human and animal studies.[21-29] The addition of collagen scaffolds into the repair has enhanced healing,[24,26,27] and a renewed interest in ACL repair has emerged. Microfracture of the ligament insertion site provides the local environment with growth factors and enhances ligament healing.[21] With an estimated 175,000 ACL reconstructions performed each year in the United States, future research will focus on ACL repair and preservation. In summary, of the available literature, proximal ligament avulsions can be repaired primarily with multiple-looped, varying-depth suture

Sgaglione NA, Lubowitz JH, Provencher MT, eds. *The Knee: AANA Advanced Arthroscopic Surgical Techniques* (pp 315-322).

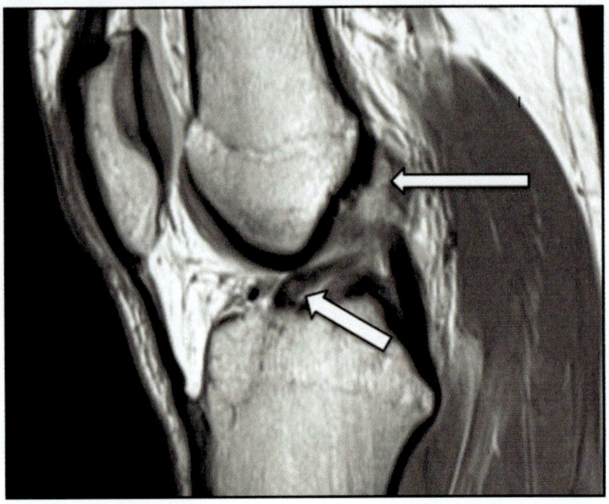

Figure 23-1. Sagittal MRI showing a proximal ACL avulsion. The long arrow marks the proximal area with edema and disorganized ligament fibers. The short arrow shows the intact distal portion of the ligament. The oblique orientation of the fibers inhibits longitudinal views of the ligament without specialized oblique MRI sequences.

repair using soft tissue graft augmentation. This maintains the native ligament's proprioceptive function, minimizes donor site morbidity, and can produce acceptable outcomes in properly selected patients.

Indications

- Indications include proximal or "off-the-wall" tears with good-quality tissue remaining.

Controversial Indications

- Controversial indications include midsubstance ruptures and distal ligament avulsions.

Pertinent Physical Findings

- Examine the knee for effusion acutely and any loss of range of motion (ROM)
- Varus/valgus stress exam
- Lachman test
- Pivot shift test (most specific[30])

Pertinent Imaging

- Plain x-rays
  - Standing anteroposterior in extension and at 30 degrees of flexion
  - Lateral view
  - Sunrise patella view
- Magnetic resonance imaging (MRI) is especially helpful in potential ligament repair situations to evaluate the location of the tear and tissue quality (Figure 23-1).

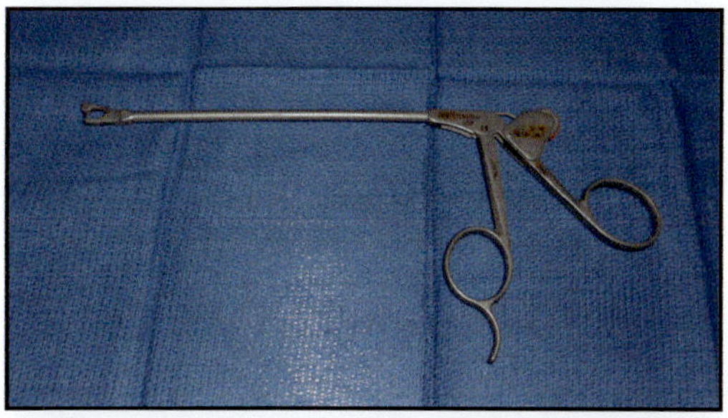

Figure 23-2. Shutt Suture Punch (Conmed) for passing and retrieving sutures.

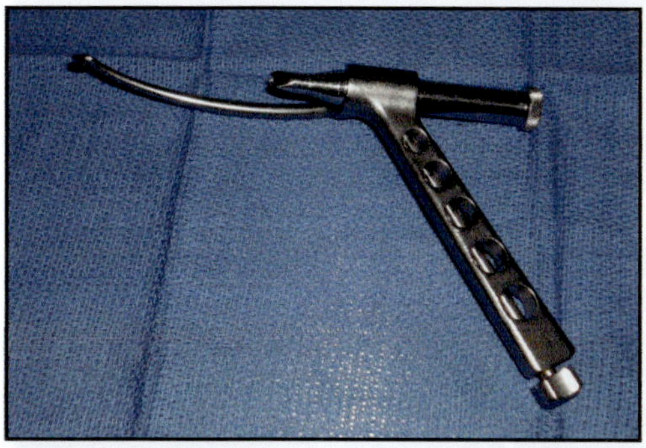

Figure 23-3. ACUFEX Rear Entry Aimer (Smith & Nephew) allows anatomic tunnel placement and protects the intact ligament fibers from the drill. The aiming arm can also be used to pull suture over the top of the lateral femoral condyle.

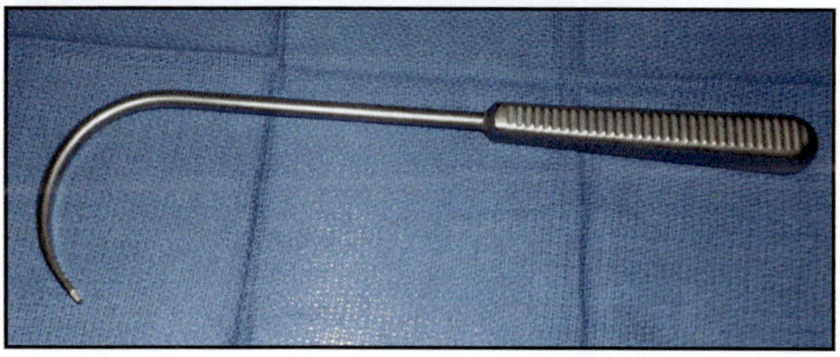

Figure 23-4. ACUFEX Rear Entry Introducer (Smith & Nephew) used to deliver passing suture through the anterolateral portal and over the top of the lateral femoral condyle.

Equipment

In addition to standard arthroscopic tools, ACL repair requires additional instruments. Suture passage can be performed with a suture punch (Figure 23-2). A cannula through one of the portals aids in preventing capsular tissue from being inadvertently captured by the sutures. A rear-entry, outside-in ACL drill guide (Figure 23-3) is useful to prevent damage to the remaining ACL tissue by the drill tip. A large curved introducer or rear-entry hook used to position the outside-in drill guide is also helpful in passing sutures over the top of the lateral femoral condyle (Figure 23-4). Varying-sized drills and ACL guides are necessary for tunnels. Drills for graft tunnels are usually smaller (6 to 8 mm) compared to standard reconstruction tunnels (9 to 11 mm). A bone pick or awl can be used to microfracture the footprint.[21] Graft fixation is completed with absorbable interference screws in the femoral and tibial tunnels to avoid cutting sutures in the tunnel.

Positioning and Portals

The patient is positioned supine on the operative table. Bony prominences should be well padded. A tourniquet is placed on the operative extremity. The contralateral leg is well padded. A leg holder is used to stabilize the femur, ensuring enough room above the knee to pass instruments

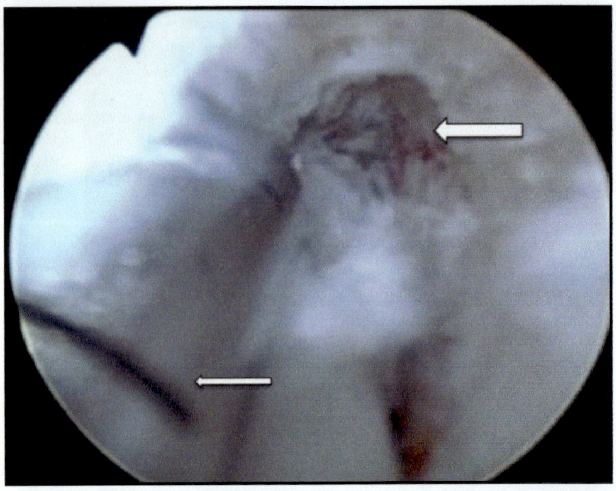

Figure 23-5. Left knee viewed from the lateral portal. The ACL is probed with a shaver (small arrow) and found to be torn from the femoral attachment (large arrow) on the lateral femoral condyle.

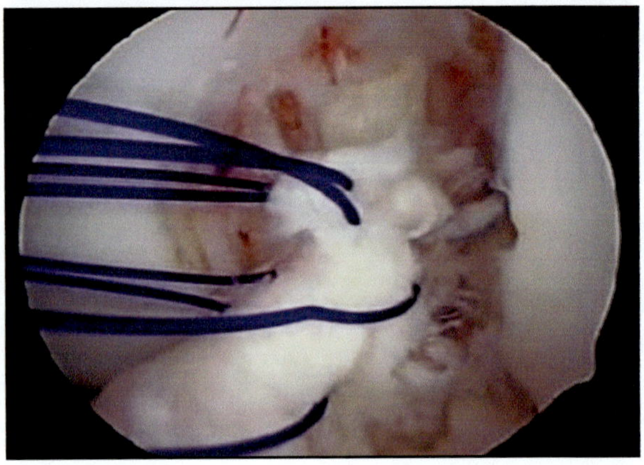

Figure 23-6. View from the lateral portal of the left knee. Multiple polydioxanone sutures are passed through the native ACL using the suture punch. The 2 ends of the suture are maintained in 2 separate groups for passage.

and sutures from inside out, and the foot of the bed is lowered. Alternatively, the foot of the bed can remain elevated, and the leg can be abducted over the side of the bed with a lateral post placed to apply valgus stress.

Step-by-Step Description of the Procedure

After careful examination under anesthesia, routine arthroscopy is performed through standard portals. The ACL is visualized and probed to assess its potential for repair (Figure 23-5). Only tears in the proximal portion of the ligament should be considered for repair. All other pathology should be corrected prior to proceeding with the ACL repair. The authors prefer a 7-mm quadriceps tendon graft, which is harvested after confirmatory arthroscopy. Four or 5 simple sutures are then placed in the ligament with an intra-articular suture device. The ends of each suture are held in 2 groups that will be passed separately (Figure 23-6). An accessory incision is made on the posterolateral aspect of the knee, and a rear-entry ACL guide is placed into the knee from the over-the-top position approximately 8 mm anterior to the back of the notch in the femoral footprint of the ACL. A guide pin is placed into the joint from outside-in and is over-reamed with a 7-mm reamer into the femoral footprint of the ACL. The rear-entry hook is then passed through the anterolateral portal into the knee and over the top of the lateral femoral condyle. A loop suture is passed into the joint with this hook and is used to pull the sutures exiting the posterior portion of the ligament over the top of the lateral femoral condyle. The anterior sutures are then pulled

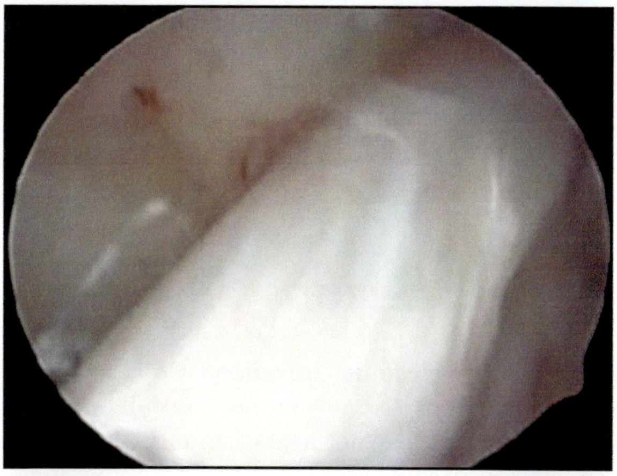

Figure 23-7. Left knee viewed from the lateral portal. The ACL sutures have been passed over the lateral femoral condyle and out the femoral tunnel holding the ACL with appropriate tension and torsion.

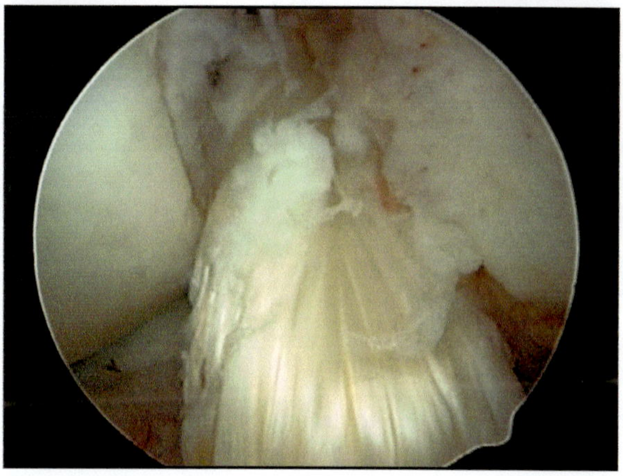

Figure 23-8. Completed ACL repair with augmentation. Left knee viewed from the medial portal. Notice the anatomic positioning, bulk of the repaired ligament and graft, and the torsion mimicking the native ACL.

through the bone tunnel using a looped suture or a wire. Pulling these 2 groups of sutures tight will pull the ligament back up to the femoral attachment, restore the footprint, and recreate the natural torsion between the 2 bundles (Figure 23-7). With the ligament pulled tight, a standard ACL guide is placed in the posterior lateral edge of the tibial footprint, and a 7-mm tunnel is reamed from outside-in. Care must be taken at this point not to disrupt an excessive amount of ACL fibers or sutures with the reamer as it pierces the tibial cortex. The previously harvested 7-mm graft is then passed through the tibial tunnel and into the femoral tunnel. The native ACL usually has to be held to the side while the graft is teased through the knee. With the knee reduced, the ACL sutures are tensioned and tied over the femoral condyle. The graft is secured in the femoral tunnel with a 7-mm interference screw. An absorbable, nonmetallic screw is used to avoid cutting the sutures in the femoral tunnel. The tibial side is then secured with an interference screw in the tibial tunnel with appropriate tension applied to the graft. The knee is carried through a full ROM to ensure there is no impingement of the graft and that the tension is appropriate (Figure 23-8). After routine closure, a sterile dressing and hinged knee brace are applied.

Postoperative Protocol

Using this technique of solid repair with augmentation, standard postoperative ACL protocols can be used. Early weightbearing and active ROM are safe. Our current protocol involves frequent icing with active straight leg leg lifts for the first 48 hours. A knee immobilizer is used for comfort.

The patient is seen in the clinic 48 hours after surgery, and large effusions can be aspirated. Active ROM is then initiated with weightbearing as tolerated using 2 crutches for the first 3 weeks. During weeks 4 to 6, the patient transitions to using a single crutch in the opposite hand once able to do a straight leg lift with no extensor lag. Stretching and strengthening are also initiated. Full weightbearing is begun at 6 weeks without crutches. Straight-line running on smooth surfaces is begun at 3 months, and cutting activities are started at 6 months.

Potential Complications

As in all extremity surgeries, complications such as bleeding, infection, or deep venous thrombosis are a small risk but may occur. Specific to this procedure, sutures may pull out from the ACL, the augmentation graft may fail, or the ligament may not heal back to the insertion. These would lead to graft failure, and persistent instability could result. If any concomitant injuries go unrecognized, stability may be affected, or further surgery may be required to address the symptomatic knee. Donor site morbidity can be significant, and graft choice must be patient dependent.

Top Technical Pearls for the Procedure

1. Use 4 or 5 sutures through the ligament to repair the proximal ACL tear.
2. Passing the sutures through a cannula in the front of the knee keeps them from becoming crossed or from pulling capsular tissue into the repair.
3. A pullout suture passed from over the lateral femoral condyle into the knee with the rear-entry hook facilitates pulling the posterior sutures over the top of the lateral femoral condyle.
4. Tunnels should be made carefully from outside-in to avoid damage to the remaining intact ACL fibers. Do not be overaggressive as the reamer reaches the cortex.
5. Use absorbable interference screws. A metal screw will cut the sutures in the ACL as they enter the femoral tunnel.

References

1. Snook GA. A short history of the anterior cruciate ligament and the treatment of tears. *Clin Orthop Relat Res.* 1983;(172):11-13.
2. Davarinos N, O'Neill BJ, Curtin W. A brief history of anterior cruciate ligament reconstruction. *Advances in Orthopedic Surgery.* 2014;(2014):706042.
3. Battle WH. Suture of the crucial ligaments. *Br Med J.* 1902;2(2189):1879.
4. Robson AW. Ruptured crucial ligaments and their repair by operation. *Ann Surg.* 1903;37(5):716-718.
5. Chahal J, Lee A, Heard W, Bach B. A retrospective review of anterior cruciate ligament reconstruction using patellar tendon: 25 years of experience. *Orthop J Sports Med.* 2013;1(3):1-7.
6. Lyman S, Koulouvaris P, Sherman S, Do H, Mandl LA, Marx RG. Epidemiology of anterior cruciate ligament reconstruction: trends, readmissions, and subsequent knee surgery. *J Bone Joint Surg Am.* 2009;91(10):2321-2328.

7. Lind M, Menhert F, Pedersen AB. Incidence and outcome after revision anterior cruciate ligament reconstruction: results from the Danish registry for knee ligament reconstructions. *Am J Sports Med.* 2012;40(7):1551-1557.
8. Barrett AM, Craft JA, Replogle WH, Hydrick JM, Barrett GR. Anterior cruciate ligament graft failure: a comparison of graft type based on age and Tegner activity level. *Am J Sports Med.* 2011;39(10):2194-2198.
9. Feagin JA Jr, Curl WW. Isolated tear of the anterior cruciate ligament: 5 year follow-up study. *Am J Sports Med.* 1976;4(3):95-100.
10. Strand T, Mølster A, Hordvik M, Krukhaug Y. Long-term follow-up after primary repair of the anterior cruciate ligament: clinical and radiological evaluation 15-23 years postoperatively. *Arch Orthop Trauma Surg.* 2005;125(4):217-221.
11. Taylor DC, Posner M, Curl WW, Feagin JA. Isolated tears of the anterior cruciate ligament: over 30-year follow-up of patients treated with arthrotomy and primary repair. *Am J Sports Med.* 2009;37(1):65-71.
12. Marshall JL, Warren RF, Wickiewicz TL. Primary surgical treatment of anterior cruciate ligament lesions. *Am J Sports Med.* 1982;10(2):103-107.
13. Sherman MF, Lieber L, Bonamo JR, Podesta L, Reiter I. The long-term followup of primary anterior cruciate ligament repair. Defining a rationale for augmentation. *Am J Sports Med.* 1991;19(3):243-255.
14. Kaplan N, Wickiewicz TL, Warren RF. Primary surgical treatment of anterior cruciate ligament ruptures: a long-term follow-up study. *Am J Sports Med.* 1990;18(4):354-358.
15. Higgins RW, Steadman JR. Anterior cruciate ligament repairs in world class skiers. *Am J Sports Med.* 1987;15(5):439-447.
16. Frank CB, Jackson DW. The science of reconstruction of the anterior cruciate ligament. *J Bone Joint Surg Am.* 1997;79(10):1556-1576.
17. Murray MM. Effect of the intra-articular environment on healing of the ruptured anterior cruciate ligament. [Invited Editorial, electronic]. *J Bone Joint Surgery (Am).* August 2001.
18. Fujimoto E, Sumen Y, Ochi M, Ikuta Y. Spontaneous healing of acute anterior cruciate ligament (ACL) injuries—conservative treatment using an extension block soft brace without anterior stabilization. *Arch Orthop Trauma Surg.* 2002;122(4):212-216.
19. Andersson C, Odensten M, Gillquist J. Knee function after surgical or nonsurgical treatment of acute rupture of the anterior cruciate ligament: a randomized study with a long-term follow-up period. *Clin Orthop Relat Res.* 1991;(264):255-263.
20. Sandberg R, Balkfors B, Nilsson B, Westlin N. Operative versus non-operative treatment of recent injuries to the ligaments of the knee. A prospective randomized study. *J Bone Joint Surg Am.* 1987;69(8):1120-1126.
21. Gobbi A, Bathan L, Boldrini L. Primary repair combined with bone marrow stimulation in acute anterior cruciate ligament lesions: results in a group of athletes. *Am J Sports Med.* 2009;37(3):571-578.
22. Joshi SM, Mastrangelo AN, Magarian EM, Fleming BC, Murray MM. Collagen-platelet composite enhances biomechanical and histologic healing of the porcine anterior cruciate ligament. *Am J Sports Med.* 2009;37(12):2401-2410.
23. Vavken P, Fleming BC, Mastrangelo AN, Machan JT, Murray MM. Biomechanical outcomes after bio-enhanced anterior cruciate ligament repair and anterior cruciate ligament reconstruction are equal in a porcine model. *Arthroscopy.* 2012;28(5):672-680.
24. Murray MM, Spindler KP, Ballard P, Welch TP, Zurakowski D, Nanney LB. Enhanced histologic repair in a central wound in the anterior cruciate ligament with a collagen-platelet-rich plasma scaffold. *J Orthop Res.* 2007;25(8):1007-1017.
25. Murray MM, Spindler KP, Abreu E, et al. Collagen-platelet rich plasma hydrogel enhances primary repair of the porcine anterior cruciate ligament. *J Orthop Res.* 2007;25(1):81-91.
26. Murray MM, Spindler KP, Devin C, et al. Use of a collagen-platelet rich plasma scaffold to stimulate healing of a central defect in the canine ACL. *J Orthop Res.* 2006;24(4):820-830.
27. Murray MM, Fleming BC. Use of a bioactive scaffold to stimulate anterior cruciate ligament healing also minimizes posttraumatic osteoarthritis after surgery. *Am J Sports Med.* 2013;41(8):1762-1770.
28. Konda E, Yasuda K, Yamanaka M, Minami A, Tohyama H. Effects of administration of exogenous growth factors on biomechanical properties of the elongation-type anterior cruciate ligament injury with partial laceration. *Am J Sports Med.* 2005;33(2):188-196.

29. Pascher A, Steinert AF, Palmer GD, et al. Enhanced repair of the anterior cruciate ligament by in situ gene transfer: evaluation in an in vitro model. *Mol Ther.* 2004;10(2):327-336.
30. Katz JW, Fingeroth RJ. The diagnostic accuracy of ruptures of the anterior cruciate ligament comparing the Lachman test, the anterior drawer sign, and the pivot shift test in acute and chronic knee injuries. *Am J Sports Med.* 1986;14(1):88-91.

Please see videos on the accompanying website at www.routledge.com/9781617119996

24

Anterior Cruciate Ligament Graft Choices and Harvest Techniques

David A. Abrutyn, MD and Peter R. Kurzweil, MD

Indications

The goal of anterior cruciate ligament (ACL) reconstruction is to produce a stable, functional knee that allows the patient to return to his or her preinjury level of activity while minimizing comorbidities and postinjury arthritis. Over the past 2 decades, multiple reports have compared various graft choices and outcomes.[1-8] The heterogeneity of surgical techniques (ie, tunnel placement, graft fixation, and rehabilitation protocol) makes comparison of the outcomes of the different graft choices difficult.

In addition, numerous variables and factors contribute to the success and outcome of ACL reconstruction, namely additional injuries at the time of ACL (ie, chondral, meniscal, or multiligamentous) injury, patient anatomy (ie, constitutional varus, narrow notch, small ACL footprint), surgical technique, graft fixation, rehabilitation protocol, and time of release to sport activities.[9-13] Therefore, not all ACL injuries or reconstructions are the same.

The ideal graft choice in ACL reconstruction remains elusive. Grafts can be autograft or allograft tissue. For autografts, the 3 prevalent choices include bone patellar tendon bone (BPTB), hamstring tendons (HT), or quadriceps tendon (QT; with or without a patellar bone plug). Allograft tissue can be procured from the BPTB, hamstring, tibialis anterior, Achilles, or posterior tibialis, as well.

Autografts are the most widely used method for ACL reconstructions worldwide. Maletis et al[14] reported 57.6% use of autografts in primary ACL reconstructions in a community-based registry. Globally, it seems that hamstring autograft is the most widely used autograft. The Danish Registry reports usage of the hamstring autograft 85% of the time.[15] In Sweden, 96.1% of ACL reconstructions in 2011 used hamstring autograft.[16] The Norwegian Registry documented 76.7% usage of hamstring autograft for ACL reconstructions in 2012.[17]

Hamstring autografts seem to be preferred to obviate the comorbidities associated with BPTB harvest, such as anterior knee pain, kneeling pain, loss of extension, quadriceps weakness, and the development of osteoarthritis.[5,18-20] The evolution of fixation of the hamstring tendon on the femoral and tibial sides has made analyzing the literature difficult. Several studies have suggested

Sgaglione NA, Lubowitz JH, Provencher MT, eds. *The Knee: AANA Advanced Arthroscopic Surgical Techniques* (pp 323-337).

a higher revision rate with hamstring autograft; however, when graft fixation and technique are the same, the results—subjective and objective—appear similar.[9,18,21-23] Taylor et al[23] reported similar results in army cadets with 2-year follow-ups using HT and patellar tendon (PT) autografts. Laxdal et al[20] compared PT to 3- and 4-stranded HT with interference fixation on the femoral and tibial sides and found no difference in functional outcome or knee laxity; the HT group had less pain with knee-walking. However, Lidén et al[24] reported no difference in objective or subjective outcomes, including kneeling pain, with 7-year follow-up. Pinczewski et al[21] reported excellent results with PT and HT autografts at 10-year follow-up; however, there were decreased donor-site symptoms and less radiographic osteoarthritis in the HT group. Aglietti et al[9] also reported no difference at 2 year follow-up between HT and PT when technique and fixation methods were identical. Several meta-analyses have sought to independently analyze the literature. The 2011 Cochrane review found no difference between the 2 graft choices for long-term functional outcome; however, they found that PT grafts were more likely to result in statically stable knees but were also more likely to develop anterior knee pain.[7]

QT autograft has recently been advocated as a viable alternative to HT and PT. The tendon can be harvested with or without a patellar bone plug. There is versatility with respect to the length and diameter of the tendon that is harvested. Sasaki et al[25] demonstrated that the QT restores knee kinematics under cadaveric testing conditions. Lund et al[26] compared QT to BPTB in a prospective randomized study. They reported similar anterior knee stability and subjective outcomes in both groups; however, there was less donor site morbidity in the QT group.[26]

Allograft tissue is widely used because its availability has increased over the past decade. Allografts potentially eliminate the comorbidities associated with autograft harvest and decrease surgical time. However, concern remains about delayed graft incorporation, disease transmission, and the integrity of the mechanical properties based on the sterilization methods used.[27-30] In analyzing the survivorship of allograft tissue, it is imperative to understand the procurement technique and sterilization method used. Krych et al[29] found no significant difference in graft failure rate, postoperative laxity, or patient-reported outcomes in comparing nonirradiated ACL reconstruction to autografts in a systemic review. Park et al[31] also found superior results comparing nonirradiated allografts to those using low-dose (< 2.5 Mrad) irradiated allografts. Krych et al[29] performed a meta-analysis of PT autograft vs allograft. When irradiated and chemically processed grafts were excluded, no significant differences were found. These studies suggest that the use of nonirradiated allografts are equivalent to autografts and are appropriate alternatives.

Graft choice depends on several factors. The authors tend to favor autografts for younger patients because the growing literature suggests fewer long-term failures when using one's own tissue. For athletes who participate in contact and collision sports, the authors' bias has been toward using PT autografts. For people who tend to kneel or crawl for a living (such as plumbers or carpet installers), the authors typically steer these patients toward HT autografts. There is a growing trend toward using QT autografts, although the authors have little experience with this option. If a surgeon is doing fewer than 20 ACLs per year, it is probably best to stick to one autograft only. The authors tend to favor fresh-frozen allografts for multiligament cases, revisions, and in patients older than 40 years.

Controversial Indications

Two variables may explain the increased early failure rate of HT autografts, including the size of the graft and timing of return to play. The size of the quadrupled hamstring has been reported to effect outcome. Mariscalco et al[32] found that HT autografts greater than 8 mm in diameter had a 0.0% revision rate at 2 years compared to 7.0% with grafts 8 mm in diameter or smaller. This suggests that HT autografts less than 8 mm in diameter may need to be augmented with nonirradiated allograft tissue to increase the diameter of the graft size. However, the Norwegian Registry data found no correlation between graft size and failure.[17]

The results from the Danish Registry found a 3.8-fold increased relative risk of revision 1 year after ACL reconstruction using HTs compared to BPTB. However, patient-reported outcome measures, the Tegner score, and Knee Injury and Osteoarthritis Outcome Score subscores of sports and activities of daily living were higher for HT grafts 1 year postoperatively compared to BPTB.[33] This suggests that consideration should be given to delaying return to sport with HT autografts. Furthermore, Taylor et al[23] found that 75% of their hamstring reruptures were in the first year. The combination of patients subjectively feeling better sooner after hamstring ACL reconstruction and the documented weakness of knee flexion after hamstring harvest may correlate with early graft rerupture if patients return to sports too soon.

In addition, if an anatomic ACL reconstruction is performed through an independent (ie, low medial portal) femoral tunnel, there can be an increased incidence of graft tunnel mismatch with BPTB autograft. The total length from the femoral tunnel to the tibial tunnel is reduced with an anatomic ACL technique; therefore, surgeons should be prepared to fix the bone plug outside of the tibial tunnel (ie, staples).

ACL surgeons need to be comfortable with the various graft choices and surgical techniques and should individualize the surgery based on patient needs and expectations. Graft choice should be considered in the context of surgeon preference, patient anatomy, patient age (ie, open growth plates), prior surgical procedures, donor site morbidity, graft incorporation, and patient choice. Consideration should be given to augmenting hamstring autografts less than 8 mm and prolonging return to play based on the graft choice and/or fixation methods.

In the authors' practice, if the HT graft is less than 8 mm, they augment the autograft tissue with gracilis or semitendinosus nonirradiated allograft tissue. Furthermore, they try to delay return to sports for at least 9 months with anatomic ACL reconstructions.

Harvest Techniques

Hamstring Tendon Autograft

Equipment

- #5 Ethibond suture x2 to secure tendon ends
- Hemostat
- HT graft harvester; open or closed

Step-by-Step Description of the Procedure

The patient is placed in the supine position with a tourniquet secured around the proximal thigh. The authors typically use a lateral side post during ACL reconstructions; however, a thigh holder may be used as well. Antibiotics with 2 g of cefazolin (or 600 mg of clindamycin, if the patient is allergic to penicillin) are given within 30 minutes of incision. A time-out is called and the lower extremity, marked preoperatively, is identified by the team. An examination under anesthesia is then performed and documented. The leg is then prepped and draped in the usual sterile fashion.

The proposed portals are marked and infiltrated with 0.25% to 0.5% bupivacaine with epinephrine. The tibial incision is marked one thumb breadth (approximately 2 cm) medial to the tibial tubercle (Figure 24-1). This is consistently the location of the semitendinosus and gracilis tendons. The authors generally do not infiltrate the tibial incision prior to harvest as to not disrupt the tissue planes and allow for an easier dissection. The skin flaps are injected with local anesthetic after the harvest is completed.

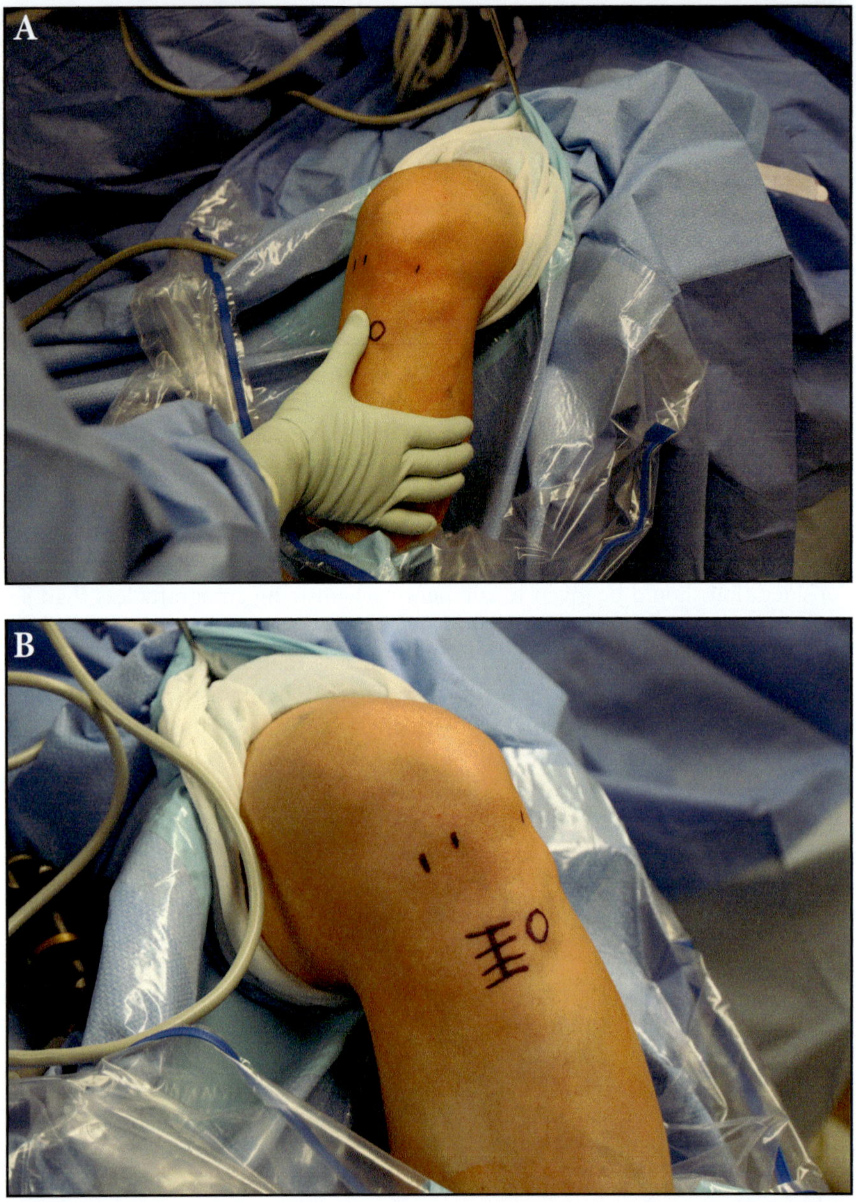

Figure 24-1. (A, B) demonstrate the typical location of pes anserinus one thumb's breadth medial to the tibial turbecle.

The leg is exsanguinated, and the tourniquet is inflated. A 3-cm longitudinal incision is made about 1 cm medial to the tibial tubercle (Figure 24-2). The soft tissue is dissected down to the sartorial fascia. A sponge can be used to sweep posteromedially to bluntly dissect and further expose the fascia. Typically, the semitendinosus and gracilis tendons can be easily palpated digitally. Forceps are used to grab the tendons with the sartorial fascia to try and elevate them off the superficial medial collateral ligament (MCL) which lies just beneath the 2 tendons (Figure 24-3). The tendons are sharply dissected off their insertion on the tibia. Again, care is used to protect the superficial MCL. A Metzenbaum scissor is then used to separate the sartorial fascia from the 2 tendons. The fascia is splint longitudinally.

The tendons can now be visualized on their posterior surfaces and distinguished from each other. The Metzenbaum scissors are used to split the 2 tendons. The 2 tendons can then be individually sutured with a #2 Ethibond suture (Figure 24-4). Once the 2 tendons are secured, they

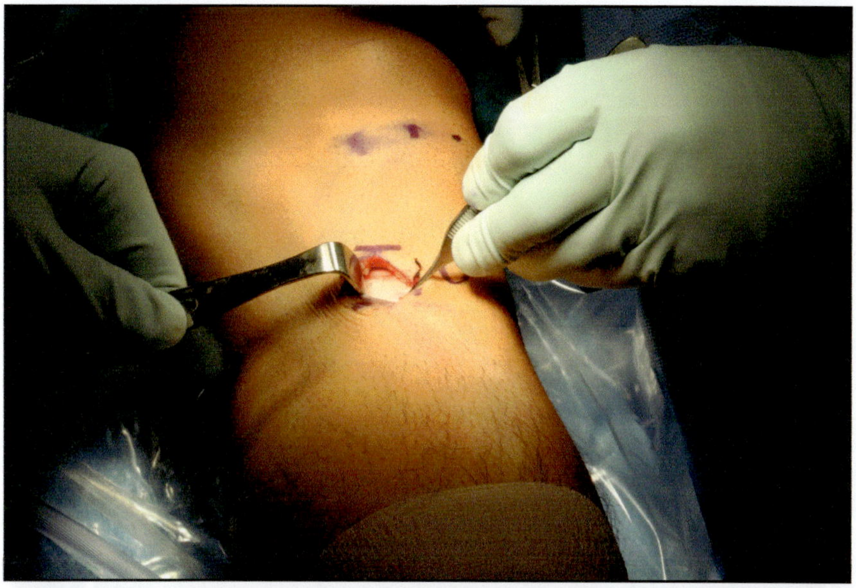

Figure 24-2. The sartorial fascia is exposed.

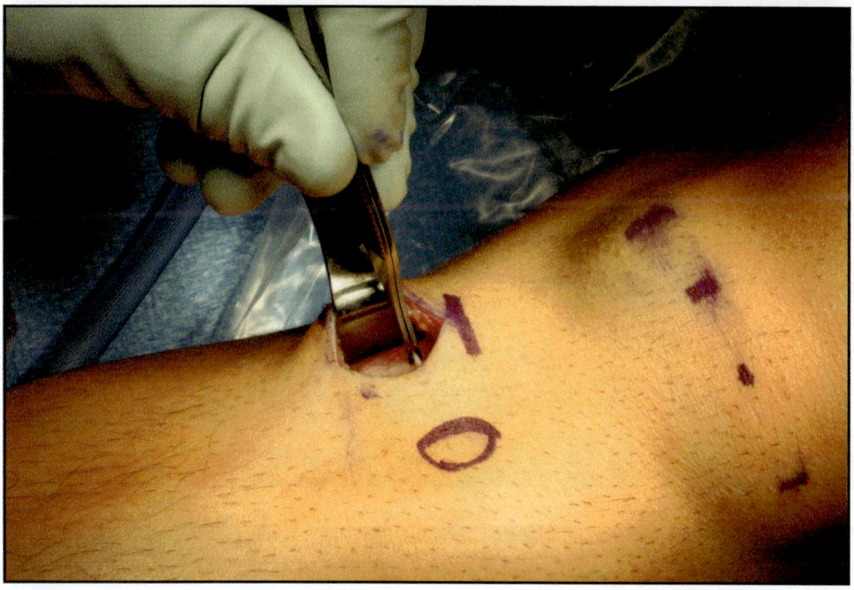

Figure 24-3. Forceps are used to lift the sartorial fascia and underlying hamstring tendons away from the superfical MCL, which lies immediately beneath the semitendinosus and gracilis.

need to be separated and released of their proximal adhesions. This is a critical step; if the tendons are prematurely harvested before the extraneous strands of tendon are released, they could easily be amputated prematurely. A simple test is to pull on the individual tendons; if there is any dimpling of the calf, additional calf adhesions need to be released. Releasing the adhesions can be done digitally or cut under direct visualization with scissors. Sometimes it is necessary to blindly insert a curved hemostat to retrieve a posterior calf adhesion and deliver it into the wound. The adhesion can then be sharply cut with a scalpel over the hemostat.

Once all the proximal adhesions are released and there is no further dimpling around the posterior calf with pulling on the tendons, the hamstrings are ready for harvest. The leg is flexed 90 degrees to protect the saphenous nerve. A closed-loop harvester is placed over the tendon, and a hemostat is wrapped around the suture. A push-pull technique is used and the hamstrings are sequentially harvested (Figure 24-5).

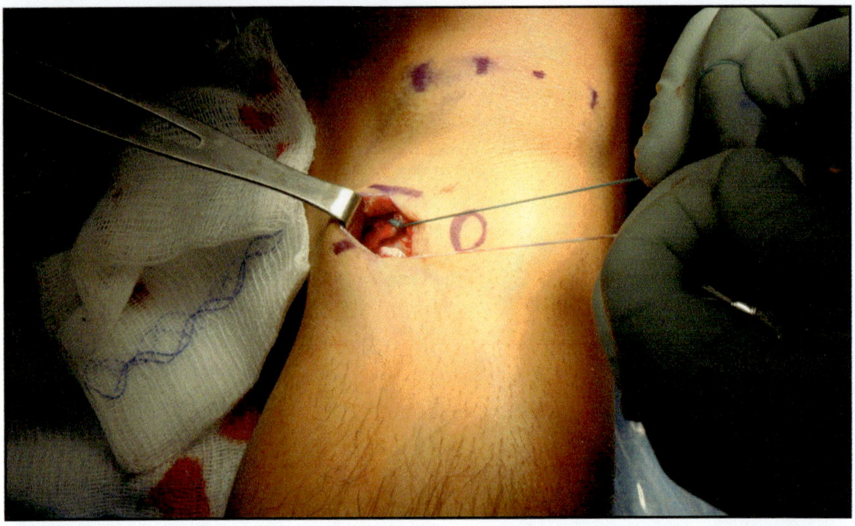

Figure 24-4. The 2 tendons are individually secured with nonabsorbable suture.

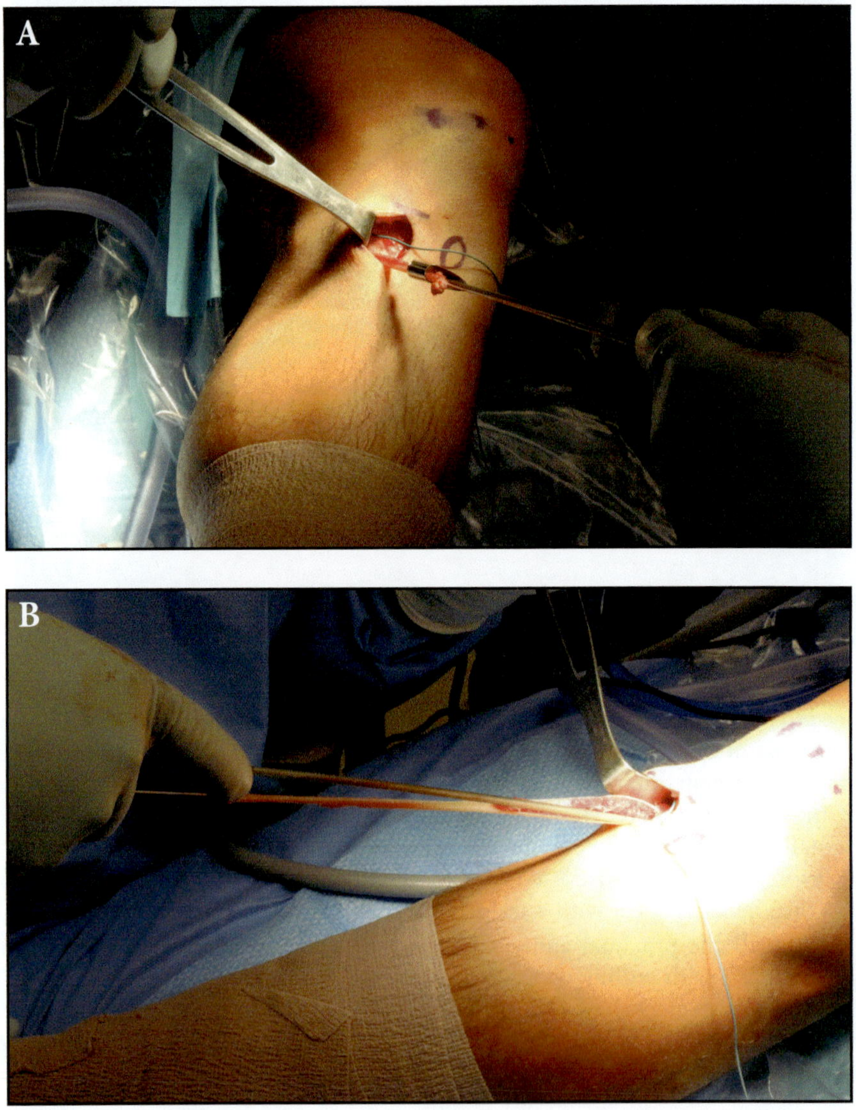

Figure 24-5. (A, B) A push-pull technique is used to sequentially harvest the hamstring tendons.

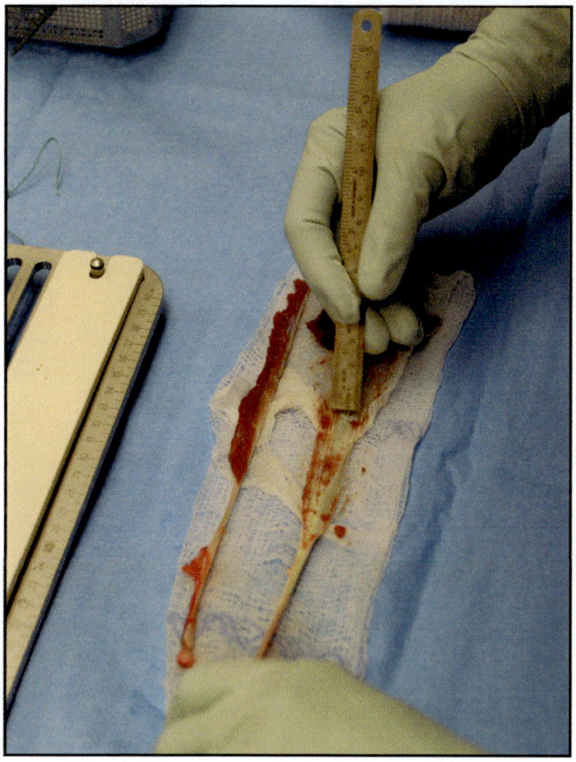

Figure 24-6. The soft tissue and muscle are removed from the tendons with a metal ruler.

The tourniquet is deflated after the hamstrings have been successfully harvested. The grafts are brought to the back table and prepared. The muscle is removed from the tendon sharply or bluntly with the back end of a metal ruler or Cobb elevator (Figure 24-6). The hamstrings are each folded over a #5 Ethibond suture and passed through a tunnel sizer to determine the appropriate tunnel diameter for the quadrupled HT graft. If the graft diameter is less than 8 mm, the authors consider augmenting with nonirradiated allograft tissue. The tibial footprint is measured with an arthroscopic ruler, and if the diameter of the quadrupled autograft tendons is less than 60% of the tibial footprint, allograft is also considered to augment the graft construct.

The graft ends are then whip stitched with #5 Ethibond suture for a length of 30 mm on each end. A Krackow- or Bunnel-type stitch is typically used (Figure 24-7). Once the tendon ends have been sutured, they are placed under tension with a graft harvester, and a moist sponge is wrapped around the tendons until they are needed for graft passage.

Top Technical Pearls for the Procedure

1. Tendons can be found one thumb breadth medial to the tibial tubercle. The incision should start at this level and proceed distal.
2. After developing full-thickness skin flaps, insert a 4-by-4 cm gauze to sweep tissue medially. This will develop a tissue plane and expose the sartorial fascia.
3. Use forceps to elevate the sartorial fascia and tendons away from the superficial MCL.
4. Pull on the tendons individually. If there is dimpling of the calf, there are calf adhesions that must be removed.
5. Harvest the tendons individually with the leg in a figure-4 position and the knee bent 90 degrees.

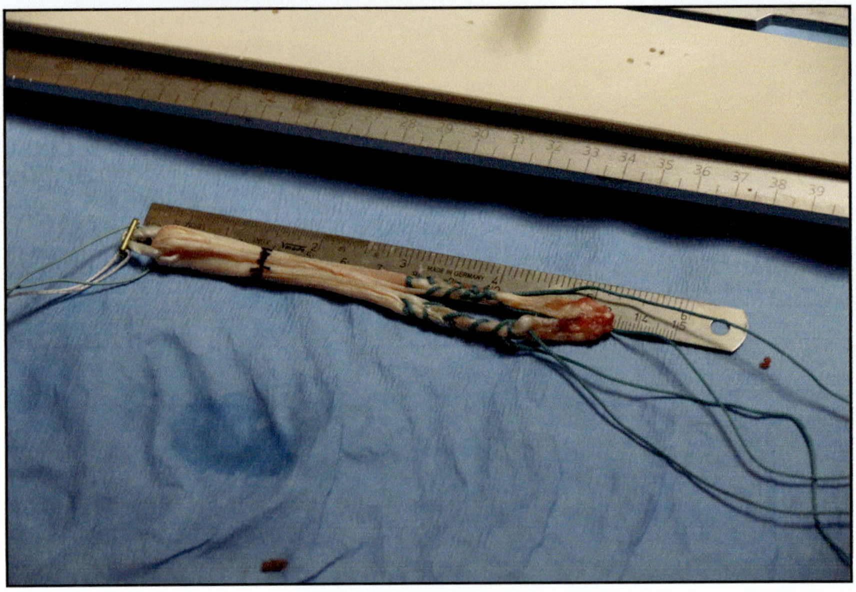

Figure 24-7. Final preparation of the hamstring tendon passed through a closed-loop EndoButton (Smith & Nephew) demonstrating Krackow stitches distally in each tendon.

Bone Patellar Tendon Bone

Equipment

- Oscillating saw with a 10-by-25-mm blade
- Towel clamp
- #5 Ethibond suture x5
- Curved osteotome

Step-by-Step Description of the Procedure

The leg is exsanguinated, and the tourniquet is inflated. A vertical longitudinal incision is made from the level of the inferior pole of the patella extending distally to the level of the tibial tubercle (Figure 24-8). Skin flaps are developed to establish a mobile window, and the soft tissue is dissected down to the paratenon. This is sharply elevated, and care is used to protect it for later repair. The paratenon tends to adhere to the tendon distally, and careful attention is needed to elevate it freely.

Once the tendon is exposed, Army Navy retractors are placed superiorly above the patella, and the knee is flexed to put the tendon under tension. The middle third of the tendon is marked, and a double-bladed scalpel (or 2 passes with a single scalpel) is used to sharply incise the central one-third of the PT. As the knife is brought distally, the mobile window follows it to facilitate exposure.

Electrocautery can be used to define the border of the tendon on the tibia. An oscillating saw is used to create a rectangular bone graft. The sides are cut first, and then the transverse cut is marked distally. A small curved osteotome is used to free the bone plug.

Alternatively, a hollow cannulated oscillating saw (Stryker) can be used. These come in sizes 9 to 12 mm. The cut is started distally on the tibia at a steep angle. Once the cortex is breached, the saw angle is gently decreased as the saw is advanced. As the saw advances toward the bone-tendon junction, it may be necessary to increase the size of the saw blade to avoid damaging the tendon (Videos 1 and 2).

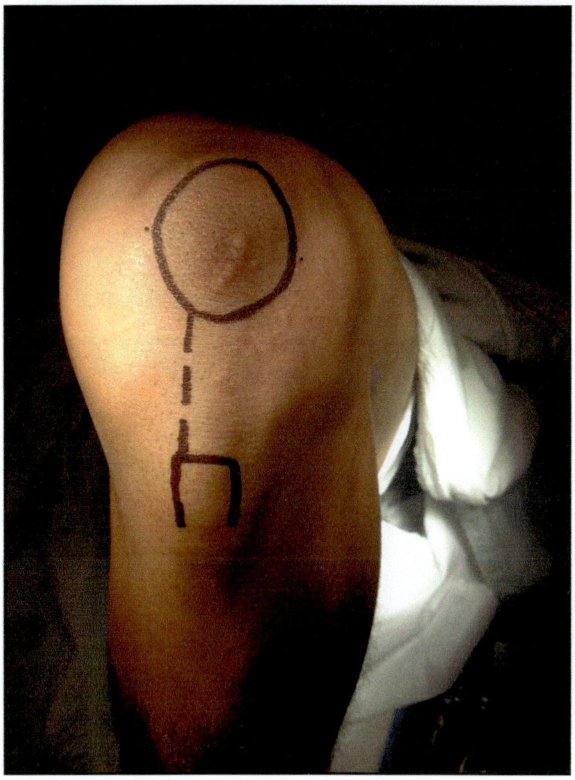

Figure 24-8. The incision is marked for BPTB starting at the distal aspect of the patella and extending distally over the tibial tubercle.

Once the tibial bone plug has been successfully harvested, the PT is freed of the fat pad, which is typically most adherent closer to its proximal insertion. A towel clamp is placed on the tibial bone plug to pull the patella into the mobile window while retracting proximally. The patellar bone plug is outlined with electrocautery. A triangular graft may be taken starting on either side and moving proximally. The saw can be used to free the bone proximally. A small curved osteotome can be used to release the bone plug. A mallet should be avoided to prevent articular cartilage damage to the patella. Alternatively, the circular oscillating saw can be used to harvest the patellar bone plug.

With the BPTB graft free, it is prepared on the back table (Figure 24-9). A rongeur is used to size the bone plugs to the desired diameter. All bone should be saved for later bone grafting of the patellar defect. The femoral bone plug is made 20 mm, and the tip is bulleted to facilitate passage into the femoral tunnel, particularly if a low medial portal is used for femoral tunnel creation. When preparing the graft, it is best to trim the bone rather than the soft tissue to make it slide through the desired tunnel diameter spacer.

A single drill hole is placed close to the tip, and a #2 Ethibond suture is passed with a Keith needle. The bone-tendon junction is marked with a marking pen, and an additional vertical mark is placed on the cancellous side of the bone plug to help with orientation during arthroscopic implantation.

Three drill holes—oriented at different angles—are made in the tibial bone plug. High-strength #2 Ethibond suture is again passed with a Keith needle (Figure 24-10).

The graft is then placed under tension on the graft board, and a moist sponge is wrapped around the graft for the duration of the case.

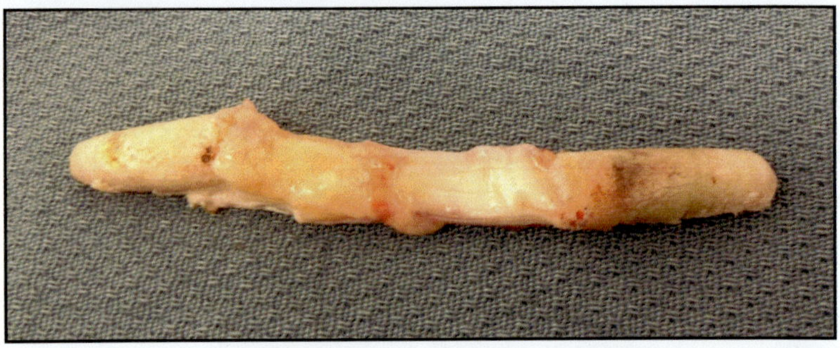

Figure 24-9. The typical graft after it is prepared on the back table. Note the beveled edges of the bone plug.

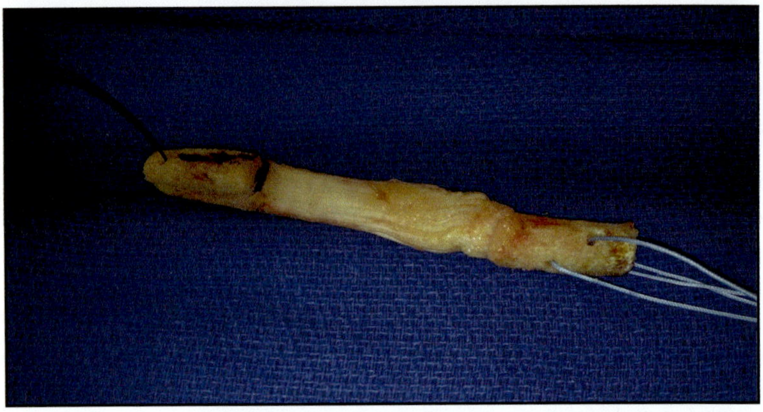

Figure 24-10. Three drill holes are made at different angles and #2 Ethibond sutures are passed.

Top Technical Pearls for the Procedure

1. Create a mobile window to enable a shorter incision.
2. Harvest the tibial side first, then pull the graft into the wound with a towel clamp on the tibial bone plug.
3. Cut the PT under slight tension with the knee in flexion over a bump.
4. Avoid overpenetrating the PT to minimize bleeding from the retropatellar fat pad.
5. Use a core drill when creating the tibial tunnel for the ACL reconstruction, and use the bone from the core drill to bone graft the harvest sites on the patella and tibia.

Quadriceps Tendon Graft

Equipment

- Army Navy retractors
- Oscillating saw 10-by-25-mm blade
- One-quarter-inch osteotome
- #5 Ethibond suture x3

Step-by-Step Description of the Procedure

The patient is placed supine, and a tourniquet is placed on the proximal thigh. A lateral post is placed. A small vertical incision is made approximately 1 cm above the superior pole of the patella. The incision is typically 4 to 5 cm in length. Soft tissue flaps are elevated, and the paratenon is

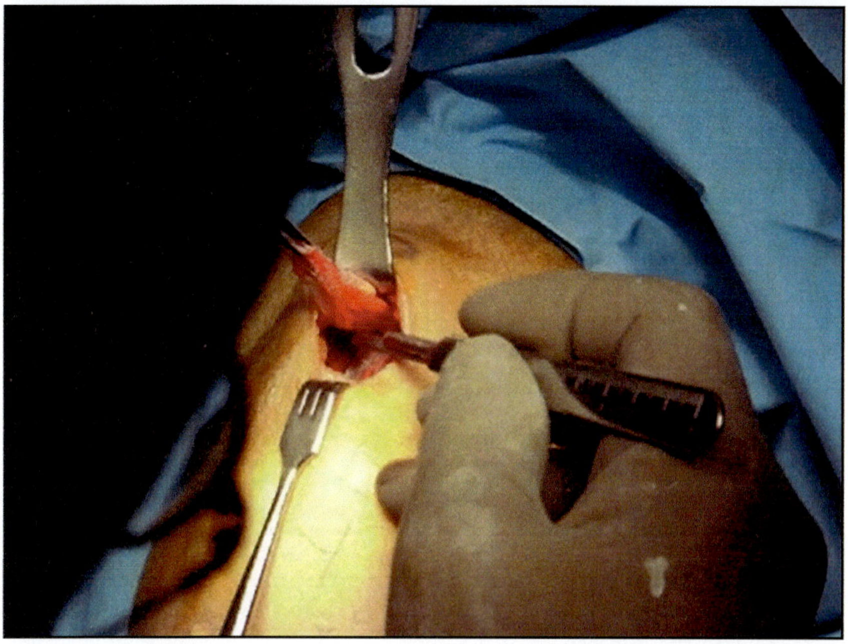

Figure 24-11. The QT is first incised medially to avoid penetration into the suprapatellar pouch. (Reprinted with permission from Walter Shelton, MD.)

exposed. Army Navy retractors can be placed, and the soft tissue window is easily mobilized to obtain visualization proximally and distally. A 9- or 10-mm-wide graft can be obtained from the central third of the QT. The tendon can be measured with a ruler in a proximal to distal direction to ensure at least a length of 80 mm can be obtained. With the QT exposed, the medial side of the quadriceps is typically incised first; this can be started proximally and extended to the superior pole of the patella. Care must be taken to avoid penetration of the scalpel into the suprapatellar pouch (Figure 24-11). This is typically avoided medially and will allow the surgeon to get a sense of the depth of the QT thickness. If the suprapatellar pouch is violated, it can be sutured closed to prevent extravasation of fluid during the arthroscopic portion of the procedure.

Once the medial incision is made, a ruler is used to measure a 10-mm width to mark the starting point of the lateral incision. A transverse incision is made in the QT, starting at the proximal extent of the medial incision and connecting to the starting point of the lateral extent of the tendon. Forceps are used to stabilize the tendon proximally, and the lateral incision is made extending distally. Care is taken to avoid penetration of the suprapatellar pouch.

At this point, depending on the length of the tendinous portion and surgical preference, the tendon harvest can be amputated from the superior pole of the patella if only a soft tissue graft is desired.

Alternatively, a bone plug from the superior pole of the patella can be obtained from the central portion of the patella. This is typically 10 mm in width and 20 mm in length. The patella is marked and sharply outlined with a scalpel. A small oscillating saw is used to a depth of 10 mm. A small one-quarter-inch osteotome can be used to liberate the bone plug. Care is taken to avoid entrance into the suprapatellar pouch.

With the graft harvested, with or without a bone plug, it is prepared on the back table. The soft tissue ends are divided into 2 limbs; this is between the vastus intermedius and the rectus femoris. This is a consistent finding, with a fatty stripe defining the 2 tendinosis limbs. These limbs can be used for a double-bundle reconstruction or, more commonly, for a single-bundle reconstruction. If a single-bundle technique is used, leave a total of 50 mm of the tendon intact (if there is no bone plug harvested) or 30 mm of the tendon (plus an additional 20-mm bone plug). This accounts for the femoral and the intra-articular portion of the graft (Figure 24-12).

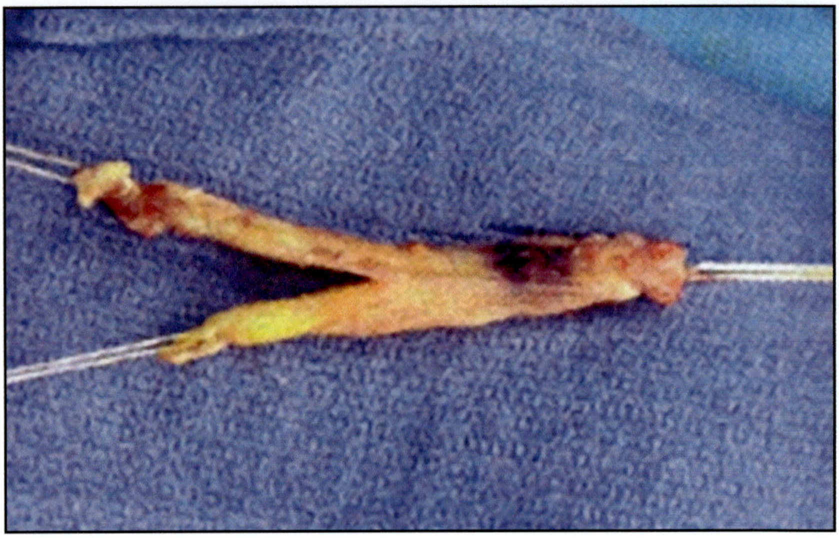

Figure 24-12. Final preparation of the QT demonstrating that 2 limbs of the tendon can be used in a double- or single-bundle technique. (Reprinted with permission from Walter Shelton, MD.)

The 2 limbs of the graft are then whip stitched with nonabsorbable suture. If a bone plug is obtained, a drill hole is made in the mid-aspect of the bone plug to pass a nonabsorbable suture for graft passage.

Please refer to Table 24-1 to compare the pros and cons of the various graft choices.

Top Technical Pearls for the Procedure

1. Develop a mobile window to enable shortening the incision.
2. Close the defect in the QT before proceeding with the arthroscopic portion.
3. Slight flexion of the knee allows the blade to be pushed proximally, facilitating the splitting of the fibers of the tendon.
4. Bone graft the patellar defect if the bone plug was harvested with the QT.
5. With experience, one can harvest a QT graft leaving a deep layer to avoid penetration into the suprapatellar capsule/joint.

Table 24-1. Comparison of Graft Choices

GRAFT CHOICE	PRO	CON
Bone patellar tendon bone	▶ Bone healing in tunnels ▶ Improved stability	▶ Anterior knee pain ▶ Kneeling pain ▶ Risk of patellar fracture ▶ Fixed length of tendon ▶ Potential loss of extension ▶ Quadriceps weakness ▶ Increased risk of osteoarthritis
Hamstring	▶ Minimal donor site morbidity ▶ Cosmesis	▶ Variable diameter ▶ Soft tissue healing in bone ▶ Hamstring weakness
Quadriceps tendon	▶ Large graft ▶ Used with or without a bone plug ▶ Minimal donor site morbidity	▶ Risk of patellar fracture ▶ Quadriceps weakness
Allograft	▶ No donor site morbidity ▶ Various tissue sources available	▶ Sterilization technique weakens the graft ▶ Healing in bone tunnels is slower ▶ Variability in donor source ▶ Theoretical risk of disease transmission

References

1. Biau DJ, Katsahian S, Kartus J, et al. Patellar tendon versus hamstring tendon autografts for reconstructing the anterior cruciate ligament: a meta-analysis based on individual patient data. *Am J Sports Med.* 2009;37(12):2470-2478.
2. Corry IS, Webb JM, Clingeleffer AJ, Pinczewski LA. Arthroscopic reconstruction of the anterior cruciate ligament. A comparison of patellar tendon autograft and four-strand hamstring tendon autograft. *Am J Sports Med.* 1999;27(3):444-454.
3. Forster MC, Forster IW. Patellar tendon or four-strand hamstring? A systemic review of autografts for anterior cruciate ligament reconstruction. *Knee.* 2005;12(3):225-230.
4. Freedman KB, D'Amato MJ, Nedeff DD, Kaz A, Bach BR Jr. Arthroscopic anterior cruciate ligament reconstruction: a metaanalysis comparing patellar tendon and hamstring tendon autografts. *Am J Sports Med.* 2003;31(1):2-11.
5. Goldblatt JP, Fitzsimmons SE, Balk E, Richmond JC. Reconstruction of the anterior cruciate ligament: meta-analysis of patellar tendon versus hamstring tendon autograft. *Arthroscopy.* 2005;21(7):791-803.

6. Kraeutler MJ, Bravman JT, McCarty EC. Bone-patellar tendon-bone autograft versus allograft in outcomes of anterior cruciate ligament reconstruction: a meta-analysis of 5182 patients. *Am J Sports Med.* 2013;41(10):2439-2448.
7. Mohtadi NG, Chan DS, Dainty KN, Whelan DB. Patellar tendon versus hamstring tendon autograft for anterior cruciate ligament rupture in adults. *Cochrane Database Syst Rev.* 2011;(9):CD005960.
8. Spindler KP, Kuhn JE, Freedman KB, Matthews CE, Dittus RS, Harrell FE Jr. Anterior cruciate ligament reconstruction autograft choice: bone-tendon-bone versus hamstring: does it really matter? A systemic review. *Am J Sports Med.* 2004;32(8):1986-1995.
9. Aglietti P, Giron F, Buzzi R, Biddau F, Sasso F. Anterior cruciate ligament reconstruction: bone-patellar tendon-bone compared with double semitendinosus and gracilis tendon grafts. A prospective, randomized clinical trial. *J Bone Joint Surg Am.* 2004;86(10);2143-2155.
10. Andernord D, Björnsson H, Petzold M, et al. Surgical predictors of early revision surgery after anterior cruciate ligament reconstruction: results from the Swedish National Knee Ligament Register on 13,102 patients. *Am J Sports Med.* 2014;42(7):1574-1582.
11. Barrett AM, Craft JA, Replogle WH, Hydrick JM, Barrett GR. Anterior cruciate ligament graft failure: a comparison of graft type based on age and Tegner activity level. *Am J Sports Med.* 2011;39(10):2194-2198.
12. Borchers JR, Pedroza A, Kaeding C. Activity level and graft type as risk factors for anterior cruciate ligament graft failure: a case-control study. *Am J Sports Med.* 2009;37(12):2362-2367.
13. Maletis GB, Inacio MC, Desmond JL, Funahashi TT. Reconstruction of the anterior cruciate ligament: association of graft choice with increased risk of early revision. *Bone Joint J.* 2013;95(5):623-628.
14. Maletis GB, Inacio MC, Funahashi TT. Analysis of 16,192 anterior cruciate ligament reconstructions from a community-based registry. *Am J Sports Med.* 2013;41(9):2090-2098.
15. Lind M, Menhert F, Pedersen AB. The first results from the Danish ACL reconstruction registry: epidemiologic and 2 year follow-up results from 5,818 knee ligament reconstructions. *Knee Surg Sports Traumatol Arthrosc.* 2009;17(2):117-124.
16. Ahldén M, Samuelsson K, Sernert N, Forssblad M, Karlsson J, Kartus J. The Swedish National Anterior Cruciate Ligament Register: a report on baseline variables and outcomes of surgery for almost 18,000 patients. *Am J Sports Med.* 2012;40(10):2230-2235.
17. Persson A, Fieldsgaard K, Gjertsen JE, et al. Increased risk of revision with hamstring tendon grafts compared with patellar tendon grafts after anterior cruciate ligament reconstruction: a study of 12,643 patients from the Norwegian Cruciate Ligament Registry, 2004-2012. *Am J Sports Med.* 2014;42(2):285-291.
18. Aune AK, Holm I, Risberg MA, Jensen HK, Steen H. Four-strand hamstring tendon autograft compared with patellar tendon-bone autograft for anterior cruciate ligament reconstruction. A randomized study with two-year follow-up. *Am J Sports Med.* 2001;29(6):722-728.
19. Ibrahim SA, Al-Kussary IM, Al-Misfer AR, Al-Mutairi HQ, Ghafar SA, El Noor TA. Clinical evaluation of arthroscopically assisted anterior cruciate ligament reconstruction: patellar tendon versus gracilis and semitendinosus autograft. *Arthroscopy.* 2005;21(4):412-417.
20. Laxdal G, Kartus J, Hansson L, Heidvall M, Ejerhed L, Karlsson J. A prospective randomized comparison of bone-patellar tendon-bone and hamstring grafts for anterior cruciate ligament reconstruction. *Arthroscopy.* 2005;21(1):34-42.
21. Pinczewski LA, Lyman J, Salmon LJ, Russell VJ, Roe J, Linklater J. A 10-year comparison of anterior cruciate ligament reconstructions with hamstring tendon and patellar tendon autograft: a controlled, prospective trial. *Am J Sports Med.* 2007;35(4)564-574.
22. Roe J, Pinczewski LA, Russell VJ, Salmon LJ, Kawamata T, Chew M. A 7-year follow-up of patellar tendon and hamstring tendon grafts for arthroscopic anterior cruciate ligament reconstruction: differences and similarities. *Am J Sports Med.* 2005;33(9):1337-1345.
23. Taylor DC, DeBardino TM, Nelson BJ, et al. Patellar tendon versus hamstring tendon autografts for anterior cruciate ligament reconstruction: a randomized controlled trial using similar femoral and tibial fixation methods. *Am J Sports Med.* 2009;37(10):1946-1957.
24. Lidén M, Ejerhed L, Sernert N, Laxdal G, Kartus J. Patellar tendon or semitendinosus tendon autografts for anterior cruciate ligament reconstruction: a prospective, randomized study with a 7-year follow-up. *Am J Sports Med.* 2007;35(5):740-748.
25. Sasaki N, Farraro KF, Kim KE, Woo SL. Biomechanical evaluation of the quadriceps tendon autograft for anterior cruciate ligament reconstruction: a cadaveric study. *Am J Sports Med.* 2014;42(3):723-730.

26. Lund B, Nielsen T, Faunø P, Christiansen SE, Lind M. Is quadriceps tendon a better graft choice than patellar tendon? A prospective randomized study. *Arthroscopy.* 2014;30(5):593-598.
27. Asselmeier MA, Caspari RB, Bottenfield S. A review of allograft processing and sterilization techniques and their role in transmission of the human immunodeficiency virus. *Am J Sports Med.* 1993;21(2):170-175.
28. Jackson DW, Grood ES, Goldstein JD, et al. A comparison of patellar tendon autograft and allograft used for anterior cruciate ligament reconstruction in the goat model. *Am J Sports Med.* 1993;21(2):176-185.
29. Krych AJ, Jackson JD, Hoskin TL, Dahm DL. A meta-analysis of patellar tendon autograft versus patellar tendon allograft in anterior cruciate ligament reconstruction. *Arthroscopy.* 2008;24(3):292-298.
30. Shelton WR, Papendick L, Dukes AD. Autograft versus allograft anterior cruciate ligament reconstruction. *Arthroscopy.* 1997;13(4):446-449.
31. Park SS, Dwyer T, Congiusta F, Whelan DB, Theodoropoulos J. Analysis of irradiation on the clinical effectiveness of allogenic tissue when used for primary anterior cruciate ligament reconstruction. *Am J Sports Med.* 2014;43(1):226-235.
32. Mariscalco MW, Flanigan DC, Mitchell J, et al. The influence of hamstring autograft size on patient-reported outcomes and risk of revision after anterior cruciate ligament reconstruction: a Multicenter Orthopaedic Outcomes Network (MOON) Cohort Study. *Arthroscopy.* 2013;29(12):1948-1953.
33. Rahr-Wagner L, Thillemann TM, Pedersen AB, Lind M. Comparison of hamstring tendon and patellar tendon grafts in anterior cruciate ligament reconstruction in a nationwide population-based cohort study: results from the Danish Registry of Knee Ligament Reconstruction. *Am J Sports Med.* 2013;42(2):278-284.

Please see videos on the accompanying website at www.routledge.com/9781617119996

25

Single-Bundle Anterior Cruciate Ligament Reconstruction

John C. Richmond, MD; Jonathan R. Maher, MD; and
Umer R. Dasti, MD

Introduction

In the 1970s and early 1980s, anterior cruciate ligament (ACL) reconstruction was performed with open surgical techniques. The development of the arthroscope and its widespread adoption led to the evolution of the arthroscopically assisted ACL reconstruction and, subsequently, the transtibial endoscopic technique. Transtibial drilling of the femoral socket for ACL reconstruction can result in suboptimal placement of the femoral socket. Suboptimal placement puts the ACL graft in a sagittal plane within the joint, which may not fully eliminate rotatory instability of the knee. Howell et al[1] recognized and described this graft placement as a clinical problem. They demonstrated that the ACL needs to be in the coronal plane of the knee and described the coronal angle in the frontal plane, which is the angle described by the axis of the joint line and the axis of the tibial tunnel (Figure 25-1). If this coronal angle is more than 75 degrees, it results in a more vertical graft and has a higher incidence of laxity and/or graft failure. The authors described a tibial start point for the tibial tunnel, which reproducibly produces a coronal angle less than 70 degrees.[2]

Use of the medial portal, as a technique to more accurately place the femoral socket within the femoral footprint of the ACL, has returned to current reconstructive techniques. Independent drilling of the femoral socket, not constrained by the tibial tunnel, can also be facilitated by using outside-in instrumentation in which placement of the guide or starter pin is done through an additional portal or incision placed superolaterally. Use of the medial portal technique requires positioning the knee so it can be flexed to 120 degrees in order to ensure an adequate length of the femoral socket (Figure 25-2). It is also facilitated by having flexible reamers and/or guide pins available to assist in placement of the instrumentation in such a way to avoid injury to the medial femoral condyle articular surface. Using an outside-in technique also requires specialized instrumentation to facilitate performance.

With the transtibial technique, the external start point of the guide pin into the tibia influences the locations where the femoral socket can be placed. Attention to the start point is a key step if one undertakes a transtibial technique. The definition of a reproducible start point has been identified as the intersection between the anterior edge of the medial collateral ligament (MCL) and the

Sgaglione NA, Lubowitz JH, Provencher MT, eds. *The Knee: AANA Advanced Arthroscopic Surgical Techniques* (pp 339-353).

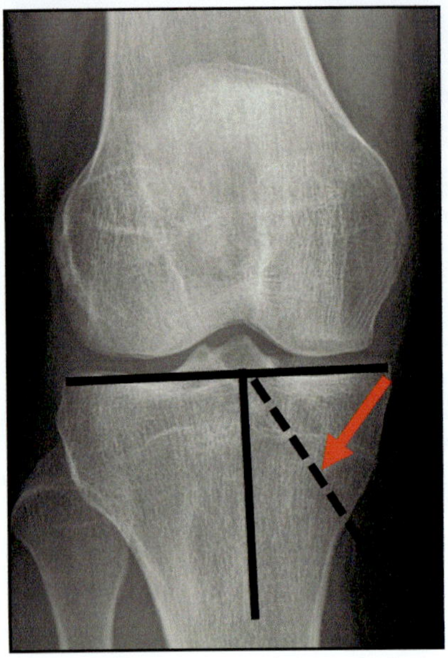

Figure 25-1. AP x-ray of the right knee illustrating the coronal angle (red arrow) as described by Howell et al.[1]

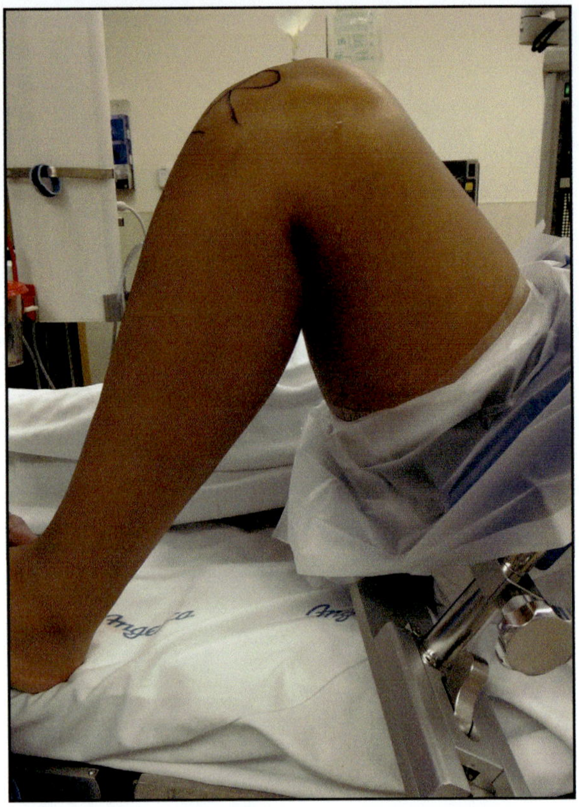

Figure 25-2. Left leg positioned in a leg holder in such a way as to facilitate flexion to 120 degrees for drilling of the femoral socket and fixation of the graft in the femoral socket.

superior border of the sartorius fascia or gracilis tendon. In the authors' study, this start point reproducibly yielded a coronal angle of 70 degrees or less, allowing the surgeon to consistently place the femoral socket within the ACL footprint.[2] Nevertheless, it tends to lead to a socket that is slightly more proximally placed within the femoral footprint compared to independent drilling techniques. Consequently, the authors only use this technique for bone patellar tendon bone (BPTB) grafts. The transtibial technique results in a femoral socket that is typically longer. This increased tunnel length allows the bone block to be recessed within the femoral socket, therefore reducing the chance of developing a graft-tunnel-length mismatch on the tibia. In order to use the transtibial technique for BPTB grafts, one must rotate the graft such that the tendinous portion is in the more distal region of the femoral socket and the screw is placed in the most proximal region of the socket, resulting in a graft that is well centered within the femoral footprint.

The choice of graft material in ACL reconstruction has potential significance. Autograft tissues are most commonly used. Allograft tendons are also reasonable alternatives. Recently, some information has been presented that irradiated allografts lead to inferior results, particularly in younger athletes.[3] The most commonly used autografts are BPTB and hamstring tendons (quadruple semitendinosus and gracilis). Quadriceps tendon is less commonly used but is a reasonable graft choice. Each graft material has potential advantages and disadvantages. Meta-analyses comparing autologous patellar tendon to hamstrings demonstrated that there are distinct differences in the outcomes. BPTB tendon grafts have been demonstrated to result in a higher percentage of clinically stable knees and a greater likelihood of athletes returning to preinjury athletic performance.[4-6] This outcome difference is not without cost because there is a greater incidence of

Table 25-1. Algorithm for Anterior Cruciate Ligament Graft Selection

GRAFT	INDICATIONS
Bone-tendon-bone autograft	High-demand young athletes (high school, college, professional) Revision of failed soft tissue grafts
Quadrupled hamstring autograft	Recreational athletes younger than 40 years High-demand young athletes with patellar tendon problems
Quadriceps tendon autograft	High-demand young athletes with inadequate patellar tendons and hamstring tendons
Allograft tendons	Recreational athletes older than 40 years Multiligament-injured knees Augment smaller hamstring autografts

anterior knee pain and quadriceps weakness in the patellar tendon group. One of the potential issues with hamstring grafts is the diameter of the graft. Recent data suggest that grafts that are 8 mm or less in diameter have a higher failure rate than larger grafts.[7] There is no single way to predict the potential graft diameter preoperatively that is completely reproducible. The patient's height can be used as a preoperative predictor of potential hamstring graft diameter.[8] For patients who end up with a graft diameter of 8 mm or less, the authors have recently started augmenting the autograft tissue with an additional allograft hamstring tendon to bring the diameter up to 9 mm or greater. To date, no data confirm whether this will improve results.

One variable that has been defined in the use of allografts is whether the tissue has been irradiated. Nonirradiated or low-dose irradiated grafts that are not treated with harsh chemicals probably give the best results.[9] Any surgeon using allograft tissues for ACL reconstruction should be cognizant of the processing techniques of the available allografts in his or her institution prior to selecting allograft tissue for use in ACL reconstruction.

The authors developed an algorithm that they use for graft selection based on the patient's age and athletic demands (Table 25-1). Autologous BPTB graft remains the authors' preference for younger, high-demand athletes. This includes competitive high school, intercollegiate, and professional athletes. For less-demanding athletes, the authors prefer a quadrupled hamstring autograft. This would typically be for recreational athletes younger than 40 years. It also includes younger, more athletic patients if their patellar tendons are so long as to result in a graft–tunnel mismatch. Tendon length can be determined by the preoperative magnetic resonance imaging (MRI) scan. As previously noted, the authors augment these hamstrings with an additional hamstring allograft if the diameter is less than 8 mm in females and 8 mm or less in males. Finally, allograft as an isolated tissue in the authors' practice is reserved for patients older than 40 years old or special situations (revision, multiligament injuries, or patient preference).

Indications

- Functional instability in an ACL-deficient knee
- Acute ACL tear in a young, active athlete
- Multiligament-injured knee with an ACL tear

Controversial Indications

No consensus exists as to the optimal technique or graft selection for ACL reconstruction. Single-bundle ACL reconstruction remains the most widely used technique, but double-bundle techniques have been proposed, potentially resulting in better fill of the ACL footprints on the femur and tibia and as a means of having a more anatomic configuration of the graft. Biomechanical analyses and comparative clinical outcome studies evaluating single- vs double-bundle techniques have been inconsistent. Due to the added complexity and cost of double-bundle techniques, single-bundle ACL reconstruction is currently the most widely performed.

Pertinent Physical Findings

- Anterior drawer
- Lachman examination
- Pivot shift

The history remains a reliable means of identifying a patient with a likely ACL tear. The majority of ACL injuries occur through noncontact events. History of a noncontact injury with an accompanying pop followed by immediate swelling is a suggestive history. Clinical evaluation, through examination of the joint, is best done early after injury. On the field or a sideline evaluation of the injured athlete before there is significant swelling and/or pain can be helpful. The most commonly performed tests are the Lachman, anterior drawer, and pivot shift. The Lachman is the most sensitive test. The subtleties of slightly increased translation or soft end point on the Lachman examination are indicative of ACL injury. Partial ACL tears occur with a similar history of injury but have more subtle physical findings. The Lachman test is performed with the patient supine and his or her muscles relaxed. The knee joint should be gently flexed to 30 degrees. In the face of acute injury, placing the knee over a soft pillow can be of benefit to relax the patient's hamstrings. A large hemarthrosis with acute pain from injury can make this examination more difficult. Aspiration of the hemarthrosis with instillation of local anesthetic may facilitate the examination early on but is only suggested in those cases when the patient is in acute pain from a tense hemarthrosis. The Lachman test is performed with the examiner's hands positioned proximal and distal to the knee joint with alternate anterior pull on the tibia while maintaining posterior force on the femur. The examiner should estimate the amount of translation in millimeters and the feel of the end point. If the anterior translation has a soft feel, this indicates an acute ACL tear. Increased translation of 5 mm or more when compared to the contralateral knee indicates a complete ACL tear.

The pivot shift phenomenon can be difficult to elicit in a painful knee, but it has the highest specificity for a complete ACL tear. There are a myriad of ways to perform this test. The use of an instrumented laxity tester, such as the KT-1000, can be of benefit in identifying subtly increased translation in the face of an acute injury.

Pertinent Imaging

- Plain x-rays (anteroposterior and lateral)
- MRI

Plain x-rays are an appropriate imaging modality to start the evaluation of the acute or chronic sports-injured knee. Although an ACL injury cannot be seen with this modality, a fracture, particularly a tibial spine avulsion or a Segond fracture, may be identified. The imaging modality of choice for identifying an ACL injury is MRI. This modality, if the patient is appropriately positioned, will identify subtle damage to the ACL. MRI has the additional benefit of being able to identify bone bruising in an acute injury. The typical bruise pattern of posterolateral tibia and anterolateral femur is highly suggestive of a complete ACL tear. MRI is also beneficial in identifying associated injuries, such as meniscal tears and additional ligament damage.

Preoperative Planning

It has become routine to delay treatment of the acute ACL tear until that time when the patient has regained full extension, near full flexion, and resolution of the acute hemarthrosis. There is no specific time frame for this, but early reconstruction in a joint that lacks full motion is associated with risk of postoperative stiffness requiring additional surgery. Early physical therapy post injury, to assist in the reduction of swelling and regaining motion while maintaining muscle strength, is appropriate and encouraged. This therapy period allows the surgeon and patient to select a surgery date and technique that is appropriate. For younger student athletes, delaying the surgery to a period of vacation has been associated with better performance in school for that semester.[10] Surgical timing should be discussed with the patient and the parents because a rush to reconstruct may facilitate a quicker return to sports but may compromise the student athlete's ability to get into the college of his or her choice if his or her grades suffer.

ACL reconstruction is readily accomplished in an outpatient surgery center. A potential reason to do this type of procedure in a full-service hospital is for a medical comorbidity. Although spinal or general anesthesia can be used, supplementation with peripheral nerve blocks (typically femoral nerve) assists with postoperative pain management.

Equipment

A multitude of orthopedic equipment manufacturers have ACL reconstruction trays that contain the instruments necessary to complete the procedure. There are subtle differences in the design of these, and the surgeon should be familiar with the equipment available at the selected surgery center and should be comfortable that he or she can perform the procedure as planned with the available equipment. The use of flexible instrumentation for medial portal techniques facilitates the procedure and can be protective of the articular cartilage. The use of a leg holder or positioning posts is beneficial. Medial portal techniques often require that the knee be flexed more than 110 degrees.

Positioning and Portals

The patient should be positioned supine with a leg holder or lateral post (see Figure 25-2).

Step-by-Step Description of the Procedure

Using the medial portal technique for soft tissue ACL reconstruction requires the knee to be flexed 110 to 120 degrees to be able to accurately place the guide pins through the medial portal and ensure adequate length of the femoral socket (see Figure 25-2). This technique is best used for soft tissue grafts (autologous quadruple hamstring or quadriceps tendon grafts and soft tissue allografts). The joint should always be examined for laxity (cruciate and collaterals) prior to

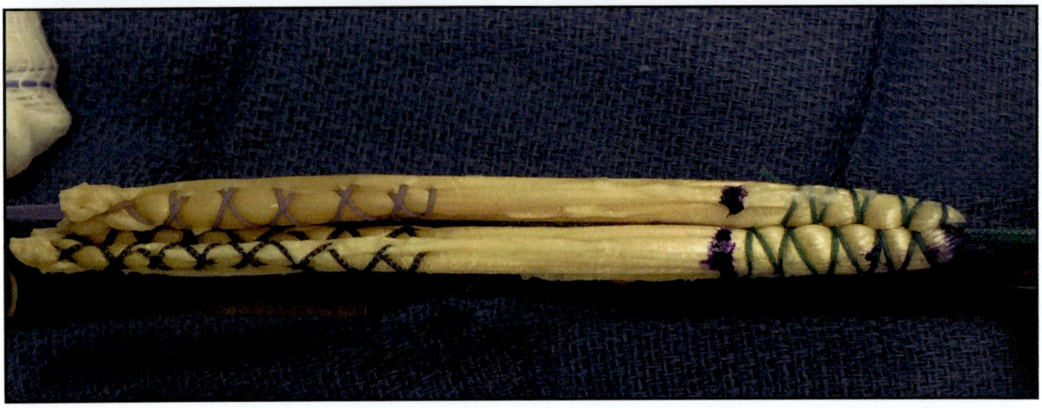

Figure 25-3. Soft tissue allograft after preparation being kept under tension on the back table, prior to insertion. The Roman sandal weave is to the right.

commencing the surgery. The authors prefer to harvest autograft tendons prior to arthroscopic examination of the joint if a complete ACL tear can be established based on the MRI scan and the presence of a pivot shift under anesthesia. If the pivot shift cannot be identified and the MRI did not clearly demonstrate a complete ACL tear, then the authors routinely arthroscope the joint to confirm that there is a complete ACL tear prior to harvesting the graft. In any case, the authors prefer to have the graft prepared on the back table while simultaneously preparing the joint. There are a myriad of fixation techniques for soft tissue ACL grafts. They generally fall into the category of suspensory (where the fixation is on the cortex) or aperture (where the fixation is within the tunnel). Although there is no consensus within the literature as to which is preferable, it has been the authors' practice to use interference-type intratunnel fixation for soft tissue allografts. The authors' preference for interference devices is to use a permanent material so that there is no potential issue with breakdown products from an absorbable interference screw and for formation of a cavitary lesion as the screws resorb. Therefore, the senior author (JCR) uses femoral and tibial Intrafix devices (DePuy Mitek). These devices are made out of permanent medical grade plastics, are exceedingly inert, and facilitate compression of the graft to the largest circumference of the socket.

Simultaneous graft preparation on the back table is accomplished with a preparation board that maintains the graft under tension while the various sutures are applied. With the authors' technique using femoral Intrafix, they use a "Roman sandal" suture that is passed around the middle of the graft while baseball sutures are placed in the ends of the graft. The resulting construct is shown in Figure 25-3. Sizing of the graft is done very early after the autologous tendons have been skeletonized or the allograft has been thawed. If the autologous hamstring tendons are sized smaller than 8 mm for females or 8 mm or less in males, the authors add an allograft hamstring tendon to them. The authors always keep the graft under tension on the back table with the hope of reducing creep in the construct during fixation and tensioning. This tension is maintained for the entire time once the graft is prepped, prior to insertion.

Complete diagnostic evaluation of the joint is the first arthroscopic portion of the procedure. Visualizing the popliteus tendon through the lateral gutter is the authors' start point. The gutters and the suprapatellar pouch should be carefully inspected for loose bodies. Laxity of the collaterals should be evaluated while arthroscoping the medial and lateral compartments. Prior to graft insertion, it is important to carefully probe the menisci to identify any potentially unstable meniscal tear that might need treatment. Once the graft has been inserted and secured, repair or removal of damaged menisci is more difficult to perform because the laxity prior to reconstruction facilitates meniscal surgery.

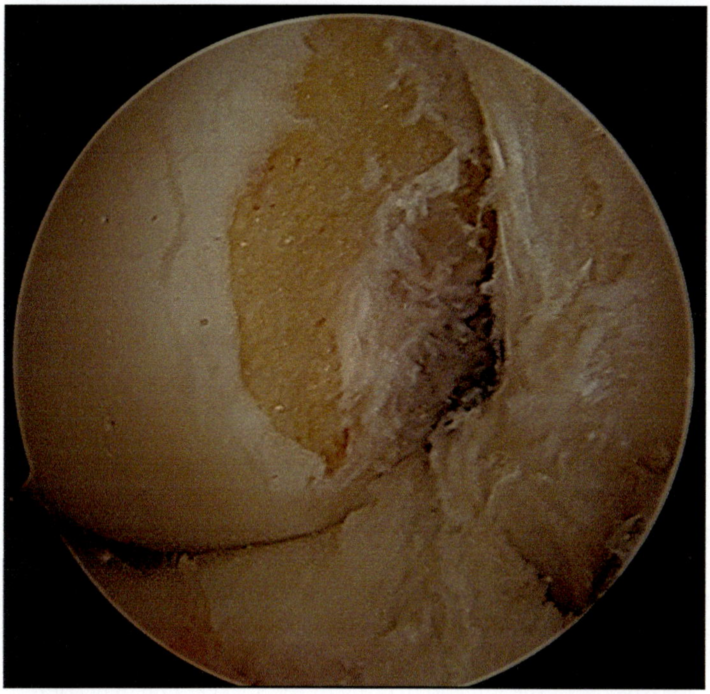

Figure 25-4. Medial portal view of the femoral footprint of the ACL in a right knee flexed to 90 degrees.

Minimal preparation of the notch is required in most acute ACL tear situations. Nevertheless, one should carefully inspect for a narrow notch, which necessitates performance of a notchplasty (Video). The authors prefer to preserve remnants of the ACL on the tibia and femur. The femoral remnant can serve as a landmark for placement of the guide pins on the femur (Figure 25-4), while the tibial remnant, which the authors often preserve at 8 mm in length, can act as a neurologic active envelope for the ACL graft, theoretically improving proprioception following ACL reconstructive surgery.[11]

Prior to drilling the tibial tunnel, it is essential to resect adequate fat pad such that the fat will not impinge into the notch and obscure the surgeon's view (Video). The authors resect the distal fat pad such that the intrameniscal ligament can be readily visualized. Once the fat pad is removed and the medial tibial flare has been exposed, the authors select an entry site for the drill guide on the anteromedial tibial surface that is just at the superior border of the sartorius fascia. When one is using the medial portal technique, it is not necessary to use the anterior edge of the MCL as an additional guide for locating the start point, and the authors prefer to use a start point closer to the tibial tubercle. Use of a commercial tibial ACL guide is encouraged for placing the tibial guide pin. The guide facilitates accurate placement of the guide pin and can reduce the risk of injury to the articular surface. The tip of this guide should be placed at the anatomical center of the ACL on the tibia, which should be midway between the medial and lateral extents of the ACL attachment and located in the anteroposterior plane at the most posterior attachment of the anterior horn of the lateral meniscus. The accurate position of the guide pin should be ascertained before overdrilling it. If the guide pin is more than a few millimeters distant from anatomic center of the ACL, it should be replaced prior to reaming. If the guide pin is within 2 mm of the optimal position, it can be slightly moved by initially overdrilling with a smaller cannulated drill. The guide pin should always be stabilized with a hemostat when it is being overdrilled so that the premature breakthrough of the drill that occurs anterior to the pin does not result in anterior migration of the tunnel. If one overdrills the 2.4-mm guide pin with a 4.5-mm cannulated drill, the guide can be displaced 1 mm in any direction by using the hemostat to push it or pull it to the appropriate position intra-articularly. If one overdrills initially with a 6-mm cannulated drill, then one can displace the guide pin 2 mm in the appropriate direction to center the guide pin in the anatomic tibial footprint of the ACL. When one is planning to use the tibial Intrafix device for a tibial fixation, the tibial tunnel should be drilled to the same diameter as the graft. The authors routinely drill the tibial tunnel prior to the femoral socket so that the tibial tunnel can be used to evacuate the bone debris from drilling the femoral socket and therefore improve visualization through that step.

Leaving a millimeter of femoral footprint for the ACL in place prior to determining the femoral start point for the guide pin can be beneficial. The authors find that it is most helpful to think of the knee in the 90-degree flexed position. The footprint is ovoid with the long axis being on the proximal to distal line of the femur and the shorter axis being in the anterior to posterior line (see Figure 25-4). Routinely placing the arthroscope through the anteromedial portal to better identify the ACL footprint is of value. The position of the anteromedial portal for medial portal technique ACL reconstruction is crucial. Some have described using an accessory, more medial portal. The authors routinely use an oblique, relatively low, primary anteromedial portal that works well for the medial portal technique. They localize the position of that portal with a spinal needle before it is cut. The spinal needle needs to be able to reach back to the ACL femoral attachment with the knee flexed to 90 degrees while being just off the articular cartilage of the medial femoral condyle. This portal placement ensures that the guide pin can be placed accurately, resulting in a femoral socket of adequate length. The medial portal technique is facilitated by having a flexible guide wire (made from nitinol) and/or flexible drills. The systems that use flexible nitinol guide pins typically do not require hyperflexion for passage of the guide pin. Because the authors prefer to pass a rigid guide pin and then immediately substitute a flexible wire for this, they use the 110- to 120-degree hyperflexed position for passage of the pin and drilling of the socket. The hyperflexed position can be disorienting and may make it difficult to ascertain whether one is in the appropriate position prior to pin passage. The authors usually mark the area in the ACL footprint that is optimal for pin passage with a shaver and/or microfracture pick prior to bringing the over-the-back femoral aimer in through the medial portal. Because the paddle of the over-the-back aimer is on articular cartilage in this position, high-offset (7.5 to 8.0 mm) aimers are optimal. Less than that will result in a tunnel that is too posterior and often too short.

Once the anatomic start point for the femoral guide pin has been determined at 90 degrees of flexion and the aimer has been positioned, it is maintained in that position while the knee is brought into hyperflexion. The guide pin is then drilled out through the lateral condyle and through the skin and immediately switched out for a flexible 2.4-mm nitinol wire (Video). With the wire in place, the knee can be moved to any position, and the location of the pin can be carefully assessed in relation to the ACL femoral footprint (Figure 25-5). This flexible pin also allows one to bend the pin away from the medial femoral condyle while the acorn drill is threaded over it. This should be done in approximately 60 to 70 degrees of flexion to minimize the risk of injury to the medial femoral condyle articular cartilage. Protection of the medial femoral condyle can also be facilitated by using a half-fluted cannulated drill or by using an accessory anterolateral portal and femoral drill guide such that the guide pin is placed into the ACL femoral footprint from outside in.

Once the cannulated acorn drill has been brought safely into the notch, the knee is brought back to the hyperflexed position. Any device that had been used to plug the tibial tunnel is then removed to facilitate drainage of fluid and bone debris from the joint. The authors typically bring a 4-mm shaver up through the tibial tunnel while drilling the femoral socket so that suction on the shaver can be used to evacuate the bone debris while drilling and watching the depth. With the femoral Intrafix system, the femoral socket needs to be a minimum of 27 mm in length, preferably 30 mm in length. In using this system, the socket should be drilled 1 mm greater in diameter than the graft was measured. Using the 7.5- to 8-mm offset over the back guide routinely generates adequate tunnel length. After the socket is drilled, all bone debris should be evacuated from the socket and the back of the joint using the shaver as a suction device. The positioning of the socket should be critically evaluated to be certain that placement was appropriate (Figure 25-6).

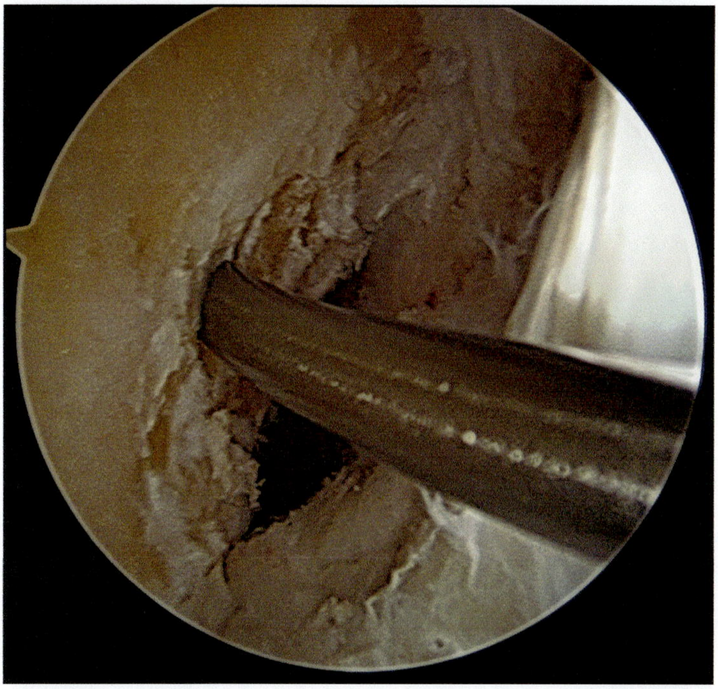

Figure 25-5. Medial portal view in a right knee flexed to 90 degrees along a nitinol wire showing the wire located centrally in the ACL femoral footprint.

The next step is to reinsert the Beath-type femoral guide pin through the medial portal and out through the femoral socket and skin. A retrieval suture is then brought into the joint and out though the femoral socket. It can then be brought down through the tibial tunnel to retrieve the graft into the femur transtibially. This is easily accomplished using the grasper up through the tibial tunnel. A #5 polyester suture is satisfactory for this step.

The graft is then retrieved transtibially up into the femur. Because the Roman sandal weave typically results in a 2-bundle construct for the femur, these should be positioned as the graft is pulled into the femur such that they reproduce the anteromedial and posterolateral bundles of the native ACL. With use of the femoral Intrafix device, there is a trial inserter, which is brought up through the medial portal in the hyperflexed position to separate the 2 arms of the graft and dilate the tunnel to accept the sheath. A small-diameter nitinol wire is inserted through this trial device before it is removed and acts as a guide wire for the femoral sheath insertion and ultimately for the femoral screw insertion. The sheath and screw come as a packaged set and should be sized according to the manufacturer's recommendations based on the measured diameter of the graft and the drill recommended for that diameter graft. The screw is then placed into the sheath over the nitinol wire. It is beneficial to remove the nitinol wire once the screw has been seated approximately three-quarters of the way so the tip of the wire will not be bent over by the screw.

Once the graft has been fixed on the femur (Figure 25-7), it should be cycled under tension prior to inserting and securing the tibial fixation device. Kleweno et al[12] demonstrated that every femoral fixation device has the potential for creep with cyclic loading. Trying to remove some of this creep through cycling the graft under tension prior to tibial fixation makes sense. Perhaps the least well-understood factor in ACL reconstruction is tensioning the graft and the position of the knee during tensioning and fixation. The authors identified that applying a maximal pull to the graft while the knee is in full extension reliably results in a high percentage of stable knees, with the added assurance that the patient will be able to regain full extension because the graft was secured in the fully extended position.[13]

After the graft has been fixed on the tibial side, the joint should be examined for laxity and range of motion to be sure the tension on the graft is appropriate and full extension and flexion

Figure 25-6. Medial portal views of the right knee of the femoral socket in (A) 90 and (B) 120 degrees of flexion demonstrating anatomic location and adequate posterior wall for interference fixation.

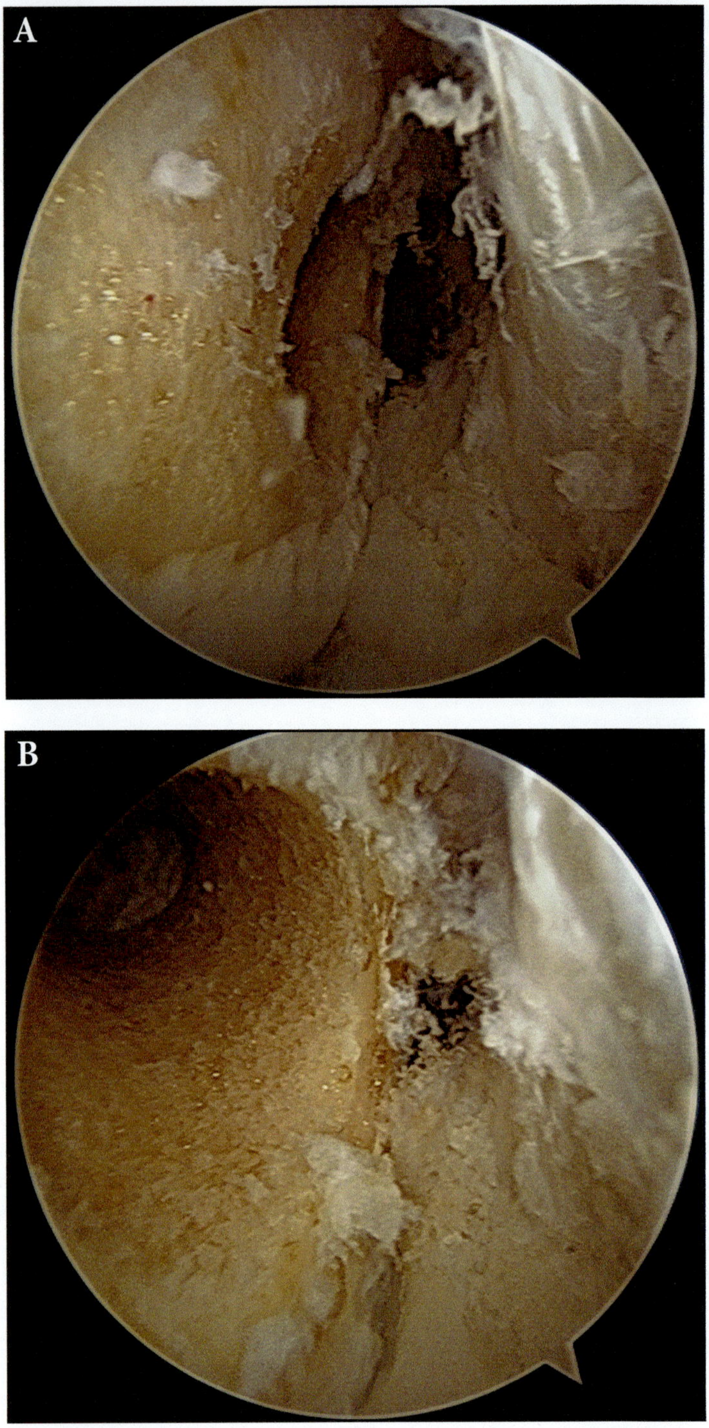

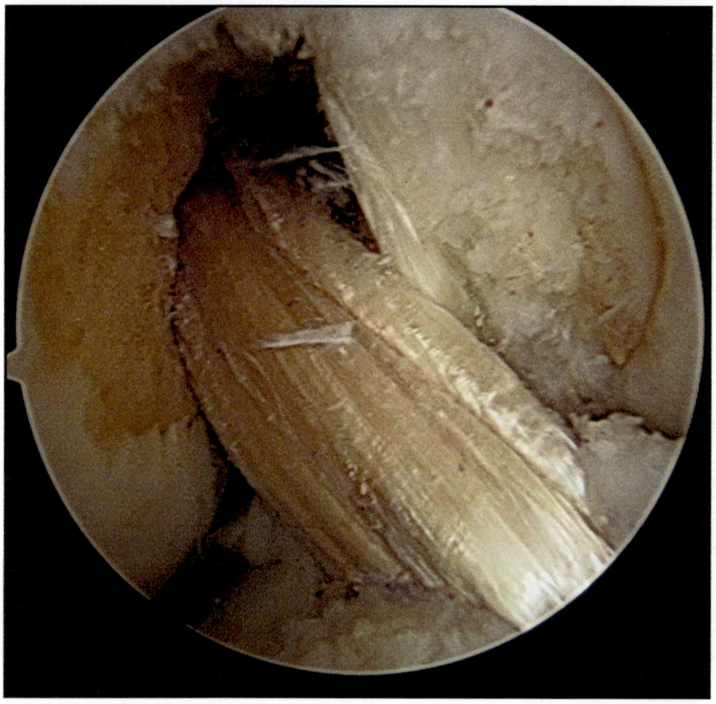

Figure 25-7. Lateral portal view of the right knee showing a graft at 90 degrees of flexion following femoral fixation demonstrating a wide triangle of space between the graft and the posterior cruciate ligament. This triangle identified by Howell et al[1] indicates the proper position of the femoral socket in the coronal plane.

are achieved. Finally, the graft should be inspected and probed to be sure there is adequate tension and no impingement (Figure 25-8). If the tension is inadequate, the tibial fixation device should be removed and the graft retensioned. If there is impingement of the graft, a notchplasty is needed.

The authors routinely use the transtibial technique when they select bone-tendon-bone autograft (or allograft) for high-demand patients. The transtibial approach results in a longer femoral socket and allows the bone block, which is harvested from the tibia, to be recessed into the femoral socket an additional 8 to 10 mm if needed. This graft positioning is beneficial when the tendinous portion of the bone-tendon-bone construct measures more than 40 mm. The authors use the preoperative MRI scan to measure the patellar tendon length prior to making a decision for graft choice. If the measured length is more than 50 mm at its shortest length, this excess length may compromise fixation because the bone block in the tibial socket may project too distally, necessitating a less-than-optimal fixation technique.

If the preoperative MRI measurement of the patellar tendon is longer than 40 mm but less than 50 mm, the authors harvest an additional 8 to 10 mm of bone from the tibia proximal to the most proximal patellar tendon fibers (Figure 25-9). This larger harvest will allow the bone block to be inserted up into the femur an additional 8 to 10 mm; therefore, the block harvested from the patella will advance that same distance into the tibia tunnel, facilitating a fixation.

As with soft tissue graft, the authors harvest the bone-tendon-bone autograft prior to preparing the joint. The assistant can prepare the graft on the back table simultaneously while the joint is prepared. The harvest of the bone-tendon-bone graft should be performed carefully. The width of the proximal patella tendon should be accurately measured prior to the harvest. For small females, the authors accept a minimum of 8 mm for the width of the graft. On preoperative evaluation of the MRI scan, if the width of the proximal patellar tendon is less than 24 mm, the patellar tendon is not an adequate source of graft. In this case, a quadriceps tendon autograft or a hamstring autograft/allograft composite may be a better choice for the graft source. The authors use an identical procedure for notch preparation with either technique. A commercial ACL tibial guide is appropriate for passage of the tibial guide wire. The MCL pes anserinus start point will

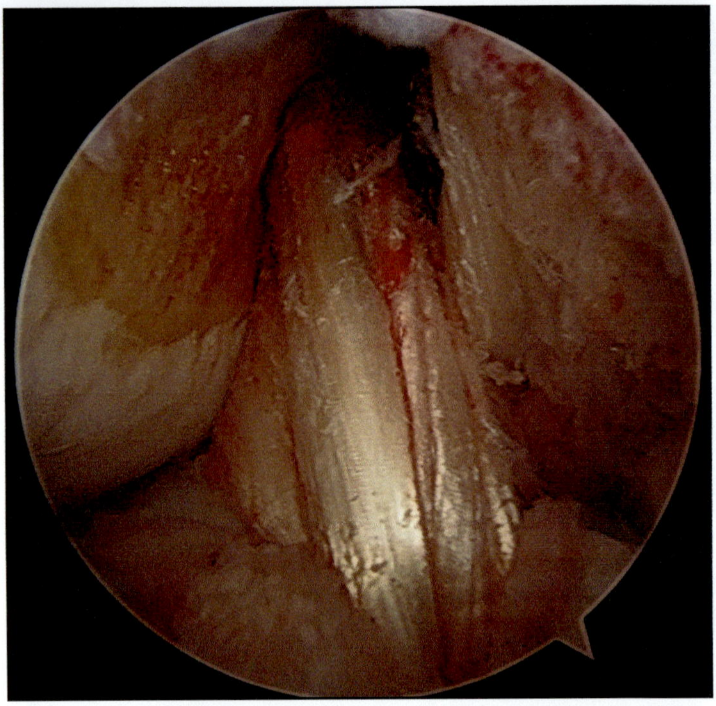

Figure 25-8. Medial portal view of the right knee graft at 90 degrees of flexion following cycling, tensioning, and fixation on the tibia.

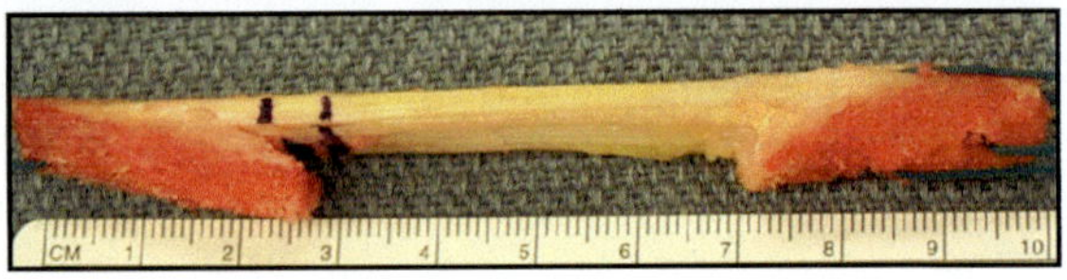

Figure 25-9. Patellar tendon graft with the bone block harvested from the tibia on the left. The additional bone harvested from the tibia proximal to the tendon attachment allows the graft to be recessed into the femur (the 8 mm marked in purple on the tendon).

give an appropriate angle for this tibial tunnel such that transtibial drilling of the femoral socket will result in anatomic positioning of the tendinous portion of the bone-tendon-bone graft on the femur. Because tensioning of the graft relies on easy sliding without resistance of the bone block within the tibial tunnel, the block should be sized so that it slides easily in the sizer.

Drilling a transtibial tunnel as outlined previously, one can accurately place a femoral Beath guide pin using a standard commercially available over-the-top–type guide. This guide is selected so that it is 2 mm more than the radius of the femoral socket that will be created. The diameter of that socket should be the diameter of the bone block harvested from the tibia measured with a snug fit. A snug fit in the femoral socket will allow use of a 7-mm cannulated titanium interference fit screw to get strong fixation.[14] Once the Beath pin has been passed through the femur and out percutaneously through the lateral thigh, it is immediately removed and replaced with a 2.4-mm nitinol wire. The nitinol wire facilitates passage of the cannulated acorn drill, specifically allowing the pin to be deformed such that the tibial tunnel is not expanded posteriorly as the drill is advanced into the joint. With this technique, the femoral socket is routinely drilled to a depth of 40 mm. This length of tunnel allows the position of the proximal bone block to be adjusted as needed within the tunnel to bring the distal bone block into the tibial tunnel and avoid a potential graft–tunnel mismatch.

Once the femoral socket is drilled and all bone debris is removed, the Beath pin is replaced for retrieval of the graft. The graft is retrieved and rotated such that the tendinous portion lies in the most distal aspect of the socket. This position is typically in the anatomic center of the ACL footprint on the femur. The bone block is then proximal within the femoral socket and the interference screw is inserted in the most proximal aspect of the socket. A commercially available notcher should be used to develop a starting position for the screw. The nitinol guide pin, over which the screw will be placed, should be inserted up into the femoral socket along with the bone block to ensure that it is parallel to the tunnel. With a snug fit of the bone block in the socket, a 7-mm diameter by 20- to 25-mm-long screw can be readily inserted, providing excellent fixation.

Because there is no creep between a titanium interference screw and the bone-tendon-bone graft, cycling the bone-tendon-bone graft prior to tibial fixation is not needed. Again, fixation of the tibial bone block in full extension is crucial to ensure that full extension will be obtainable postoperatively. External rotation of the tibial bone block by 90 degrees will reproduce the normal ACL rotation.[15]

The authors tension with the knee in full extension (including hyperextension), applying maximal tension to the graft prior to tibial fixation. Fixation in the tibial tunnel should be done with an 8- or 9-mm-diameter titanium interference screw. The length of the screw should be selected so that the tip of the screw on insertion should not impinge on the soft tissue portion of the graft. The authors routinely place the screw so that the threads abut the cancellous portion of the block and the wall of the tunnel to reduce the risk of damage to the tendinous portion of the graft.

Postoperative Protocol

Tensioning the graft in full extension facilitates the patient regaining full extension postoperatively. The authors stress this early on in the rehabilitation program and require the patient to be in an adjustable postoperative brace locked in extension for 18 hours daily, removing it only for 6 hours (in 2-hour increments) of passive motion and other exercises. While using continuous passive motion (CPM), obtaining full extension is also stressed. This position is facilitated by placing a rolled towel behind the Achilles tendon. The CPM machine should be set at a minimum of 0 degrees of extension and preferentially to 10 degrees of hyperextension. Motion is begun from 0 to 40 degrees for 2 hours 3 times a day and then increased in 5- to 10-degree daily increments until the first postoperative visit approximately 10 days postoperatively. Quadriceps setting and straight leg lifts can be of benefit in maintaining quadriceps tone during this time. It is appropriate to take some precautions to reduce the risk of thrombophlebitis or pulmonary embolism. The authors routinely use elastic compression socks on both calves for the first 2 days postoperatively and on the operated calf until the first postoperative visit. Ankle pumps are encouraged. Use of aspirin or a cyclooxygenase nonsteroidal anti-inflammatory drug may act as a mild chemoprophylactic for thrombophlebitis as well.

At the first postoperative visit, wounds are checked, the calf is examined for signs of phlebitis, and motion is ascertained. In the authors' protocol, formal physical therapy routinely begins at this point, and the brace is used only for ambulation and is locked in extension. The authors use a protocol that gradually advances strengthening exercises and progressively increases the stress on the graft. The brace is discontinued 4 weeks after surgery. The graduated rehabilitation program for strength and endurance is designed so that unopposed quadriceps contraction early on (felt to unduly strain the graft) is avoided.[16] High-risk activities are delayed until a minimum of 4.5 months after bone-tendon-bone autograft to preferably 6 to 9 months for soft tissue autograft or allografts.

Potential Complications

- Thrombophlebitis/pulmonary embolism
- Iatrogenic chondral damage

- Pain/stiffness
- Motion loss
- Infection
- Nerve/vascular injury
- Fracture
- Graft rupture
- Tunnel malposition
- Graft–tunnel mismatch

Top Technical Pearls for the Procedure

1. Have a variety of autografts and allografts available within your skill set so you can tailor graft selection to the patient's demands and his or her anatomy.
2. To use the medial portal technique, the leg must be positioned so that the knee can be flexed to 120 degrees for accurate placement of the femoral socket.
3. Resecting the fat pad to expose the intrameniscal ligament will facilitate visualization for the medial portal technique.
4. For patellar tendon autograft, harvesting an additional 8 mm of tibial bone plug proximal to the patellar tendon insertion will help avoid graft–tunnel mismatch.
5. Fix grafts in full extension with high tension force to establish good tension and maintain mobility.

References

1. Howell SM, Gittins ME, Gottlieb JE, Traina SM, Zoellner TM. The relationship between the angle of the tibial tunnel in the coronal plane and loss of flexion and anterior laxity after anterior cruciate ligament reconstruction. *Am J Sports Med.* 2001;29(5):567-574.
2. Raffo CS, Pizzarello P, Richmond JC, Pathare N. A reproducible landmark for the tibial tunnel origin in anterior cruciate ligament reconstruction: avoiding a vertical graft in the coronal plane. *Arthroscopy.* 2008;24(7):843-845.
3. Pallis M, Svoboda SJ, Cameron KL, Owens BD. Survival comparison of allograft and autograft anterior cruciate ligament reconstruction at the United States Military Academy. *Am J Sports Med.* 2012;40(6):1242-1246.
4. Goldblatt JP, Fitzsimmons SE, Balk E, Richmond JC. Reconstruction of the anterior cruciate ligament: meta-analysis of patellar tendon versus hamstring tendon autograft. *Arthroscopy.* 2005;21(7):791-803.
5. Yunes M, Richmond JC, Engels EA, Pinczewski LA. Patellar versus hamstring tendons in anterior cruciate ligament reconstruction: a meta-analysis. *Arthroscopy.* 2001;17(3):248-257.
6. Freedman KB, D'Amato MJ, Nedeff DD, Kaz A, Bach BR Jr. Arthroscopic anterior cruciate ligament reconstruction: a metaanalysis comparing patellar tendon and hamstring tendon autografts. *Am J Sports Med.* 2003;31(1):2-11.
7. Conte EJ, Hyatt AE, Gatt CJ Jr, Dhawan A. Hamstring autograft size can be predicted and is a potential risk factor for anterior cruciate ligament reconstruction failure. *Arthroscopy.* 2014;30(7):882-890.
8. Tuman JM, Diduch DR, Rubino LJ, Baumfeld JA, Nguyen HS, Hart JM. Predictors for hamstring graft diameter in anterior cruciate ligament reconstruction. *Am J Sports Med.* 2007;35(11):1945-1949.
9. Curran AR, Adams DJ, Gill JL, Steiner ME, Scheller AD. The biomechanical effects of low-dose irradiation on bone-patellar tendon-bone allografts. *Am J Sports Med.* 2004;32(5):1131-1135.

10. Trentacosta NE, Vitale MA, Ahmad CS. The effects of timing of pediatric knee ligament surgery on short-term academic performance in school-aged athletes. *Am J Sports Med.* 2009;37(9):1684-1691.
11. Lee BI, Kwon SW, Kim JB, Choi HS, Min KD. Comparison of clinical results according to amount of preserved remnant in arthroscopic anterior cruciate ligament reconstruction using quadrupled hamstring graft. *Arthroscopy.* 2008;24(5):560-568.
12. Kleweno CP, Jacir AM, Gardner TR, Ahmad CS, Levine WN. Biomechanical evaluation of anterior cruciate ligament femoral fixation techniques. *Am J Sports Med.* 2009;37(2):339-345.
13. Nabors ED, Richmond JC, Vannah WM, McConville OR. Anterior cruciate ligament graft tensioning in full extension. *Am J Sports Med.* 1995;23(4):488-492.
14. Hulstyn M, Fadale PD, Abate J, Walsh WR. Biomechanical evaluation of interference screw fixation in a bovine patellar bone-tendon-bone autograft complex for anterior cruciate ligament reconstruction. *Arthroscopy.* 1993;9(4):417-424.
15. Samuelson TS, Drez D Jr, Maletis GB. Anterior cruciate ligament graft rotation. Reproduction of normal graft rotation. *Am J Sports Med.* 1996;24(1):67-71.
16. Beynnon BD, Fleming BC, Johnson RJ, Nichols CE, Renström PA, Pope MH. Anterior cruciate ligament strain behavior during rehabilitation exercises in vivo. *Am J Sports Med.* 1995;23(1):24-34.

Please see videos on the accompanying website at www.routledge.com/9781617119996

26

Anatomic Double-Bundle Anterior Cruciate Ligament Reconstruction

Garth N. Walker, MD; James M. Bullock, MD; and
Freddie H. Fu, MD, DSc (Hon), DPs (Hon)

Introduction

Anterior cruciate ligament (ACL) rupture is a common injury worldwide. Estimates suggest an annual incidence of ACL rupture of 35 per 100,000 people of all ages, with an approximately 2- to 8-times higher risk in female than in male athletes.[1-3] Double-bundle ACL reconstruction originated from the application of research findings to an individualized surgical approach tailored to patient anatomy. Murawski et al[4] recently reported that most studies show no differences between anatomic single- and double-bundle ACL reconstruction with respect to patient-reported outcome scores and that double-bundle reconstruction may provide superior knee joint laxity outcome measurements compared with the single-bundle technique. Double-bundle ACL reconstruction is based on reconstructing the anteromedial and posterolateral bundle when ruptured. Although some studies indicate cartilage protection with ACL reconstruction, there is no definitive consensus that double-bundle reconstruction effectively prevents the development of osteoarthritis. However, it is known that the double-bundle technique and concept better restores native kinematics, and future long-term studies may potentially reveal a difference.

Indications

There are no absolute indications established for double-bundle reconstruction; however, the important factors that indicate a patient for double-bundle reconstruction include the following:

- Tear patterns include a 2-bundle complete tear, partial tears of both bundles with poor tissue integrity or laxity, and 1 bundle completely torn with other bundle partially torn with incompetent tissue.
- Native footprint size: A tibial insertion size greater than 18 mm indicates a patient for double-bundle reconstruction because, otherwise, single-bundle reconstruction will likely not restore a sufficient portion of the native ACL.

Sgaglione NA, Lubowitz JH, Provencher MT, eds. *The Knee: AANA Advanced Arthroscopic Surgical Techniques* (pp 355-371).

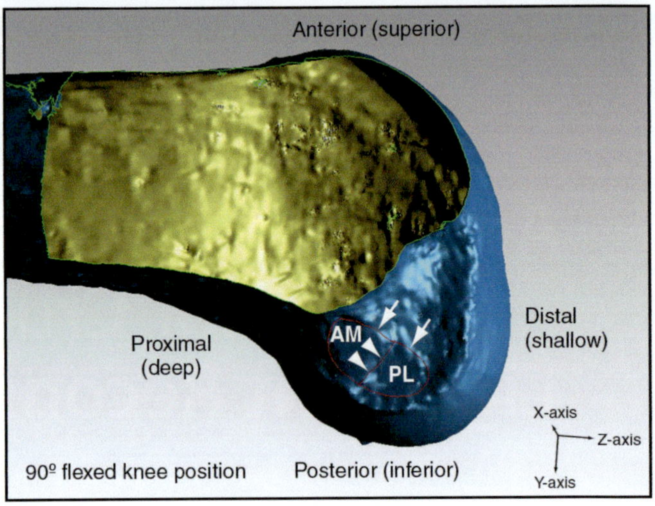

Figure 26-1. The anatomical relationship of the anteromedial (AM) and posterolateral (PL) bundles at 90 degrees of flexion. Lateral intercondylar ridge is double arrow; and bifurcate ridge is double arrowhead.

Controversial Indications

Controversial indications for double-bundle reconstruction may arise when native insertion site measurements fall between 14 and 18 mm. In this case, double-bundle surgery is indicated depending on other parameters, such as notch morphology. A narrow notch may provide ideal drilling only for single-bundle placement, although a notch morphology that can house drilling sufficient for 2 grafts may provide enough area for double-bundle placement.

Contraindications

Relative contraindications for double-bundle ACL reconstruction include the following[5]:

- ACL tibial insertion size less than 14 mm (better suited for anatomic single-bundle reconstruction)
- Open physes
- Severe bone bruising over the lateral femoral condyle due to risk of possible fracture
- Narrow (< 14 mm) or shallow notch (< 14 mm) can lead to inability to appropriately drill femoral tunnels and cause impingement, respectively
- Severe arthritic changes (grade 3 or greater)
- Multiligamentous injuries (due to likely need for other tunnels and risk of tunnel convergence/overlap and associated fracture risk)

Anatomy

The ACL originates from the medial aspect of the lateral femoral condyle (femoral origin) and inserts between the medial and lateral tibial spines (tibial insertion site). To remain consistent, this chapter refers to positional relationships with the knee located in the anatomic position or full knee extension. Arthroscopic evaluation of the ACL typically occurs with the knee flexed to 90 degrees (Figure 26-1). For this reason, the anatomically anterior border of the ACL will appear arthroscopically as the superior border. Similarly, the anatomically posterior extent of the ACL will appear as the arthroscopic inferior border when the knee is flexed to 90 degrees (see Figure 26-1).

The femoral insertion site or ACL origin is located at the posterior aspect of the medial wall of the lateral femoral condyle. The length of the femoral footprint of the ACL is 17.7 ± 1.2 mm, and the width is 9.9 ± 0.8 mm. The surface of the origin of the 2 bundles is not flat, and there is variable slope of each origin. The femoral attachment of the anteromedial bundle forms an angle with the posterolateral bundle of 27.6 ± 8.8 degrees. The average length of the femoral anteromedial bundle is 9.8 ± 0.8 mm, and the average length of the femoral posterolateral bundle is 7.3 ± 0.5 mm. The anatomically anterior (arthroscopically superior) border of the femoral origin of the ACL is defined by an important bony landmark referred to as the lateral intercondylar ridge (see Figure 26-1). The lateral bifurcate ridge, another important osseous landmark, delineates the anteromedial and posterolateral insertion areas, with the anteromedial proximal and posterolateral distal to this landmark. Ferretti et al[6] arthroscopically visualized the lateral bifurcate ridge in 81% of patients undergoing ACL reconstruction, with variable prominence of the ridge.

In its midportion, the ACL tapers to a thinner diameter, similar to an hourglass shape. The cross-sectional area of the insertion sites are 3 to 3.5 times larger than the cross-sectional area of the ligament's midsubstance.[7] The ACL fibers fan out and insert on the center of the tibial plateau, between the tibial spines consistent with their 2 given names: anteromedial and posterolateral bundles. The length of the tibial insertion site and its area has been described with tremendous variability across studies; the authors feel that is due to varying measurement and dissection techniques in addition to use of cadaveric specimen of varying ages. The authors recognize that there is patient-to-patient variability, and they have found the length of the tibial insertion site to range from 9 to 25 mm, with the majority between 14 and 18 mm.[8] It is important to realize that the course of the anteromedial and posterolateral bundles is distinct. This is evident from the embryological stage, with fetal anatomical and histological studies demonstrating the 2 bundles and a septum between the bundles.[9] The bundles are parallel near full extension but have different orientations as the knee approaches 90 degrees of flexion (Figure 26-2).[10]

Cadaveric study has shown that the length of each bundle changes throughout the arc of flexion-extension, with the bundles being longer toward extension as opposed to 90 degrees of flexion (see Figure 26-2). Therefore, avoidance of overconstraint of the knee in reconstruction is one reason the bundles should be tensioned in 0 and 20 to 30 degrees for the posterolateral and anteromedial bundles, respectively.

Biomechanics

The anteromedial bundle functions more to limit anteroposterior (AP) translation, and the posterolateral more so facilitates rotation within a controlled range.[11] In addition, many studies have tried to describe the exact functional role of the anteromedial and posterolateral bundles in terms of AP translation. A recent study evaluated in vivo kinematics of the anteromedial and posterolateral bundles. Fifteen knees were examined sequentially during surgery before reconstruction, after fixation of the posterolateral bundle, and after fixation of the posterolateral and anteromedial bundles.[12] They discovered that isolated posterolateral bundle reconstruction improved AP and rotational laxity and that the addition of the anteromedial bundle further improved laxity parameters.[12]

The anteromedial and posterolateral bundles do not remain isometric throughout a full functional range of motion (ROM).[10] Each bundle of native ACL is exposed to varying degrees of tension at various flexion angles. The anteromedial bundle is slightly more isometric than the posterolateral bundle, remaining taut throughout a greater ROM. In contrast, the posterolateral bundle is taut with the knee in extension and is lax when the knee is flexed. Logically, the contribution of the posterolateral bundle to knee stability becomes increasingly important under greater degrees of tension or near full extension.[13-15]

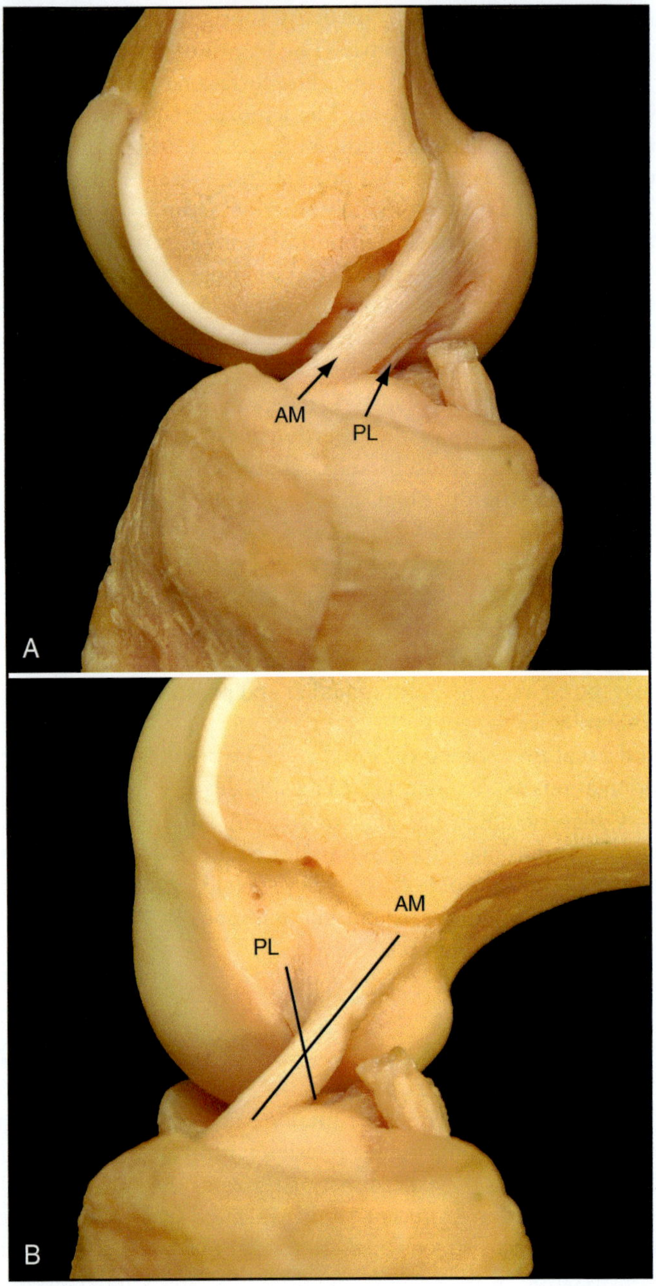

Figure 26-2. (A) Cadaveric knee specimen in full extension. (B) Cadaveric knee specimen in flexion. AM, anteromedial; PL, posterolateral.

Patient History

Before understanding double-bundle ACL reconstruction indications, a surgeon must know when to recommend ACL surgery in general. To master the indications, the provider must take a thorough history and perform a physical examination. It is important for the physician to inquire about the mechanism of injury and consider all possible associated pathologies. While obtaining the history and physical examination listen for key words such as pop, pivot, and swelling, which are commonly reported with ACL rupture.[16]

Distinguishing acute from chronic ACL injury is important because of the increased likelihood of associated injuries in the chronic setting. Acute cases typically present with a clear mechanism of injury and reported symptoms, whereas chronic cases can present with great variability in complaints due to secondary injuries or may present with recurrent instability. Recurrent instability or giving way associated with pain and/or limitation of activity and sports typically leads to presentation in chronic cases. Secondary injury in chronic cases may include meniscal tear (usually medial) or cartilage damage, leading to further pain and complaints.

Different injury mechanisms place varying strains on the anteromedial and posterolateral bundles that manifest as various, documented rupture patterns (Figure 26-3). Two distinct injury mechanisms of the ACL have been classically described by Muller et al,[17] including hyperextension trauma with resultant stretch of the ACL over the anterior intercondylar notch roof and moderate extension trauma, during which the anteromedial bundle is taut and a valgus and/or external rotation force is applied. Based on the variable tension patterns exhibited at different positions of knee flexion, the authors have seen various 2-bundle injury patterns and isolated anteromedial or isolated posterolateral bundle injuries. Isolated posterolateral bundle injury occurs when stress is applied at or near full extension. In greater degrees of flexion (30 to 60 degrees), isolated anteromedial bundle injury can occur (see Figure 26-3).

During surgery, the authors recommend detailed dissection of the remnant ACL as an important first step prior to proceeding with the reconstructive portion of ACL surgery due to the prevalence of partial tears to the ACL during injury. Zantop et al[18] studied 121 consecutive patients and found that 25% of patients had partial tears, with 12% having no injury to the posterolateral bundle. The other 75% had complete tears of both bundles. Single-bundle augmentation is performed when appropriate according to the specific injury pattern.[19] Preservation of intact native tissue has distinct advantages, including preservation of the microvasculature and proprioceptive fibers. Isolated reconstruction of the anteromedial or posterolateral bundle alone requires an awareness of such injury patterns and more precise pre- and intraoperative diagnostic assessment of the injury pattern to equip physicians with the proper knowledge to approach surgery.

Pertinent Physical Findings

Mastery of the physical examination is important. Acutely, the physician should do the following:

- Inspect for any effusion or swelling around the knee followed by palpation of the joint for tenderness.
- Evaluate active and passive ROM with palpation to assess for the presence of loose bodies.
- Evaluate for associated ligamentous or meniscal injury.
- Begin the clinical evaluation by observing the gait pattern and overall limb alignment.
- Compare all examination aspects to the contralateral (healthy) knee.
- For assessment of ACL integrity, the pertinent tests to master are the Lachman, anterior drawer, and pivot shift tests.
- The pivot shift test is the most specific but may be limited in the acute setting due to guarding and should be avoided if displaced meniscal tear is suspected.
- At the authors' institution, they also use the KT-2000 for additional objective analysis.

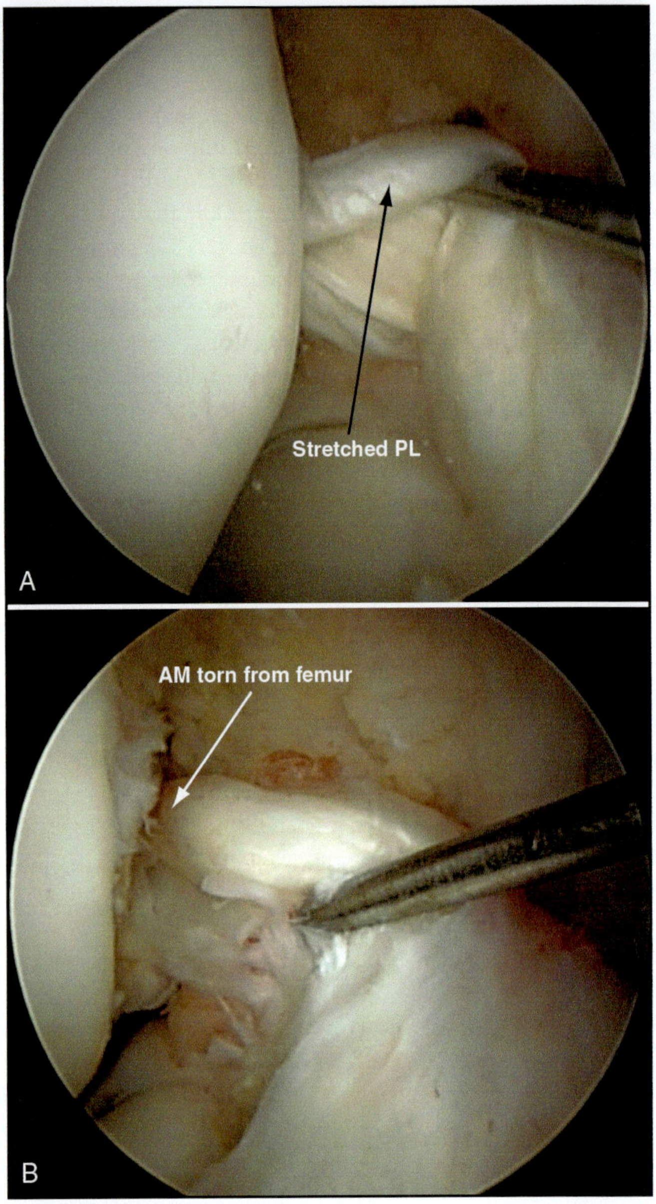

Figure 26-3. (A, B) Rupture pattern due to hyperextension and moderate extension trauma. AM, anteromedial; PL, posterolateral.

Pertinent Imaging

X-Rays

- The physician should first order plain x-rays.
- The authors' recommended sequence includes flexion weightbearing PA (both knees), flexion lateral, and Merchant views (both knees) to evaluate for fracture or other osseous abnormality.
- In most cases of acute ACL injury, the x-ray will be negative, but it is still necessary to obtain it.
- Plain x-rays allow the surgeon to evaluate for malalignment, joint space narrowing, and other signs of early degenerative arthritis.

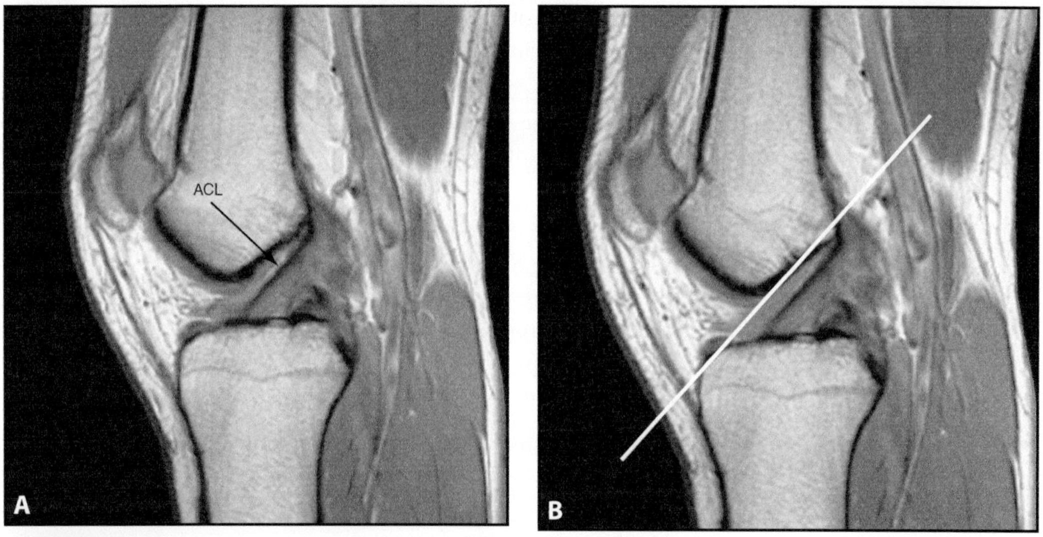

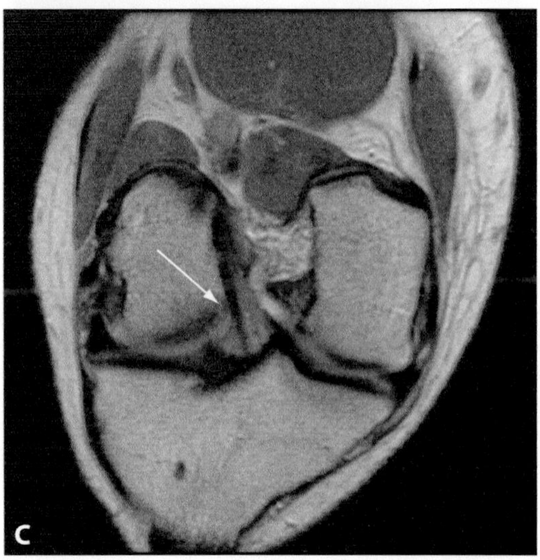

Figure 26-4. (A) Coronal. (B) Sagittal. (C) Coronal oblique, which is taken in coronal oblique plane consistent with white line seen in B.

- The Segond fracture, or lateral tibial rim avulsion of the meniscotibial ligament, is considered pathognomonic for ACL injury and should be screened as well.
- In the chronic setting or revision cases, long-cassette limb alignment studies are also useful to determine if any significant malalignment is associated with recurrent instability.

Advanced Imaging

The most important imaging modality is magnetic resonance imaging (MRI), which is highly sensitive for evaluating tears.

- High-resolution MRI with dedicated ACL sequences greatly increases the sensitivity.
- Standard MRI protocols consist of sagittal, coronal, and axial T1- and T2-weighted images.
- With standard basic protocols, it can be difficult to evaluate both functional bundles, so the authors recommend using special MRI protocols that also include sagittal oblique and coronal oblique imaging (Figure 26-4). These additional sequences help to clearly delineate both bundles by viewing them in the plane of the ACL fibers, providing greater detail.[20]

- These sequences improve specificity and sensitivity of evaluating complete and partial tears.[21] The surgeon should also evaluate for associated ligament, cartilage, or meniscal injury and bone bruise patterns.
- From the MRI, preparation to individualize the surgery can be achieved by measuring the ACL insertion site size, ACL length, ACL angle, and the quadriceps and patellar tendon size for graft possibilities.
- The general patient population insertion site size tends to be between 9 and 18 mm.[8]
- Because each patient's anatomy is different and varies on a spectrum, these measurements allow the physician to predict the appropriate intraoperative decisions best suited for the anatomically placed ACL and estimate the appropriate graft size.[20,22]
- In revision cases, computed tomography (CT) scan is valuable to help determine tunnel placement and the proper measurements needed for preoperative planning.[23,24]
- The authors also obtain 3-dimensional reconstructions of these CT scans when performed and find them helpful in planning and explaining findings to the patient (see Figure 26-4).

Equipment

- Articulated bed (with foot piece that can flex sufficiently to allow knee flexion to at least 120 degrees)
- Well-leg holder and arthroscopic limb holder
- Well-padded tourniquet
- 30-degree arthroscope
- Malleable arthroscopic ruler
- Standard knee arthroscopic ACL instrumentation
- ACL tip guide
- Flexible and straight guide wires and reamers/drills
- Heavy braided suture for graft passage
- Suspensory fixation devices (EndoButton; Smith & Nephew)
- Interference screw fixation devices (Biosure PK screws; Smith & Nephew)
- Mini C-arm for intraoperative fluoroscopy

Step-by-Step Description of the Procedure

Positioning and Examination Under Anesthesia

Various anesthesia options can be used, depending on anesthesiologist, patient, and surgeon preferences. These include general anesthesia with or without a regional nerve block or spinal anesthesia. In addition, when a regional nerve block is used with general anesthesia, it may be performed pre- or postoperatively. Once anesthesia has been induced, the first step is a thorough examination under anesthesia. The injured knee and contralateral normal knee are examined for ROM and laxity. A thorough knee examination is done to evaluate collateral, posterolateral corner ligament integrity, and posterior cruciate ligament status. Specific to the ACL, the authors perform the anterior drawer, Lachman, and pivot shift tests. The examination under anesthesia findings are compared to the measurements from the in-office examination. The pivot shift test

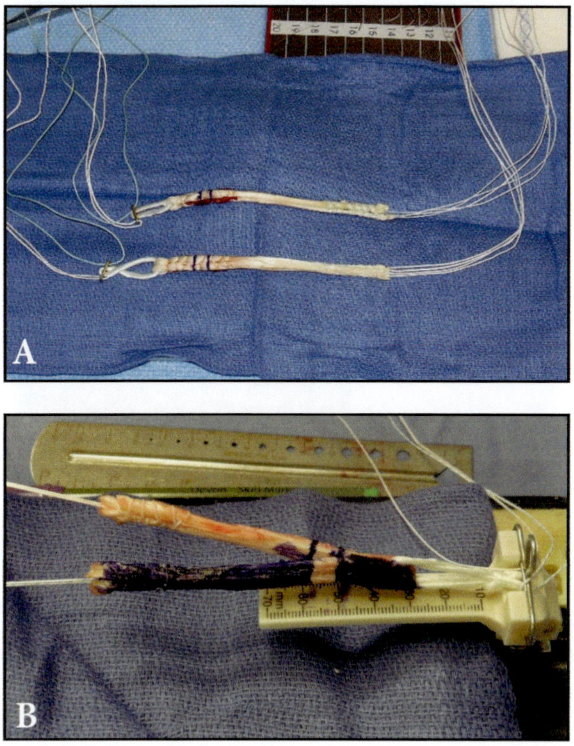

Figure 26-5. (A) Anteromedial and posterolateral bundle graft preparation. (B) Prepared quadriceps tendon graft with bone block.

is often better appreciated in the examination under anesthesia because there is no guarding and it is more sensitive.[25]

Once examination under anesthesia is performed, the supine patient is brought distally on the bed to the point where the knees are beyond the articulation in the bed where the foot portion will be flexed. This facilitates adequate maximal flexion to at least 120 degrees when the foot piece of the bed is maximally flexed. The nonoperative lower extremity is secured in a padded well-leg holder in the lithotomy position to safely facilitate access to the operative knee from the medial side. A well-padded tourniquet is applied in the proximal portion of the thigh of the operative extremity, and the extremity is secured in an arthroscopic leg holder with the post at the level of the tourniquet.

Graft Choice and Preparation

The graft options for double-bundle reconstruction fall into 2 main categories, including soft tissue and soft tissue with bone block. The authors use hamstring autograft or allograft for all soft tissue grafts (Figure 26-5). With the autograft, the authors typically use the semitendinosus graft doubled for the anteromedial bundle and the gracilis doubled (or tripled) for the posterolateral bundle. If the autograft size is inadequate, the surgeon should have allograft options readily available for supplementation and should discuss this possibility with the patient preoperatively. For the quadriceps with patellar bone block, the authors split the soft tissue portion for the 2 bundles and maintain the bone block for the femoral origin side.[26] The authors take preoperative measurements to ensure that the thickness of the quadriceps tendon and quality are appropriate for proper incorporation. They also measure patellar thickness and length to ensure it is large enough to accommodate bone block harvest with low risk of fracture (see Figure 26-5).

Various factors influence graft choice. The authors recommend autograft tissue in younger patients, especially those involved in high-risk sport/activity. The main limitation on autograft

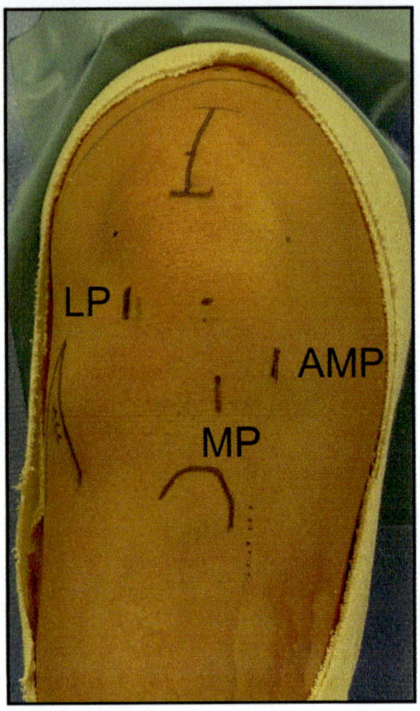

Figure 26-6. Three-portal placement of the knee. AMP, anteromedial portal; LP, lateral portal; MP, medial portal.

tissue is potential inadequate size. The surgeon should be prepared to supplement if necessary with all soft tissue grafts. The preoperative measurement of quadriceps tendon size, patellar thickness, and length from the MRI can help avoid that issue with the quadriceps harvest (see Figure 26-5). Allograft tissue has the advantage of having a predetermined size prior to incision and the possibility of prep before incision for efficiency. However, drawbacks include delayed vascularization, potential reaction or disease transmission, increased cost, and lack of availability/variable supply. The authors do not recommend allograft in younger patients (< 35 years) in high-risk sports with suitable autograft options.

The authors typically use the EndoButton continuous loop for suspensory femoral fixation (method detailed in the femoral fixation discussion), but several options are available. For the soft tissue grafts, the authors prepare both ends of each graft with #2 Ticron whip stitched sutures with appropriate tensioning throughout suturing. The portion of the graft to go within the femoral tunnel is sutured and marked at the appropriate depth for full seating and an additional 7 mm to allow for the EndoButton to totally exit the tunnel and flip. The tunnel must also be drilled to a depth at least 7 mm beyond the desired length of the graft in the tunnel to allow the EndoButton to flip. If the authors use a fibrin clot, it is sutured into the graft using resorbable nonbraided clear suture on the femoral side of the intra-articular portion of the graft.

Portal Placement and Diagnostic Arthroscopy

The order of graft harvest/preparation and diagnostic arthroscopy will depend on the surgeon's examination findings and graft choice.

Appropriate portal placement is critical in performing thorough diagnostic arthroscopy and for accurate tunnel placement/drilling. The authors use and recommend 3 portals for that reason (Figure 26-6).[27] The first portal is the lateral portal, which is more accurately a high lateral portal created above Hoffa's fat pad, and is created with an 11-blade scalpel. This high lateral portal will give a good overview of ACL anatomy within the notch. Subsequently, the central portal and accessory medial portal are created with 18-gauge needle localization under direct visualization. The central portal is adjacent to the patellar tendon on the medial edge or transpatellar at times in the distal one-third of the notch just above the joint line and intermeniscal ligament. The central portal facilitates looking straight at the ACL and both insertion sites and is also used for

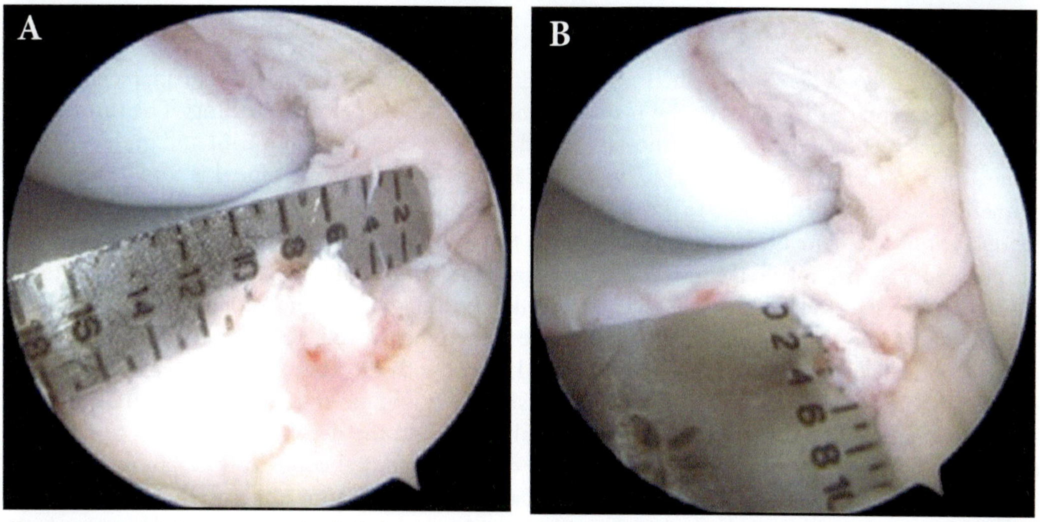

Figure 26-7. (A) Measurement of AP length of ACL tibial insertion (~ 18 mm in this patient, indicating double-bundle ACL reconstruction). (B) Measurement of the diameter of the posterolateral tibial insertion (7 mm in this patient).

measuring the ACL dimensions. The medial portal is created more medially above the joint line with a direct trajectory of the spinal needle to the ACL femoral origin. The medial portal should be slightly proximal to the central portal and should allow sufficient clearance of medial femoral condyle cartilage for passage of instruments to avoid iatrogenic cartilage injury. The medial portal is used for drilling femoral tunnels and for best viewing of the AP profile of the medial wall of the lateral femoral condyle. The portal size should also facilitate easy passage of the scope and necessary equipment without tissue trauma. All 3 knee compartments are examined in diagnostic arthroscopy to evaluate for associated injuries to cartilage or menisci and pathology addressed as indicated.

The ACL injury pattern is thoroughly evaluated because there is variability in ACL rupture patterns,[18] and this must be respected in determining reconstruction needs. All 3 portals are used to evaluate the origin and insertion sites of the ACL. The native femoral origin is best seen via the central and medial portals. Prior to preparing the medial wall of the lateral femoral condyle, any remaining soft tissue at the origin is carefully probed, and the outline of the soft tissue is preserved when using the arthroscopic shaver and radiofrequency thermal device (Arthrocare). The osseous landmarks are also examined and include the lateral intercondylar ridge and bifurcate ridge. Osseous and soft tissue landmarks are useful for determining the native origin site.[6,28] The tibial insertion site is best seen from the lateral portal, and appreciating the entire footprint for both bundles is critical to placement of the tunnels. Placing the leg in a figure-4 position can better demonstrate the posterior extent of the posterolateral bundle insertion, and a probe can be used when remnant tissue exists to facilitate visualization. When remnant tissue is present, the surgeon may sharply dissect the tissue to get a good overview of the entire footprint. The native ACL dimensions are measured with a malleable arthroscopic ruler (Smith & Nephew) and compared to the MRI measurements (Figure 26-7). The authors measure the entire ACL origin, insertion footprint, and individual bundles. Notch dimensions are also critical and are measured because a narrow notch (< 14 mm) will not facilitate drilling of 2 tunnels. The pre- and intraoperative data are used to determine final reconstruction technique respecting the double-bundle concept.

Tunnel Placement and Drilling

Once the femoral origin and tibial insertion site positions and dimensions are appreciated, the next step is to mark the center of the planned tunnels and then perform drilling. The tunnel size will vary between patients because they are based on the size of their footprint and graft size, but typically, the anteromedial tunnel is 7 to 8 mm and the posterolateral tunnel is 5 to 7 mm. The tunnel sizes are planned to be 1 to 2 mm smaller in diameter than the native bundle sizes to allow for an appropriate bone bridge of 2 mm between the 2 tunnels on the tibial and femoral sides.

The femoral posterolateral tunnel is created first. With the arthroscope in the central portal, a Steadman awl is introduced via the accessory medial portal and is advanced 3 mm into the center of the posterolateral bundle. A flexible guide wire is then introduced, seated in the pilot hole from the awl, and advanced through the lateral femoral cortex with the knee flexed. Knee hyperflexion in femoral tunnel drilling is more critical when using a straight pin to avoid posterior trajectory. A small incision is made at the wire exit over lateral thigh, and the depth gauge is used to measure the length from the lateral cortex to medial wall of lateral femoral condyle. The cannulated flexible reamer is then advanced over the guide wire approximately 7 mm more shallow than the full length of the guide wire in the bone to avoid lateral blow out, but the aim is to achieve at least 20 mm of graft depth in the tunnel. The EndoButton drill is used to perforate the lateral cortex for passage of the fixation device later on the femoral side.

The tibial tunnels are then created, with the posterolateral bundle being created first. A sharp vertical 3- to 4-cm incision is made over the proximal portion of the anteromedial tibia 2 cm below the joint line and 1 to 2 cm medial to the tibial tubercle. Full-thickness soft tissue flaps are created. The arthroscope is placed in the lateral portal, and an ACL tip guide set at 45 degrees is inserted into the joint through the medial portal and placed at the marked center of the posterolateral bundle. The tip guide drill sleeve is advanced until it is secured against the anteromedial cortex of the tibia, anterior to the superficial medial collateral ligament. The straight 3.2-mm guide wire is advanced to the center of the tip of the guide in the center of the bundle. Next, the guide is set at 55 degrees, and the tip is centered in the anteromedial bundle. Externally, the starting points are planned 2 cm apart so that both tibial tunnels maintain an adequate bony bridge on the tibial cortex. The drill sleeve is secured, and the guide wire is advanced to the center of the anteromedial bundle. Both guide pins are advanced further into the joint, and the knee is taken to full extension to ensure there is no impingement with the roof of the notch and planned graft–tunnel position. The tibial tunnels are then drilled over guide wires approximately 1 to 2 mm smaller than planned final size and sequentially dilated in 0.5-mm increments up to the final desired size.

The femoral anteromedial tunnel center is identified with the arthroscope viewing from the central portal, and the Steadman awl is used to make the pilot hole. Femoral anteromedial tunnel guide wire placement and reaming may take place through 3 sites (via the accessory medial portal, transtibially through the posterolateral tibial tunnel, or transtibially through the anteromedial portal). However, the authors have found that for true anatomic placement, the accessory medial portal will nearly always (> 95%) produce the desired starting point. Drilling the femoral anteromedial tunnel through the posterolateral tibial tunnel will work in some (~ 50%) cases, whereas it is rare (~ 10%) for the transtibial through the anteromedial tibial tunnel to work, and it runs the risk of creating a high femoral anteromedial tunnel. Whichever option is chosen, the most important factors are anatomic, divergent tunnels that maximize tunnel length. Dilation of the femoral tunnel to the desired diameter can then be performed, and an EndoButton drill bit is used to perforate lateral cortex for fixation device passage.

Graft Passage, Tensioning, and Fixation

Looped suture at the ends of the flexible drill guide wires or on the ends of a Beath pin are passed through the medial portal and up through the femoral posterolateral tunnel, and then the distal end is retrieved with a suture retriever through the tibial posterolateral tunnel. The same is done for the anteromedial tunnel with another looped suture. As an extra precaution, the authors typically use different colored sutures to facilitate keeping track of tunnels and grafts as a supplement to direct visualization. The posterolateral graft is the first reconstructed bundle that is passed and is secured on the femoral side. Once that is examined, the anteromedial bundle is passed. Appropriate position of the EndoButton fixation devices on the lateral cortex is confirmed visually by observing intra-articular graft position when tugging on each graft and also fluoroscopically to see the button seated on the lateral cortex. The grafts are cycled with tension if no fibrin clot was used. If a fibrin clot was used, the authors do not cycle the knee to avoid extrusion of the clot from within the grafts.

The tibial fixation of the posterolateral bundle is performed at 0 degrees, and the anteromedial bundle fixation is done at 20 to 30 degrees in keeping with their position of maximal tightness from biomechanical studies. The leg is placed on an adjustable-height Mayo stand for stability during tibial fixation. Various fixation devices may be used, such as interference screws, suture post cortical fixation, staples, etc. The authors prefer interference screw fixation for the tibial side and routinely use nonabsorbable biocompatible interference screws. The screw size should be the same as the tunnel diameter or 1 mm wider in diameter for good fit. Final arthroscopic inspection is performed to evaluate graft position, ensure there is no impingement at full extension, and probe the graft to confirm good tension. This final inspection of the graft uses the same principles emphasized throughout the case of carefully analyzing the femoral origin and tibial insertion sites and is done from all 3 portals for the best overview. Sterile dressings are applied after incision closure. A foot-to-thigh dressing for gentle compression and a cool pack are applied. Finally, a hinged knee brace locked in extension is applied.

Double-Bundle Anterior Cruciate Ligament Reconstruction With Quadriceps Tendon With Bone Block

The main differences between the authors' quadriceps tendon bone block technique and the all soft tissue graft technique are detailed later in this chapter. The femoral tunnel is created to respect the double-bundle concept; therefore, the center of the femoral tunnel is placed in the center of the entire ACL femoral footprint at the border between the anteromedial and posterolateral bundles at the bifurcate ridge (Figure 26-8).

The tibial tunnels are created next in the same fashion as described previously. The Beath pin with looped suture is passed through the femoral tunnel via the medial portal and is viewed from the lateral portal. The looped suture is used to shuttle passage sutures for the EndoButton that was prepared on bone block side of graft. The bone block prepared with the EndoButton is then passed through the medial portal, pulled into the femoral tunnel, and appropriately seated. The fixation device position on the lateral femoral cortex is confirmed per the previous fashion. The authors prepare their quadriceps tendon bone block grafts with the posterolateral bundle marked with blue ink for easy visualization. They ensure that the split soft tissue portions of the graft are appropriately oriented, with the posterolateral inked bundle more distal in the posterolateral region of the femoral origin for direct trajectory into posterolateral tunnel (see Figure 26-8).

The same goes for ensuring proper anatomic orientation of the anteromedial bundle, which is not marked with ink. The sutures for the posterolateral and anteromedial soft tissue portions of the graft are retrieved and pulled through the respective tibial tunnels. The posterolateral portion is passed first into the knee joint from the medial portal and then pulled down into the posterolateral tibial tunnel. Then, the anteromedial portion is pulled down into the anteromedial tibial tunnel. Tibial fixation is performed as previously described (Figure 26-9).

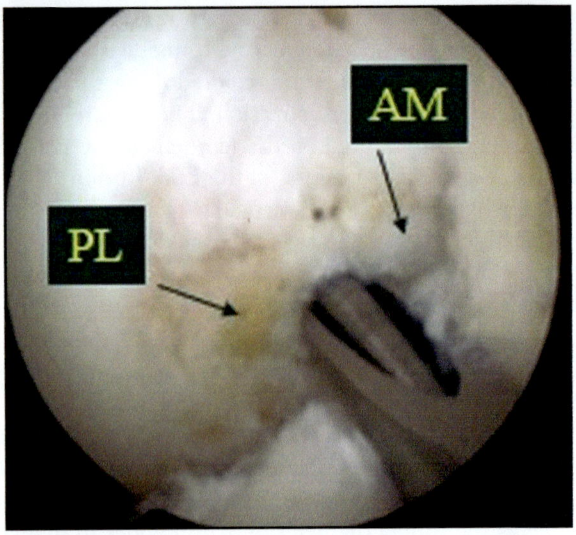

Figure 26-8. Femoral tunnel for quadriceps graft with a guide wire in the anatomic position between the 2 bundles to respect the double-bundle anatomic concept despite use of 1 tunnel on the femoral side. AM, anteromedial; PL, posterolateral.

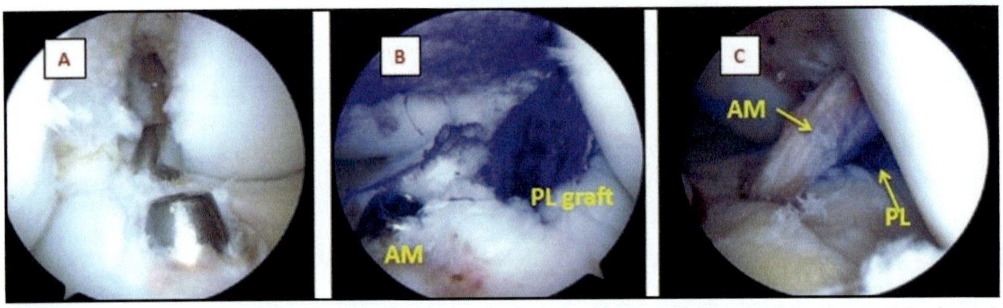

Figure 26-9. (A) View from the medial portal of a single femoral tunnel for bone block and 2 tibial tunnels with dilators in place. (B) Dilator in the anteromedial (AM) tunnel and posterolateral (PL) graft already passed. (C) Both bundles passed from the femoral bone block into their respective tibial tunnels in anatomic double-bundle positions. (B) and (C) are viewed from lateral portal.

Postoperative Protocol

The rehabilitation protocol for double-bundle ACL reconstruction is the same as for anatomic single-bundle ACL reconstructions. The brace remains locked in extension for the first 7 days for ambulation with crutches. If no meniscal repair was performed, the patient is allowed to bear weight with the brace and crutches immediately once the regional nerve block has worn off. The patient is instructed to perform heel slides and active isometric quadriceps strengthening starting on postoperative day 1. If available, a continuous passive motion machine is also used from the day of surgery starting at 0 to 45 degrees and is advanced 5 to 10 degrees daily as tolerated. By approximately 6 weeks, the patient is weaned off of the crutches and brace. Gradual progression through the phases of rehabilitation continues under the supervision of a therapist over the next several months. Initial emphasis in the first 3 months is on swelling control, ROM, and quadriceps strengthening, particularly with closed chain kinetic activities. After 3 months, noncutting, higher-intensity activity may commence if appropriate strength and motion are present. This may include straight-line jogging/running, cycling, and swimming. With good progress, controlled functional training may ensue with introduction of controlled cutting activities and more explosive work. Return to sports follows successful completion of functional testing and sport-specific training, with an emphasis on gradual return to sport activity in controlled training environments. If the patient successfully completes the aforementioned measures, full competitive participation is then allowed.

Typically, athletes return at approximately 9 ± 2 months. It can sometimes take up to 1 year for an athlete to be ready, and the authors emphasize the importance of avoiding premature return to minimize reinjury risk. An array of information factors into the decision to clear an athlete for return to sport and includes painless activity with no effusion, ligament stability on clinical examination, no concerning subjective reports, minimum 85% quadriceps strength vs the contralateral knee, and passing of the required functional tests. If there is any concern prior to return to sport or if the time for return to sport is earlier than typical, the authors do not hesitate to obtain an MRI to evaluate healing. Pertinent to the double-bundle reconstruction, the posterolateral bundle seems to demonstrate more prolonged increased signal intensity than the anteromedial bundle, so close attention needs to be given to the 2 bundles because they may potentially heal at different rates.[24] The clinical examination before clearance must include evaluation of AP and rotatory ligament integrity to evaluate the anteromedial and posterolateral bundles, respectively.

Potential Complications

Similar to single-bundle ACL reconstruction, double-bundle ACL reconstruction poses several risks to the patient. The most common risk is iatrogenic injury due to the provider's technical skill, tunnel placement resulting in flexion and extension issues, misdiagnosis, poor fixation, or mismanagement of preoperative preparation and postoperative protocol. Other less common complications include saphenous nerve injury, fibrosis, hardware failure, patellar failure, and wound infection.

Conclusion

Single-bundle reconstruction has served as the mainstay for ACL reconstruction surgery for decades, but with improved understanding of the native ACL anatomy and biomechanical function, more sophisticated techniques have been developed to restore normal kinematics and aim to potentially prevent the development of early osteoarthritis. Anatomic single-bundle reconstruction is one of these techniques, but in some patients with sufficiently large ACL footprints and ideal notch morphology, the double-bundle technique is needed to maximally restore the native anatomy. Although the anatomic double-bundle technique has not been widely adopted, early clinical and imaging evaluation is promising.[23,29,30]

To fully comprehend the double-bundle concept and technique, surgeons should have an intimate understanding of the native anatomy and measurements to appropriately understand when double-bundle ACL reconstruction may be indicated. More prospective randomized controlled trials are necessary to further evaluate the overall clinical benefit of double-bundle ACL reconstruction, but currently, early studies suggest improved kinematic function and have motivated future exploration.[31]

Top Technical Pearls for the Procedure

1. Portal placement: Use 3 portals. High lateral portal for viewing: Keep it high enough to avoid the Hoffa's fat pad and to give best overview of the entire ACL. Accessory medial portal: Optimal placement is under direct visualization above the meniscus, and allowing clearance from the medial femoral condyle for drilling is critical to avoiding iatrogenic injury.
2. Native footprint and measurements: It is critical to appreciate the native anatomy and know the dimensions of the native footprint to determine if a patient is indicated appropriately for double-bundle reconstruction. Use osseous and soft tissue landmarks when available as a guide. Notch morphology and dimensions are also a key component.
3. Tunnels: Maintain an appropriate bony bridge between tunnels.
4. Graft size: Be prepared to supplement soft tissue autografts with allograft if necessary and discuss this beforehand with the patient.
5. Graft passage and fixation: Mark the posterolateral bundle with ink so that it is distinguishable. Pass the posterolateral bundle first, then the anteromedial bundle. Respect the biomechanical function of the 2 bundles by fixing the posterolateral bundle at 0 degrees and the anteromedial bundle at 20 to 30 degrees of flexion.

References

1. Gianotti SM, Marshall SW, Hume PA, Bunt L. Incidence of anterior cruciate ligament injury and other knee ligament injuries: a national population-based study. *J Sci Med Sport.* 2009;12(6):622-627.
2. Hootman JM, Dick R, Agel J. Epidemiology of collegiate injuries for 15 sports: summary and recommendations for injury prevention initiatives. *J Athl Train.* 2007;42(2):311-319.
3. Agel J, Arendt EA, Bershadsky B. Anterior cruciate ligament injury in national collegiate athletic association basketball and soccer: a 13-year review. *Am J Sports Med.* 2005;33(4):524-530.
4. Murawski CD, van Eck CF, Irrgang JJ, Tashman S, Fu FH. Operative treatment of primary anterior cruciate ligament rupture in adults. *J Bone Joint Surg Am.* 2014;96(8):685-694.
5. Muller B, Hofbauer M, Wongcharoenwatana J, Fu FH. Indications and contraindications for double-bundle ACL reconstruction. *Int Orthop.* 2013;37(2):239-246.
6. Ferretti M, Ekdahl M, Shen W, Fu FH. Osseous landmarks of the femoral attachment of the anterior cruciate ligament: an anatomic study. *Arthroscopy.* 2007;23(11):1218-1225.
7. Harner CD, Baek GH, Vogrin TM, Carlin GJ, Kashiwaguchi S, Woo SL. Quantitative analysis of human cruciate ligament insertions. *Arthroscopy.* 1999;15(7):741-749.
8. Kopf S, Musahl V, Tashman S, Szczodry M, Shen W, Fu FH. A systematic review of the femoral origin and tibial insertion morphology of the ACL. *Knee Surg Sports Traumatol Arthrosc.* 2009;17(3):213-219.
9. Ferretti M, Levicoff EA, Macpherson TA, Moreland MS, Cohen M, Fu FH. The fetal anterior cruciate ligament: an anatomic and histologic study. *Arthroscopy.* 2007;23(3):278-283.
10. Wang JH, Kato Y, Ingham SJ, et al. Measurement of the end-to-end distances between the femoral and tibial insertion sites of the anterior cruciate ligament during knee flexion and with rotational torque. *Arthroscopy.* 2012;28(10):1524-1532.
11. Amis AA. The functions of the fibre bundles of the anterior cruciate ligament in anterior drawer, rotational laxity and the pivot shift. *Knee Surg Sports Traumatol Arthrosc.* 2012;20(4):613-620.
12. Kopf S, Musahl V, Bignozzi S, Irrgang JJ, Zaffagnini S, Fu FH. In vivo kinematic evaluation of anatomic double-bundle anterior cruciate ligament reconstruction. *Am J Sports Med.* 2014;42(9):2172-2177.
13. Buoncristiani AM, Tjoumakaris FP, Starman JS, Ferretti M, Fu FH. Anatomic double-bundle anterior cruciate ligament reconstruction. *Arthroscopy.* 2006;22(9):1000-1006.

14. Gabriel MT, Wong EK, Woo SL, Yagi M, Debski RE. Distribution of in situ forces in the anterior cruciate ligament in response to rotatory loads. *J Orthop Res.* 2004;22(1):85-89.
15. Sakane M, Fox RJ, Woo SL, Livesay GA, Li G, Fu FH. In situ forces in the anterior cruciate ligament and its bundles in response to anterior tibial loads. *J Orthop Res.* 1997;15(2):285-293.
16. Wagemakers HP, Luijsterburg PA, Boks SS, et al. Diagnostic accuracy of history taking and physical examination for assessing anterior cruciate ligament lesions of the knee in primary care. *Arch Phys Med Rehabil.* 2010;91(9):1452-1459.
17. Muller W. *Form, Function, and Ligament Reconstruction.* Berlin, Germany: Springer; 1982.
18. Zantop T, Brucker PU, Vidal A, Zelle BA, Fu FH. Intraarticular rupture pattern of the ACL. *Clin Orthop Relat Res.* 2007;(454):48-53.
19. Siebold R, Fu FH. Assessment and augmentation of symptomatic anteromedial or posterolateral bundle tears of the anterior cruciate ligament. *Arthroscopy.* 2008;24(11):1289-1298.
20. Araujo P, van Eck CF, Torabi M, Fu FH. How to optimize the use of MRI in anatomic ACL reconstruction. *Knee Surg Sports Traumatol Arthrosc.* 2013;21(7):1495-1501.
21. Starman JS, Vanbeek C, Armfield DR, et al. Assessment of normal ACL double bundle anatomy in standard viewing planes by magnetic resonance imaging. *Knee Surg Sports Traumatol Arthrosc.* 2007;15(5):493-499.
22. Hofbauer M, Muller B, Murawski CD, van Eck CF, Fu FH. The concept of individualized anatomic anterior cruciate ligament (ACL) reconstruction. *Knee Surg Sports Traumatol Arthrosc.* 2014;22(5):979-986.
23. Basdekis G, Christel P, Anne F. Validation of the position of the femoral tunnels in anatomic double-bundle ACL reconstruction with 3-D CT scan. *Knee Surg Sports Traumatol Arthrosc.* 2009;17(9):1089-1094.
24. Miyawaki M, Hensler D, Illingworth KD, Irrgang JJ, Fu FH. Signal intensity on magnetic resonance imaging after allograft double-bundle anterior cruciate ligament reconstruction. *Knee Surg Sports Traumatol Arthrosc.* 2014;22:1002-1008.
25. Donaldson WF III, Warren RF, Wickiewicz T. A comparison of acute anterior cruciate ligament examinations. Initial versus examination under anesthesia. *Am J Sports Med.* 1985;13(1):5-10.
26. Rabuck SJ, Musahl V, Fu FH, West RV. Anatomic anterior cruciate ligament reconstruction with quadriceps tendon autograft. *Clin Sports Med.* 2013;32(1):155-164.
27. Araujo PH, van Eck CF, Macalena JA, Fu FH. Advances in the three-portal technique for anatomical single- or double-bundle ACL reconstruction. *Knee Surg Sports Traumatol Arthrosc.* 2011;19(8):1239-1242.
28. Tsukada S, Fujishiro H, Watanabe K, et al. Anatomic variations of the lateral intercondylar ridge: relationship to the anterior margin of the anterior cruciate ligament. *Am J Sports Med.* 2014;42(5):1110-1117.
29. Sun R, Chen BC, Wang F, Wang XF, Chen JQ. Prospective randomized comparison of knee stability and joint degeneration for double- and single-bundle ACL reconstruction [published online ahead of print March 22, 2014]. *Knee Surg Sports Traumatol Arthrosc.*
30. Zaffagnini S, Bruni D, Marcheggiani Muccioli GM, et al. Single-bundle patellar tendon versus non-anatomical double-bundle hamstrings ACL reconstruction: a prospective randomized study at 8-year minimum follow-up. *Knee Surg Sports Traumatol Arthrosc.* 2011;19(3):390-397.
31. Irrgang JJ, Tashman S, Moore C, Fu FH. Challenge accepted: description of an ongoing NIH-funded randomized clinical trial to compare anatomic single-bundle versus anatomic double-bundle ACL reconstruction. *Arthroscopy.* 2012;28(6):745-747.

Please see videos on the accompanying website at www.routledge.com/9781617119996

27

Arthroscopic All-Inside Anterior Cruciate Ligament Reconstruction

Patrick A. Smith, MD

Introduction

All-inside anterior cruciate ligament (ACL) reconstruction was first described in 1995 by Morgan.[1] Initially, the procedure was performed using a bone-hamstring-bone composite graft and was fixated with metal interference screws. Subsequently, in 2006, Lubowitz[2] published a technical note on no-tunnel all-inside ACL reconstruction based on drilling the femoral and tibial sockets transtibially with use of the RetroCutter (Arthrex). The RetroCutter is a proprietary device that serves as a retroreamer (Figure 27-1). It consists of a specialized, cannulated guide pin that is drilled into the joint from a small tibial skin incision capturing the RetroCutter, which is reverse threaded on its guide. Drilling in forward, the socket is reamed to the desired depth, preserving the tibial cortex. Then, the RetroCutter is brought back in the joint and the drill reversely engages the RetroCutter back onto the guide for removal from the joint. Fixation with the Lubowitz technique was accomplished by an absorbable RetroScrew (Arthrex) interference screw for the femur and an absorbable RetroScrew placed at the aperture of the tibial socket from inside the joint with the Retro Screwdriver (Arthrex) that was cannulated to allow passage of a suture to pull the screw onto the driver to then be secured against the graft. In 2007, Smith[3] described a modification of Lubowitz's technique, drilling the femoral socket through the anteromedial portal with absorbable TransFix (Arthrex) cross-pin fixation. One inherent advantage of this change for the single-bundle all-inside approach relates to drilling the femoral socket through the anteromedial portal because many studies have shown better localization of the femoral socket through anteromedial portal drilling as opposed to transtibial femoral drilling, particularly to avoid vertical graft placement.[4-7] This procedure was soon modified for a double-bundle construct.[8]

The next development in the evolution of all-inside ACL reconstruction is related to the FlipCutter (Arthrex; Figure 27-2). The FlipCutter is a pin and reamer in 1 unit; the 3.5-mm pin is drilled in the desired center of the socket and, then, with a simple mechanism, is flipped to become a reamer. After completing the reaming process, it is reflipped for removal and a suture is passed through the pin tract for later graft passage. In essence, this unique device replicated drilling the femoral socket like a 2-incision outside-in approach.[9,10] It also represents an alternative to

Sgaglione NA, Lubowitz JH, Provencher MT, eds. *The Knee: AANA Advanced Arthroscopic Surgical Techniques* (pp 373-388).

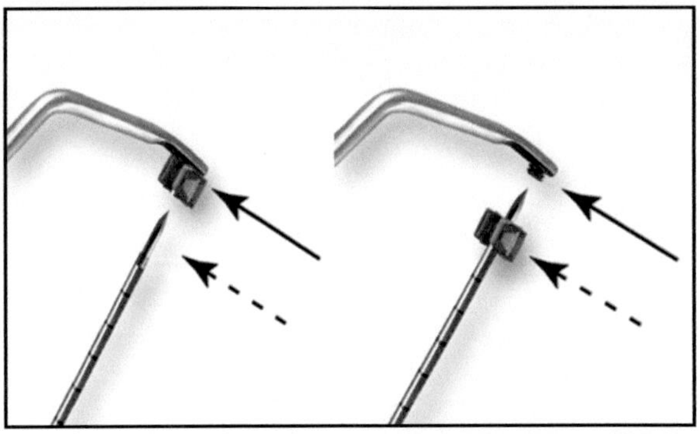

Figure 27-1. The RetroCutter is reverse threaded on the guide, and when the RetroCutter guide pin (Arthrex) is drilled in forward, the threads on this pin engage the RetroCutter and it becomes threaded on the pin to perform the retroreaming. The process to deliver the RetroCutter back on the guide occurs with drilling the pin back through the guide and then reversing the drill.

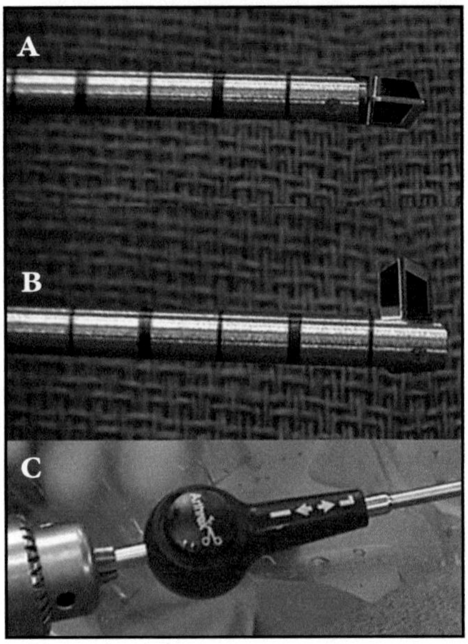

Figure 27-2. The FlipCutter is a unique pin reamer. When the blue trigger (C) is squeezed and pushed forward, the drill pin is flipped for reaming (B). Squeezing and sliding the trigger the other way unflips it for removal as a simple pin (A) after reaming.

drilling the femoral socket from the anteromedial portal, which can be challenging, particularly because it allows drilling the femoral socket at 90 degrees of knee flexion for easy arthroscopic visualization.[6] The FlipCutter has a special guide sleeve that is malleted 7 mm into the cortex prior to reaming the socket, which ensures this amount of bone bridge for suspensory cortical fixation as the reamer is stopped at this point as the socket is retroreamed. The FlipCutter is also used to create the tibial socket, and specific centering guides (Arthrex) are available for both the femur and tibia.

The final technological step in facilitating progression of the all-inside technique to the GraftLink related to the development of the TightRope (Arthrex), which allows for suspensory cortical fixation (Figure 27-3). The TightRope is an adjustable continuous loop device. It is based on a proprietary suture loop construct with a #5 polyethylene suture spliced on itself to create 2 shortening strands that, when tightened, provide fixation against a metal button suspended on the femoral or tibial cortex. The shortening sutures can be threaded either way through the button. The TightRope Reverse Tensioning (RT) device is preferred; RT refers to the direction the white shortening sutures are pulled, which can be used on the femur or the tibia. The TightRope button is 3-by-12 mm in dimension. It passes through a 3.5-mm hole via an attached blue #2 FiberWire passing suture (Arthrex) and is self-flipping. There is also a TightRope Attachable Button System (ABS) (Arthrex) construct, which consists of a 2-holed cortical button 12 mm long and 8 mm wide that can be attached to the loop of a No Button TightRope (Arthrex) to create the TightRope

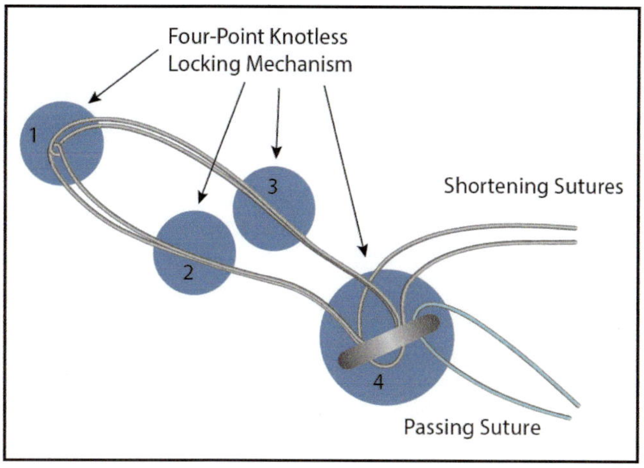

Figure 27-3. The TightRope device consists of a #5 polyethylene suture spliced onto itself and passed through a 12-by-3-mm button. It has 4 points of fixation. As the shortening loops are pulled in an alternating fashion, the graft positioned in the loop between the button and the point marked 1 will be compressed between the 2 spliced limbs marked 2 and 3. Fixation also occurs between 1 and the suture limb 4 through the button, which is suspended on the cortex as the loop is tightened.

mechanism—commonly done on the tibial side—and then the loop is shortened to this button for fixation. There are 4 points of fixation, including 2 points of friction where the suture is spliced, 2 linked loops that are interconnected, and suture against the eyelet of the button (Figure 27-3).

TightRope suspensory cortical fixation has been studied biomechanically. Petre et al[11] showed that the ultimate failure strength of the TightRope fixation device on the femur was 859 N tested in porcine bone with 2.74 mm of cyclic displacement after 1000 cycles. They concluded that the TightRope possessed the necessary biomechanical properties for soft tissue femoral fixation for ACL reconstruction. Smith and DeBerardino[12] compared the strength of the TightRope in a continuous loop GraftLink construct to interference screw fixation on the tibia in porcine bone. They found that average ultimate load to failure of tibial suspensory fixation for the all-inside GraftLink continuous loop construct was 1012 N, which was significantly different compared to the tibial interference screw group at 612 N ($P < .001$). The stiffness of the continuous loop construct at 165 N/mm and cyclic displacement of 2.5 mm was not statistically significant compared to the interference group (193 N/mm and 1.9 mm, respectively).[12] They concluded that tibial fixation of the TightRope was satisfactory for the normal loads placed on the ACL with activities of daily living.[13-17]

The GraftLink construct refers to single soft tissue tendon—commonly a semitendinosus autograft—quadrupled and linked together by sutures on each end of a TightRope loop (Figure 27-4).[18] It is created by placing a TightRope RT loop on one end (for the femur) of a graft prep station and a TightRope RT or a No Button TightRope loop on the other end (for the tibia). A semitendinosus tendon is passed through the tibial TightRope loop first, and then the 2 free ends are passed through the TightRope RT loop on the femoral end in opposite directions. The 2 free ends are then sutured together with a #0 TigerLoop (Arthrex) suture in a SpeedWhip pattern, and this suture is used to bury the free tissue ends of the graft on the inside of the outer graft loop on the tibial side to create a quadrupled construct.[19] The graft is placed under tension, and then 4 #0 FiberWire (Arthrex) sutures are placed on each end of the construct passing the needle through all 4 tendons and then wrapping each suture end around the 4 tendons prior to tying the knot, thereby securely incorporating all 4 loops for linkage. The author routinely leaves in place the 2 free 0 TigerLoop sutures on the tibial side used to initially suture the graft ends together so he can tie them later to the tibial button for backup fixation here. Graft preparation is shown in the surgery video.

In all-inside ACL reconstruction, it is essential that the depth of socket creation for the femur and tibia, along with the intra-articular ACL distance, is greater than the final graft length. This is critical so the graft does not bottom out in the sockets because, otherwise, it would be lax. The author routinely uses an intra-articular measuring device (Arthrex) to determine the ACL

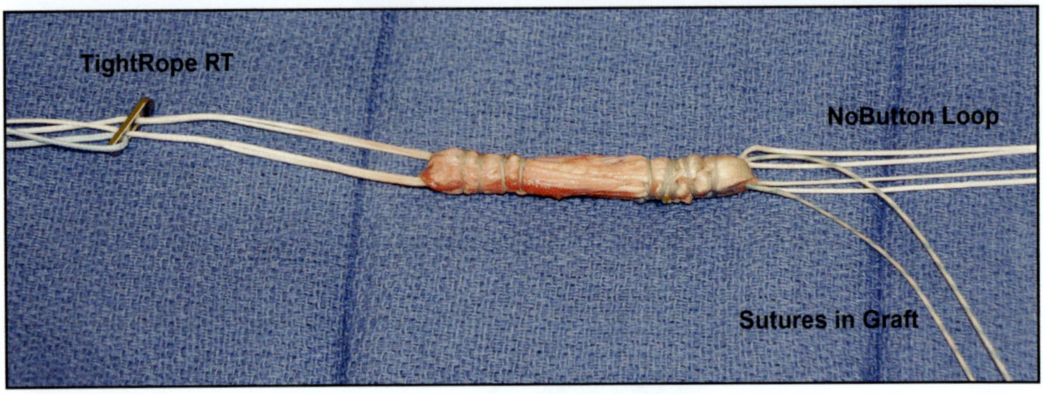

Figure 27-4. A final GraftLink construct with a TightRope RT loop on one end and a No Button loop on the other end. Note the two 0 TigerLoop sutures free on the tibial side, which represents the suture that attached the 2 free tendon ends here to complete the quadrupling of the graft. They will be incorporated with the tibial button to be tied here for backup fixation.

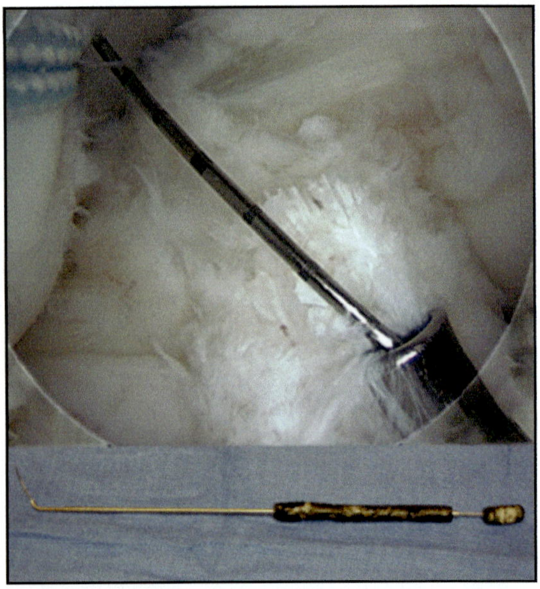

Figure 27-5. The intra-articular measuring device has a small sliding ruler that retracts. Each mark is 2 mm from the bulb tip placed at the femoral socket aperture, and the curve at the base, which is placed at the tibial socket site, represents 7 mm of distance. This a right knee viewing from the anterolateral portal with the device placed through the anteromedial portal.

distance, and the depth of reaming for the femoral and tibial sockets is easily known (Figure 27-5). It is the author's approach to overream the tibia by 5 mm to allow for adequate graft tensioning, which ensures the graft will not be too long. Typically, his graft lengths are a minimum of 63 mm and a maximum of 75 mm in length, whereas the intra-articular distance is usually in the range of 23 to 26 mm. Generally, he then has at least 20 mm of graft in both the femoral and tibial sockets.

All-Inside Advantages

Less postoperative pain is an evidence-based advantage of all-inside ACL reconstruction. This was shown first in a Level 1 randomized controlled trial with allograft comparing all-inside reconstruction to a full tibial tunnel.[20] It was then proven again using semitendinosus autograft with the GraftLink technique.[21] Given the trend for outpatient surgery and accelerated rehabilitation after ACL reconstruction, less postoperative pain is an advantage for patients.

All-inside ACL reconstruction is suitable for any patient deemed an appropriate surgical candidate because it is flexible from the standpoint of graft selection. At this time, the author's preferred graft is a semitendinosus autograft harvested through a small popliteal incision.[22] A recent study of 60 of the author's patients showed an average graft diameter of 9.0 mm and length of 70.3 mm with this minimally invasive, single-incision, posterior hamstring harvest technique.[23] Analyzed for sex, average female graft length was 68.1 mm with an average final graft diameter of 8.6 mm compared to grafts of 71.7 and 9.3 mm, respectively, in males. In both sexes, patient height and weight were strongly correlated to the final construct diameter ($r = 0.60$ and $r = 0.56$) and length ($r = 0.47$ and $r = 0.44$), respectively. Also, in this study, the amount of graft in the femoral socket averaged 22.4 and 23.7 mm in the tibial socket with the all-inside GraftLink technique.

Alternative grafts are amendable to the all-inside technique. Folding the tibial bone plug and suturing it to the tendon to shorten the length allows the patellar tendon bone-tendon-bone graft to be used in an all-inside reconstruction. Quadriceps tendon autografts (with or without bone) can be used with a technique of securing the tendinous ends to the TightRope loops. Soft tissue allografts also work well. In this chapter, the outside-in approach with the FlipCutter is described first with an allograft. The anteromedial portal approach is then done with a semitendinosus autograft. Instructive videos for both techniques are provided.

Indications

- ACL tears in active individuals with functional instability
- Any age is suitable because all-epiphyseal GraftLink can be done in children, avoiding the growth plates
- Autograft hamstring with quadrupled semitendinosus
- Soft tissue allograft quadrupled semitendinosus or anterior/posterior tibialis for larger graft
- Revision cases: Suspensory fixation on the femur and tibia facilitates fixation
- Most minimally invasive technique if pain is an issue for the patient

Pertinent Physical Findings

- Lachman test at 30 degrees of flexion (very sensitive for ACL tears)
- Pivot shift test: Indicative of the rotational instability from an ACL tear putting one at risk of giving way with twisting or pivoting activities (with sports and activities of daily living[24,25])
- Valgus and varus stress testing at 30 degrees of flexion (important to determine the need for associated extra-articular surgery)
- Dial test to rule out associated posterolateral corner instability

Pertinent Imaging

X-Rays

- Bilateral weightbearing anteroposterior views in full extension and posteroanterior Rosenberg views in flexion
- Lateral weightbearing of the affected knee

- Bilateral sunrise (Merchant) views
- Valgus and varus stress films if needed in full extension and 30 degrees of flexion
- Alignment hip to ankle weightbearing films if concerned about possible need for associated osteotomy

Magnetic Resonance Imaging

- Evaluate cartilage integrity and subchondral bone edema
- Status of menisci
- Evaluate extent of any collateral ligament injury

Equipment

GraftLink Preparation (Video)

- Graft Preparation Station to secure TightRope devices
- TightRope RT for femoral fixation
- TightRope No Button for tibial fixation
- 0 FiberLoop suture for free ends of quadrupled graft
- 0 FiberWire suture to link graft limbs (4 on each side)

Anteromedial Portal Approach

- CaliBlator (Arthrex)
- Measuring pin for femoral intraosseous distance used with offset guide
- Low-profile reamer for anteromedial drilling of the femoral socket
- RetroCutter for creating a tibial socket with a special guide and sleeve
- RetroCutter cannulated guide pin
- Intra-articular measuring device
- PassPort cannula (Arthrex)
- Looped-tip wire
- 0 FiberWire suture to create a luggage tag passing suture for the No Button loop
- Free #2 FiberStick (Arthrex) suture as a shuttle for the tibia
- ABS button for No Button TightRope

FlipCutter Approach

- CaliBlator
- FlipCutter for the femoral and tibial sockets
- 6-9 femoral guide (Arthrex) for the FlipCutter
- #2 FiberStick in a red tube as a femoral shuttling suture
- PassPort cannula
- Intra-articular measuring device
- Tibial guide for the FlipCutter

- #2 TigerStick (Arthrex) in a red tube as a tibial shuttling suture
- 0 FiberWire suture to create luggage tag passing suture for the No Button loop
- ABS button for the No Button TightRope

Positioning and Portals

The author prefers the patient to be in a supine position with the foot supported on the bed by a foot holder of a leg-positioning device to allow for flexion of the knee as necessary. A lateral thigh post is also used to support the thigh in flexion, which allows positioning to be hands free. A shorter, removable lateral post is placed just above the knee to serve as a fulcrum for valgus positioning to assess and treat medial compartment pathology; it is then removed. A tourniquet is not used. This positioning approach easily allows access to the popliteal region for the minimally invasive single posterior incision semitendinosus harvest. The author prefers to use an arthroscopic pump (Arthrex) set at 40 mm of inflow run through the scope, so a superior portal is not necessary.

Step-by-Step Description of the Procedure

Outside-In Approach With a FlipCutter for the Femur and Tibia

The illustrated case is a right knee done with a sterile, prefabricated soft tissue Allograft GraftLink (LifeNet Health) 70 mm in length and 10.5 mm in diameter. The Allograft GraftLink is assembled on the back table, placing a TightRope RT on the femoral side and a No Button Loop on the tibial side. There are 2 free suture ends in the tibial side of the graft that are left in place to use on the tibial side for backup fixation. The femoral socket is localized by use of a CaliBlator device, which allows for distance measurement from the proximal articular cartilage margin near the over-the-top position to the distal articular surface margin using accepted referencing based on a 90-degree knee flexion arthroscopic view (Figure 27-6). This device is calibrated in 2-mm increments, and the author uses data from the meta-analysis done by Piefer et al[26] to localize the femoral socket center point approximately 43% of the distance from the proximal articular cartilage landmark at the over-the-top position. In addition, the author strives for the posterior socket margin to be 2 mm from the posterior lateral femoral articular surface as the CaliBlator has a 7-mm bend for this purpose. The CaliBlator is also a radiofrequency device that allows for simple marking of this determined point. There are different aiming guides that can be used to drill the FlipCutter from the lateral femur to this centering point in the joint, but the author prefers the 6-9 guide. The inner diameter of this guide positioned on the femur from the anterolateral portal represents a 6-mm-diameter socket, and the outer guide is 9 mm, which allows for a good visual reference as to where the femoral socket will be located (Figure 27-7). In terms of orientation for drilling with the FlipCutter, the guide is positioned 60 degrees perpendicular to the femoral anatomic axis and 20 degrees relative to the transepicondylar axis (Figure 27-8).[27]

An inherent advantage of the FlipCutter technique is that the femoral socket can easily be lengthened by changing the guide sleeve angle to be more vertical in the coronal plane, which cannot be done with anteromedial portal drilling of the femoral socket. Prior to drilling, the femoral intraosseous distance can be measured off the guide sleeve. It is helpful to predrill with a stiffer 3.5-mm pin to prevent migration of the FlipCutter; then, the guide sleeve is tapped in the outer cortex 7 mm, followed by drilling with the FlipCutter. As noted previously, the author's preferred femoral socket position is slightly proximal to the center position, referring to the point

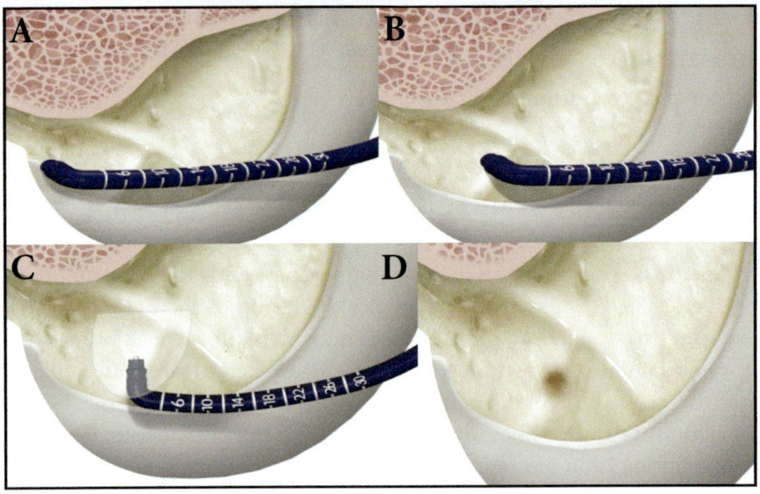

Figure 27-6. The CaliBlator simplifies direct measurement by allowing the surgeon to arthroscopically measure the femur (and tibia) while also marking the desired guide pin location for reference. This schematic model shows a left knee viewing from the anteromedial portal while marking the centering point for the femoral reaming using the CaliBlator from the anterolateral portal. (A) Shows measurement from proximal over-the-top articular cartilage margin to distal femoral articular surface margin. (B) Based on (A) measurement determining the point approximately 43% distance from the proximal over-the-top articular cartilage margin. (C) Referencing the B point with the 7-mm curve of the CaliBlator ensures 2 mm distance from posterior lateral condyle articular surface with a 10-mm socket. This mark (D) can then be referenced with either placement of a FlipCutter guide (Arthrex) through the anterolateral portal or by using a standard guide pin and low-profile reamer (Arthrex) drilling through the anteromedial portal.

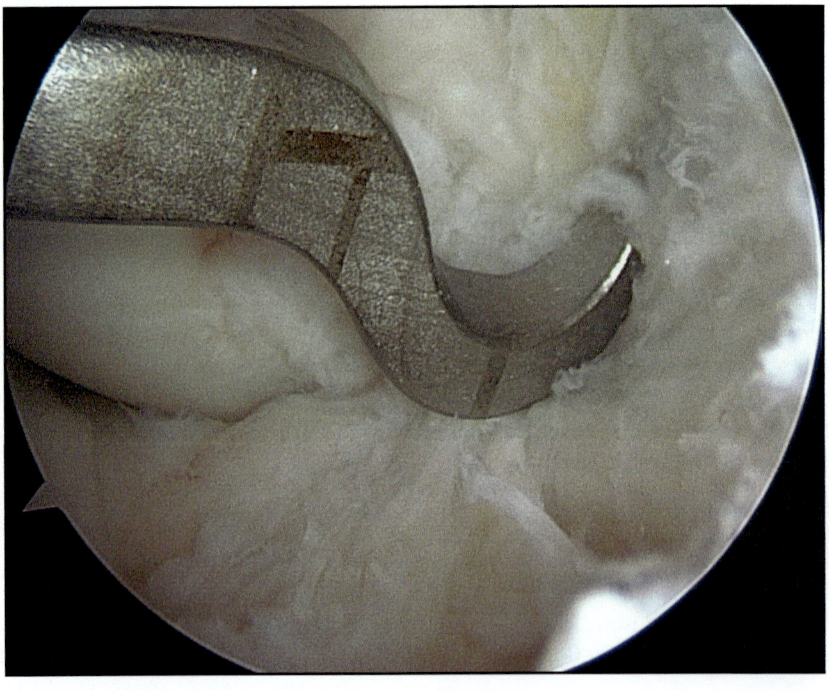

Figure 27-7. The 6-9 guide is shown here for a right knee viewing from the anteromedial portal as the guide is positioned on the femoral ACL footprint from the anterolateral portal. The inner diameter represents a 6-mm socket and the outer a 9-mm socket, with the FlipCutter drilled outside-in to the center of the guide. The knee is at 90 degrees of flexion.

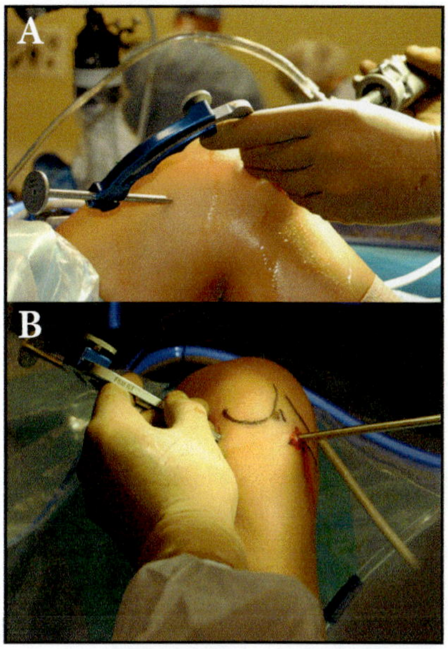

Figure 27-8. The FlipCutter guide is oriented for this right knee with the tip of the 6-9 guide in the anterolateral portal positioned on the femur intra-articularly. The angle of the guide is 20 degrees in the transepicondylar axis (A) and 60 degrees in the coronal plane (B). The knee is at 90 degrees of flexion.

between the native posterolateral and anteromedial ACL bundles, so he favors a bit toward the anteromedial attachment on the femur by referencing approximately 43% of the distance from the proximal articular cartilage margin to the distal articular surface margin. After the femoral socket is drilled, a #2 FiberStick in its red sheath is passed through the 3.5-mm drill hole and is retrieved on the joint side and docked outside the joint to be the passing suture for the graft into the femoral socket later on (Figure 27-9).

Prior to creating the tibial socket, the intra-articular distance for the ACL graft is measured with the intra-articular measuring device. This distance is then added to the depth of the femoral socket created and referenced to the length of the GraftLink construct to determine the desired depth of the tibial socket. The next step is reaming the tibial socket. Again, the FlipCutter is used with the tibial aiming device. The author's preferred position is just anteromedial to the normal ACL center. In most cases, there are native ACL fibers from the tibial footprint here still present that can be used for orientation. The one constant landmark to reference is the anterior horn of the lateral meniscus, and the author strives for approximately three-quarters of the tibial socket to be anterior to the posterior margin of the anterior horn attachment point, representing more of an anteromedial bundle attachment location on the tibia. The CaliBlator can also be used to mark the desired centering point for the tibial socket to facilitate positioning the tibial aiming device. Just as with the femur, the tibial intraosseous distance is measured to know the limit of tibial socket depth. The guide pin is predrilled with the stiffer 3.5-mm pin, and then the guide sleeve is tapped in 7 mm through the tibial cortex. The FlipCutter pin is drilled in to the joint and flipped to retro-ream the tibial socket, always leaving a 7-mm bone bridge on the tibial cortex to ensure suspensory cortical fixation with the TightRope. This tibial socket depth is generally at least 5 mm greater than the desired graft length in the tibia, which allows for graft tensioning so that the graft does not bottom out. Final tibial socket position is still well within the tibial footprint, even with this slightly more anteromedial position (Figure 27-10).

On the tibial side, a #2 TigerStick suture in its red sheath is passed into the joint. Prior to retrieving this tibial socket suture, the author always places a PassPort cannula in the anteromedial portal to prevent a soft tissue bridge during graft passage, which can be disruptive to the flow of the procedure if it were to occur.

Graft passage is straightforward. The FiberStick suture—"F" for femur—is pulled out of the PassPort cannula, followed by the TigerStick suture—"T" for tibia. First, the TightRope RT

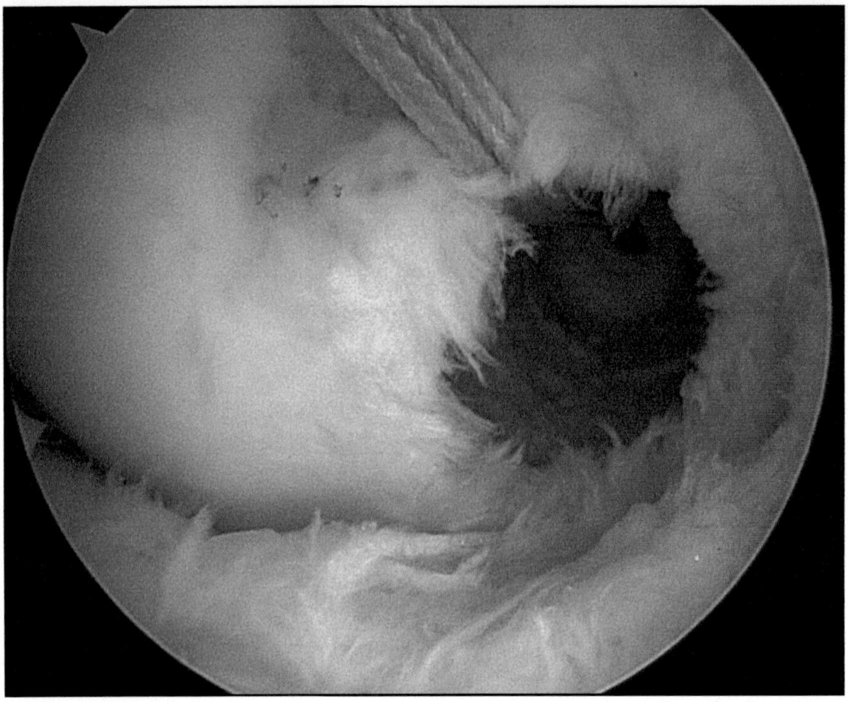

Figure 27-9. The femoral socket is seen with the FiberStick docking suture in place. This is an arthroscopic view from the anterolateral portal for a right knee at 90 degrees of flexion. The author's optimal position is just proximal to the true ACL center, favoring more toward the anteromedial bundle attachment than the posterolateral attachment point in the proximal/distal orientation. The posterior margin of the femoral socket should ideally be 2 mm from the posterior lateral femoral condyle articular surface.

sutures are passed in the femoral socket via the blue passing suture on the button, along with the white shortening sutures. The intraosseous distance is marked on the shortening sutures with methylene blue as a guide for when the button should flip outside the lateral femoral cortex. It is usually easy to feel when the button flips. The graft is then hoisted into the femoral socket by alternatively pulling the 2 shortening sutures until the graft is fully seated to the expected depth in the femoral socket, again, marked on the graft with methylene blue. At this point, the author always cycles the knee 20 times and, if necessary, retensions the TightRope femoral sutures to eliminate any potential cyclic displacement or creep in the fixation here.

On the tibial side, when using the No Button TightRope, which the author finds easier than the TightRope RT here, it is important to protect the loop during passage. A simple luggage tag–type suture with a 0 FiberWire is placed at the base of the loop. Then, this suture and the 2 free suture ends from the tibial side of the GraftLink construct are passed through the TigerWire loop and pulled out of the small anterior tibial incision. This of course is through the PassPort cannula also passing the graft into the tibial socket. Now, the shortening strands are delivered out with the No Button loop, and the 0 FiberWire suture is removed from the loop. The ABS button (12-by-8 mm) is assembled to the No Button loop to create a regular TightRope, and the shortening sutures are pulled in an alternating fashion down toward the tibia. Before final seating of the button down to the bone, the sutures in the tibial end of the graft are passed in the slots of the button, and the knee is brought to full extension to avoid overconstraining the joint, and the shortening sutures are secured to the button. The knee is cycled again to eliminate any potential cyclic displacement with the TightRope, and then the shortening sutures are retightened in full

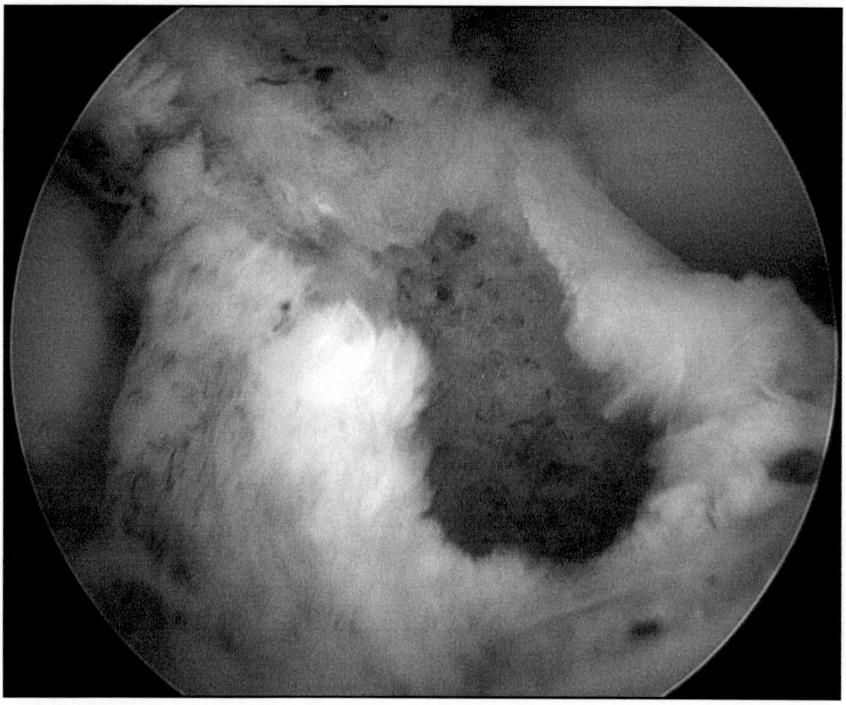

Figure 27-10. The final tibial socket for a right knee as viewed from the anterolateral portal is shown completely within the native tibial footprint. The author's optimal position is just anteromedial to the center of the ACL with approximately one-quarter of the tibial socket behind the anterior horn of the lateral meniscus.

extension and tied down to the button. The tibial graft sutures are then tied to the button for backup fixation. Final graft position is checked arthroscopically to make sure there is no notch impingement, especially in hyperextension (Figure 27-11). The author does not routinely perform a notchplasty because he rarely sees impingement after all-inside ACL reconstruction. Plus, in his experience of second-look ACL reconstruction after a notchplasty has been done, it always grows back with fibrocartilage, thereby defeating its purpose.

Anteromedial Portal

This case is a right knee GraftLink ACL reconstruction done with a quadrupled semitendinosus autograft harvested from a single posterior incision. Given the flexibility of the all-inside technique, drilling the femur through the anteromedial portal works well and is a known and comfortable approach for many surgeons. This is facilitated by use of low-profile reamers (Arthrex) to avoid iatrogenic injury to the medial femoral condyle. Furthermore, the author has found it unnecessary to create an accessory anteromedial portal because a low anteromedial portal allows for full accessibility of the femoral ACL footprint. Also, as mentioned previously with the FlipCutter technique, the author rarely performs femoral notchplasty.

The author's optimal femoral socket location is slightly proximal to the center of the native anteromedial and posterolateral bundles, which favors a bit toward the anteromedial bundle attachment. This is consistent with the Piefer meta-analysis study and a center point 43% of the distance from the proximal femoral articular margin landmark to the distal lateral femoral articular margin.[26] This can easily be determined with a ruler measuring technique, and the CaliBlator radiofrequency device works well to find this point. The author's goal is for the most posterior margin of the femoral socket to be 2 mm from the posterior femoral articular surface margin. An

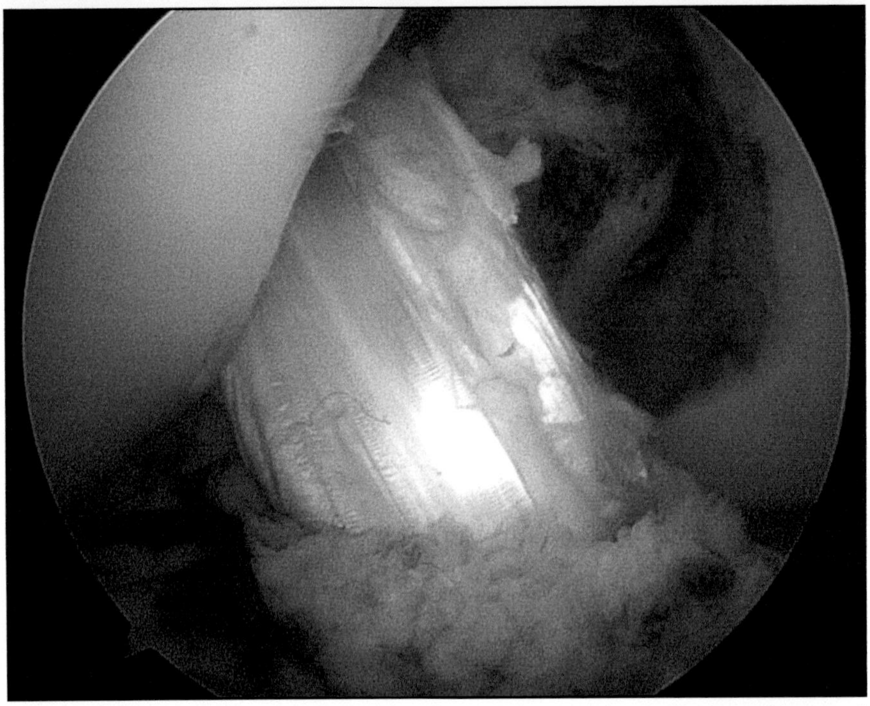

Figure 27-11. Final ACL graft position. Quadrupled GraftLink soft tissue prefabricated allograft for a right knee as viewed from the anterolateral portal. Note the native ACL fibers around the base of the new graft, confirming optimal position within the tibial footprint.

offset guide (Arthrex) placed through the anteromedial portal also works well to find this point. It is critical after creating the femoral socket centering point to check its position and view it from the anteromedial portal to verify proper location.

To create the femoral socket for the GraftLink construct with TightRope suspensory fixation, it is necessary to measure the femoral intraosseous distance. After determining the femoral socket centering position as outlined previously, a special spade tip measuring pin (Arthrex) that also acts like a depth gauge is drilled from the anteromedial portal, usually at approximately 120 degrees of flexion to allow for easy determination of the femoral intraosseous distance. The low-profile reamer matching the graft diameter is then passed carefully in a vertical orientation through the anteromedial portal, avoiding the medial femoral condyle articular surface, and the femoral socket is reamed to the appropriate depth. This depth is based on the intraosseous distance and the desired amount of graft in the femoral socket given the length of the GraftLink construct, with the key being preserving the lateral femoral cortex for the TightRope fixation. Generally, the author does not have less than 20 mm of graft in the femoral socket with this technique. A #2 FiberStick suture is then docked here to pull the graft up into the femur later.

The next step is measuring the intra-articular distance from the femoral socket margin to the proposed tibial socket aperture with the special intra-articular measuring device. Usually, this distance is in the range of 23 to 26 mm. Now, with the known depth of the created femoral socket, the intra-articular distance, and the length of the graft, the desired length of the tibial socket is determined. As with the femur, the tibial intraosseous is measured so as to know the limit of the tibial socket depth that can be drilled while preserving the tibial cortex for the TightRope fixation. As described with the FlipCutter technique, the tibial socket depth is generally created 5 mm longer than the expected graft length in the socket to allow room for graft tensioning.

The author prefers using the RetroCutter to create the tibial socket because it is so accurate visually to place the RetroCutter matching the graft diameter right where you want the tibial socket to be, although the FlipCutter also works well. Through a small tibial incision, the RetroCutter guide sleeve is placed down to the bone, and the cannulated RetroCutter pin is drilled forward into the joint, capturing the RetroCutter that is reverse threaded on the guide. In forward drilling mode, the RetroCutter reams the tibial socket to the desired depth. It is then brought back in the joint and, when reengaging the guide, is switched to reverse to deliver the RetroCutter back onto the guide for removal. At this time, the small pin within the RetroCutter pin is removed to open the cannulation, and a passing wire is easily passed into the joint. A PassPort cannula is placed in the anteromedial portal to retrieve this wire, and then a #2 TigerStick suture is folded in half and a simple loop knot is created, and one end of this suture is passed out of the small tibial incision. This suture will be used to shuttle the tibial end of the graft and the No Button TightRope loop, which the author prefers over the TightRope RT for fixation on the tibial side into the tibial socket.

The graft is first passed into the femur by retrieving the FiberStick docking suture through the PassPort cannula. The TightRope RT blue passing and white shortening sutures are passed through this FiberStick loop and are shuttled out the small lateral pin incision. The shortening sutures have been marked with the femoral intraosseous distance to facilitate the expected flipping of the button on the lateral femoral cortex, which can usually be felt. Pulling on the graft outside the PassPort cannula confirms button flippage with no pullback. Next, the graft is hoisted in the femoral socket by alternating pulling on the white TightRope shortening sutures. The expected graft depth in the femoral socket is marked with methylene blue as a guide. After the graft is seated fully in the femur, the knee is always cycled 20 times at this point to make sure there is no slippage or creep with the femoral TightRope fixation; if necessary, the femoral shortening sutures can be retensioned.

To facilitate shuttling of the No Button TightRope loop out the small tibial incision, as described with the FlipCutter technique, a 0 FiberWire luggage tag–type suture is placed at the base of the loop. This suture, along with the sutures in the tibial end of the GraftLink construct, are then passed through the PassPort cannula via the #2 TigerStick with the loop into the tibial socket pulling the graft in the socket in the process. The No Button loop and shortening sutures are delivered now out the small tibial incision. The 0 FiberWire suture is removed from the No Button loop, and the ABS button is attached to convert to a regular TightRope. The 2 sutures in the tibial end of the graft are passed through the slots in the button, and then the white shortening sutures are pulled in an alternating fashion to the button for fixation bringing the knee into full extension so as not to overconstrain the joint. As on the femoral side, the knee is cycled 20 times to eliminate any potential creep with the tibial fixation, and then the shortening sutures are pulled taut again and tied to the ABS button and the sutures in the tibial end of the graft are tied to the button for backup fixation.

Postoperative Protocol

For the FlipCutter technique and the anteromedial portal technique, the author generally begins early motion with use of a continuous passive motion machine in the recovery room. Formal outpatient physical therapy is started the next day with the first dressing change, and initiation of quadriceps exercises with quadriceps sets progressing to straight leg raises when there is no extensor lag. Patellar mobilization is emphasized to avoid infrapatellar scarring or contraction. The exercise bicycle is usually started at 10 to 14 days. Weightbearing off crutches is allowed once the patient demonstrates good leg control, which typically takes 2 weeks or so. Sometimes with a difficult meniscal repair (ie, in the white-white zone), the author keeps the patient nonweightbearing for the first 3 weeks and limits knee flexion to 90 degrees for the first 2 weeks to minimize rollback stress on the repair site. Closed chain exercises are initiated once the patient is fully weightbearing at 3 to 4 weeks. Running is allowed by 3 months, and return to sport is delayed at least until 6 months postoperatively and is based on functional testing results at that time along with completion of ACL prevention-type exercises conducted by the physical therapist.

Potential Complications

All-inside ACL reconstruction is a safe and reproducible procedure with a short learning curve. However, as with any surgery, anything can happen. Potential complications could include a problem with anesthesia or a postoperative infection. Prophylactic antibiotics are always administered intravenously right before the incision is made. Deep venous thrombosis can occur and, generally, any patient felt to be an increased risk for deep venous thrombosis is placed on aspirin 325 mg twice daily beginning the night of surgery and is continued until the patient is fully weightbearing.[28]

Relative to the steps of the procedure itself, one potential complication would be if the final graft length is longer than the sum of the femoral and tibial socket depths and the intra-articular graft distance. In that circumstance, the graft could not be tensioned and still would be lax. The bailout would be to remove the tibial ABS button so that the tibial end of the graft could be pulled out of the tibial socket and out of the PassPort cannula where a new suture could be passed through the loop of the graft. Then, the FlipCutter or the RetroCutter could be used to create a full tibial tunnel in the location of the socket. The graft would then be pulled back into the joint by way of a passing wire or suture to be fixated in the full tibial tunnel with an interference screw backed up by a distal PushLock (Arthrex) or SwiveLock (Arthrex).

Another possible complication that could occur on the femoral or tibial side would be inadvertent creation of a full tunnel by violating the cortex during the reaming process. This could happen on the femur with the anteromedial portal drilling technique and on the tibia using the RetroCutter. This would not occur with the FlipCutter technique because the 7-mm depth stop on the guide sleeve protects the cortical bridge of bone here. The bailout on the femoral side would be use of an extender button (Arthrex) that allows the TightRope button to fit within it and, because it is longer at 20 mm, it can span a larger femoral cortical hole while also providing adequate fixation. On the tibial side, the bailout is the extender button if a regular TightRope is used here or a larger, circular 14-mm-diameter ABS button to cover the larger cortical hole and provide suspensory fixation.

A final complication would be securing the TightRope fixation with the knee in flexion because, in the author's experience, the TightRope fixation is secure and at time zero on the operating table; these knees are clinically tight on stress testing with Lachman, pivot shift, and anterior drawer tests. Therefore, the author always brings the knee out to full extension (or hyperextension if present) before final fixation of the graft. His concern would be if the graft was fixed at 20 degrees of flexion, the knee could be overconstrained and the patient may not achieve full extension, which would be a definite postoperative complication.

Top Technical Pearls for the Procedure

1. With the all-inside technique, it is necessary to make sure the sum of the depth of the femoral and tibial sockets and the intra-articular ACL distance between the sockets is at least 5 mm greater than the final length of the graft. This ensures that the graft will not bottom out at the base of the tibial socket, which would leave it lax and unable to be tensioned at the time of final fixation.
2. Use of a cannula (such as the PassPort) in the anteromedial portal is critical during suture—and subsequent—graft passage. If one tethers the anterior fat pad soft tissues with a passing suture, this may make passage of the graft difficult. This tissue is tenacious and traps the sutures securely and will make for a frustrating experience near the end of the case, which compounds the angst of this potential problem.
3. It is helpful to mark the shortening sutures for the femoral TightRope with the measured femoral socket intraosseous distance with methylene blue from the base of the button to facilitate the self-flipping of the button as it exits the femoral drill hole. In this way, the button will sit flush against the bone with no intervening soft tissue.
4. Using a passing suture for the No Button Loop as it is passed into the tibial socket is important to avoid iatrogenic damage to the TightRope prior to assembling the ABS button to this TightRope for the definitive tibial fixation step. The 0 FiberWire simple luggage tag suture works well for this purpose.
5. Always cycle the knee after securing first the femoral Tight Rope to make sure there is no creep, and tension the shortening sutures again here if necessary. The same holds true on the tibial side; cycle the knee after first securing the shortening sutures to the ABS button here and tension again. This final tibial fixation step should always be done with the knee in full extension to avoid being too tight with the graft and risk a permanent loss of full knee extension.

Acknowledgments

Dr. Smith would like to thank Jordan Bley for his assistance in writing and editing this chapter.

References

1. Morgan CD. The all-inside ACL reconstruction. In: Morgan CD, ed. *Operative Technique Manual.* Naples, FL: Arthrex; 1995.
2. Lubowitz JH. No-tunnel anterior cruciate ligament reconstruction: the transtibial all-inside technique. *Arthroscopy.* 2006;22(8):900.e1-900.e11.
3. Smith PA. An alternative method for "all-inside" anterior cruciate ligament reconstruction. *Arthroscopy.* 2007;23(4):451.
4. Alentorn-Geli E, Samitier G, Alvarez P, Steinbacher G, Cugat R. Anteromedial portal versus transtibial drilling techniques in ACL reconstruction: a blinded cross-sectional study at two- to five-year follow-up. *Int Orthop.* 2010;34(5):747-754.
5. Bedi A, Musahl V, Steuber V, et al. Transtibial versus anteromedial portal reaming in anterior cruciate ligament reconstruction: an anatomic and biomechanical evaluation of surgical technique. *Arthroscopy.* 2011;27(3):380-390.

6. Lubowitz JH. Anteromedial portal technique for the anterior cruciate ligament femoral socket: pitfalls and solutions. *Arthroscopy.* 2009;25(1):95-101.
7. Duffee A, Magnussen RA, Pedroza AD, Flanigan DC, Group M, Kaeding CC. Transtibial ACL femoral tunnel preparation increases odds of repeat ipsilateral knee surgery. *J Bone Joint Surg Am.* 2013;95(22):2035-2042.
8. Smith PA, Schwartzberg RS, Lubowitz JH. No tunnel 2-socket technique: all-inside anterior cruciate ligament double-bundle retroconstruction. *Arthroscopy.* 2008;24(10):1184-1189.
9. Gill TJ, Steadman JR. Anterior cruciate ligament reconstruction the two-incision technique. *Orthop Clin North Am.* 2002;33(4):727-735.
10. Wright RW. Two-incision anterior cruciate ligament reconstruction. *J Knee Surg.* 2014;27(5):343-346.
11. Petre BM, Smith SD, Jansson KS, et al. Femoral cortical suspension devices for soft tissue anterior cruciate ligament reconstruction: a comparative biomechanical study. *Am J Sports Med.* 2013;41(2):416-422.
12. Smith PA, DeBerardino TM. Tibial fixation properties of a continuous-loop ACL hamstring graft construct with suspensory fixation in porcine bone [published online ahead of print October 27, 2014]. *J Knee Surg.*
13. Morrison JB. The mechanics of the knee joint in relation to normal walking. *J Biomech.* 1970;3(1):51-61.
14. Shelburne KB, Pandy MG. Determinants of cruciate-ligament loading during rehabilitation exercise. *Clin Biomech (Bristol, Avon).* 1998;13(6):403-413.
15. Shelburne KB, Pandy MG. A dynamic model of the knee and lower limb for simulating rising movements. *Comput Methods Biomech Biomed Engin.* 2002;5(2):149-159.
16. Shelburne KB, Pandy MG, Anderson FC, Torry MR. Pattern of anterior cruciate ligament force in normal walking. *J Biomech.* 2004;37(6):797-805.
17. Noyes FR, Butler DL, Grood ES, Zernicke RF, Hefzy MS. Biomechanical analysis of human ligament grafts used in knee-ligament repairs and reconstructions. *J Bone Joint Surg Am.* 1984;66(3):344-352.
18. Lubowitz JH, Ahmad CS, Anderson K. All-inside anterior cruciate ligament graft-link technique: second-generation, no-incision anterior cruciate ligament reconstruction. *Arthroscopy.* 2011;27(5):717-727.
19. White KL, Camire LM, Parks BG, Corey WS, Hinton RY. Krackow locking stitch versus locking premanufactured loop stitch for soft-tissue fixation: a biomechanical study. *Arthroscopy.* 2010;26(12):1662-1666.
20. Lubowitz JH, Schwartzberg R, Smith P. Randomized controlled trial comparing all-inside anterior cruciate ligament reconstruction technique with anterior cruciate ligament reconstruction with a full tibial tunnel. *Arthroscopy.* 2013;29(7):1195-1200.
21. Benea H, d'Astorg H, Klouche S, Bauer T, Tomoaia G, Hardy P. Pain evaluation after all-inside anterior cruciate ligament reconstruction and short term functional results of a prospective randomized study. *Knee.* 2014;21(1):102-106.
22. Franz W, Ulbrich J. A new technique for harvesting the semitendinosus tendon for cruciate ligament reconstruction. *Arthroskopie.* 2004;17(2):104-107.
23. Nuelle CW, Cook JL, Galizzi MA, Smith PA. Posterior single-incision semitendinosus harvest for a quadrupled anterior cruciate ligament graft construct: determination of graft length and diameter based on patient sex, height, weight, and body mass index. *Arthroscopy.* 2015;31(4):684-690.
24. Lane CG, Warren R, Pearle AD. The pivot shift. *J Am Acad Orthop Surg.* 2008;16(12):679-688.
25. Sanchis-Alfonso V, Baydal-Bertomeu JM, Castelli A, et al. Laboratory evaluation of the pivot-shift phenomenon with use of kinetic analysis: a preliminary study. *J Bone Joint Surg Am.* 2011;93(13):1256-1267.
26. Piefer JW, Pflugner TR, Hwang MD, Lubowitz JH. Anterior cruciate ligament femoral footprint anatomy: systematic review of the 21st century literature. *Arthroscopy.* 2012;28(6):872-881.
27. Lubowitz JH, Akhavan S, Waterman BR, Aalami-Harandi A, Konicek J. Technique for creating the anterior cruciate ligament femoral socket: optimizing femoral footprint anatomic restoration using outside-in drilling. *Arthroscopy.* 2013;29(3):522-528.
28. Ye S, Dongyang C, Zhihong X, et al. The incidence of deep venous thrombosis after arthroscopically assisted anterior cruciate ligament reconstruction. *Arthroscopy.* 2013;29(4):742-747.

Please see videos on the accompanying website at www.routledge.com/9781617119996

28

Revision Anterior Cruciate Ligament Reconstruction

Adam V. Metzler, MD; Joseph Brunkhorst, DO; and
Darren L. Johnson, MD

Introduction

Over the past few decades, the number of anterior cruciate ligament (ACL) reconstructions has increased to an estimated 250,000 per year.[1,2] Primary ACL reconstruction has been shown to be successful in restoring knee stability and function. An improved ability to identify, reconstruct, and rehabilitate these patients has led to a better understanding of the natural history and functional consequences of an ACL-deficient knee. Although current techniques are successful in restoring a large percentage of patients to competitive play,[3] the authors anticipate an ever-increasing number of patients who will present with ACL failure. There are 3 main categories of ACL reconstruction failure, including loss of motion, recurrent instability, and persistent pain.

Loss of motion can result in significant impairment and functional disability. Extension loss remains a major concern after ACL reconstruction because most patients tolerate mild flexion loss. Studies have shown that even a 5-degree loss of flexion can result in poor subjective outcomes in patients.[4,5] Multiple factors play into motion loss, and the etiology of this must be understood before proceeding with revision ACL reconstruction. Factors that can cause motion loss include improper tunnel placement, noncompliance with physical therapy, excessive graft tension, impingement, and cyclops lesions.[6-9]

Recurrent instability is most often related to technical errors. It has been estimated that 70% to 80% of ACL failures may be due to improperly placed tunnels.[10] Malpositioned tunnels can lead to excessive graft tensioning, laxity, or impingement. The 2 bony landmarks that define the femoral location of the ACL femoral insertion are the lateral intercondylar ridge and the lateral bifurcate ridge. No fibers of the ACL insert superior to the lateral intercondylar ridge. The bifurcate ridge separates the anteromedial and the posterolateral bundles of the ACL on the femoral attachment.[11] One recent study demonstrated that the native ACL femoral attachment lies at a point 50% along a line drawn from the proximal articular cartilage and the distal articular cartilage border, parallel to the tibial surface with the knee at 90 degrees of flexion.[12] Another study showed similar results in their systematic review in regard to arthroscopically measurable landmarks. They determined that the anatomic location of the ACL femoral footprint is 43% of the

Sgaglione NA, Lubowitz JH, Provencher MT, eds. *The Knee: AANA Advanced Arthroscopic Surgical Techniques* (pp 389-404).

distance from the proximal articular margin to the distal articular margins. In addition, they also showed that a rim of bone of 2.5 mm exists between the posterior ACL fibers and the posterior articular cartilage margin.[13] The tibial footprint, the larger of the 2, is more variable in description of its anatomic location, and the literature supports this variability. A recent systematic review of the tibial footprint showed that the ACL tibial footprint is 15 mm anterior to the posterior cruciate ligament (PCL) and two-fifths of the medial-lateral width of the interspinous distance, with the majority of the ACL fibers attaching anterior to the posterior margin of the lateral meniscus.[14] The authors place their tibial tunnel directly across from the midportion of the anterior horn of the lateral meniscus and as far medial as possible as not to injure the cartilage of the medial tibial plateau. Previous reports of placing the ACL tibial tunnel 5 to 6 mm anterior to the PCL produced a nonanatomic tibial ACL tunnel based on the current evidence; this is also based on the senior author's experience.[15]

The objective of anatomic single- or double-bundle reconstruction is to restore a maximum percentage of the native ACL insertion, thereby reproducing the native ACL insertion site anatomy and restoring the normal ACL kinematics and stability. It is imperative that the graft be placed at the anatomic location of native ACL to prevent clinical failure. To provide the most anatomic ACL graft placement, the current literature weighs heavily in favor of medial portal reaming, outside-in, or double-bundle ACL reconstruction.[16,17]

Recent studies have also looked at the importance of graft size with primary ACL reconstruction. One study showed that revision was performed in 1.7% of patients with grafts greater than 8 mm in diameter, 6.5% with 7.5- or 8-mm-diameter grafts, and 13.6% with grafts 7 mm or less in diameter.[18] Another study found similar results and noted that a revision was required in no patients with grafts greater than 8 mm in diameter and 7.0% with grafts 8 mm in diameter or smaller. Among patients aged 18 years or younger, revision was required in no patients with grafts greater than 8 mm in diameter and 18.3% with grafts 8 mm in diameter or smaller.[19] Thus, when doing revision ACL reconstruction, the authors believe it is imperative to use larger grafts and supplement with allograft tissue if needed to increase the overall collagen content of the graft.

The desired level of activity of the patient and the primary graft source must be considered in revision ACL surgery. It is imperative that surgeons recognize the different incorporation rates between soft tissue and bone autografts and allografts.[20,21] Appropriate rehabilitation for each graft is important, and a cookbook standard rehabilitation protocol may result in early clinical failure. Adherence to biologic principles is essential to the success of the primary and revision surgery.

Traumatic failures can occur whenever the graft is exposed to tensile loads that exceed the biomechanical strength and stiffness of the graft during a particular stage of healing and maturation. Early failures are defined as those that occur during the process of graft incorporation and remodeling (< 1 year), whereas late failures occur once the graft has matured (after 1 year).[7] Overaggressive rehabilitation, premature return to sports, and a significant reinjury can all result in traumatic failure of the primary ACL reconstruction. Although they are commonly used, accelerated rehabilitation programs may injure the immature graft or cause fixation loosening and graft failure.[22]

ACL injuries often are associated with concomitant injuries approximately 75% of the time. Failure to recognize associated injuries can result in repeat graft failure. Posterolateral corner injuries are the most commonly unrecognized concurrent injury and have been reported to be present 10% to 15% of the time.[23] The Multicenter ACL Revision Study group has shown that approximately 10% of patients have normal menisci/articular cartilage at the time of revision ACL surgery.[24] The medial collateral ligament, posterior horn of the medial meniscus, and posteromedial capsule also provide secondary stability to the ACL-deficient knee. In addition, limb alignment must be critically analyzed as well, with consideration of osteotomies as needed. Recognition and management of these concurrent issues is vital to the success of revision ACL reconstruction.

Persistent pain after ACL reconstruction can originate from a plethora of areas. Pain may be due to recurrent instability, graft site morbidity, and patellofemoral joint pain. Intra-articular sources include traumatic arthrosis, osteochondral defects, and meniscal tears. It is important to understand that if a revision ACL reconstruction is performed for pain only, poor outcomes should be expected. ACL reconstruction is an instability-reducing procedure, not a pain-reducing procedure.

Indications

- Failed primary ACL reconstruction
- Traumatic rerupture
- Loss of motion from improperly placed tunnels
- Pain only if the pain is secondary to recurrent instability episodes

Controversial Indications

- Revision ACL reconstruction in the setting of arthritis
- Revision ACL reconstruction for pain alone

Pertinent Physical Findings

Physical examination of the extremity should be comprehensive. It must include all objective and subjective tests to qualify and quantify the amount of patholaxity present as well as concomitant pathology that will affect the revision surgery, including evaluation of the ACL, menisci, posterolateral corner, and posteromedial capsule.

- The best test is examination under anesthesia, which provides the most accurate indications of pathology compared to the in-office evaluation. The examination under anesthesia must include the following:
  - Lachman test
  - Anterior drawer test
  - Posterior drawer test
  - Varus and valgus assessment
  - Posteromedial and lateral rotatory assessment

Pertinent Imaging

- Preoperative x-rays should be obtained, including standing anteroposterior, posteroanterior 45, lateral, and sunrise views. Alignment films must also be considered to rule out mechanical axis issues. Degenerative changes should be noted and discussed with the patient because many revision ACL reconstruction patients have degenerative pathology. Preoperative x-rays should be use to evaluate the hardware used, tunnel position, and expansion. Previously placed metal screws do not always need to be removed depending on their locations. If the previously placed metallic screws do not interfere with revision tunnel location, they should be left to prevent bone void defects. If hardware removal is necessary, a complete set of implant drivers and screw removal instruments must be on hand.

- Tunnels should be assessed for osteolysis and bone loss. Excessively posterior femoral tunnels from the original procedure may cause back wall blowout. When the tunnel exceeds 16 to 17 mm, the authors recommend staged bone grafting and returning in 6 months for revision ACL after the bone graft has incorporated.
- Magnetic resonance imaging (MRI) and 3-dimensional computed tomography scan may be useful tools to fully evaluate tunnel osteolysis and tunnel position. MRI is more useful in determining integrity of the graft and chondral and meniscal pathology but has limited use when metallic screws are present due to metallic artifact.

Preoperative Planning

Evaluation

A thorough preoperative evaluation is imperative when presented with a patient with a prior ACL reconstruction. It is vital to determine the cause of graft failure and what the patient's expectations for a revision ACL reconstruction are. The surgeon and the patient should have realistic expectations for revision ACL reconstruction because it has been shown that success rates of revision ACL reconstruction do not match that of primary ACL reconstruction.[25,26] For many patients, revision surgery may be considered a salvage procedure. For some patients returning to activities of daily living without instability, it could be considered a success. Return to sports or high-level activities may be unlikely and should be stressed preoperatively.[27]

History

The initial evaluation must include a careful history that addresses the nature of the primary injury and procedure, postoperative regimen, ability to return to activity, and timing of recurrent instability. The surgeon must have the operative notes from the primary surgery and, ideally, the intraoperative images to help guide the revision surgery. Information regarding the original graft, fixation type and manufacturer, and status of the menisci and articular cartilage is important in preoperative planning. Symptoms of pain and instability must be clearly differentiated because the treatment and prognosis may significantly differ. Typically, patients with symptomatic instability and objective findings of patholaxity have the highest potential for successful outcomes after revision ACL reconstruction.

Graft Selection

There is no single optimal graft option for revision ACL reconstruction, and each patient should be individualized in regard to graft choice. Studies have shown no significant difference in allograft and autograft use in the revision setting.[28,29] The authors' preferred graft choice in athletes younger than 22 years is autograft tissue, especially patellar tendon autograft. However, in less-active and lower-demand patients, allograft tissue remains an excellent option. Factors such as previous graft used, tunnel placement and enlargement, presence of patellofemoral symptoms, existing skin incision, other surgical procedures planned as part of the revision, and patient preference should be taken into account when making this decision. Allograft tissue offers several advantages that are relevant in the revision setting. Lack of donor site morbidity, decreased operative time, and smaller incision are all beneficial to the patient. For the surgeon, variable graft sizes, ability to create larger bone plugs, and increased tissue availability provides improved surgical flexibility. Bone patellar tendon bone and Achilles tendon grafts are the most commonly used allografts in the revision setting; however, slower graft incorporation and the risk of disease transmission are concerns.

Equipment

The surgeon must have all necessary equipment ready at the time of surgery. There should be no question as to what implants were used for the primary surgery and any special equipment needed for their possible removal. The authors routinely request the following for all revision surgeries:

- ACUFEX PINPOINT Anatomic ACL Guide System (Smith & Nephew)
- ACL revision REDUX system for screw removal, including broken screws (Smith & Nephew)
- Mini C-arm for localization of hardware
- Richards Staple Tray (Smith & Nephew; used in some instances for tibial-sided supplemental graft fixation in addition to interference screw)
- Large fragment set (can be used for femoral fixation in instances of posterior wall blowout of the lateral post and washer)
- Geofit screw and washer set (Mitek; used in some instances for tibial-sided supplemental graft fixation in addition to interference screw)
- ACUFEX ACL/posterior cruciate ligament drill guide system for tibial tunnel reaming (Smith & Nephew)
- Femoral head frozen allograft (if bone grafting)
- Graft Master (Smith & Nephew) when soft tissue graft is used
- Bone crimpers for shaping bone plugs
- Fully fluted reamers, acorn reamers, and single-fluted reamers
- Curette set
- Bone tamps
- Power saw and blade for harvest of patellar tendon graft
- Interference screws of surgeon's preference
- Cortical fixation button of surgeon's choice if soft tissue fixation is used
- Any special equipment needed for removal of the previous implant from the primary surgery (The authors routinely call the sales representative if they are unsure of any hardware needed for implant removal.)
- Zone-specific cannulas for inside-out meniscal repair
- Henning retractor or a pediatric half speculum for inside-out meniscal repair
- All-inside meniscal repair system of surgeon's preference
- Sterile bowl and frosted pestle for fibrin clot if needed for meniscal repair

Positioning and Portals

The patient's operative leg is placed in the ACUFEX leg holder, and the nonoperative leg is placed in a well-leg holder. The operative leg or femur should be parallel to the floor when placed in the leg holder (Figure 28-1). A high and tight anterolateral portal, a low and tight anteromedial portal, and an accessory anteromedial portal are created (Figure 28-2). The fat pad is debrided enough to allow full visualization in addition to a limited (3-mm) wall and notchplasty. Complete visualization of the ACL femoral and tibial footprints is imperative. The scope can alternate between the 3 portals for better visualization as needed. This setup allows for hyperflexion if

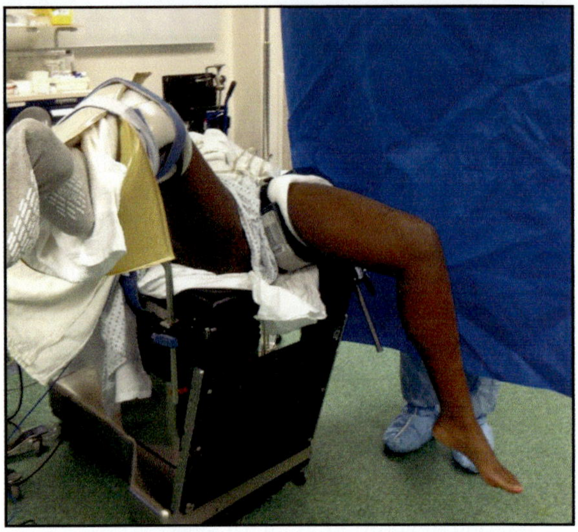

Figure 28-1. Standard arthroscopic setup for primary or revision ACL reconstruction. The left leg is in the arthroscopic leg holder. The nonoperative leg is in the well-leg holder.

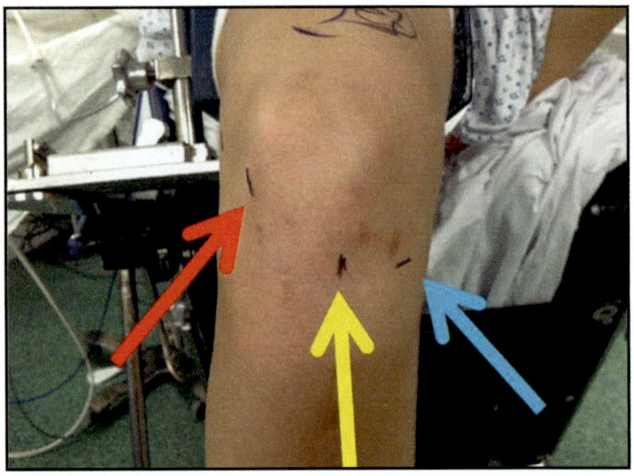

Figure 28-2. Portal placement. "High and tight" anterolateral portal (red arrow), central medial portal (yellow arrow), and accessory anteromedial portal (blue arrow).

needed for accessory medial portal femoral drilling and for complete access to the operative leg for assistants to hold retractors and perform meniscal repairs, etc (Figure 28-3).

Hardware Removal

The decision to remove or retain hardware can be one of the hardest decisions in revision ACL reconstruction. The following 2 questions should be asked: (1) Can the hardware be safely removed? (2) Does the hardware need to be removed? In general, hardware should only be removed when it interferes with the planned procedure, but the surgeon should be prepared for hardware removal in all cases. The importance of previous surgical reports and having the appropriate instrumentation available cannot be overemphasized.

Tunnel Placement

Previous tunnel position may also affect revision graft integrity and, therefore, the ability to perform a single-stage revision. For example, a transtibial primary ACL reconstruction commonly results in a posteriorly placed tibial tunnel and an anteriorly and superiorly placed femoral tunnel. In this scenario, drilling an anatomic femoral tunnel in native bone is often possible; however, it is more common that the tibial tunnel necessitates bone grafting and staged surgery. Prior tunnel

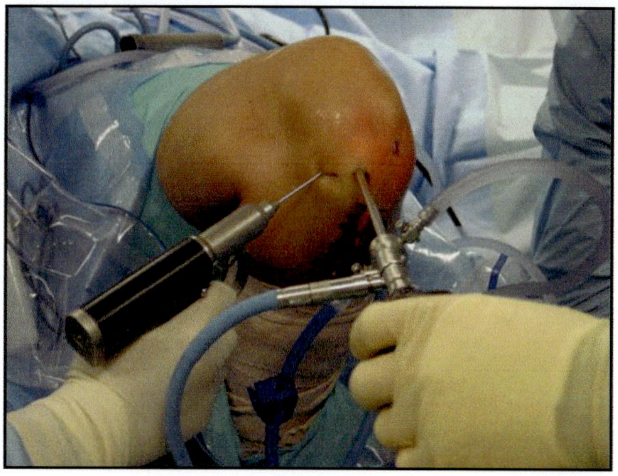

Figure 28-3. Hyperflexion reaming of the femoral portal through the accessory anteromedial portal.

position can be described as anatomically placed (entire tunnel opening is 100% in the native ACL footprint), nonanatomically placed (commonly seen in transtibial femoral tunnel drilling), or partially anatomic (overlapping). The greatest variation in tunnel placement is seen on the femur. When the femoral tunnel is nonanatomically placed, it rarely interferes with the revision tunnel placement and can be ignored, leaving the previous fixation hardware in place. Partially overlapping tunnel placement creates the most difficult scenario because the existing and revision tunnels will create a figure-8 tunnel. Often, redirection of the tunnel (diverging from the existing tunnel) can address this on the femur, allowing for adequate fixation of the new graft. In the authors' experience, outside-in femoral tunnel drilling has proven successful in this situation. A revision ACL surgeon must be comfortable with multiple techniques to reproduce anatomic tibial and femoral tunnels.

Outside-In (Two-Incision) Anterior Cruciate Ligament Revision Reconstruction

The choice of surgical technique should be guided by the preoperative plan, intraoperative findings, and comfort level with the diverse revision methods. Decisions regarding single-incision arthroscopic vs the outside-in (2-incision) technique and double- vs single-bundle ACL reconstruction must be made after vigilant considerations of all variables. Currently, the senior author prefers the outside-in (2-incision) technique for most revision ACL reconstructions and, in some instances, performs double-bundle ACL reconstruction. In cases in which the femoral tunnel is drilled vertically, the standard hyperflexion/accessory anteromedial portal drilling technique is used for femoral tunnel revision drilling. The following section describes the outside-in (2-incision) technique.

Step-by-Step Description of the Procedure

Bone Grafting

Before the start of the case, the surgeon should determine whether bone grafting needs to be performed. If significant tunnel osteolysis is noted on preoperative imaging, bone grafting and staging is performed as discussed in the following section.

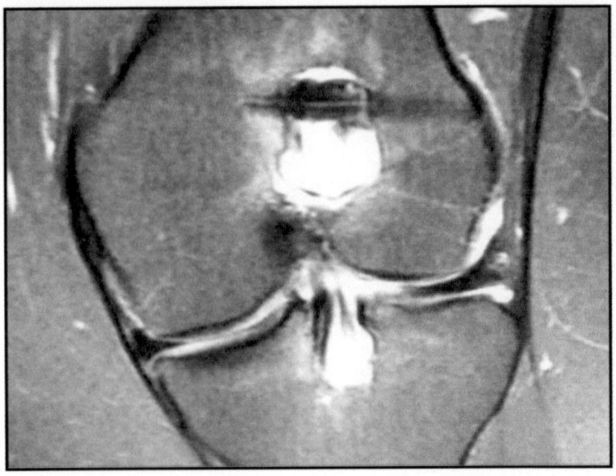

Figure 28-4. Coronal MRI showing severe tunnel osteolysis on the femoral and tibial tunnels.

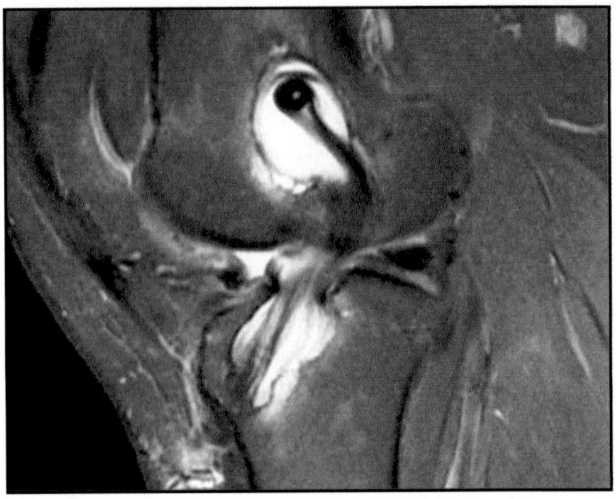

Figure 28-5. Sagittal MRI showing severe tunnel osteolysis on the femoral and tibial tunnels.

Bone Grafting Case Example

Figures 28-4 and 28-5 show significant femoral and tibial tunnel osteolysis after ACL reconstruction with the allograft and femoral cross transfixation pin. Tibial tunnel lysis measured 20 mm in diameter. The femoral tunnel lysis was 22 mm in size. Due to significant tunnel widening, a staged revision involving bone grafting of the femoral and tibial tunnels with femoral head allograft was recommended. Intraoperatively, the femoral tunnel was prepared with curettes and a shaver until bleeding bone was exposed. The femoral tunnel was measured and filled with femoral head allograft dowels that were subsequently tamped in place (Figures 28-6 through 28-8). The tibial tunnel was prepared with reamers, curettes, and a shaver. Bleeding bone was visualized, and the tunnel was filled with femoral head allograft. Figure 28-9 shows an x-ray of a separate patient who had bone grafting of his vertical, nonanatomic tunnel; the x-ray shows full incorporation of the grafted tunnel and revision hamstring ACL reconstruction. The senior author prefers to contour the bone block out of frozen femoral head allograft. An alternative option is precontoured bone dows that are commercially available.

Outside-In (Two-Incision) Technique

Once adequate visualization has been obtained with the previously described portals placed, a full diagnostic evaluation of the knee is performed. A full evaluation of the cartilage and meniscus must be performed. The menisci should be repaired if possible due to their importance as

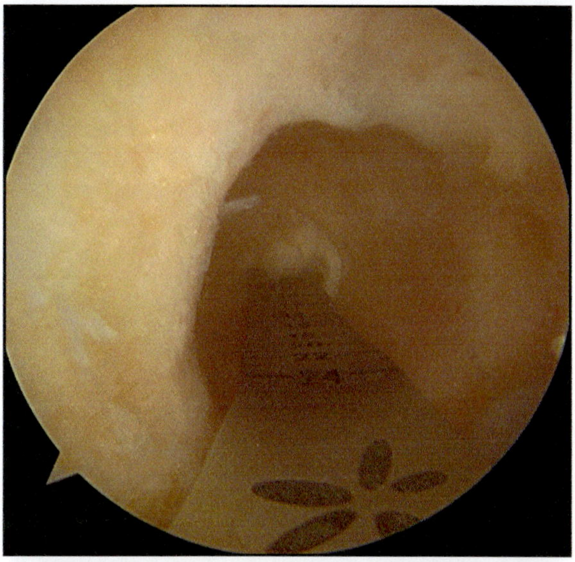

Figure 28-6. The femoral tunnel has been rereamed to good bleeding bone. View from the direct medial portal.

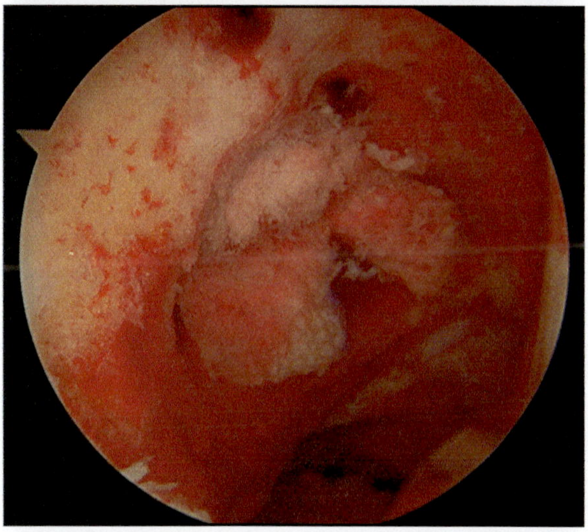

Figure 28-7. Femoral tunnel bone grafted with fresh-frozen femoral head allograft. View from the direct medial portal.

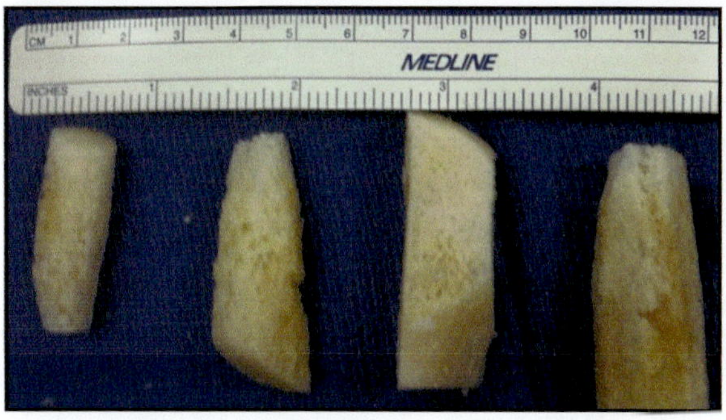

Figure 28-8. Femoral head allograft bone plugs created in the operating room using a rongeur and saw.

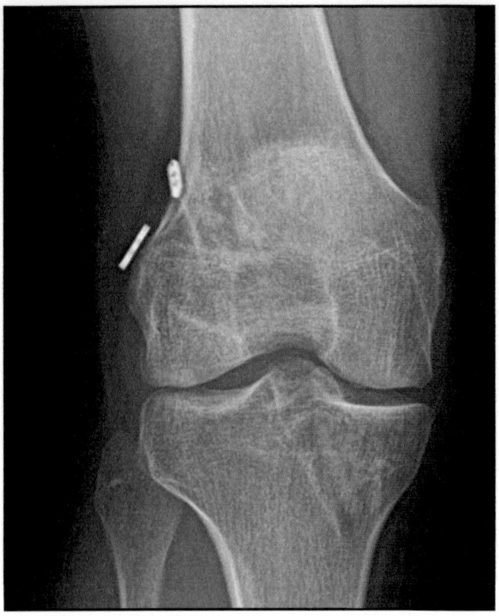

Figure 28-9. X-ray of separate patient in Figures 28-4 and 28-5 after bone grafting 6 months earlier with good allograft incorporation.

secondary stabilizers. If there is a medial or lateral drive through sign, this would indicate significant medial collateral ligament or posterolateral corner laxity and should be addressed concomitantly at the time of revision ACL reconstruction. The previous ACL graft should be debrided, and critical arthroscopic analysis of the tunnels should be done. Once all of the above has been addressed, the appropriate ACUFEX PINPOINT guide size is chosen, with options ranging from 6 to 10 mm. The scope is placed in the central medial portal, and the outside-in PINPOINT guide is placed through the anterolateral portal. The intra-articular portion of the guide is placed on the anatomic position on the medial aspect of the lateral femoral condyle. Next, the trochar is placed through the handle to mark the skin incision laterally. The starting point for the drill in general is anterior and proximal to the lateral epicondyle, except for use in skeletally immature patients. In these patients, the entrance point must be distal to the femoral physis, which is directly above the epicondyle or femoral attachment of the fibular collateral ligament. Care must be taken to maintain the intra-articular portion of the guide in the anatomic position.

The trochar is removed once the skin is marked, and a 2- to 3-cm skin incision is made in line with the iliotibial band. Skin retractors are placed, the trochar is reinserted, the iliotibial band is incised in line with its fibers, and the trochar is advanced through the guide handle abutting the lateral femoral condyle. While the guide is held firmly in place, a Beath pin is slowly advanced through the trochar and visualized with the scope, passing a few millimeters into the intercondylar notch (Figure 28-10). The guide is removed, and retractors are placed deep to the iliotibial band on each side of the Beath pin to prevent the reamer from injuring the iliotibial band. The Beath pin is grabbed with a pituitary grabber via the low anteromedial portal. The appropriately sized, fully fluted reamer is drilled in an outside-in manner while an assistant holds the Beath pin to prevent advancement. The pin and reamer are removed, the tunnel is debrided, and a plug is placed into the tunnel to prevent fluid extravasation (Figures 28-11 through 28-13). Drilling outside-in allows for a new virgin tunnel to be drilled, with tunnel convergence at the notch.

The tibial tunnel is drilled in a standard fashion. If the previously used screw can be avoided, the screw is left in place. In some cases, the screw is removed, and the tunnel is rereamed to allow for good bleeding bone. In addition, in some cases, if biocomposite screws were used in the original case, they are drilled through. It is important to start reaming with small reamers and progress up in size because previously placed screws can cause deflection of the reamers and cause nonanatomic tunnels. To pass the graft, a passing suture is looped and grabbed with a

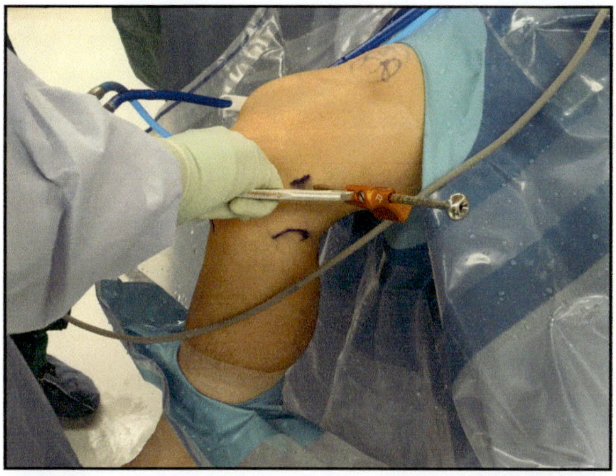

Figure 28-10. ACUFEX PINPOINT Anatomic ACL Guide System.

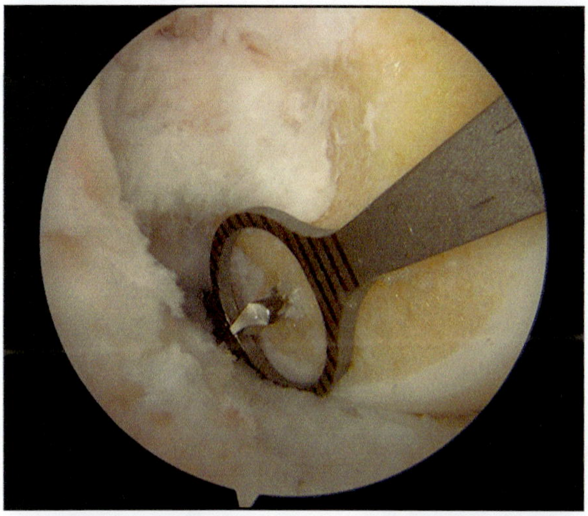

Figure 28-11. ACUFEX PINPOINT Anatomic ACL Guide System shown with the guide placed at the anatomic insertion of the femoral ACL footprint. The Beath pin can be seen advanced through the targeting circle. View from the direct medial portal.

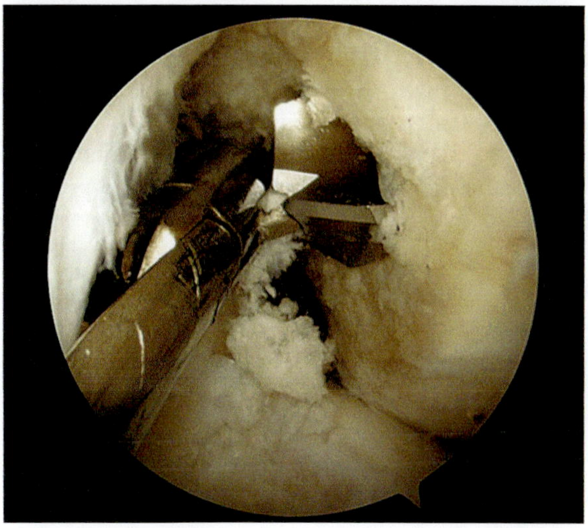

Figure 28-12. ACUFEX PINPOINT Anatomic ACL Guide System shown with the guide placed at the anatomic insertion of the femoral ACL footprint. The reamer has been advanced over the Beath pin. A pituitary grabber is used to grab the Beath pin to prevent advancement of the reamer into the notch. View from the direct medial portal.

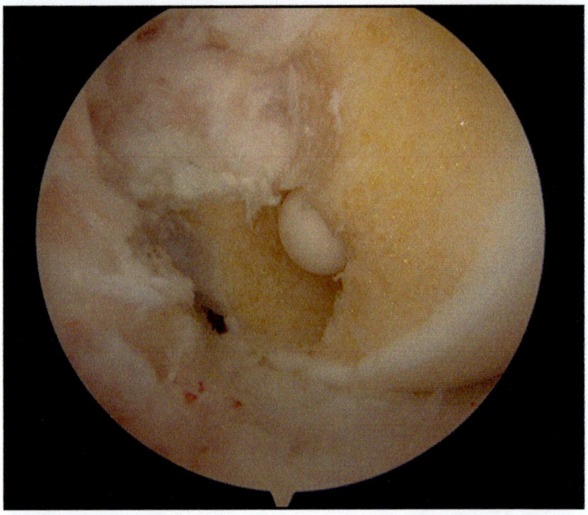

Figure 28-13. The bone plug can be seen placed from outside-in to prevent fluid extravasation. View from the direct medial portal.

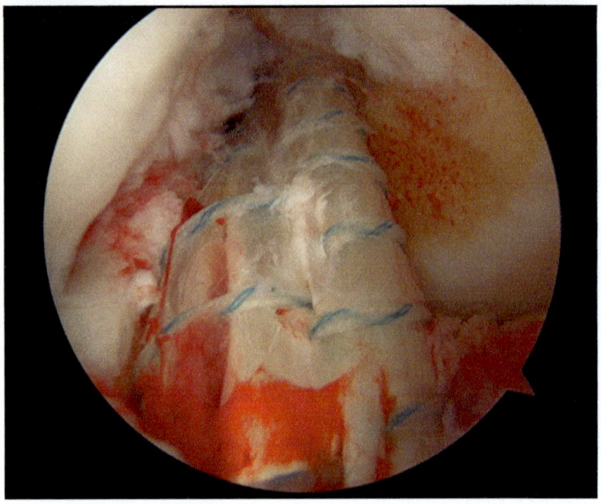

Figure 28-14. ACL graft viewed from the direct medial portal.

pituitary grabber. The passing suture is placed in a retrograde fashion through the lateral femoral condyle and passed off to another grabber through the drilled tibial tunnel. The graft can then be pulled into appropriate position (Figure 28-14). If a bone tendon bone graft is chosen, the bone plug is fixed on the femoral side with a metal screw placed from outside-in. The guide wire is placed in a retrograde manner, and the bone plug must be directly observed to prevent aberrant screw placement. The tibial side is fixed with a metal screw in the standard fashion (Figure 28-15).

If a hamstring tendon graft is used, the graft is passed in a similar manner; however, a 10-mm EndoButton (Smith & Nephew) with an Xtendobutton (Smith & Nephew) attachment is used for femoral fixation. A biocomposite screw and a staple or a screw with a spiked washer are used for tibial fixation (Figure 28-16).

Postoperative Protocol

Standard rehabilitation after revision ACL reconstruction is the same as a primary. The authors place all of their patients in a telescoping brace locked in full extension for 1 month when ambulating and weightbearing as tolerated. The brace can be unlocked for sleep at night and is removed

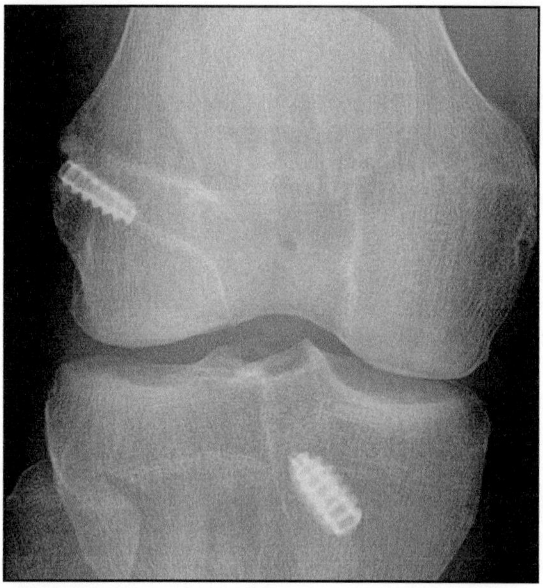

Figure 28-15. Anteroposterior x-ray showing a bone tendon bone graft fixed with metal interference screw fixation.

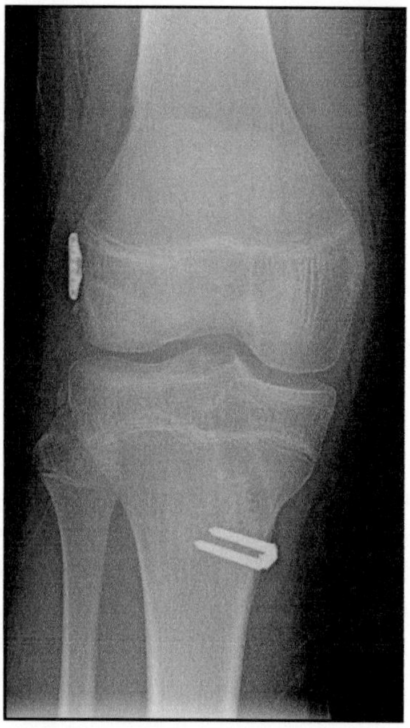

Figure 28-16. Anteroposterior x-ray showing a hamstring graft with a 10-mm EndoButton with an Xtendobutton used for femoral fixation. A biocomposite screw and a staple are used for tibial fixation.

when the patient is seated, and immediate full range of motion (ROM) is started on postoperative day 1. Formal physical therapy is started 3 to 5 days from the index procedure. At 1 month, the telescoping brace is shortened and unlocked. At 2 months, the patient is fitted with a standard off-the-shelf knee sleeve. Functional ACL braces are used for patients returning to contact sports, such as football and hockey, for the first year after the reconstruction. Patients are advised to start immediate full ROM on postoperative day 1 with quadriceps sets and straight leg raises initiated. Around 1 month, mini-squats and wall slides are started and bicycle is added. The patient in general is advised not to jog for 4 months with no running for 5 months. Sport-specific drills are initiated around 6 months, and return to sports after a revision is advised between 9 and 12 months, depending on quadriceps function. The rehabilitation protocol is adjusted depending on associated meniscal, cartilage, or alignment procedures performed.

Potential Complications

The following is an abbreviated list of the many complications that can occur with revision ACL reconstruction:

- Arthrofibrosis
- Graft rerupture
- Inability to return to play
- Lateral collateral ligament femoral insertion disruption, from outside-in reaming
- Poor graft fixation (if done in a single stage and not bone grafted or if tunnels converge)

- Lateral femoral condyle fracture (from multiple drill tunnels)
- Chronic pain
- Broken hardware or inability to remove previously placed hardware

Conclusion

As the number of primary ACL reconstructions increases, so will the number of revisions. ACL failure can be attributed to numerous factors. Loss of motion, chronic pain, and recurrent laxity are all reasons for patients to present with dissatisfaction with their primary reconstruction. It is imperative to understand the exact reason why the primary ACL reconstruction failed to ensure a successful outcome for the revision ACL reconstruction.

Return to play after revision ACL reconstruction is noted to be approximately 60%, and many of those patients will not be able to return to their previous levels of play.[26] The greatest concern is that more than 50% of patients have early radiographic findings of degenerative changes as early as 5 years after primary ACL surgery. The authors believe that the use of nonanatomic principles combined with failure to recognize associated patholaxity is the primary reason for primary ACL graft failure. The outside-in technique allows for a predictable method for revision ACL reconstruction. Adhering to anatomic reconstruction principles and addressing missed injuries to the secondary stabilizers should restore knee kinematics to as normal as possible and, therefore, improve overall outcomes. The senior author currently uses the outside-in technique on the majority of his revision ACL reconstructions.

Top Technical Pearls for the Procedure

1. If the previously placed metallic screws do not interfere with revision tunnel location, the screws should be left to prevent bone void defects.
2. Bone graft and stage if tunnel widening is greater than 16 to 17 mm.
3. Before revision surgery, the previous operative report must be available for preoperative planning.
4. Secondary stabilizer pathology must be addressed to prevent ACL graft retear.
5. When reaming through biocomposite screws, sequentially ream up starting with smaller reamers to prevent deflection of the reamer and nonanatomic tunnels.

References

1. American Orthopaedic Society for Sports Medicine. *Understanding and Preventing Noncontact ACL Injuries.* Champaign, IL; Human Kinetics; 2007.
2. Miyasaka KC, Daniel DM, Stone ML. The incidence of knee ligament injuries in the general population. *Am J Knee Surg.* 1991;4:43-48.
3. Ardern CL, Webster KE, Taylor NF, Feller JA. Return to sport following anterior cruciate ligament reconstruction surgery: a systematic review and meta-analysis of the state of play. *Br J Sports Med.* 2011;45(7):596-606.

4. Irrgang JJ, Harner CD. Loss of motion following knee ligament surgery. *Sports Med.* 1995;19(2):150-159.
5. Sachs RA, Daniel DM, Stone ML, Garfein RF. Patellofemoral problems after anterior cruciate ligament reconstruction. *Am J Sports Med.* 1989;17(6):760-765.
6. Johnson DL, Fu FH. Anterior cruciate ligament reconstruction: why do failures occur? *Instr Course Lect.* 1995;44:391-406.
7. Johnson DL, Harner CD, Maday MG, Fu FH. Revision anterior cruciate ligament surgery. In: Fu FH, Harner CD, Vince KG, eds. *Knee Surgery.* Baltimore, MD: Williams & Wilkins; 1994;1:877-895.
8. Maday MG, Harner CD, Fu FH. Revision ACL surgery: evaluation and treatment. In: Feagin JA Jr, ed. *The Crucial Ligaments: Diagnosis and Treatment of Ligamentous Injuries About the Knee.* New York, NY: Churchill-Livingstone; 1994:711-723.
9. Jackson DW, Schaefer RK. Cyclops syndrome: loss of extension following intra-articular anterior cruciate ligament reconstruction. *Arthroscopy.* 1990;6(3):171-178.
10. Wetzler MJ, Bartolozzi AR, Gillespie MJ, et al. Revision anterior cruciate ligament reconstruction. *Oper Tech Orthop.* 1996;6:181-189.
11. Fu FH, Jordan SS. The lateral intercondylar ridge—a key to anatomic anterior cruciate ligament reconstruction. *J Bone Joint Surg Am.* 2007;89(10):2103-2104.
12. Bird JH, Carmont MR, Dhillon M, et al. Validation of a new technique to determine midbundle femoral tunnel position in anterior cruciate ligament reconstruction using 3-dimensional computed tomography analysis. *Arthroscopy.* 2011;27(9):1259-1267.
13. Piefer JW, Pflugner TR, Hwang MD, Lubowitz JH. Anterior cruciate ligament femoral footprint anatomy: systematic review of the 21st century literature. *Arthroscopy.* 2012;28(6):872-881.
14. Hwang MD, Piefer JW, Lubowitz JH. Anterior cruciate ligament tibial footprint anatomy: systematic review of the 21st century literature. *Arthroscopy.* 2012;28(5):728-734.
15. Gadikota HR, Sim JA, Hosseini A, Gill TJ, Li G. The relationship between femoral tunnels created by the transtibial, anteromedial portal, and outside-in techniques and the anterior cruciate ligament footprint. *Am J Sports Med.* 2012;40(4):882-888.
16. Marchant BG, Noyes FR, Barber-Westin SD, Fleckenstein C. Prevalence of nonanatomical graft placement in a series of failed anterior cruciate ligament reconstructions. *Am J Sports Med.* 2010;38(10):1987-1996.
17. Duffee A, Magnussen RA, Pedroza AD, Flanigan DC; MOON Group, Kaeding CC. Transtibial ACL femoral tunnel preparation increases odds of repeat ipsilateral knee surgery. *J Bone Joint Surg Am.* 2013;95(22):2035-2042.
18. Magnussen RA, Lawrence JT, West RL, Toth AP, Taylor DC, Garrett WE. Graft size and patient age are predictors of early revision after anterior cruciate ligament reconstruction with hamstring autograft. *Arthroscopy.* 2012;28(4):526-531.
19. Mariscalco MW, Flanigan DC, Mitchell J, et al. The influence of hamstring autograft size on patient-reported outcomes and risk of revision after anterior cruciate ligament reconstruction: a MOON cohort study. *Arthroscopy.* 2013;29(12):1948-1953.
20. Rodeo SA, Arnoczky SP, Torzilli PA, Hidaka C, Warren RF. Tendon healing in a bone tunnel: a biomechanical and histological study in the dog. *J Bone Joint Surg Am.* 1993;75(12):1795-1803.
21. Jackson DW, Grood ES, Goldstein JD, et al. A comparison of patellar tendon autograft and allograft used for anterior cruciate ligament reconstruction in the goat model. *Am J Sports Med.* 1993;21(2):176-185.
22. Graf B, Uhr F. Complications of intra-articular anterior cruciate ligament reconstruction. *Clin Sports Med.* 1988;7(4):835-848.
23. Noyes FR. An unresolved dilemma: treatment of injuries to the posterolateral knee structures. *Am J Knee Surg.* 1993;6:95.
24. MARS Group, Wright RW, Huston LJ, et al. Descriptive epidemiology of the Multicenter ACL Revision Study (MARS) cohort. *Am J Sports Med.* 2010;38(10):1979-1986.
25. Johnson DL, Swenson TM, Irrgang JJ, Fu FH, Harner CD. Revision anterior cruciate ligament surgery: experience from Pittsburgh. *Clin Orthop Relat Res.* 1996;(325):100-109.
26. Grossman MG, El Attrache NS, Shields CL, Glousman RE. Revision anterior cruciate ligament reconstruction: three- to nine-year follow-up. *Arthroscopy.* 2005;21(14):418-423.
27. Johnson DL, Coen MJ. Revision ACL surgery. Etiology, indications, techniques, and results. *Am J Knee Surg.* 1995;8(4):155-167.

28. Getelman MH, Schepsis AA, Zimmer J. Revision ACL reconstruction: autograft vs allograft. *Arthroscopy.* 1995;11:378.
29. Noyes FR, Barber-Westin SD. Revision anterior cruciate ligament reconstruction: experience from Cincinnati. *Clin Orthop Relat Res.* 1996;(325):116-129.

Please see videos on the accompanying website at www.routledge.com/9781617119996

29

Arthroscopic Posterior Cruciate Ligament Reconstruction

Gregory C. Fanelli, MD

Introduction

This chapter addresses single- and double-bundle arthroscopic transtibial tunnel posterior cruciate ligament (PCL) reconstruction. This discussion includes physical examination, imaging studies, equipment requirements, patient positioning, surgical technique, postoperative program, potential complications, and the top technical pearls for the procedure. Isolated PCL tears are rare in the author's practice, and PCL injuries and reconstruction must always be considered in the context of the multiple-ligament injured knee.[1,2] Recognition and treatment of collateral ligament instability (posteromedial and posterolateral instability) is essential for successful PCL reconstruction.[3] Other factors that maximize the probability of a successful PCL reconstruction include strong graft material, accurate tunnel placement approximating anatomic ligament insertion sites, minimal graft bending, mechanical graft tensioning, secure graft fixation, and the appropriate postoperative rehabilitation program.[4,5] Single- and double-bundle PCL reconstruction surgical techniques are successful when evaluated with stress radiography, KT 1000 arthrometer measurements, and knee ligament rating scales. Indications for double-bundle PCL reconstruction include severe hyperextension of the knee and revision PCL reconstruction.[6] The author's long-term postsurgical results revealed successful PCL reconstruction using the arthroscopic transtibial tunnel surgical technique.[7,8]

Indications

- PCL-based multiple-ligament injured knee[4,9]
- PCL tears with articular surface and/or meniscal injuries[4,9]
- Isolated chronic PCL tear with functional instability

Sgaglione NA, Lubowitz JH, Provencher MT, eds. *The Knee: AANA Advanced Arthroscopic Surgical Techniques* (pp 405-414).

Controversial Indications

- Acute isolated PCL tear

Pertinent Physical Findings

- Tibial stepoff with the knee in 90 degrees of flexion
- Posterior drawer test
- KT 1000 knee ligament arthrometer

Because correct diagnosis of posteromedial and posterolateral instability is essential to successful PCL reconstruction, the posteromedial and posterolateral corners must be thoroughly evaluated.[4,9]

The author has observed 3 types of instability patterns in posteromedial and posterolateral knee injuries. These include type A (axial rotation instability only), type B (axial rotation instability combined with varus and/or valgus laxity with a firm endpoint), and type C (axial rotation instability combined with varus and/or valgus laxity with little or no endpoint). Thus, physical examination must include varus and valgus laxity and axial rotation instability evaluation. Varus and valgus laxity are assessed with varus and valgus stress at 0 and 30 degrees of knee flexion. Axial rotation instability is assessed with the posteromedial and posterolateral drawer tests at 90 degrees of knee flexion and the dial test at 30 and 90 degrees of knee flexion.[10,11]

In the author's experience, the axial rotation instability (type A) medial or lateral side is most frequently overlooked. It is also critical to understand that combined medial and lateral side instability of different types occurs with bicruciate and unicruciate multiple-ligament knee injuries. Examples include PCL, anterior cruciate ligament (ACL), lateral side type C, and medial side type A, or PCL, medial side type B, and lateral side type A instability patterns. Failure to recognize combined ligament instability patterns will jeopardize the success of the PCL reconstruction.[3]

Pertinent Imaging

- Plain x-rays
- Magnetic resonance imaging
- Computed tomography scans for revision surgery evaluation and evaluation of fracture dislocations
- Stress radiography[4,9,12,13]

Equipment

The Biomet Sports Medicine PCL/ACL System (Biomet Sports Medicine) includes the surgical instruments that the author uses for this surgical procedure; however, other equipment companies offer surgical instrumentation. Intraoperative radiography and C-arm image intensifiers may routinely used for this surgical procedure depending upon surgeon preference.

PCL-based reconstruction procedures are routinely performed in an outpatient setting unless specific circumstances indicate the necessity of an inpatient environment. The same experienced surgical teams are assembled for these complex surgical procedures. Experienced and familiar teams provide for a smoother operation, shorter surgical times, enhanced patient care, and a greater probability of success in these difficult surgical procedures.

Positioning and Portals

The patient is placed on the operating room table in the supine position, and after satisfactory induction of anesthesia, the operative and nonoperative lower extremities are carefully examined.[4-6,9,14-18] A tourniquet is applied to the upper thigh of the operative extremity but is not routinely inflated, and that extremity is prepped and draped in a sterile fashion. The well leg is supported by the fully extended operating room table, which also supports the surgical leg during medial- and lateral-side surgery. A lateral post is used to control the surgical extremity. An arthroscopic leg holder is not used. Pre- and postoperative antibiotics are given, and antibiotics are routinely used to help prevent infection in these time-consuming, difficult, and complex cases. Allograft tissue is prepared prior to bringing the patient into the operating room to minimize general anesthesia time for the patient. Autograft tissue is harvested prior to beginning the arthroscopic portion of the procedure.[19]

Step-by-Step Description of the Procedure

The principles of PCL reconstruction are to identify and treat all pathology, accurately place tunnels to produce anatomic graft insertion sites, use strong graft material, mechanical graft tensioning, secure graft fixation, and a deliberate postoperative rehabilitation program. Reasons for PCL reconstruction failure include failure to address associated ligament instabilities, varus osseous malalignment, and incorrect tunnel placement.[3-6,9,14-18]

The author's preferred grafts for PCL reconstruction are the Achilles tendon allograft for single-bundle PCL reconstructions and Achilles tendon (anterolateral bundle) and tibialis anterior (posteromedial bundle) allografts for double-bundle PCL reconstructions. The allograft tissue used is from the same tissue bank with the same methods of tissue procurement and preservation that provides a consistent graft of high quality. It is important for the surgeon to know the tissue bank and to obtain high-quality allograft tissue that will maximize the probability of surgical success.[5-8,14-22]

The arthroscopic instruments are inserted with gravity inflow through the superolateral patellar portal. Instrumentation and visualization are positioned through the inferomedial and inferolateral patellar portals and can be interchanged as necessary.[14,15,19] Additional portals are established as necessary. The author does not use arthroscopic fluid pumps. Exploration of the joint consists of evaluation of the patellofemoral joint, the medial and lateral compartments, medial and lateral menisci, and the intercondylar notch. The 3-zone arthroscopic evaluation technique for PCL assessment is performed and is particularly helpful for evaluation peel off lesions and bony avulsion injuries. The residual stumps of the PCL are debrided; however, the posterior (and ACL when applicable) anatomic insertion sites are preserved to serve as tunnel reference points. The notchplasty for the ACL portion of the procedure in combined PCL-ACL reconstruction cases is performed at this time.

An extracapsular, extra-articular posteromedial safety incision is made by creating an incision approximately 1.5 to 2 cm long starting at the posteromedial border of the tibia approximately 1 inch below the level of the joint line and extending distally (Figure 29-1). Dissection is carried down to the crural fascia, which is incised longitudinally. An interval is developed between the medial head of the gastrocnemius muscle and the nerves and vessels posterior to the surgeon's finger, and the capsule of the knee joint anterior to the surgeon's finger. The posteromedial safety

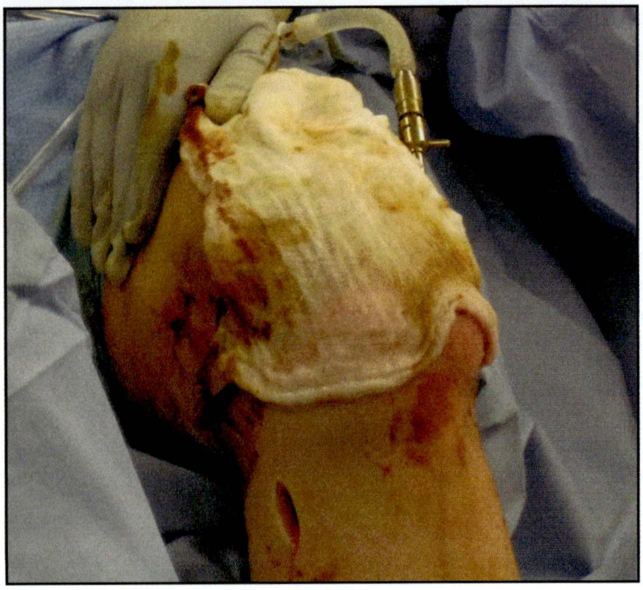

Figure 29-1. An extracapsular, extra-articular, posteromedial safety incision is made by creating an incision approximately 1.5 to 2 cm long starting at the posteromedial border of the tibia approximately 1 inch below the level of the joint line and extending distally. An interval is developed between the medial head of the gastrocnemius muscle and the nerves and vessels posterior to the surgeon's finger and the capsule of the knee joint anterior to the surgeon's finger. The posteromedial safety incision enables the surgeon to protect the neurovascular structures, confirm the accuracy of the PCL tibial tunnel, and facilitate the flow of the surgical procedure. The patient is supine on the fully extended operating table. A lateral post is used. No leg holder is used. The arthroscope is in the inferior lateral patellar portal on this left knee.

incision enables the surgeon to protect the neurovascular structures, confirm the accuracy of the PCL tibial tunnel, and facilitate the flow of the surgical procedure. The neurovascular structures of the popliteal fossa are in close proximity to the posterior capsule of the knee joint and are at risk during transtibial PCL reconstruction. The posteromedial safety incision is important for the protection of these structures.

The curved over-the-top PCL instruments (Biomet Sports Medicine) are used to sequentially lyse adhesions in the posterior aspect of the knee and elevate the capsule from the posterior tibial ridge. This will allow accurate placement of the PCL/ACL drill guide and correct placement of the tibial tunnel.

The arm of the PCL/ACL guide (Biomet Sports Medicine) is inserted through the inferior medial patellar portal (Figure 29-2). The tip of the guide is positioned at the inferior lateral aspect of the PCL anatomic insertion site. This is below the tibial ridge posterior and in the lateral aspect of the PCL anatomic insertion site. The bullet portion of the guide contacts the anteromedial surface of the proximal tibia at a point midway between the posteromedial border of the tibia and the tibial crest anterior at or just below the level of the tibial tubercle. This will provide an angle of graft orientation such that the graft will turn 2 smooth 45-degree angles on the posterior aspect of the tibia. The tip of the guide, in the posterior aspect of the tibia, is confirmed with the surgeon's finger through the extracapsular, extra-articular posteromedial safety incision. Intraoperative anteroposterior and lateral x-rays may also be used; however, the author does not routinely use intraoperative x-rays. When the PCL/ACL guide is positioned in the desired area, a blunt spade-tipped guide wire is drilled from anterior to posterior. The surgeon's finger confirms the position of the guide wire through the posterior medial safety incision.

The appropriately sized standard cannulated reamer is used to create the tibial tunnel. The surgeon's finger through the extracapsular, extra-articular posteromedial incision is monitoring the position of the guide wire. When the drill is engaged in bone, the guide wire is reversed with the blunt end pointing posterior for additional patient safety. The drill is advanced until it comes to the posterior cortex of the tibia. The chuck is disengaged from the drill, and completion of the tibial tunnel is performed by hand.

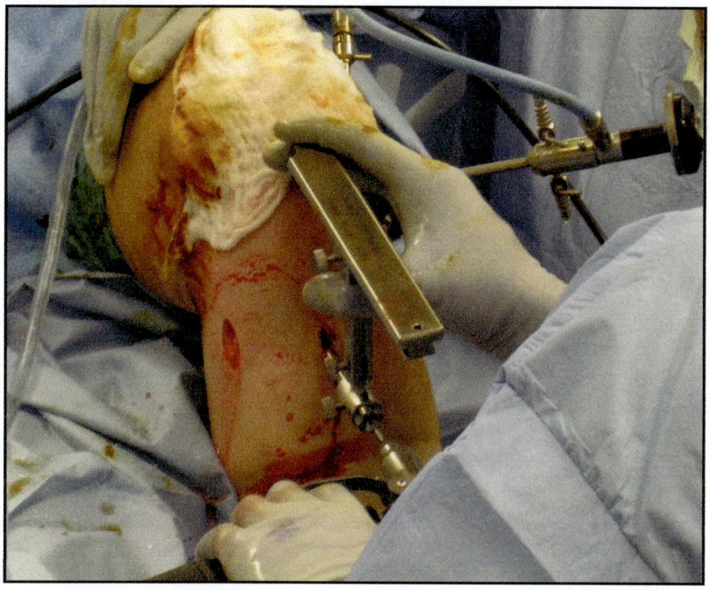

Figure 29-2. The arm of the PCL/ACL guide is inserted through the inferior medial patellar portal. The tip of the guide is positioned at the inferior lateral aspect of the PCL anatomic insertion site. The bullet portion of the guide contacts the anteromedial surface of the proximal tibia at a point midway between the posteromedial border of the tibia and the tibial crest anterior at or just below the level of the tibial tubercle. The patient is supine on the fully extended operating table. A lateral post is used. No leg holder is used. The arthroscope is in the inferior lateral patellar portal on this left knee.

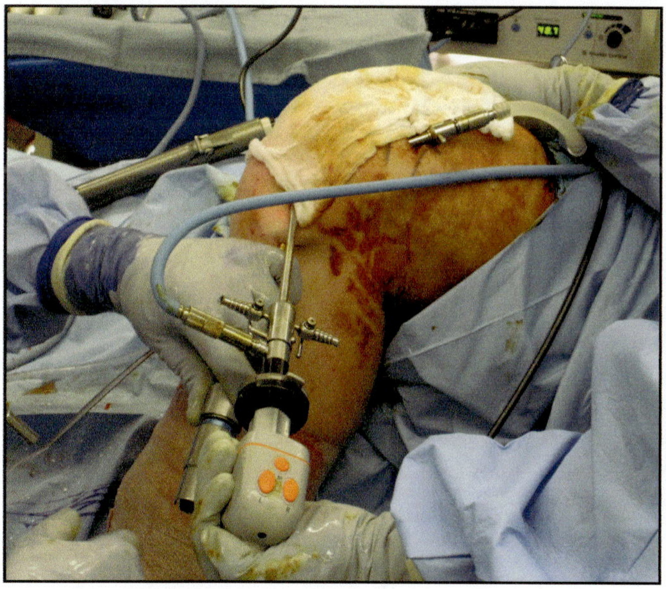

Figure 29-3. The PCL single- or double-bundle femoral tunnels are made from inside-out using the low anterior lateral patellar arthroscopic portal. The surgical knee is in 90 to 110 degrees of flexion during femoral tunnel creation. Femoral tunnel creation from inside-out provides a greater margin of safety between the PCL femoral tunnels and the medial femoral condyle articular surface. In addition, a more accurate placement of the PCL femoral tunnels is possible because the double-bundle aimer or endoscopic reamer can be placed on the anatomic footprint of the anterior lateral or posterior medial PCL insertion site under direct visualization. The patient is supine on the fully extended operating table. A lateral post is used. No leg holder is used. The arthroscope is in the inferior lateral patellar portal on this left knee.

The PCL single- or double-bundle femoral tunnels are made from inside-out using the double-bundle aimers, or an endoscopic reamer can be used as an aiming device (Biomet Sports Medicine). The appropriately sized double-bundle aimer or endoscopic reamer is inserted through a low anterior lateral patellar arthroscopic portal to create the PCL anterior lateral bundle femoral tunnel with the surgical knee in 90 to 110 degrees of knee flexion (Figure 29-3). The double-bundle aimer or endoscopic reamer is positioned directly on the footprint of the femoral anterior lateral bundle PCL insertion site. The appropriately sized guide wire is drilled through the aimer or endoscopic reamer, through the bone, and out of a small skin incision. Care is taken to prevent compromise of the articular surface. The double-bundle aimer is removed, and the endoscopic

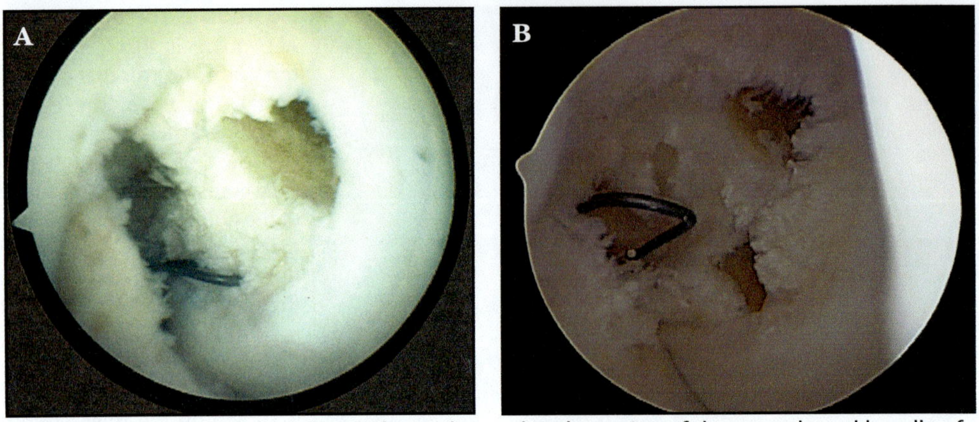

Figure 29-4. (A) A single-bundle PCL femoral tunnel in the region of the anterolateral bundle of the PCL. (B) Double-bundle PCL reconstruction tunnels approximating the anatomic insertion sites of the anterolateral and posteromedial bundles of the PCL. The patient is supine on the fully extended operating table. A lateral post is used. No leg holder is used. The arthroscope is in the inferior lateral patellar portal on this right knee.

reamer is used to drill the anterior lateral PCL femoral tunnel from inside to outside. When the surgeon chooses to perform a double-bundle double femoral tunnel PCL reconstruction, the same process is repeated for the posterior medial bundle of the PCL. Care must be taken to ensure that there will be an adequate bone bridge (approximately 5 mm) between the 2 femoral tunnels prior to drilling. This is accomplished using the calibrated probe and direct arthroscopic visualization of the PCL femoral anatomic insertion sites (Figure 29-4).

The author prefers the surgical technique of PCL femoral tunnel creation from inside to outside for 2 reasons. There is a greater distance and margin of safety between the PCL femoral tunnels and the medial femoral condyle articular surface using the inside to outside method. In addition, a more accurate placement of the PCL femoral tunnels is possible because one can place the double-bundle aimer or endoscopic reamer on the anatomic footprint of the anterior lateral or posterior medial PCL insertion site under direct visualization.

A Magellan suture retriever (Biomet Sports Medicine) is introduced through the tibial tunnel into the joint and is retrieved through the femoral tunnel. The traction sutures of the graft material are attached to the loop of the Magellan suture retriever, and the graft is pulled into position. The graft material is secured on the femoral side using a bioabsorbable interference screw for primary aperture opening fixation, and a polyethylene ligament fixation button is used for backup fixation (Figure 29-5).

The cyclic dynamic method of graft tensioning using the Biomet graft tensioning boot is used to tension the PCL and ACL grafts.[23] Tension is placed on the PCL graft distally using the Biomet graft-tensioning boot (Biomet Sports Medicine). Tension is gradually applied with the knee in 0 degrees of flexion (full extension), reducing the tibia on the femur (Figure 29-6). This restores the anatomic tibial stepoff. The knee is cycled through a full range of motion (ROM) multiple times to allow pretensioning and settling of the graft. The process is repeated until there is no further change in the torque setting on the graft tensioner. The knee is placed in 70 to 90 degrees of flexion, and fixation is achieved on the tibial side of the PCL graft with a bioabsorbable interference screw and backup fixation with a bicortical screw and spiked ligament washer or polyethylene ligament fixation button (Figure 29-7).

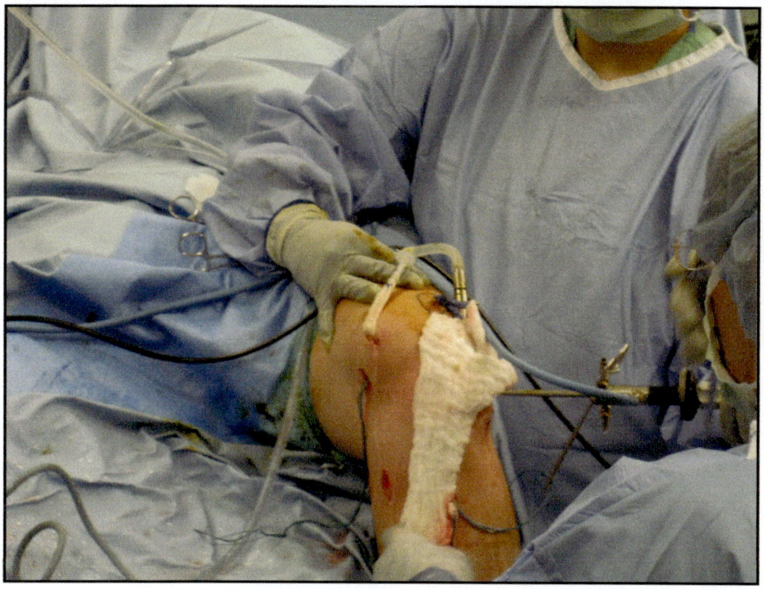

Figure 29-5. Achilles tendon allograft passage is shown reconstructing the anterolateral bundle of the PCL in a double-bundle PCL reconstruction. Note the ligament fixation button that will serve as cortical suspensory backup fixation. The patient is supine on the fully extended operating table. A lateral post is used. No leg holder is used. The arthroscope is in the inferior lateral patellar portal on this left knee.

Postoperative Protocol

The knee is maintained in full extension for 3 to 5 weeks nonweightbearing. Progressive ROM begins during postoperative weeks 3 through 5. Progressive weightbearing occurs at the beginning of postoperative weeks 3 through 5. Progressive closed kinetic chain strength training, proprioceptive training, and continued motion exercises are initiated slowly, beginning at postoperative week 12. Return to sports and heavy labor occurs after the 9th to 12th postoperative month when sufficient strength, ROM, and proprioceptive skills have returned. Functional bracing may be used at the surgeon's discretion. It is important to carefully observe these complex knee ligament injury patients and get a feel for the personality of the knee. The surgeon may need to make adjustments and individualize the postoperative rehabilitation program as necessary. Careful and gentle ROM under general anesthesia is a useful tool in the treatment of these complex cases and is used as necessary. Pre- and postoperative antibiotics are given, and antibiotics are routinely used to help prevent infection in these time-consuming, difficult, and complex cases.[19,24-27]

Potential Complications

Potential complications include injury to the posterior neurovascular structures of the knee, articular surface damage during tunnel creation, osteonecrosis, peroneal nerve injury during posterolateral reconstruction, infection, problematic wound healing, deep venous thrombosis, postoperative fracture, arthrofibrosis, persistent laxity, compartment syndrome, and physeal injury.[28-30]

Conclusion

The goals leading to successful PCL reconstruction include identification and treatment of associated pathology, such as posterolateral instability, posteromedial instability, and lower-extremity malalignment. The use of strong graft material, properly placed tunnels as closely as possible to the approximate PCL insertion sites, and minimization of graft bending also enhance

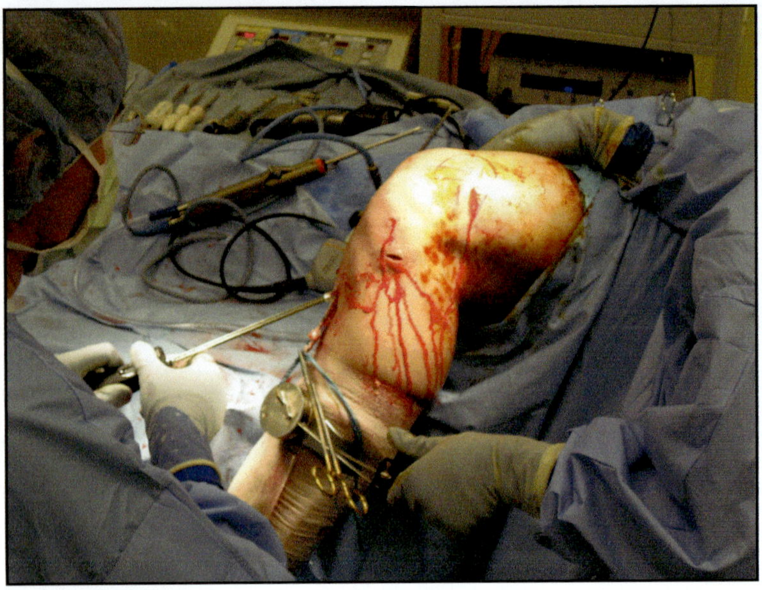

Figure 29-6. The cyclic dynamic method of graft tensioning using the Biomet graft tensioning boot is used to tension the PCL graft. Tension is gradually applied with the knee in 0 degrees of flexion (full extension), reducing the tibia on the femur. This restores the anatomic tibial stepoff. The knee is cycled through a full ROM multiple times to allow pretensioning and settling of the graft. The process is repeated until there is no further change in the torque setting on the graft tensioner. The knee is placed in 70 to 90 degrees of flexion, and fixation is achieved on the tibial side of the PCL graft with a bioabsorbable interference screw and backup fixation with a bicortical screw and spiked ligament washer or polyethylene ligament fixation button. The patient is supine on the fully extended operating table. A lateral post is used. No leg holder is used. The arthroscope is in the inferior lateral patellar portal on this left knee.

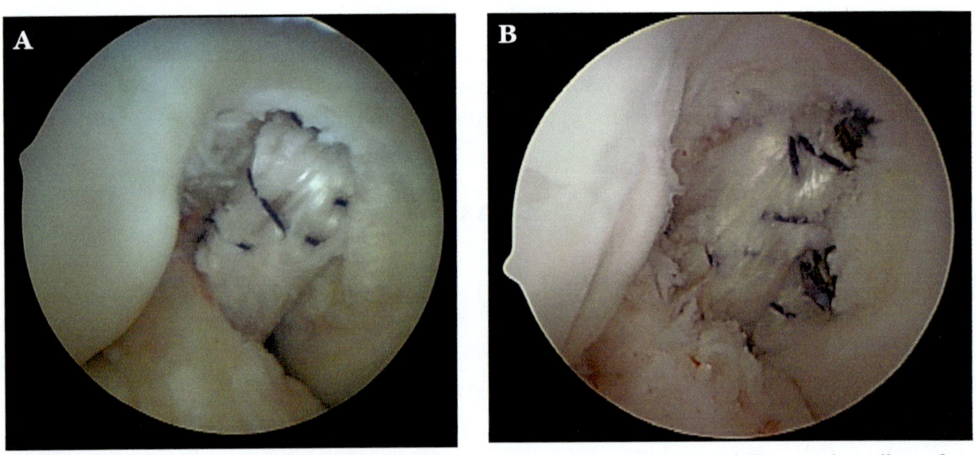

Figure 29-7. (A) Single- and (B) double-bundle PCL reconstructions. An Achilles tendon allograft is used for the anterolateral bundle of the PCL in both reconstructions. A tibialis anterior allograft is used for the posteromedial bundle PCL reconstruction in double-bundle PCL reconstructions. The patient is supine on the fully extended operating table. A lateral post is used. No leg holder is used. The arthroscope is in the inferior lateral patellar portal on this right knee.

the probability of PCL reconstruction success. In addition, mechanical graft tensioning, secure PCL graft fixation, and an appropriate postoperative rehabilitation program are also necessary ingredients for PCL reconstruction success. Single- and double-bundle PCL reconstruction surgical techniques are successful when evaluated with stress radiography, KT 1000 arthrometer measurements, and knee ligament rating scales. Indications for double-bundle PCL reconstruction include severe hyperextension of the knee and revision PCL reconstruction. The author's postsurgical results reveal successful PCL reconstruction using the arthroscopic transtibial tunnel surgical technique using allograft tissue.[5-8,15,17-22]

Top Technical Pearls for the Procedure

1. Identify and treat all pathology (posterolateral instability, posteromedial instability, alignment) using anatomic graft insertion sites
2. Posteromedial safety incision
3. Mechanical graft tensioning
4. Secure fixation
5. Appropriate postoperative rehabilitation program

References

1. Fanelli GC. Posterior cruciate ligament injuries in trauma patients. *Arthroscopy.* 1993;9(3):291-294.
2. Fanelli GC, Edson CJ. Posterior cruciate ligament injuries in trauma patients: part II. *Arthroscopy.* 1995;11(5):526-529.
3. Noyes FR, Barber-Westin SD. Posterior cruciate ligament revision reconstruction, part 1: causes of surgical failure in 52 consecutive operations. *Am J Sports Med.* 2005;33(5):646-654.
4. Fanelli GC, Beck JD, Edson CJ. Current concepts review: the posterior cruciate ligament. *J Knee Surg.* 2010;23(2):61-72.
5. Fanelli GC, Beck JD, Edson CJ. Arthroscopic double-bundle posterior cruciate ligament reconstruction surgical technique. *J Knee Surg.* 2010;23(2):89-94.
6. Fanelli GC, Beck JD, Edson CJ. Single compared to double-bundle PCL reconstruction using allograft tissue. *J Knee Surg.* 2012;25(1):59-64.
7. Fanelli GC, Edson CJ. Surgical treatment of combined PCL-ACL medial and lateral side injuries (global laxity): surgical technique and 2- to 18-year results. *J Knee Surg.* 2012;25(4):307-316.
8. Fanelli GC, Sousa PL, Edson CJ. Long-term followup of surgically treated knee dislocations: stability restored, but arthritis is common. *Clin Orthop Relat Res.* 2014;472(9):2712-2717.
9. Fanelli GC, Giannotti BF, Edson CJ. The posterior cruciate ligament arthroscopic evaluation and treatment. *Arthroscopy.* 1994;10(6):673-688.
10. Fanelli GC, Feldman DD. Management of combined anterior cruciate ligament/posterior cruciate ligament/posterolateral complex injuries of the knee. *Oper Tech Sports Med.* 1999;7(3):143-149.
11. Fanelli GC, Harris JD. Late medial collateral ligament reconstruction. *Tech Knee Surg.* 2007;6(2):99-105.
12. Malone JW, Verde F, Weiss D, Fanelli GC. MR imaging of knee instability. *Magn Reson Imaging Clin N Am.* 2009;17(4):697-724.
13. Staubli HU. Stress radiography: measurements of knee motion limits. In: Daniel D, ed. *Knee Ligaments: Structure, Function, Injury, and Repair.* New York, NY: Raven Press; 1990:461-480.
14. Fanelli GC. *Rationale and Surgical Technique for PCL and Multiple Knee Ligament Reconstruction.* 3rd ed. Warsaw, IN: Biomet Sports Medicine; 2012.

15. Fanelli GC. Surgical treatment of combined PCL-ACL medial and lateral side injuries (global laxity): acute and chronic. In: Fanelli GC, ed. *The Multiple Ligament Injured Knee. A Practical Guide to Management.* 2nd ed. New York, NY: Springer-Verlag; 2013:281-301.
16. Fanelli GC, Boyd J. How I manage PCL injuries. *Oper Tech Sports Med.* 2009;17(3):175-193.
17. Fanelli GC, Beck JD, Edson CJ. Double bundle posterior cruciate ligament reconstruction: surgical technique and results. *Sports Med Arthrosc Rev.* 2010;18(4):242-248.
18. Fanelli GC, Beck JD, Edson CJ. Arthroscopic double-bundle posterior cruciate ligament reconstruction. *J Knee Surg.* 2010,23(2):89-94.
19. Fanelli GC. The multiple ligament injured knee: what I have learned. In: Fanelli GC, ed. *The Multiple Ligament Injured Knee. A Practical Guide to Management.* 2nd ed. New York, NY: Springer-Verlag; 2013:3-14.
20. Fanelli GC, Edson CJ. Combined posterior cruciate ligament-posterolateral reconstructions with Achilles tendon allograft and biceps femoris tendon tenodesis: 2- to 10-year follow-up. *Arthroscopy.* 2004;20(4):339-345.
21. Fanelli GC, Edson CJ. Arthroscopically assisted combined anterior and posterior cruciate ligament reconstruction in the multiple ligament injured knee: 2- to 10-year follow-up. *Arthroscopy.* 2002;18(7):703-714.
22. Fanelli GC, Edson CJ, Orcutt DR, Harris JD, Zijerdi D. Treatment of combined anterior-posterior cruciate ligament medial lateral side injuries of the knee. *J Knee Surg.* 2005;18(3):240-248.
23. Fanelli GC. Mechanical graft tensioning in multiple ligament knee surgery. In: Fanelli GC, ed. *The Multiple Ligament Injured Knee. A Practical Guide to Management.* 2nd ed. New York, NY: Springer-Verlag; 2013:323-330.
24. Fanelli GC. Posterior cruciate ligament rehabilitation: how slow should we go? *Arthroscopy.* 2008;24(2):234-235.
25. Edson CJ, Fanelli GC, Beck JD. Rehabilitation after multiple-ligament reconstruction of the knee. *Sports Med Arthrosc Rev.* 2011;19(2):162-166.
26. Edson CJ, Fanelli GC, Beck JD. Postoperative rehabilitation of the posterior cruciate ligament. *Sports Med Arthrosc Rev.* 2010;18(4):275-279.
27. Edson CJ, Fanelli GC. Postoperative rehabilitation of the multiple ligament injured knee. In: Fanelli GC, ed. *The Multiple Ligament Injured Knee. A Practical Guide to Management.* 2nd ed. New York, NY: Springer-Verlag; 2013:437-442.
28. Fanelli GC, Monahan TJ. Complications of posterior cruciate ligament reconstruction. *Sports Med Arthrosc Rev.* 1999;7(4):296-302.
29. Fanelli GC, Monahan TJ. Complications in posterior cruciate ligament and posterolateral corner surgery. *Oper Tech Sports Med.* 2001;9(2);96-99.
30. Fanelli GC, Orcutt DR. Complications posterior cruciate ligament reconstruction. *Sports Med Arthrosc Rev.* 2004;12(3):196-201.

Please see videos on the accompanying website at www.routledge.com/9781617119996

30

Arthroscopic All-Inside Posterior Cruciate Ligament Reconstruction

Nathan Jacobson, MD; Robby Sikka, MD;
Ryan Dunlay, MD; and Joel Boyd, MD

Introduction

The primary function of the posterior cruciate ligament (PCL) is to prevent posterior tibial translation, and a secondary function is to restrict the rotation of the knee.[1] Only by understanding the anatomy and function of the PCL is it possible to attempt anatomic reconstruction and restoration of proper stability and kinematics to the knee. Consequently, significant research has gone into accurately describing the PCL. Current descriptions of the PCL describe a continuum of fibers that can be delineated into 2 separate bundles, including the anterolateral and the posteromedial bundles. Tension in these 2 bundles differs during range of motion (ROM), with the anterolateral bundle experiencing more tension during flexion and the posteromedial bundle experiencing more tension during extension.[1-7] However, in normal ROM, Papannagari et al[4] demonstrated synergistic function of the 2 bundles because both experienced an increase in length, with degrees of flexion ranging from 0 to 120 degrees using dual-orthogonal fluoroscopic imaging.

The femoral and tibial footprints have been described using multiple anatomical references in an attempt to allow accurate footprint identification and reconstruction. The average femoral footprint has been measured at 209 ± 33.82 mm^2 (anterolateral, 118 ± 23.95 mm^2; posteromedial 90 ± 16.13 mm^2) and the tibial footprint at 243 ± 38.2 mm^2 (anterolateral, 93.1 ± 16.6 mm^2; posteromedial, 150.8 ± 31.0 mm^2).[5-7] Specific identification of the centers of the anterolateral and posteromedial bundles has been extensively studied in reference to local anatomical landmarks to facilitate accurate reconstruction of the individual bundles.

The tibial insertion of the PCL is predominantly within the posterior PCL or intercondylar facet, which is a relatively flat area bordered anteriorly by the posterior horn of the medial meniscus and posteriorly by the posterior cortex of the tibia.[8] Edwards et al[3] and Takahashi et al[9] measured the distance from the medial tibia to the centers of the anterolateral and posteromedial bundles and reported them as a percentages of the width of the tibial plateau, averaging $48\% \pm 4\%$[3] and 51%,[9] respectively, for the anterolateral bundle and $48\% \pm 5\%$[3] and 50%[9] for the posteromedial bundle. The center of the PCL insertion can reproducibly be identified 7 mm anterior to the

Sgaglione NA, Lubowitz JH, Provencher MT, eds. *The Knee: AANA Advanced Arthroscopic Surgical Techniques* (pp 415-434).

posterior cortex of the tibia.[8] The anterolateral bundle inserts at the superolateral portion of the facet, and the posteromedial bundle is upon the inferomedial portion.[5]

Femoral footprints have shown greater variability than tibial footprints. Femoral tunnel placement during reconstruction has proven to have a significant impact on the function of the PCL, as demonstrated by multiple investigators.[1,6,7,10,11] When varying the femoral tunnel location, Mannor et al[10] demonstrated that the tension of the graft was subsequently altered and the biomechanical properties of the knee were changed. Markolf et al[11] also investigated the biomechanical effects of tunnel placement; they used 10 cadaveric knees to test the effect of 5 mm of displacement (medial and lateral) of the femoral footprint and found that the medially displaced graft was subjected to greater forces at knee flexion angles greater than 5 degrees. These studies underline the importance of establishing the proper anatomic position for the femoral footprint of the PCL and have been the focus of multiple studies. Takahashi et al[9] measured the distances from the center of the anterolateral (9.6 mm) and posteromedial (10.6 mm) bundles from the articular cartilage, using a line drawn parallel to Blumensaat's line. Conversely, Morgan et al[12] measured the centers of the anterolateral and posteromedial bundles at 13 ± 0.5 mm and 8 ± 0.5 mm, respectively, posterior to the medial articular cartilage-intercondylar wall interface and 13 ± 0.5 mm and 20 ± 0.5 mm, respectively, inferior to the articular cartilage-intercondylar roof interface. Lopes et al[6] coined the term *medial intercondylar ridge* after identifying an osseous prominence just proximal to the femoral footprint of the PCL in 18 of 20 (90%) cadaver specimens. In addition, in 8 of 20 (40%) of the specimens, they identified and named an osseous bridge dividing the anterolateral and posteromedial bundles the medial bifurcate ridge.[6] These anatomical landmarks may be of great utility in proper anatomic intraoperative footprint identification.

Controversy remains in regard to the degree in which function can be restored through various surgical techniques. Gill et al[13] showed that under normal physiologic loads, single-bundle reconstruction restores the anteroposterior laxity of the PCL at flexion angles up to 90 degrees. In addition, Gill et al[13] showed a nonstatistically significant reduction of external rotation in single-bundle repaired knees. However, the success of single-bundle reconstruction in restoring the rotational component of PCL function is a matter of contention. In studies by Race et al,[14] Harner et al,[15] and Whiddon et al,[16] in vitro double-bundle PCL reconstruction more closely restored the function of the native PCL. Wijdicks et al[17] also demonstrated significantly less internal rotation with double-bundle repair at angles of 90 degrees or greater. However, Bergfeld et al[18] found no definitive advantage of double-bundle repair.

Indications[19-23]

- Multiligamentous knee injury
- Avulsion fractures
- Decrease in tibial stepoff greater than 8 mm
- Chronic functional instability
- Failed conservative management

Controversial Indications[23]

- Grade I and II PCL injuries
- Isolated complete PCL injuries

Pertinent Physical Findings[1-3]

Tests to be performed include the following:

- Posterior drawer test: Posterior displacement of the tibia 0 to 5 mm is grade I; 6 to 10 mm is grade II; and greater than 10 mm is grade III posterior drawer.
- Quadriceps active test: The patient is in the supine position with the knee being evaluated flexed to 90 degrees, and he or she then contracts his or her quadriceps muscle. In the PCL-deficient knee, the tibia is reduced from its posteriorly subluxed position (posterior sagittal sign), translating anteriorly due to the pull of the quadriceps.
- Full ligamentous and ROM examination for the injured and contralateral knees: This is performed to help identify a baseline/normal knee examination if possible and determine concomitant injuries.

Pertinent Imaging

- Stress x-rays[24,25]: Obtaining lateral x-rays of the knee while performing a posterior drawer test allows for direct measurement of the displacement of the tibia from the reduced anterior position and the posterior subluxed position. Posterior displacement of 8 mm indicates complete PCL disruption, and displacement of greater than 12 mm indicates that additional structures have been compromised in the posterior lateral corner of the knee.
- Magnetic resonance imaging: Can aid when the patient is guarding and evaluate the remaining structures of the knee for concomitant injuries that would need to be addressed concomitantly to produce a stable knee.

Equipment

- TightRope Attachable Button System (ABS; Arthrex)
- GraftLink
- Anatomic Contour PCL Guide (Arthrex)
- FlipCutter (Arthrex)
- #2 FiberStick (Arthrex)
- 30-degree scope
- Leg holder

Step-by-Step Description of the Procedure

All-Inside Technique

The goals of PCL reconstruction have remained consistent: accurately reconstruct normal anatomy by placing the PCL within the original footprint, reestablish stability, and restore knee ROM and proper knee function. The all-inside PCL reconstruction technique has multiple advantages over open tibial inlay techniques. By using smaller incisions, the all-inside technique is less invasive and can avoid additional operative time through use of arthroscopically assisted placement of the tibial tunnel.[26] This less-invasive approach is particularly useful in multiligamentous reconstructions by preventing spacing issues between incisions and limiting the additional surgical trauma of the reconstruction to the already traumatized knee. The all-inside technique allows the surgeon to avoid a posterior incision and popliteal fossa dissection, the drilling of the tibia is done using a FlipCutter that allows drill progression/advancement to be directed away from the posterior neurovascular structures, and less bone is removed by creation of a tibial socket as opposed to the traditional full-length transtibial tunnel. Furthermore, the creation of a tibial socket limits the potential for graft migration. Lubowitz and Konicek[27] demonstrated that retrograde socket drilling is more accurate than antegrade drilling in a cadaveric study in which a 3.5-mm tibial socket drilled in a retrograde fashion was significantly more accurate than a 2.4-mm tibial socket drilled in an antegrade fashion.

Reconstruction strengths have been found comparable between the all-inside and open inlay techniques.[28,29] In a cadaveric model, Zehms et al[28] demonstrated that arthroscopic double-bundle PCL inlay reconstruction performed with an all-inside techniques provided comparable stability to its open counterpart. In addition, Kim and Park[29] demonstrated less than 3 mm of side-to-side difference in posterior translation after double-bundle PCL reconstruction using an all-inside inlay technique.

With the open tibial inlay technique, there is concerning evidence that clinical laxity may be created as a result of the posterior capsulotomy that is required during the open exposure. Using 14 cadaveric knees, Ritchie et al[30] demonstrated that after posteromedial capsular sectioning, there was an average increase of 0.59 mm of posterior translation. Park et al[31] similarly found that posterior capsule violation increased posterior translation by 0.97 mm at 0 degrees of flexion and 0.94 mm at 120 degrees of knee flexion. These increases in laxity are relatively small but must be kept in mind when the goal is to increase restraint and return stability to the PCL-deficient knee.

Visualization is facilitated by usage of the posteromedial portal. With all-inside techniques, the surgeon has the ability to fully visualize the distal extent of the PCL tibial insertion through the posteromedial portal while not working around and retracting the posterior neurovascular structures. This improves visualization and facilitates proper footprint identification and, thus, tunnel placement for anatomic PCL reconstruction. Although there is no conclusive clinical outcomes evidence to support the superiority of the all-inside PCL reconstruction technique when compared to the open counterpart, there are major benefits to the surgeon.

Patient Positioning

The patient is placed supine on the operating table. Once adequate anesthesia is achieved, the operative leg is prepped and draped (Figure 30-1A). The operative limb is at 90 degrees in an arthroscopic leg holder. The well leg is placed in a leg holder that keeps the well leg flexed and abducted to keep it out of the way. This gives the surgeon posteromedial access for the posteromedial portal (Figures 30-1B and 30-1C.)

A soft tissue graft is prepared by folding the TightRope ABS implant and stitching the tails together with #2 FiberLoop (Arthrex) after quadrupling the graft (GraftLink Technique Video). The graft is prepared to the appropriate length, and the ends can be tapered with a stitch to ease graft passage.

An accessory posteromedial portal may first be localized with a spinal needle. Once established, a 2-cm incision is made, and a screw-in cannula is placed under direct visualization in an outside-in fashion. An alternative approach would be to make use of the knee obturator device for posterior portals and create the posteromedial portal in an inside-out fashion (Figure 30-2).

The soft tissue remaining on the PCL footprint is gently debrided with a shaver and/or a radiofrequency ablator device placed through the posteromedial portal to expose the full extent of the PCL footprint on the tibia (Figure 30-3). Care should be taken to protect the neurovascular structures that lie just posterior to the capsule by keeping a device facing the posterior tibia.

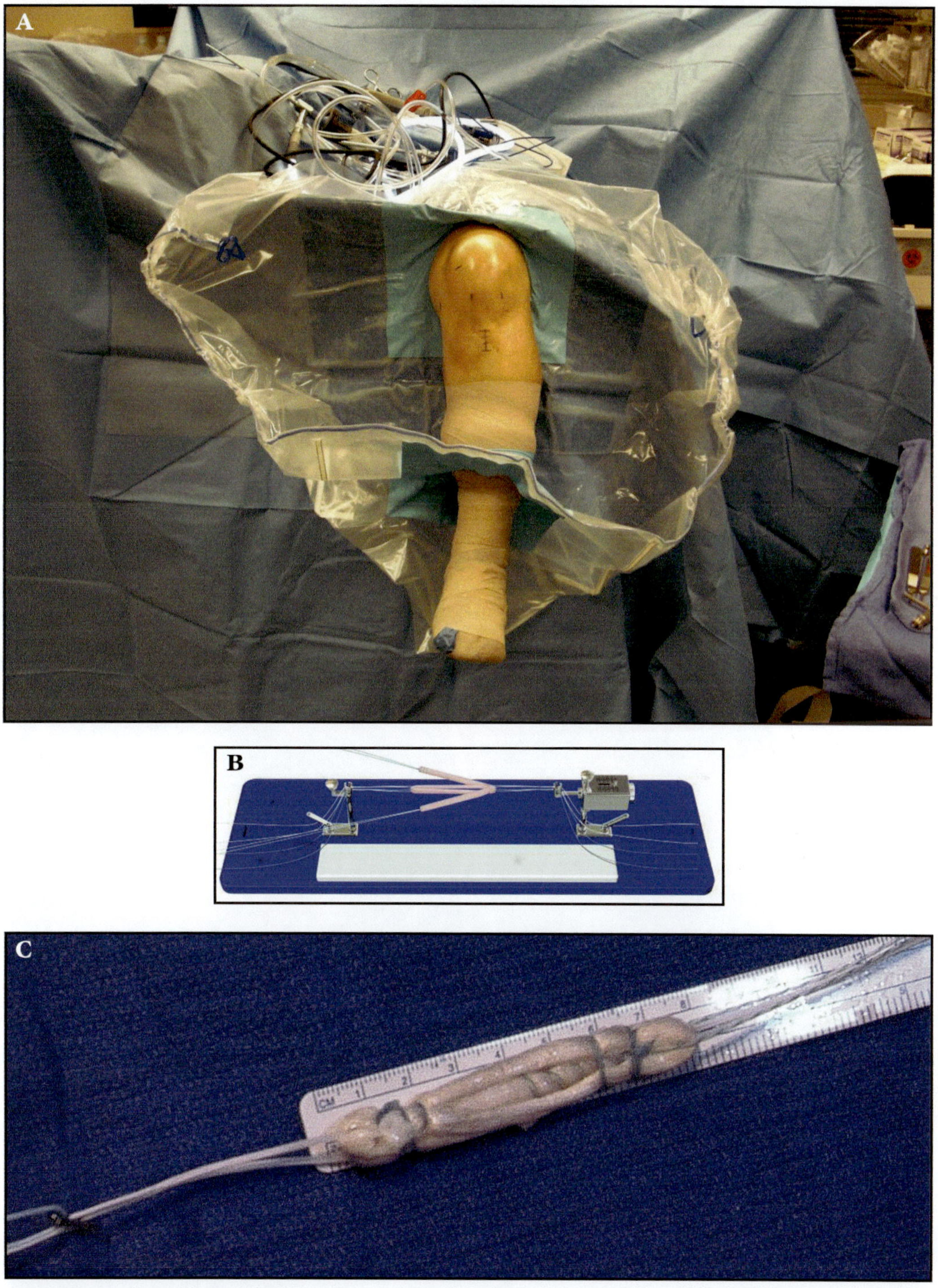

Figure 30-1. (A-C) Patient positioning and graft preparation using the TightRope ABS and GraftLink technique.

The mammillary bodies at the posterior aspect of the tibia can be palpated through the posteromedial portal to confirm anatomic placement. The PCL should be positioned directly between these 2 bodies and distal on the tibia. The side-specific Anatomic Contour PCL Guide is placed

Figure 30-2. (A) The accessory posteromedial portal can be placed in an inside-out fashion. With the arthroscope in the posterior medial compartment through transcondylar visualization, the soft spot between the medial collateral ligament and the medial head of the gastrocnemius and semimembranosus can be identified. (B, C) Using this window, a knee obturator device grasper can be used to deliver the cannula into the knee joint.

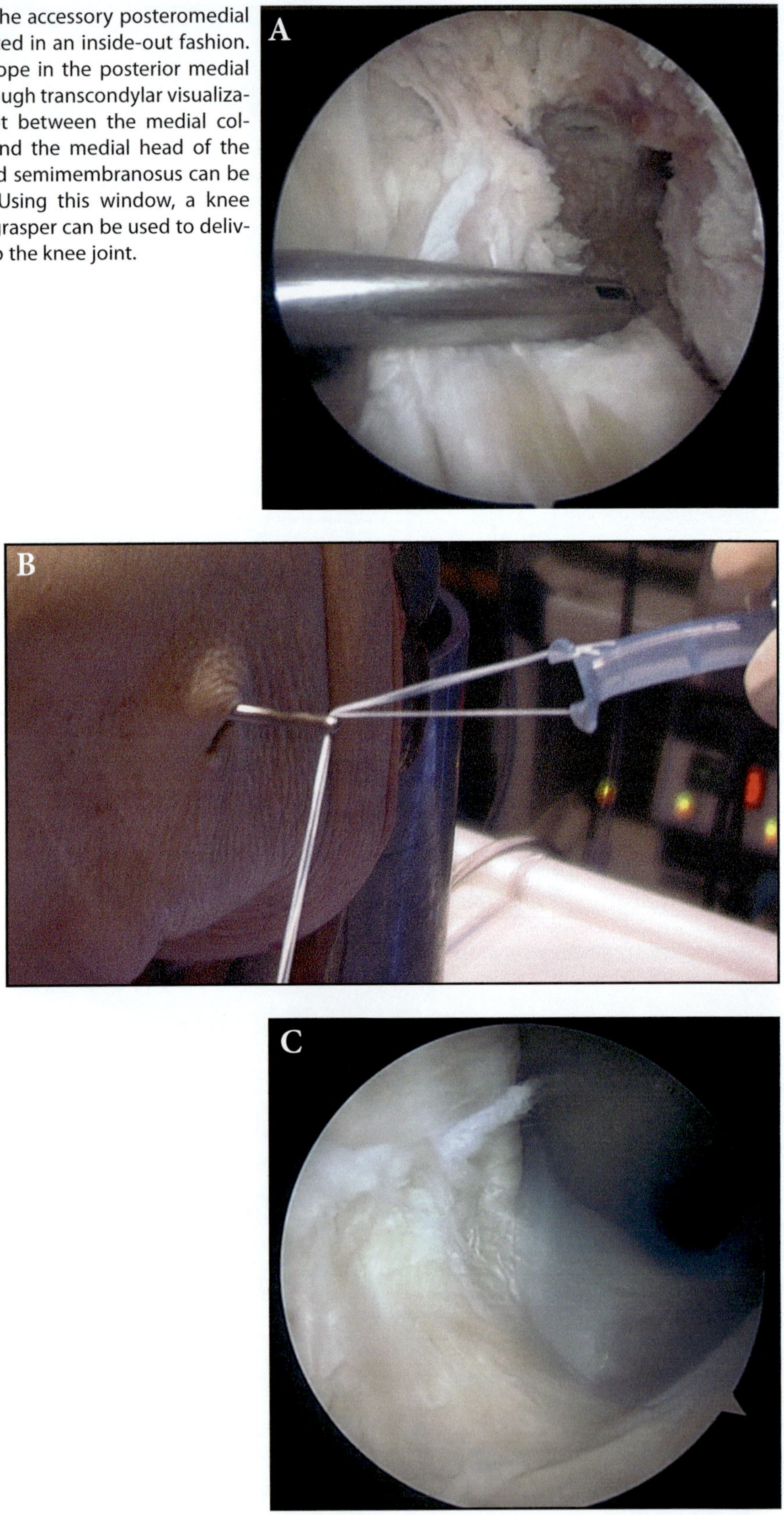

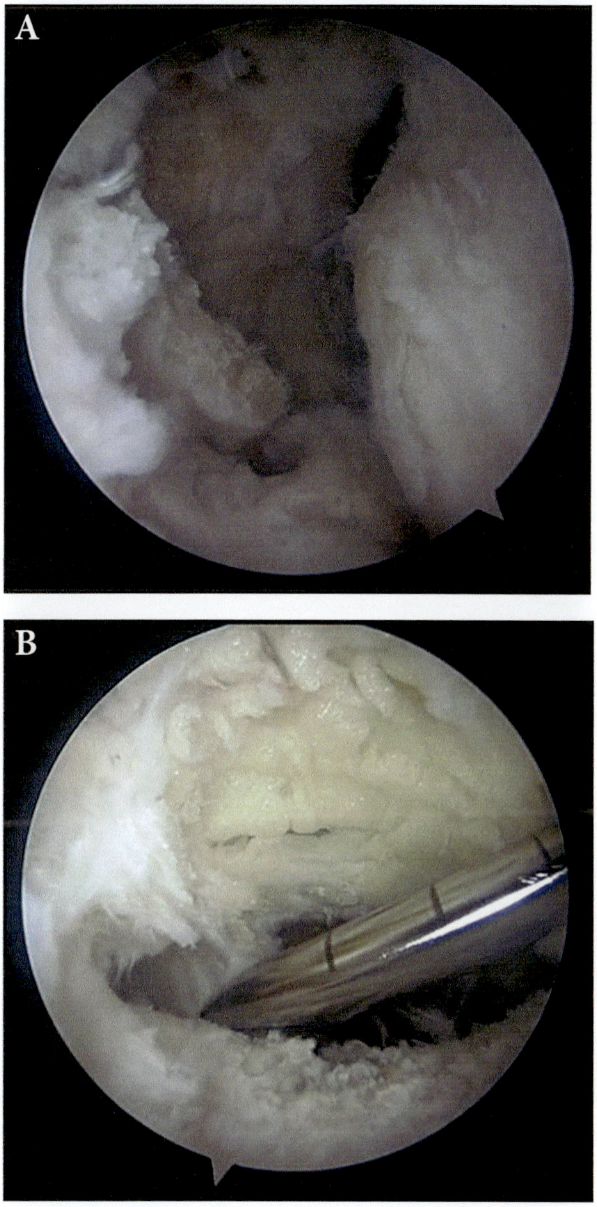

Figure 30-3. (A, B) The PCL footprint is cleared of all remaining tissue to allow for placement of the PCL guide.

over the back of the tibia through the anteromedial portal and positioned between the mammillary bodies (Figure 30-4). The arthroscope can be placed in the posteromedial portal to best visualize the footprint. Fluoroscopic guidance may be used to confirm correct positioning of the posterior guide in the over-the-top position and assist with drill trajectory. When in position, the marking hook will guide the FlipCutter to the ideal location and angle for transtibial PCL reconstruction (Figure 30-5). A small 2- to 3-cm incision is made in this location, and the guide is gently tapped to confirm that it is in cortical bone (Figure 30-6). Before drilling the FlipCutter, note the osseous length as read by the drill sleeve markings as it enters the guide handle (see Figure 30-6).

Place the FlipCutter into the drill sleeve and move the rubber grommet back to a distance equal to the interosseous length (Figure 30-7). This will give an indication of drill depth. With the arthroscope in the posteromedial portal, drill the FlipCutter until it is visualized just in the joint. Remove the guide and confirm that the FlipCutter is in the center of the PCL footprint (Figure

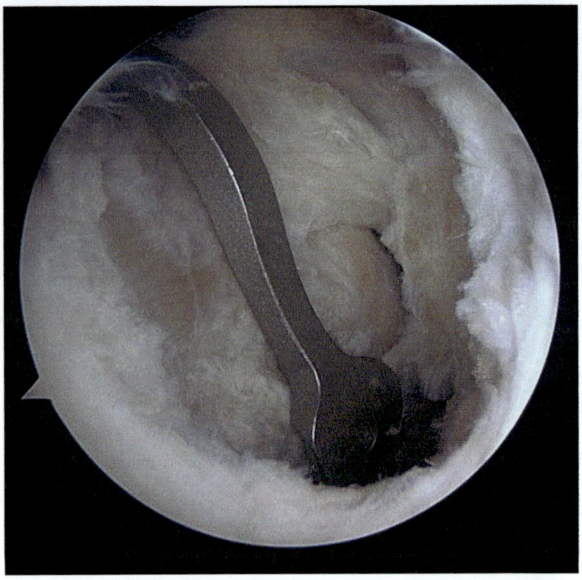

Figure 30-4. The Anatomic Contour PCL Guide is placed through the anteromedial portal over the back of the tibia and is positioned between the mammillary bodies.

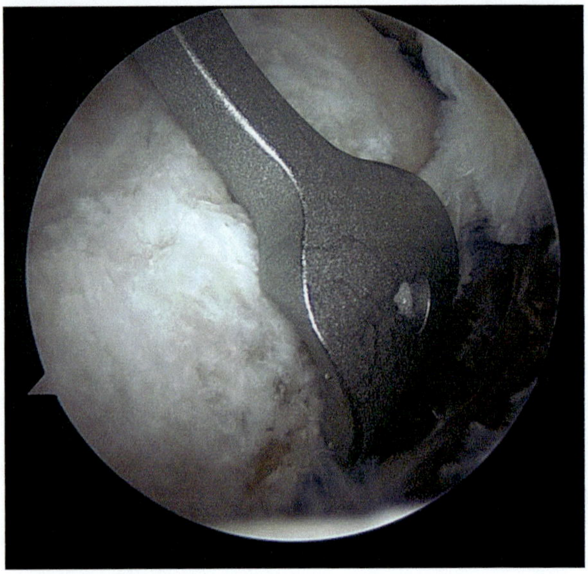

Figure 30-5. The marking hook is used to guide the FlipCutter to the ideal location and angle for drilling the tibial socket.

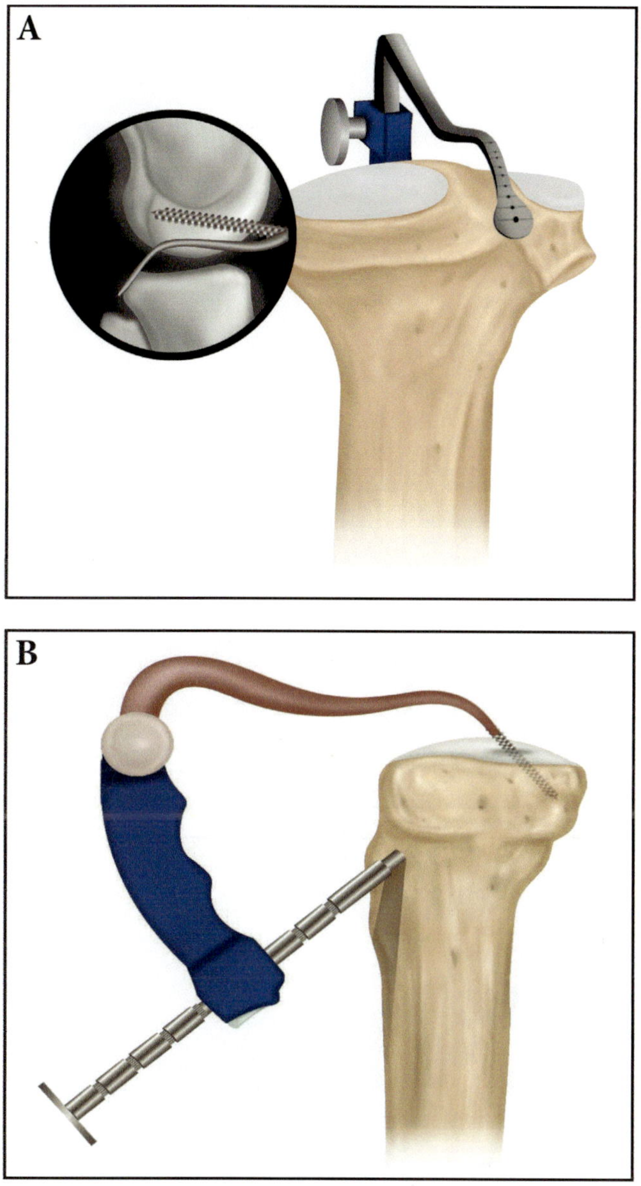

Figure 30-6. (A, B) The guide is tapped down to make sure it is seated in bone before drilling. The osseous length is determined off of the drill sleeve. (Figures redrawn from original Arthrex images with permission from Arthrex.)

30-8). Tap in the Stepped Drill Sleeve and slide down the rubber grommet until it is flush with the drill guide. Flipcut the socket to a depth of at least 20 mm, as indicated by the distance on the drill sleeve. After completing the socket, unflip the FlipCutter and remove it from the drill sleeve. Place a #2 FiberStick up the sleeve and into the joint for future graft passage (Figure 30-9). Retrieve the suture using an arthroscopic grasper through the medial portal.

Place the arthroscope back into the anterolateral portal and visualize the femoral footprint of the PCL (Figure 30-10). Place the All-Inside PCL Femoral Guide (Arthrex) in the center of the anterolateral bundle. Drill the FlipCutter from outside-in, and flipcut the socket to a depth of at least 20 mm as indicated by the distance on the drill sleeve. Place a #2 FiberStick down the sleeve and into the joint for future graft passage. Alternatively, the femoral socket can be drilled with a standard reamer from inside-out, and a Beath pin (Arthrex) can be used to pass the suture retrograde for future graft passage. This technique may be used if interference screw fixation is chosen on the femoral side.

Figure 30-7. (A, B) The rubber grommet is used to mark the drill sleeve to the proper depth for the osseous tunnel. (Figures redrawn from original Arthrex images with permission from Arthrex.)

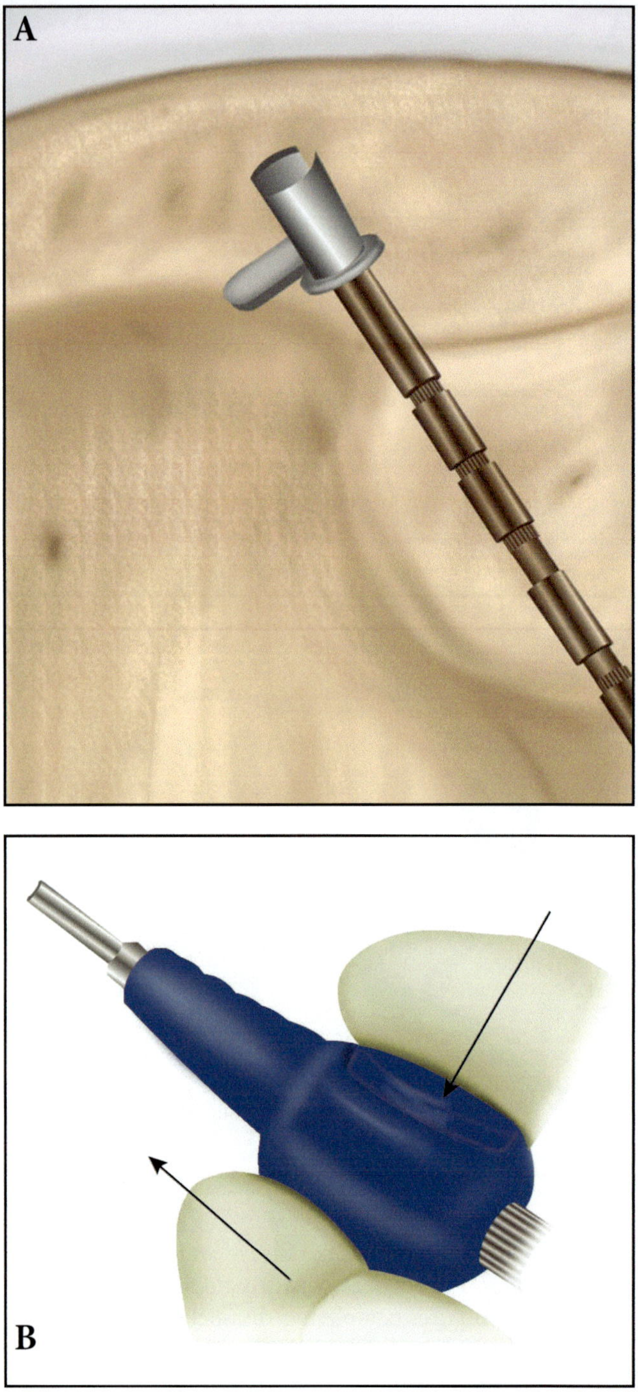

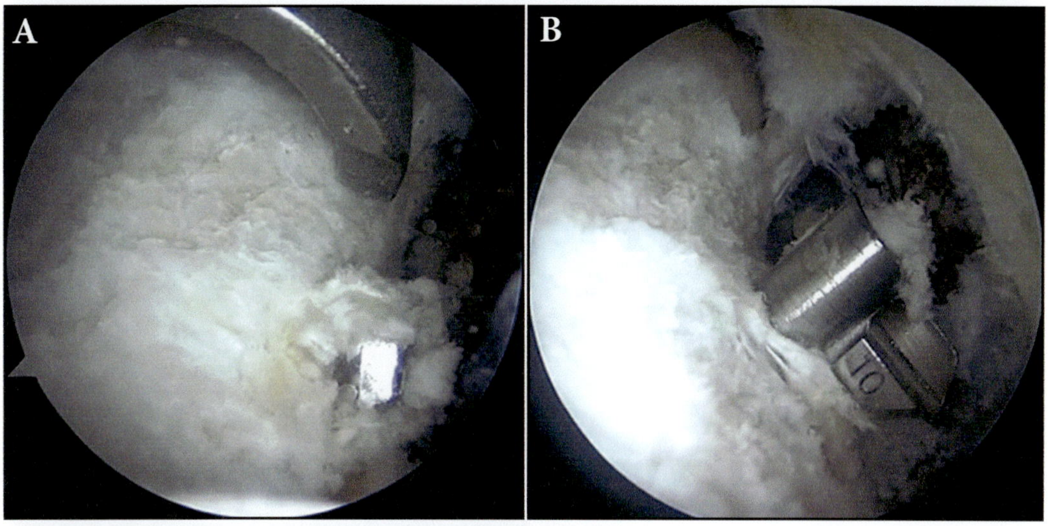

Figure 30-8. (A, B) Confirm that the FlipCutter is in the center of the PCL footprint before drilling.

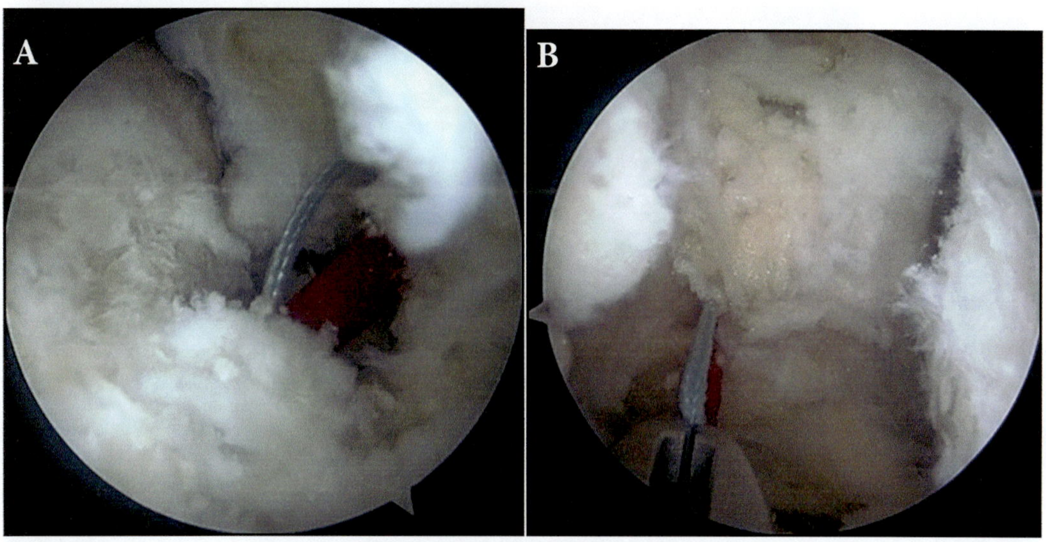

Figure 30-9. (A, B) Thread a #2 FiberStick into the joint for use with graft passage.

The #2 FiberStick sutures are retrieved through the anteromedial portal. Care should be taken to avoid a suture bridge (Figure 30-11). The graft is introduced through the portal, and the TightRope ABS is passed into the tibia using the passing/safety suture so that the tibial TightRope is not inadvertently shortened (Figure 30-12). The graft is advanced all the way to the bottom of the tibial socket by pulling on the inner loop of the implant without shortening the loop (Figure 30-13). The #2 suture with the attached button is next retrieved from the femoral socket, and the graft is pulled into the femoral socket. The femoral end of the graft can be tensioned with the knee at 90 degrees of flexion (Figure 30-14). The graft is tensioned on the tibial side at 90 degrees, supporting the foot to eliminate gravity and anterior drawer. The free TightRope button is applied, and the graft is tensioned (Figure 30-15). Once the femoral and tibial sides are secured and tensioned, a knot may be tied over the button to act as another form of fixation. Alternatively, the excess suture can be used for further backup fixation or the excess cut for removal.

Figure 30-10. (A-D) The femoral footprint of the PCL.

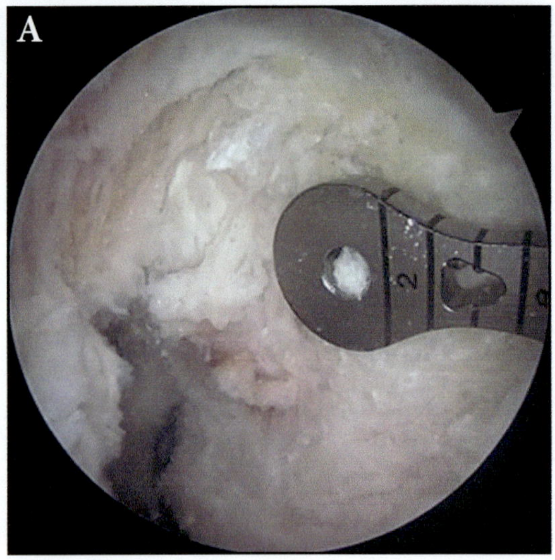

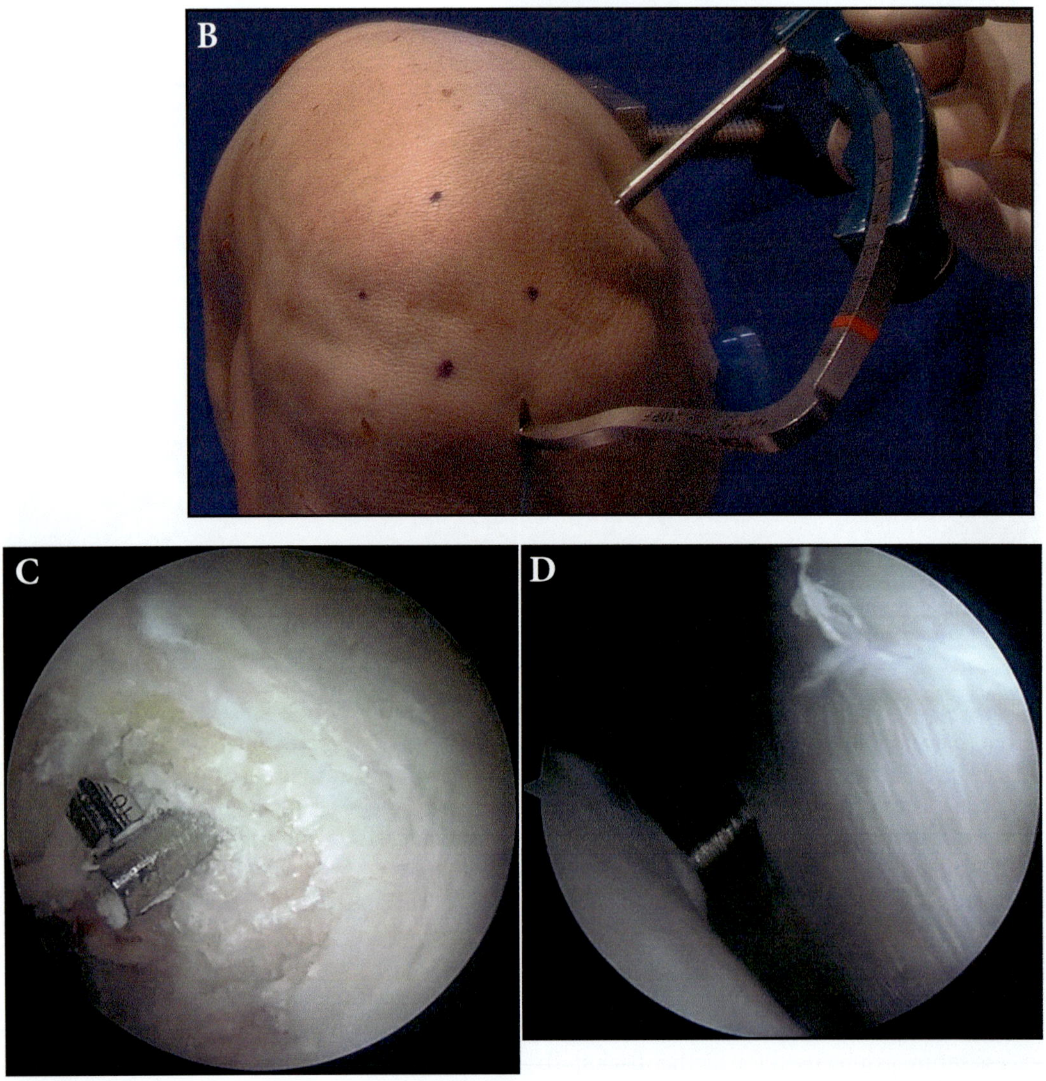

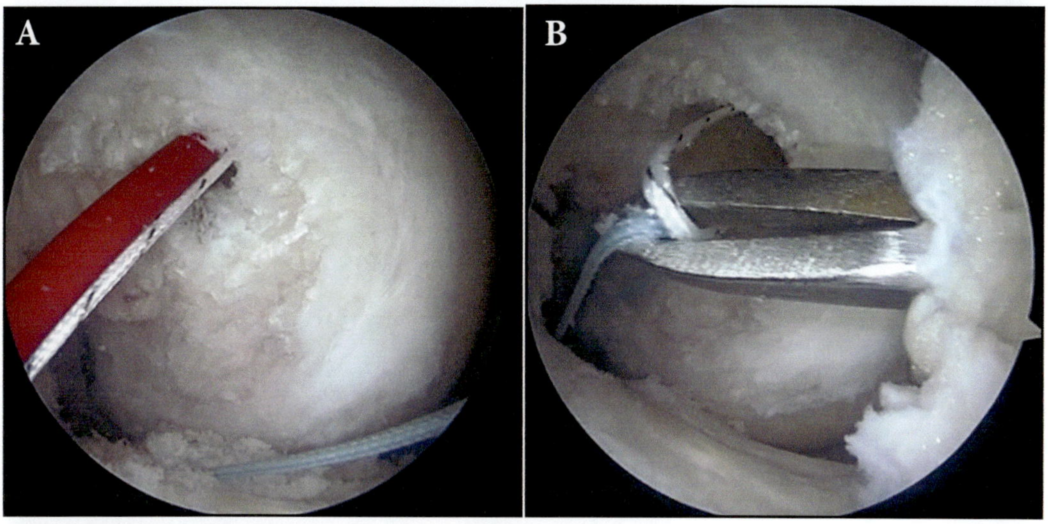

Figure 30-11. (A, B) Passing sutures.

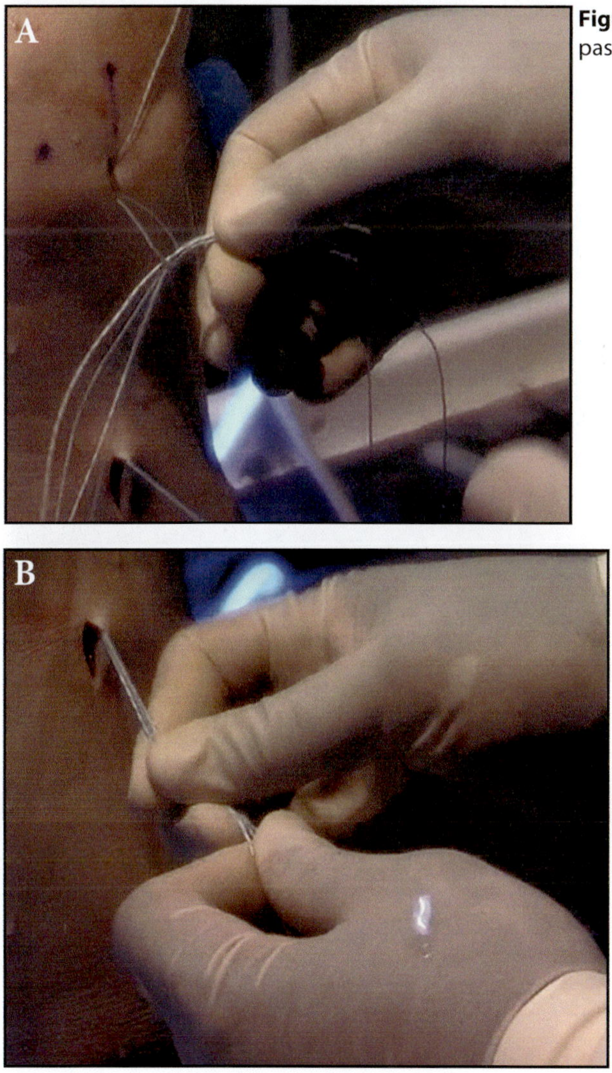

Figure 30-12. (A, B) A suture passer is used to pass the TightRope into the tibial socket.

Figure 30-13. (A, B) The inner loop of the implant is used to seat the graft in the tibial socket.

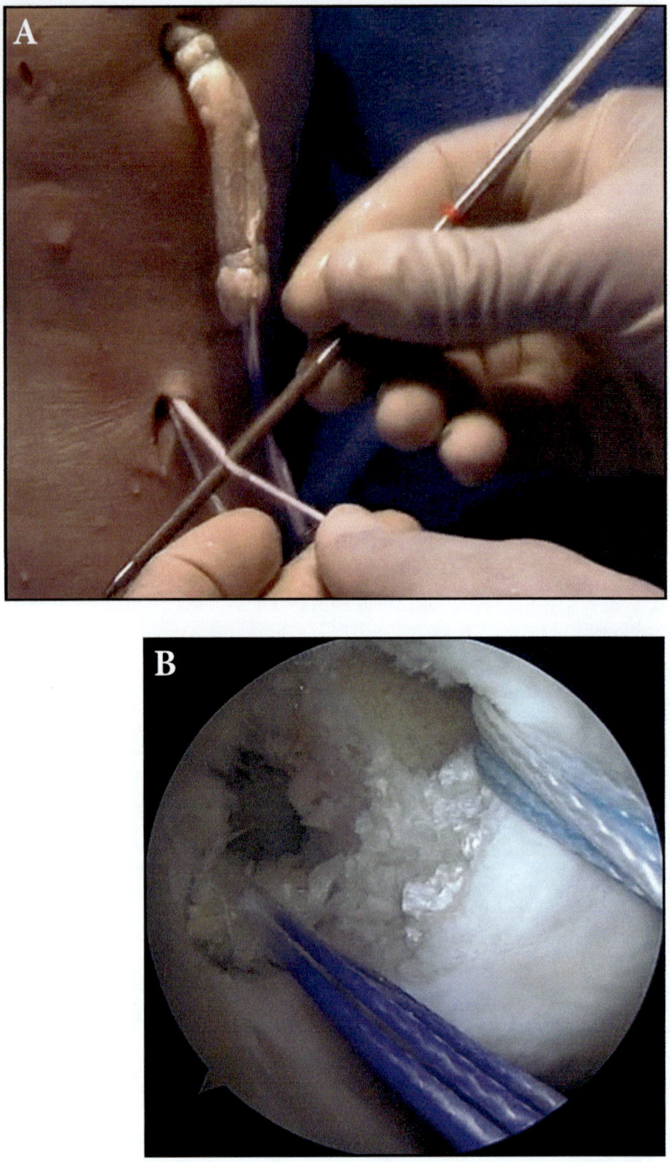

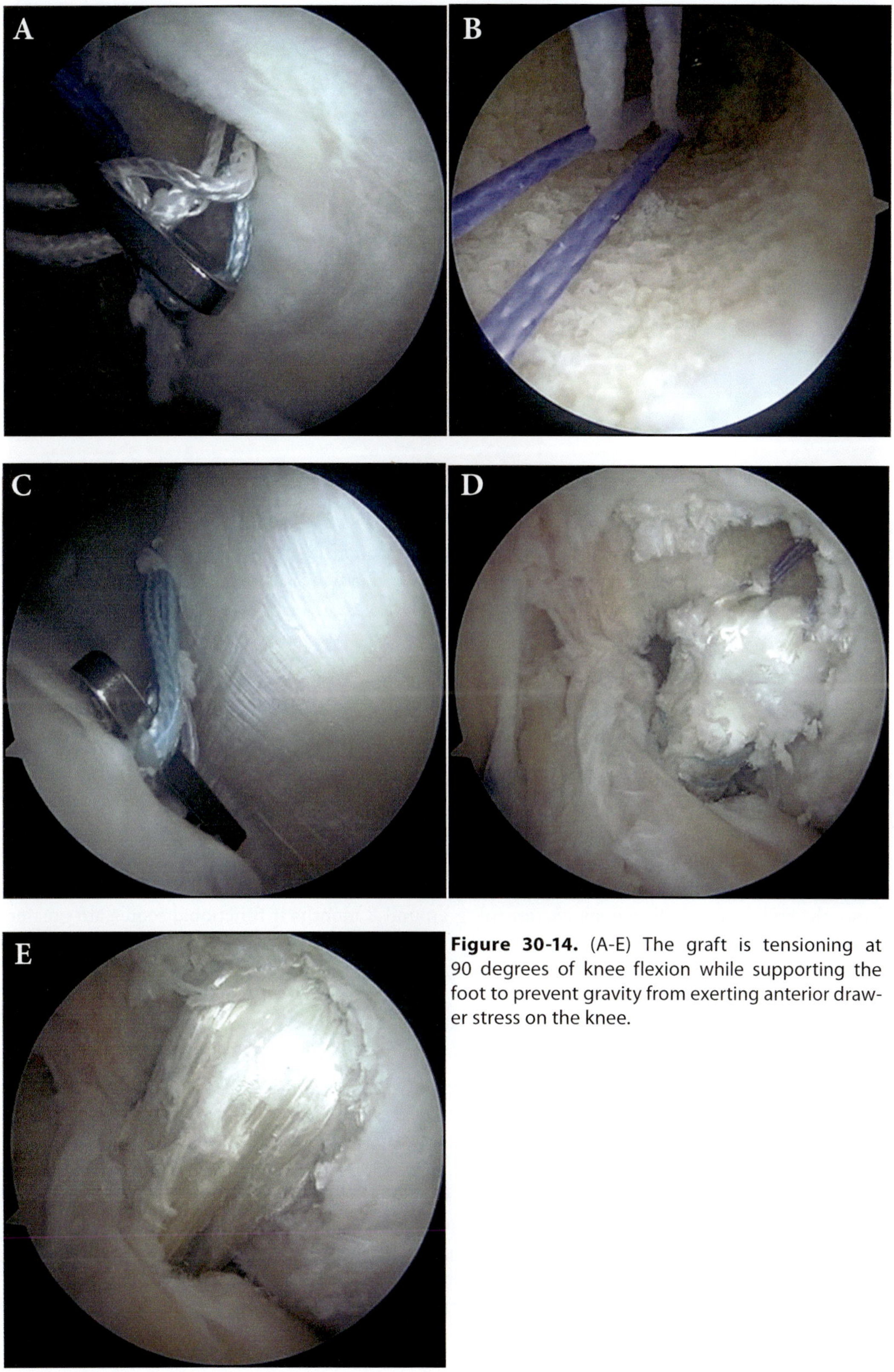

Figure 30-14. (A-E) The graft is tensioning at 90 degrees of knee flexion while supporting the foot to prevent gravity from exerting anterior drawer stress on the knee.

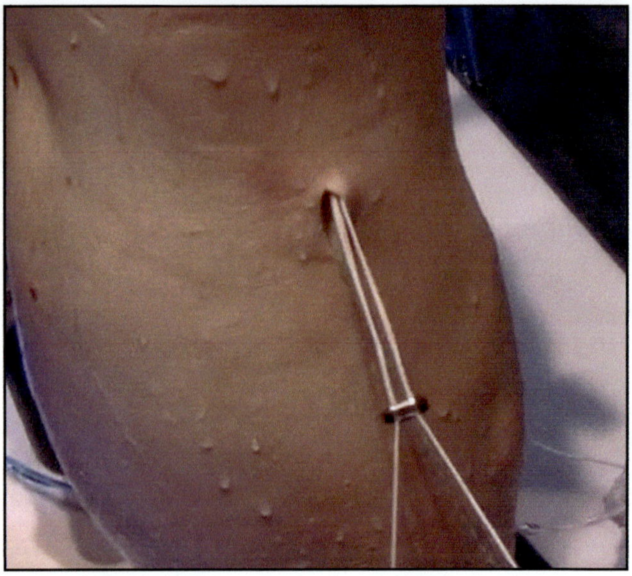

Figure 30-15. The TightRope button is applied.

A cold compressive dressing is placed atop the wound, and the patient is placed in a knee immobilizer until quadriceps function adequately returns. The patient is typically made weightbearing as tolerated with ROM as tolerated.

Postoperative Protocol

General follow-up intervals are 2 weeks, 6 weeks, 3 months, 6 months, and 1 year. The patient starts physical therapy immediately after surgery with the goal of providing edema control and restoration of ROM. Physical therapy progresses to closed chain strengthening of the involved leg with a focus on quadriceps strength at 6 to 8 weeks. The targeted time frame for sport-specific rehabilitation is 4 to 5 months, with the addition of more plyometric-based rehabilitation at 6 to 7 months. The goal for return to play varies by sport, with noncontact sports returning around 6 months and contact/collision sports returning around 8 months if functional scores are greater than 80% of the contralateral uninjured leg.

Potential Complications

Common complications may include knee pain and instability. The saphenous nerve can be injured with accessory posterior medial portal placement. Li et al[32] reported 1 patient with anterior knee pain, 2 with parasthesias that resolved in 6 months, and 1 with arthrofibrosis that required arthroscopic lysis of adhesions and manipulation. Wu et al[33] also reported a case of arthrofibrosis. Zhao et al[34] reported 5 patients with medial knee discomfort with flexion. This was corrected 1 year postoperatively by removing the tape knots and mini-plate of the femoral fixation. Hardware removal and complex regional pain syndrome has also been described in a few patients.[33,35,36] Although rare, injury to the popliteal neurovascular structures is possible when not adhering to meticulous posterior compartment arthroscopic techniques and must be mentioned for completeness.

Table 30-1. Studies of All-Inside, Single-Bundle Posterior Cruciate Ligament Reconstruction Within the Past 10 Years

Author	Year	No. of Patients	Minimum Follow-Up	Graft Tendon	IKDC Grade (%)				Lysholm
					A	B	C	D	
Lin et al[37]	2013	25	36	Q	16	68	16	0	92
		34	36	H	35	59	6	0	94
Boutefnouchet et al[35]	2013	15	12	H	67	27	6	0	91
Kim et al[38]	2009	8	24	A	—	—	—	—	87
Li et al[32]	2009	15	24	H	53	20	20	7	85
Zhao and Huangfu[34]	2007	21	24	H	52	24	19	5	83
		22	24	H[a]	64	27	9	0	92
Wu et al[33]	2007	22	60	Q	23	64	13	0	89
MacGillivray et al[39]	2006	13	24	Q and A	—	—	—	—	81
Seon and Song[40]	2006	21	24	H	—	—	—	—	91
Chan et al[36]	2006	20	36	H	25	60	10	5	93

A, Achilles; H, hamstring; IKDC, International Knee Documentation Committee; Q, quadriceps.

[a]7-strand graft.

Outcomes

The degree to which all-inside single-bundle reconstructions can restore proper knee function is not clearly elucidated in the literature. The results from multiple recent outcome studies on all-inside, single-bundle PCL reconstruction are summarized in Table 30-1.[32-40] In general, when using Lysholm and International Knee Documentation Committee scores, outcomes are satisfactory and postoperative restoration of function is obtained. Long-term follow-up studies using Lysholm scores by Wu et al[33] and Boutefnouchet et al[35] found 86% and 93% of patients had good or excellent scores at a minimum of 60-month follow-up and 4.1 years, respectively. In a systematic review of arthroscopic single-bundle transtibial PCL reconstruction, Kim et al[41] concluded that this technique can improve posterior knee laxity by one grade, with 75% of patients reaching normal or near normal outcomes.

The debate between all-inside, single-, and double-bundle reconstruction in the clinical setting is ongoing. Yoon et al[42] found that double-bundle reconstruction using an Achilles tendon allograft had no subjective difference but yielded a better International Knee Documentation Committee score and objective stability than single-bundle. In contrast, Wang et al[43] found no difference in clinical outcomes between patients treated with single- vs double-bundle PCL reconstruction with semitendinosus and gracilis tendon grafts. Similarly, Fanelli et al[44] found no difference between single- and double-bundle reconstruction in regard to Lysholm, Tegner, or Hospital for Special Surgery ratings. In a study comparing PCL reconstruction via arthroscopic tibial inlay single-bundle, arthroscopic tibial inlay double-bundle, and conventional transtibial single-bundle techniques, Kim et al[38] demonstrated that between the tibial inlay groups, the double-bundle group had a statistically significant difference in mean side-to-side difference. In another study of patients requiring concurrent reconstruction of the lateral collateral ligament and popliteus tendon, Kim et al[45] found no significant difference between single- and double-bundle PCL reconstruction in regard to posterior translation, posterolateral rotary instability, and International Knee Documentation Committee and Lysholm knee scores. Ultimately, the all-inside, single-bundle reconstruction technique exhibits satisfactory outcomes compared to the double-bundle reconstruction technique for isolated and multiligamentous PCL injury.

Top Technical Pearls for the Procedure

1. Proper graft preparation is necessary for the all-inside technique (TightRope ABS and GraftLink techniques).
2. The surgeon should be comfortable with placement of the accessory posteromedial portal.
3. The mammillary bodies should be palpated to accurately identify the correct tibial footprint/tunnel location.
4. Tension the graft at 90 degrees of knee flexion while supporting the foot to prevent gravity from exerting anterior drawer stress on the knee.
5. Graft fixation is achieved by proper tensioning of the TightRope.

References

1. Voos JE, Mauro CS, Wente T, Warren RF, Wickiewicz TL. Posterior cruciate ligament: anatomy, biomechanics, and outcomes. *Am J Sports Med.* 2012;40(1):222-231.
2. Race A, Amis AA. The mechanical properties of the two bundles of the human posterior cruciate ligament. *J Biomech.* 1994;27(1):13-24.
3. Edwards A, Bull AM, Amis AA. The attachments of the fiber bundles of the posterior cruciate ligament: an anatomic study. *Arthroscopy.* 2007;23(3):284-290.
4. Papannagari R, DeFrate LE, Nha KW, et al. Function of posterior cruciate ligament bundles during in vivo knee flexion. *Am J Sports Med.* 2007;35(9):1507-1512.
5. Forsythe B, Harner C, Martins CA, Shen W, Lopes OV Jr, Fu FH. Topography of the femoral attachment of the posterior cruciate ligament. Surgical technique. *J Bone Joint Surg Am.* 2009;91(suppl 2 pt 1):89-100.
6. Lopes OV Jr, Ferretti M, Shen W, Ekdahl M, Smolinski P, Fu FH. Topography of the femoral attachment of the posterior cruciate ligament. *J Bone Joint Surg Am.* 2008;90(2):249-255.
7. Tajima G, Nozaki M, Iriuchishima T, et al. Morphology of the tibial insertion of the posterior cruciate ligament. *J Bone Joint Surg Am.* 2009;91(4):859-866.
8. Moorman CT III, Murphy Zane MS, Bansai S, et al. Tibial insertion of the posterior cruciate ligament: a sagittal plane analysis using gross, histologic, and radiographic methods. *Arthroscopy.* 2008;24(3):269-275.
9. Takahashi M, Matsubara T, Doi M, Suzuki D, Nagano A. Anatomical study of the femoral and tibial insertions of the anterolateral and posteromedial bundles of human posterior cruciate ligament. *Knee Surg Sports Traumatol Arthrosc.* 2006;14(11):1055-1059.
10. Mannor DA, Shearn JT, Grood ES, Noyes FR, Levy MS. Two-bundle posterior cruciate ligament reconstruction. An in vitro analysis of graft placement and tension. *Am J Sports Med.* 2000;28(6):833-845.

11. Markolf KL, McAllister DR, Young CR, McWilliams J, Oakes DA. Biomechanical effects of medial-lateral tibial tunnel placement in posterior cruciate ligament reconstruction. *J Orthop Res.* 2003;21(1):177-182.
12. Morgan CD, Kalman VR, Grawl DM. The anatomic origin of the posterior cruciate ligament: where is it? Reference landmarks for PCL reconstruction. *Arthroscopy.* 1997;13(3):325-331.
13. Gill TJ, DeFrate LE, Wang C, et al. The biomechanical effect of posterior cruciate ligament reconstruction on knee joint function. Kinematic response to simulated muscle loads. *Am J Sports Med.* 2003;31(4):530-536.
14. Race A, Amis AA. PCL reconstruction. In vitro biomechanical comparison of "isometric" versus single and double-bundled "anatomic" grafts. *J Bone Joint Surg Br.* 1998;80(1):173-179.
15. Harner CD, Janaushek MA, Kanamori A, Yagi M, Vogrin TM, Woo SL. Biomechanical analysis of a double-bundle posterior cruciate ligament reconstruction. *Am J Sports Med.* 2000;28(2):144-151.
16. Whiddon DR, Zehms CT, Miller MD, Quinby JS, Montgomery SL, Sekiya JK. Double compared with single-bundle open inlay posterior cruciate ligament reconstruction in a cadaver model. *J Bone Joint Surg Am.* 2008;90(9):1820-1829.
17. Wijdicks CA, Kennedy NI, Goldsmith MT, et al. Kinematic analysis of the posterior cruciate ligament, part 2: a comparison of anatomic single- versus double-bundle reconstruction. *Am J Sports Med.* 2013;41(12):2839-2848.
18. Bergfeld JA, Graham SM, Parker RD, Valdevit AD, Kambic HE. A biomechanical comparison of posterior cruciate ligament reconstructions using single- and double-bundle tibial inlay techniques. *Am J Sports Med.* 2005;33(7):976-981.
19. Shelbourne KD, Clark M, Gray T. Minimum 10-year follow-up of patients after an acute, isolated posterior cruciate ligament injury treated nonoperatively. *Am J Sports Med.* 2013;41(7):1526-1533.
20. Parolie JM, Bergfeld JA. Long-term results of nonoperative treatment of isolated posterior cruciate ligament injuries in the athlete. *Am J Sports Med.* 1986;14(1):35-38.
21. Boynton MD, Tietjens BR. Long-term followup of the untreated isolated posterior cruciate ligament-deficient knee. *Am J Sports Med.* 1996;24(3):306-310.
22. Dejour H, Walch G, Peyrot J, Eberhard P. The natural history of rupture of the posterior cruciate ligament [in French]. *Rev Chir Orthop Réparatrice Appar Mot.* 1988;74(1):35-43.
23. Sekiya JK, Whiddon DR, Zehms CT, Miller MD. A clinically relevant assessment of posterior cruciate ligament and posterolateral corner injuries. Evaluation of isolated and combined deficiency. *J Bone Joint Surg Am.* 2008;90(8):1621-1627.
24. Margheritini F, Mancini L, Mauro CS, Mariani PP. Stress radiography for quantifying posterior cruciate ligament deficiency. *Arthroscopy.* 2003;19(7):706-711.
25. Schulz MS, Steenlage ES, Russe K, Strobel MJ. Distribution of posterior tibial displacement in knees with posterior cruciate ligament tears. *J Bone Joint Surg Am.* 2007;89(2):332-338.
26. Noyes FR. *Noyes' Knee Disorders: Surgery, Rehabilitation, Clinical Outcomes.* Philadelphia, PA: Saunders Elsevier; 2009.
27. Lubowitz JH, Konicek J. A 3.5-mm-diameter anterior cruciate ligament tibial retrograde socket drilling pin is more accurate than a 2.4-mm-diameter pin. *Arthroscopy.* 2011;27(5):666-671.
28. Zehms CT, Whiddon DR, Miller MD, et al. Comparison of a double bundle arthroscopic inlay and open inlay posterior cruciate ligament reconstruction using clinically relevant tools: a cadaveric study. *Arthroscopy.* 2008;24(4):472-480.
29. Kim SJ, Park IS. Arthroscopic reconstruction of the posterior cruciate ligament using tibial-inlay and double-bundle technique. *Arthroscopy.* 2005;21(10):1271.
30. Ritchie JR, Bergfeld JA, Kambic H, Manning T. Isolated sectioning of the medial and posteromedial capsular ligaments in the posterior cruciate ligament-deficient knee. Influence on posterior tibial translation. *Am J Sports Med.* 1998;26(3):389-394.
31. Park SE, Stamos BD, DeFrate LE, Gill TJ, Li G. The effect of posterior knee capsulotomy on posterior tibial translation during posterior cruciate ligament tibial inlay reconstruction. *Am J Sports Med.* 2004;32(6):1514-1519.
32. Li B, Wen Y, Wu H, Qian Q, Wu Y, Lin X. Arthroscopic single-bundle posterior cruciate ligament reconstruction: retrospective review of hamstring tendon graft versus LARS artificial ligament. *Int Orthop.* 2009;33(4):991-996.
33. Wu CH, Chen AC, Yuan LJ, et al. Arthroscopic reconstruction of the posterior cruciate ligament by using a quadriceps tendon autograft: a minimum 5-year follow-up. *Arthroscopy.* 2007;23(4):420-427.

34. Zhao J, Huangfu X. Arthroscopic single-bundle posterior cruciate ligament reconstruction: retrospective review of 4- versus 7-strand hamstring tendon graft. *Knee*. 2007;14(4):301-305.
35. Boutefnouchet T, Bentayeb M, Qadri Q, Ali S. Long-term outcomes following single-bundle transtibial arthroscopic posterior cruciate ligament reconstruction. *Int Orthop*. 2013;37(2):337-343.
36. Chan YS, Yang SC, Chang CH, et al. Arthroscopic reconstruction of the posterior cruciate ligament with use of a quadruple hamstring tendon graft with 3- to 5-year follow-up. *Arthroscopy*. 2006;22(7):762-770.
37. Lin YC, Chen SK, Liu TH, Cheng YM, Chou PP. Arthroscopic transtibial single-bundle posterior cruciate ligament reconstruction using patellar tendon graft compared with hamstring tendon graft. *Arch Orthop Trauma Surg*. 2013;133(4):523-530.
38. Kim SJ, Kim TE, Jo SB, Kung YP. Comparison of the clinical results of three posterior cruciate ligament reconstruction techniques. *J Bone Joint Surg Am*. 2009;91(11):2543-2549.
39. MacGillivray JD, Stein BE, Park M, Allen AA, Wickiewicz TL, Warren RF. Comparison of tibial inlay versus transtibial techniques for isolated posterior cruciate ligament reconstruction: minimum 2-year follow-up. *Arthroscopy*. 2006;22(3):320-328.
40. Seon JK, Song EK. Reconstruction of isolated posterior cruciate ligament injuries: a clinical comparison of the transtibial and tibial inlay techniques. *Arthroscopy*. 2006;22(1):27-32.
41. Kim YM, Lee CA, Matava MJ. Clinical results of arthroscopic single-bundle transtibial posterior cruciate ligament reconstruction: a systematic review. *Am J Sports Med*. 2011;39(2):425-434.
42. Yoon KH, Bae DK, Song SJ, Cho HJ, Lee JH. A prospective randomized study comparing arthroscopic single-bundle and double-bundle posterior cruciate ligament reconstructions preserving remnant fibers. *Am J Sports Med*. 2011;39(3):474-480.
43. Wang CJ, Weng LH, Hsu CC, Chan YS. Arthroscopic single- versus double-bundle posterior cruciate ligament reconstructions using hamstring autograft. *Injury*. 2004;35(12):1293-1299.
44. Fanelli GC, Beck JD, Edson CJ. Single compared to double-bundle PCL reconstruction using allograft tissue. *J Knee Surg*. 2012;25(1):59-64.
45. Kim SJ, Jung M, Moon HK, Kim SG, Chun YM. Anterolateral transtibial posterior cruciate ligament reconstruction combined with anatomical reconstruction of posterolateral corner insufficiency: comparison of single-bundle versus double-bundle posterior cruciate ligament reconstruction over a 2- to 6-year follow-up. *Am J Sports Med*. 2011;39(3):481-489.

Please see videos on the accompanying website at www.routledge.com/9781617119996

31

Tibial Inlay Posterior Cruciate Ligament Reconstruction

Austin Crow, MD; James Starman, MD; Adam Wilson, MD; and Mark Miller, MD

Introduction

The posterior cruciate ligament (PCL) is critical for stability of the knee. The PCL stabilizes the knee against posterior translation of the tibia with respect to the femur and against external rotation of the knee.[1-8] Insufficiency of the PCL can result in clinically noticeable instability and pain. However, PCL injuries are relatively infrequent when compared to other soft tissue injuries in the knee, with PCL injuries accounting for less than 1% to 16% of knee injuries.[9-11] Traditionally, PCL injuries have garnered significantly less attention than anterior cruciate ligament (ACL) injuries. Interest in PCL reconstruction has increased recently as surgeons have noted an increased incidence of unrecognized PCL instability.[9,10] Although most patients are able to tolerate a PCL-deficient knee, interest has increased in the altered biomechanics seen with a PCL-deficient knee.[8,10] Therefore, significant controversy remains with when and how to best address PCL injuries. The goal of PCL reconstruction is to reduce or eliminate pathologic laxity and the resultant wear in the medial and patellofemoral compartments.[6]

In order to understand and treat PCL injuries, a familiarity with the anatomy is necessary. The PCL originates from the medial femoral condyle and consists of 2 bundles, including an anterolateral bundle, which is tight in flexion, and a posteromedial bundle, which is tight in extension. The PCL inserts on the central, posterior tibia 1.0 to 1.5 cm distal to the joint line.[2,8,12-15] The femoral origin of the PCL is intra-articular, whereas the tibial insertion of the ligament is at the capsular junction at the proximal tibia. In addition, the meniscofemoral ligaments (ligaments of Humphrey and Wrisberg) run from the lateral meniscus to the medial femoral condyle, inserting anterior or posterior to the PCL, respectively, which can remain intact after a PCL injury and provide minimal residual posterior stability of the knee.

The method of PCL reconstruction has been controversial and has undergone significant evolution over time. Original techniques for PCL reconstruction involved transosseous tunnels in the femur and the tibia. This resulted in an anteroinferior to posterosuperior tibial tunnel. This method is popular today but has been challenged due to concerns resulting from the biomechanics of the technique. The transtibial tunnel has proven over time to result in difficult graft passage,

Sgaglione NA, Lubowitz JH, Provencher MT, eds. *The Knee: AANA Advanced Arthroscopic Surgical Techniques* (pp 435-447).

requiring the graft to bend over a significant angle around the posterior tibia. This angle, deemed the killer turn, has also been shown to be a cause of graft failure.[8,10,15-17]

In the majority of situations, the authors prefer the more recently developed tibial inlay technique. The tibial inlay technique provides a more anatomic reconstruction of the tibial insertion of the PCL and avoids the killer turn. Traditionally, the tibial inlay technique has involved an open approach to the posterior knee but continues to undergo advances, with some authors advocating an all-arthroscopic technique.[10,11,17] Since its introduction, the tibial inlay technique has proven to be a durable method for PCL reconstruction.[8] This technique is discussed in depth in this chapter.

Indications

Historical treatment for the majority of PCL injuries has been nonoperative with bracing and early range of motion and quadriceps strengthening. Nonoperative management remains the mainstay of treatment for isolated grade I and II PCL injuries, both acute and chronic. However, continued knee instability has been increasingly recognized and has resulted in orthopedic surgeons developing broader indications for surgical management of PCL injuries.[4-7,18,19] Currently, there is controversy over the timing of this procedure, but the authors believe that injuries with concomitant posterolateral corner injuries should be reconstructed within 2 weeks due to improved ability to identify the anatomy, particularly the peroneal nerve, prior to abundant scar formation.

Indications[4-7,18,20]

- Acute grade III PCL injuries
- Chronic grade III PCL injuries with symptomatic instability after a failed nonoperative treatment course
- PCL injury in conjunction with bony avulsion injuries and posterolateral corner injuries
- PCL injury as part of a multiligamentous injury, specifically a grade II or higher medial collateral ligament injury or an ACL rupture

Relative Indications

- Grade II injury in a young, active patient with symptomatic instability after attempted nonoperative management

Contraindications

- Patients with a prior history of vascular procedures in the extremity because the relevant anatomy becomes distorted and unpredictable

Pertinent Physical Findings

Diagnosis and treatment of PCL injuries begins with a thorough history and physical examination. Unlike ACL injuries, which are most commonly the result of a noncontact mechanism, PCL injuries typically present from a more direct mechanism. Typical mechanisms for isolated PCL injuries are a posteriorly directed force on the proximal tibia, dashboard injuries, or during active quadriceps contraction with knee hyperflexion. PCL injuries more frequently occur with high-energy mechanisms resulting in multiligamentous injuries. The most common pattern of multiligamentous injuries involves rupture of the ACL, PCL, and posterolateral corner.[4-8,18,19]

Patients with PCL insufficiency often continue to participate in activities and complain of an aching sensation or subtle instability during activities. They will often report increased difficulty with stairs, particularly with descent.[4-8,18]

Physical Findings[4-8,18]

- Best test: Posterior drawer test (Figure 31-1)
  - 90% sensitive and 99% specific
  - Performed with the knee in 90 degrees of flexion
  - PCL injuries are graded I to III with grade I defined as 5 mm of posterior translation of the tibia, grade II as 6 to 10 mm, and grade III as greater than 10 mm. This is best accomplished by placing the thumbs on the anterior joint line and documenting the translation of the tibia in reference to the femoral condyles. Grade III PCL injuries are rarely isolated, and a high suspicion for other ligamentous injuries must be suspected when a grade III posterior drawer is noted.
- Posterior sag test
- Godfrey test
- Prone drawer test
- Quadriceps active test
- Dynamic posterior shift
- Dial test to assess for posterolateral instability: The dial test should be performed with the patient prone. Asymmetry of external rotation of the feet should be looked for at 30 and 90 degrees of knee flexion. A positive test at 30 degrees only indicates an isolated posterolateral corner injury, whereas a positive dial test at 30 and 90 degrees indicates combined PCL and posterolateral corner injuries. Additional maneuvers to diagnose posterolateral instability include varus laxity, the external rotation recurvatum test, posterolateral and posteromedial drawer tests, and the reverse pivot shift.[18]

Pertinent Imaging

Plain X-Rays

- Assess for any bony avulsion
- Assess for concomitant tibial plateau fracture or fibular head fracture

Stress X-Rays

- Quantify the extent of the injury
- Performed by the physician in the imaging suite by application of a posteriorly directed force at the level of the proximal tibia
- The authors use the Telos system, which applies 15 decaNewtons (daN) of force, to obtain stress x-rays. The extent of posterior instability is determined by recording the degree of posterior translation of the tibial plateau in relation to the femoral condyles (Figure 31-2).
- The authors also obtain varus stress x-rays to assess the lateral joint opening because increased widening of the lateral joint has been found to correlate with posterolateral corner injuries.[21]

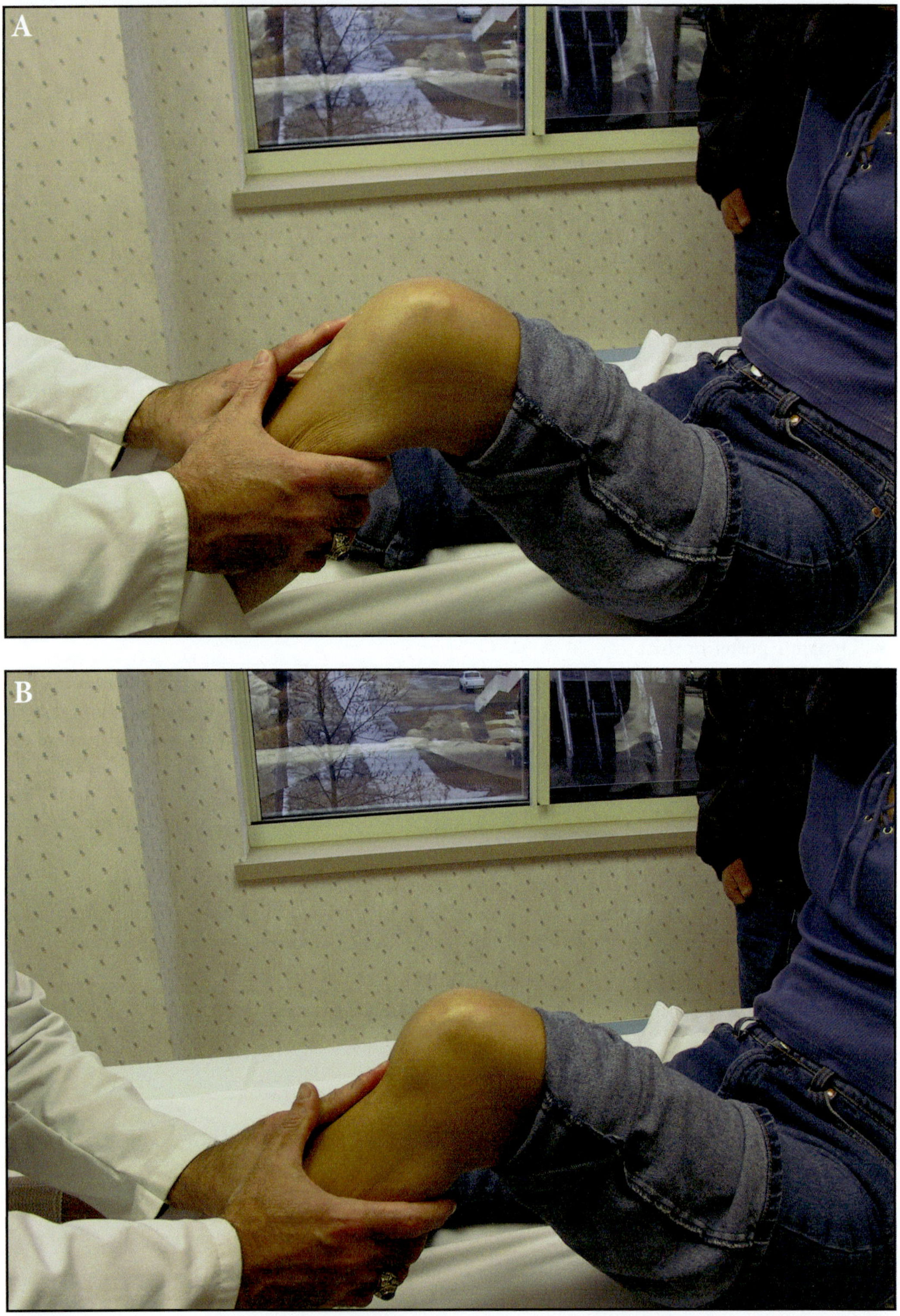

Figure 31-1. The posterior drawer test. (A) The knee should be flexed to 90 degrees with the tibia in neutral rotation and centered under the knee. (B) A posterior force should be applied, and the amount of translation relative to the femoral condyles should be noted. Grade I injuries will have less than 5 mm, grade II will have 6 to 10 mm, and grade III will have greater than 10 mm of posterior translation.

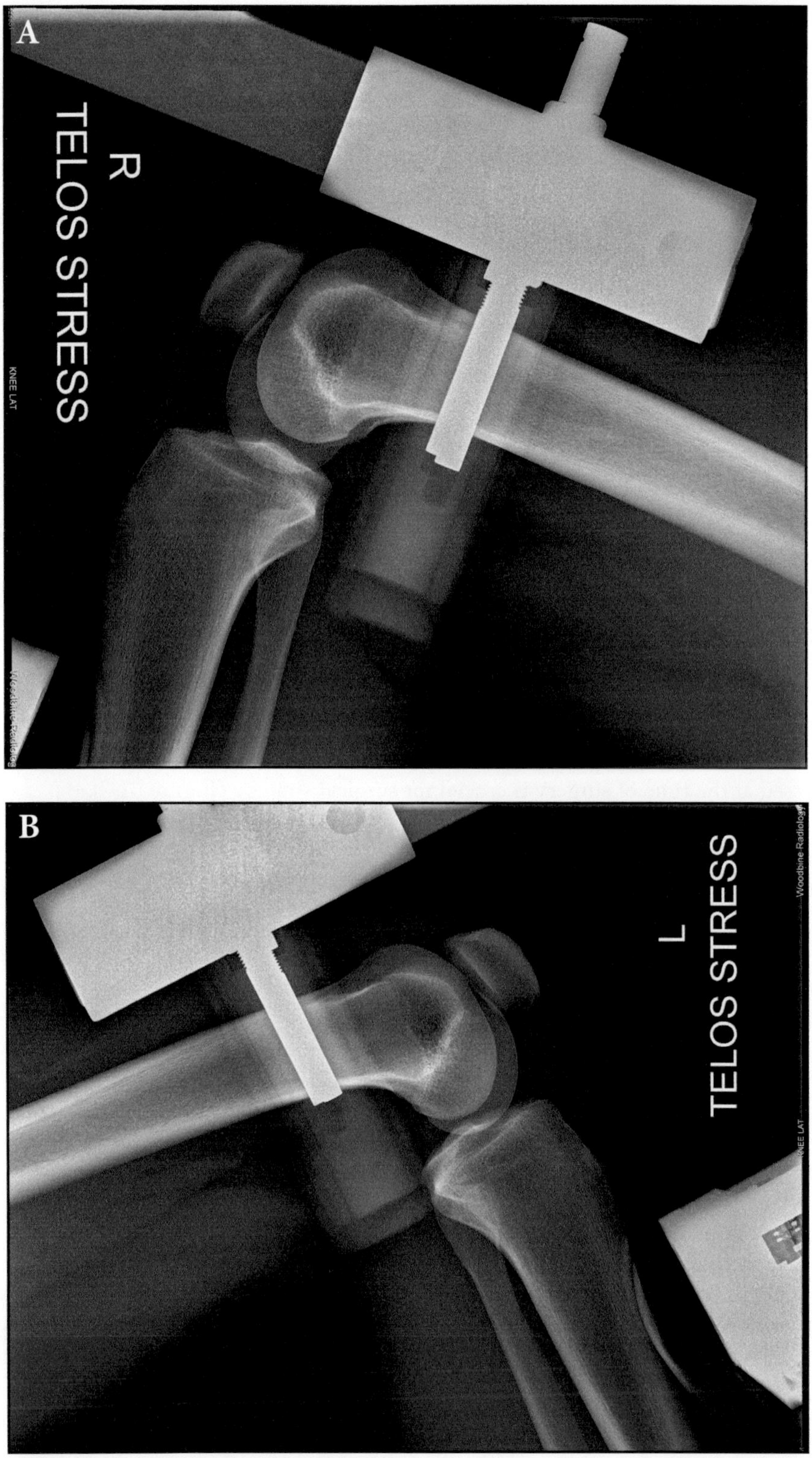

Figure 31-2. Telos stress x-rays. Both knees are radiographed with the Telos system applying 15 daN of force, and the side-to-side difference in posterior tibial translation is measured. (A) The uninjured knee will have minimal translation, (B) whereas the PCL-injured leg will have increased translation.

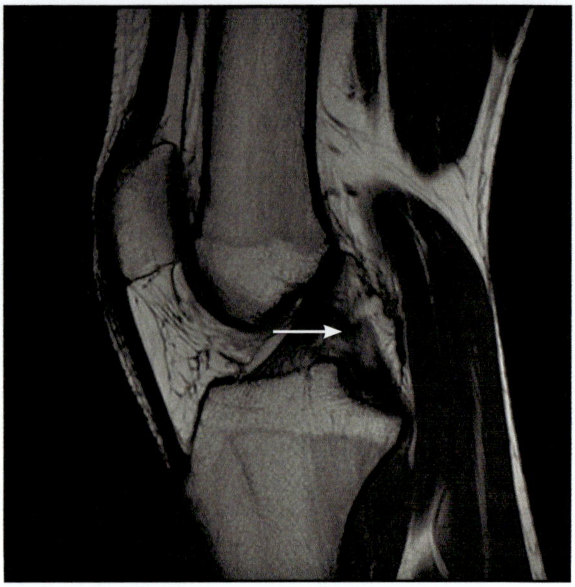

Figure 31-3. Magnetic resonance image of a PCL-injured knee. In a grade III PCL injury, complete disruption of the ligament will be observed on sagittal sequences. Close attention should be paid to the other structures of the knee because associated ligamentous, meniscal, and articular injuries are common.

Magnetic Resonance Imaging

- Confirm suspected ligamentous injury
- Diagnosis suspected concomitant injuries to the knee
- This is essential for preoperative planning. Awareness of additional injuries needing to be addressed at the time of surgery is crucial for surgical strategy (Figure 31-3).[22]

Equipment

Because this is a combined open and arthroscopic procedure, it is important to have standard equipment for both available. Similar to many relatively complex cases, there are often specific instruments, implants, and pans that do not necessarily need to be open at the beginning of the case but should be readily available. It is also important to have a reliable implant technician to assist with any issues related to equipment or implants.

A standard knee arthroscopy (with 30- and 70-degree arthroscopes) and major orthopedic pan should be open at the beginning of the case, in addition to the equipment for bone patellar tendon bone autograft harvest. Solid or cannulated screws should be available for the tibial inlay fixation (the authors prefer 4.5-mm cannulated screws with washers). Preferred fixation for the femoral side is a titanium interference screw, but alternative fixation, such as a cortical suspensory device, should be available. Luque wires can be used to pass the graft. Femoral PCL guides are used for femoral tunnel placement. Round or oval burrs are used to create the trough in tibia. Several 3/32-in guide pins should be open and are used for retraction and femoral tunnel placement. A Shantz pin with a T-handle should be available and is used to apply an anterior drawer on the tibia when the PCL graft is fixed.

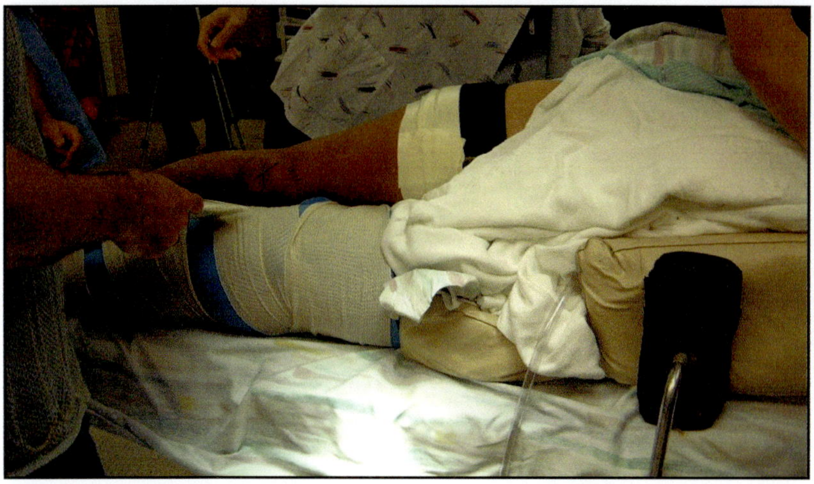

Figure 31-4. Lateral decubitus positioning. The patient is in the lateral decubitus position with the injured side up and thorough padding of the down leg. The patient can be supported by hip positioning posts or a bean bag.

Positioning and Portals

Once the patient is intubated and under anesthesia, it is essential to perform a thorough examination of the knee to rule out associated ACL, posteromedial, or posterolateral injuries. After completing the examination under anesthesia, the authors position the patient in the lateral decubitus position with the injured leg up (Figure 31-4). It is important to pad the contralateral leg and all other extremities and use an axillary roll. A bean bag is used to hold the patient in position; with obese patients, hip positioners are used to augment the bean bag. The authors use a nonsterile tourniquet but do not use a leg holder on the thigh. The authors place the operative foot and leg into a bracketed leg holder, which helps position the leg during the anterior portions of the procedure (Figure 31-5).

Step-by-Step Description of the Procedure

The authors adapted this technique shortly after the report by Berg and have modified it over the years.[5,23] The authors combined this technique with the posterior approach previously described by Burks and Shaffer[24] and have subsequently made further modifications.

The PCL graft can be fixed directly into a trough at its tibial origin, and an anatomic PCL reconstruction can be accomplished. The authors have shown that the approach is safe because the popliteal artery is retracted by the medial head of the gastrocnemius well out of the surgical field.[25,26] The authors have also eliminated the problems associated with repositioning the patient during this procedure by placing the patient in the lateral decubitus position and rotating the leg at the hip to access the front of the knee.[27]

For patients with an acute combined injury (within 2 weeks), the authors usually begin with an egress incision in the center of their planned corner incision to prevent iatrogenic compartment syndrome. Next, they harvest a generous (11- to 12-mm) central one-third bone-patellar tendon-bone graft and prepare it on the back table. They prefer to use the tibial portion of the graft for the tibial inlay and make it rectangular and approximately 20 to 25 mm in length. The patellar portion of the graft is "bulleted" and is fashioned to be approximately 18 mm in length. This smaller size facilitates easier graft passage into the femoral tunnel. The graft is placed under tension on a graft board during the next portions of the procedure.

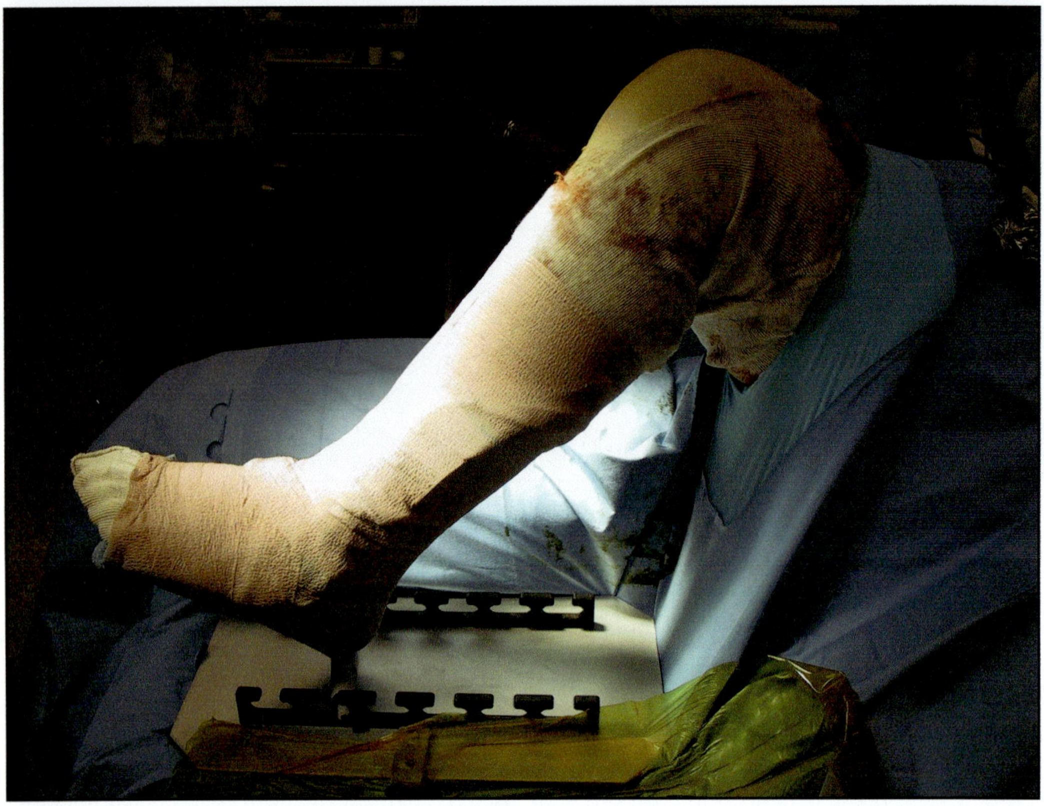

Figure 31-5. Positioning during arthroscopy. The up leg can be placed in a bracketed leg holder and can be easily positioned for the arthroscopic portion of the case.

Arthroscopy is then performed, and the injured PCL is debrided with a basket and a shaver. If there are intact fibers (including meniscofemoral ligaments), the authors try to retain them whenever possible. ACL laxity may be normal, and this pseudolaxity will resolve when an anterior drawer is applied.[28]

The femoral tunnel is drilled from outside-in. A subvastus approach is made through an incision in Langer's lines, and a guide is used to place a 3/32-in guide pin high in the notch (at approximately 1:30 on the clock face for a right knee) and 6 to 8 mm from the articular surface (Figure 31-6). The authors have found that the outside-in approach reduces the amount of graft bend into the femoral tunnel (the critical corner).[29-31] The tunnel is overdrilled with the appropriate cannulated drill and bone graft from the drill flutes is collected for later placement in the patellar harvest site. The posterior aspect of the tunnel is rasped to reduce graft abrasion. A looped 18-gauge Luque wire is then positioned arthroscopically through the tunnel and into the posterior aspect of the knee.

The authors then place the leg onto a Mayo stand and prepare for the tibial inlay approach. The surgeon sits on an operative stool and uses a headlight to directly approach the popliteal fossa. An incision is made in the popliteal crease, and the gastrocnemius fascia is incised. A hockey stick incision is made in the fascia (but not in the skin as originally described by Burks and Shaffer[24]). The medial head of the gastrocnemius is identified and bluntly mobilized. The tendinous portion of this large muscle is on the deep surface. The medial head of the gastrocnemius is mobile and can be retracted laterally, past the midline. This muscle can be held in place with 3/32-in pins that can be bent and used as retractors. The muscle belly of the popliteus is identified, and a posterior arthrotomy is made at its superior border. This can be enlarged with Mayo scissors, and the pre-placed Luque wire is retrieved. The PCL fossa is palpated and electrocautery, a rongeur, and a burr

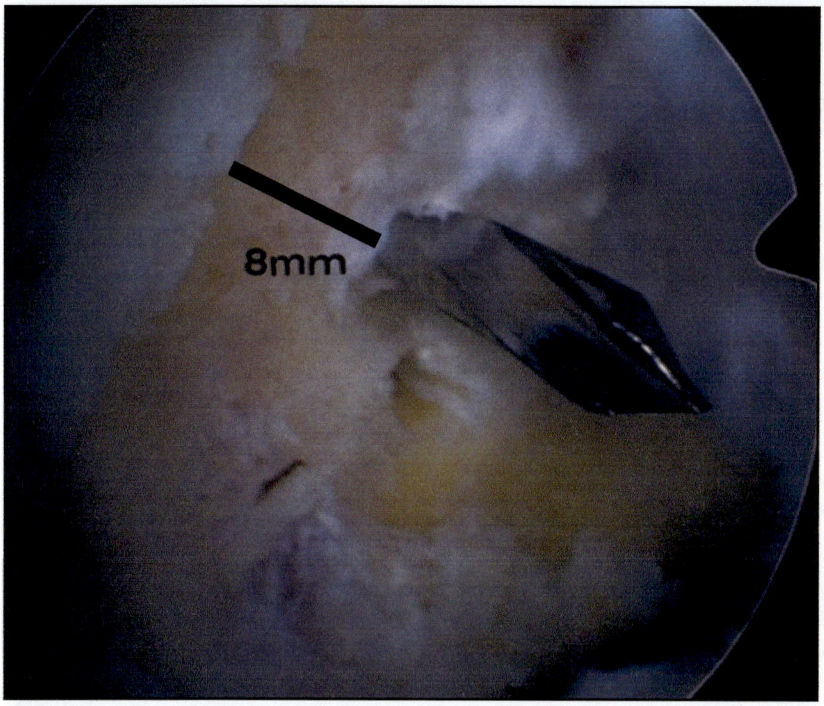

Figure 31-6. Femoral guide pin placement. Viewed through the anterolateral arthroscopic portal, the femoral guide pin can be placed with a PCL guide and should be high in the notch (at approximately a 1:30 position on a right knee) and 6 to 8 mm from the articular margin. This position can be confirmed by direct measurement or intraoperative fluoroscopy.

are used to create a trough that matches the dimensions of the graft (Figure 31-7). The graft is then brought up to the operative field and secured to the drapes (safety net). The patellar portion of the graft is pulled into the knee (and hopefully directly into the femoral tunnel), and the tibial portion is inlayed into the trough. The authors secure the graft with 4.5-mm cannulated screws. These screws are serially drilled, measured, and placed to secure the graft into the trough. It is helpful to clamp the guide wires at the anterior portion of the tibia prior to drilling to help with screw placement.

The knee is then placed back into the bracketed knee holder, and the graft is arthroscopically visualized. If the patellar bone block did not get delivered into the femoral tunnel, it is passed at this point. Sometimes it is necessary to toggle the graft with a right angle clamp to facilitate passage. Once it is in the tunnel, the knee is cycled to eliminate any kinking, and the graft is fixed in the femur with a 9-by-20-mm metal interference screw. An anterior drawer force is placed on the tibia while the graft is fixed. A Shantz pin with a T-handle from the external fixation set can be useful for this purpose (Figure 31-8). The patient is examined on the table to ensure the posterior tibial laxity has been corrected and the remaining portions of the case are completed prior to standard closure.

Postoperative Protocol

Initial Postoperative Period

Patients should be placed into an external hinged knee brace that is locked in full extension for the first 2 weeks. Fifty percent partial weightbearing with crutches should be used for the first 4 to 6 weeks, with subsequent progression to weightbearing as tolerated. Under the direction of a physical therapist, passive range of motion exercises from 0 to 90 degrees should be started; it is essential that these ROM exercises be done in the prone position to avoid early stress on the reconstruction. Quadriceps sets and edema control are also used in the early time period.

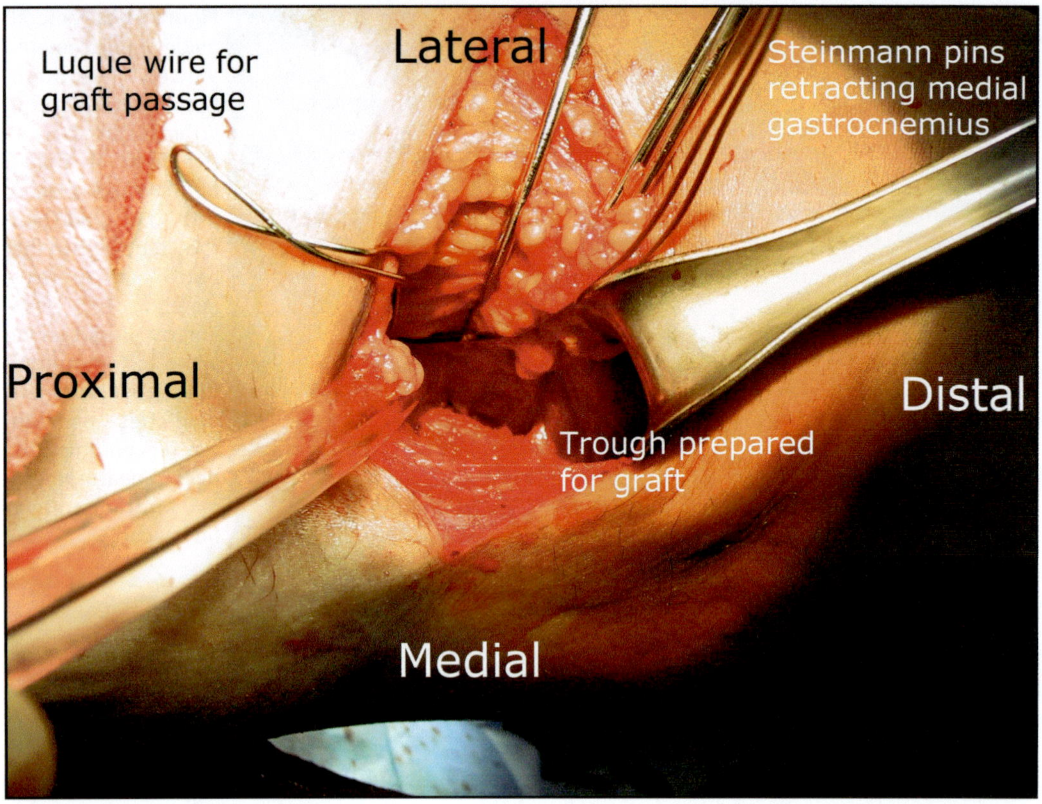

Figure 31-7. Tibial inlay trough. A left knee viewed in the lateral position after the posterior approach has been performed. The posterior tibia is well exposed, with 2 to 3 Steinmann pins acting as self-retainers to retract the medial head of the gastrocnemius. The trough is placed in the PCL fossa at the superior border of the popliteus muscle.

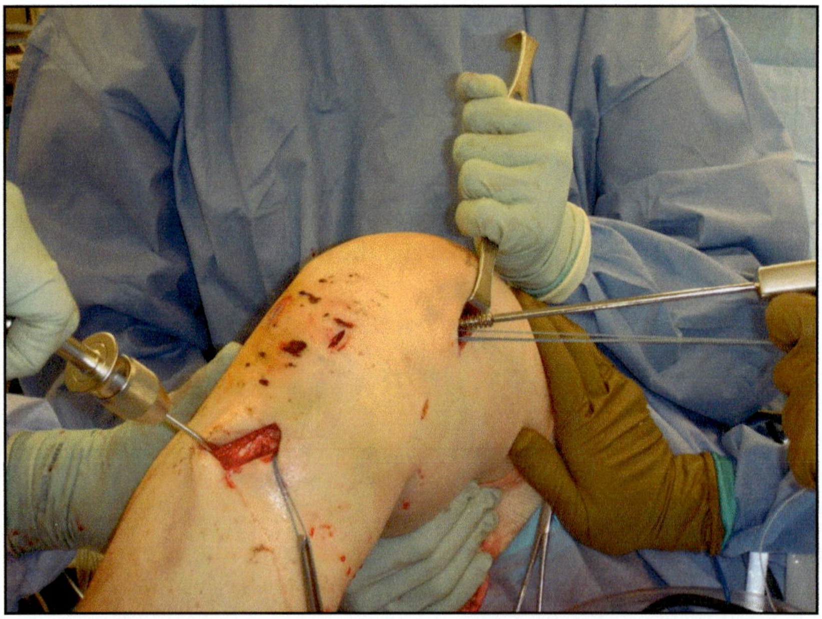

Figure 31-8. Placement of femoral fixation. A left knee with the knee held by the bracketed leg holder. The final step in graft fixation is the placement of an outside-in interference screw. The Shantz pin is in the proximal tibia, which facilitates an anterior drawer force to reduce any pseudolaxity prior to definitive fixation of the graft.

Progressive Physical Therapy

At the 4- to 6-week mark, the patient may begin full weightbearing and focused quadriceps strengthening with straight leg raises and progression to closed chain terminal knee extension exercises at 8 weeks. No hamstring strengthening should be performed until 3 months postoperatively. Jogging on a treadmill may begin at 10 to 12 weeks postoperatively, but running should be avoided for 4 to 6 months. Plyometrics and sport-specific activities may begin at 16 weeks postoperatively. Return to sport is typically 6 to 9 months depending on the strength and dynamic control of the limb.

Potential Complications

As with any surgical intervention, infection is always a concern. In a lengthy procedure such as this and with multiple steps and numerous instruments being used, the infection rate is higher than other arthroscopic procedures. A review of the American Board of Orthopaedic Surgery database from 2003 to 2009 showed the arthroscopic procedure with the highest complication rate was PCL reconstruction at 20.1%, with infection being the most common.[32] Because there are so many instruments and assistants used in this surgery, the surgeon must be diligent in observing sterile technique and ensuring the additional operating room staff remain sterile throughout the case.

The most severe, and certainly most dreaded, complication following PCL reconstruction is neurovascular injury. Mastery of the anatomy in the posterior knee is mandatory when performing the tibial inlay technique. Consider reviewing the anatomy or performing a cadaveric dissection prior to a PCL reconstruction to help decrease the risk of this complication. The risk of vascular injury can also be decreased by performing careful dissection during the posterior approach because anomalous branches of the genicular arteries can result in significant intra- and postoperative bleeding.

Excess pressure can develop in the soft tissue due to extravasation of the arthroscopic fluid, especially in the setting of a multiligament injury with significant capsular injury. It is important to manually check the pressure in the thigh and leg with intermittent palpation throughout the case.

Early arthrofibrosis and late laxity can be seen after this procedure. If early loss of motion is noted, lysis of adhesions and manipulation under anesthesia may be necessary. Late laxity can be multifactorial but can best be avoided with meticulous surgical technique and treating any concomitant ligamentous injuries, especially frequently overlooked posterolateral corner disruptions.

Top Technical Pearls for the Procedure

1. Special care should be given to padding the down leg to ensure there is no pressure on the peroneal nerve as it crosses the fibular neck (see Figure 31-4).
2. Have multiple options for fixation of your graft, especially on the femoral side, and consider backup fixation.
3. Use a probe or marked instrument to measure guide pin placement before overdrilling the femoral tunnel. In addition, intraoperative fluoroscopy can be used to assess tunnel placement.
4. The knee should be cycled multiple times with the graft under tension, prior to final graft fixation to remove any residual laxity.
5. Use a Shantz pin in the proximal tibia to place an anterior drawer force during final graft fixation; the knee should be in 90 degrees of flexion (see Figure 31-8).

References

1. Salim, R, Fogognolo F, Kfuri M Jr. A new simplified onlay technique for posterior cruciate ligament reconstruction. *J Knee Surg.* 2014;27(4):289-294.
2. Benedetto KP, Hoffelner T, Osti M. The biomechanical characteristics of arthroscopic tibial inlay techniques for posterior cruciate ligament reconstruction: in vitro comparison of tibia graft tunnel placement. *Int Orthop.* 2014;38(11):2363-2368.
3. Curry Rde P, Mestriner MB, Kaleka CC, Severino NR, de Oliveira VM, Camargo OP. Double-bundle PCL reconstruction using autogenous quadriceps tendon and semitendinous graft: surgical technique with 2-year follow-up clinical results. *Knee.* 2014;21(3):763-768.
4. Whiddon DR, Zehms CT, Miller MD, Quinby JS, Montgomery SL, Sekiya JK. Double compared with single-bundle open inlay posterior cruciate ligament reconstruction in a cadaver model. *J Bone Joint Surg Am.* 2008;90(9):1820-1829.
5. Berg EE. Posterior cruciate ligament tibial inlay reconstruction. *Arthroscopy.* 1995;11(1):69-76.
6. Miller MD, Bergfeld JA, Fowler PJ, Harner CD, Noyes FR. The posterior cruciate ligament injured knee: principles of evaluation and treatment. *Instr Course Lect.* 1999;48:199-207.
7. Miller MD, Johnson DL, Harner CD, Fu FH. Posterior cruciate ligament injuries. *Orthop Rev.* 1993;22(11):1201-1210.
8. Voos, JE, Mauro CS, Wente T, Warren RF, Wickiewicz TL. Posterior cruciate ligament: anatomy, biomechanics, and outcomes. *Am J Sports Med.* 2012;40(1):222-231.
9. Dennis MG, Fox JA, Alford JW, Hayden JK, Bach BR Jr. Posterior cruciate ligament reconstruction: current trends. *J Knee Surg.* 2004;17(3):133-139.
10. Panchal HB, Sekiya JK. Open tibial inlay versus arthroscopic transtibial posterior cruciate ligament reconstructions. *Arthroscopy.* 2011;27(9):1289-1295.
11. Nancoo TJ, Lord B, Yasen SK, Smith JO, Risenbury MJ, Wilson AJ. Transmedial all-inside posterior cruciate ligament reconstruction using a reinforced tibial inlay graft. *Arthrosc Tech.* 2013;2(4):e381-e388.
12. Lee DW, Jang HW, Lee YS, et al. Clinical, functional, and morphological evaluations of posterior cruciate ligament reconstruction with remnant preservation: minimum 2-year follow-up. *Am J Sports Med.* 2014;42(8):1822-1831.
13. Lee YS, Jung YB. Posterior cruciate ligament: focus on conflicting issues. *Clin Orthop Surg.* 2013;5(4):256-262.
14. Lee SH, Jung YB, Lee HJ, Jung HJ, Kim SH. Remnant preservation is helpful to obtain good clinical results in posterior cruciate ligament reconstruction: comparison of clinical results of three techniques. *Clin Orthop Surg.* 2013;5(4):278-286.
15. Stannard JP. Anatomic posterior cruciate ligament reconstruction with allograft. *J Knee Surg.* 2010;23(2):81-87.
16. Laupattarakasem W, Boonard M, Laupattarakasem P, Kosuwon W. Tibial inlay technique using hamstring graft for posterior cruciate ligament reconstruction and remnant revision. *Arthrosc Tech.* 2013;2(1):e1-e7.
17. Weber AE, Bissell B, Wojtys EM, Sekiya JK. Is the all arthroscopic tibial inlay double-bundle PCL reconstruction a viable option in multiligament knee injuries? *Clin Orthop Relat Res.* 2014;472(9):2667-2679.
18. Montgomery SR, Johnson JS, McAllister DR, Petrigliano FA. Surgical management of PCL injuries: indications, techniques, and outcomes. *Curr Rev Musculoskelet Med.* 2013;6(2):115-123.
19. Ettinger, M, Buermann S, Calliess T, et al. Tibial inlay press-fit fixation versus interference screw in posterior cruciate ligament reconstruction. *Orthop Rev (Pavia).* 2013;5(4):e35.
20. Richter D, Wascher DC, Schenck RC Jr. A novel posteromedial approach for tibial inlay PCL reconstruction in KDIIIM injuries: avoiding prone patient positioning. *Clin Orthop Relat Res.* 2014;472(9):2680-2690.
21. Gwathmey FW Jr, Tompkins MA, Gaskin CM, Miller MD. Can stress radiography of the knee help characterize posterolateral corner injury? *Clin Orthop Relat Res.* 2012;470(3):768-773.
22. Mariani PP, Adriani E, Bellelli A, Maresca G. Magnetic resonance imaging of tunnel placement in posterior cruciate ligament reconstruction. *Arthroscopy.* 1999;15(7):733-740.
23. Bergfeld JA, McAllister DR, Parker RD, Valdevit AD, Kambic HE. A biomechanical comparison of posterior cruciate ligament reconstruction techniques. *Am J Sports Med.* 2001;29(2):129-136.

24. Burks RT, Shaffer JJ. A simplified approach to the tibial attachment of the posterior cruciate ligament. *Clin Orthop Relat Res.* 1990;(254):216-219.
25. Miller MD, Kline AJ, Gonzales J, Beach WR. Vascular risk associated with a posterior approach for posterior cruciate ligament reconstruction using the tibial inlay technique. *J Knee Surg.* 2002;15(3):137-140.
26. Cohen SB, Boyd L, Miller MD. Vascular risk associated with posterior cruciate ligament reconstruction using the arthroscopic transtibial tunnel technique. *J Knee Surg.* 2004;17(4):211-213.
27. Johnson DH, Fanelli GC, Miller MD. PCL 2002: indications, double-bundle versus inlay technique and revision surgery. *Arthroscopy.* 2002;18(9 suppl 2):40-52.
28. Fanelli GC, Giannotti BF, Edson CJ. The posterior cruciate ligament arthroscopic evaluation and treatment. *Arthroscopy.* 1994;10(6):673-688.
29. Handy MH, Blessey PB, Miller MD. Measurement of the tibial tunnel/graft angle and the graft/femoral tunnel angle in posterior cruciate ligament reconstruction: a cadaveric study comparing two techniques for femoral tunnel placement. *Arthroscopy.* 2003;19(5):129-130.
30. Handy MH, Blessey PB, Kline AJ, Miller MD. The graft/tunnel angles in posterior cruciate ligament reconstruction: a cadaveric comparison of two techniques for femoral tunnel placement. *Arthroscopy.* 2005;21(6):711-714.
31. Schoderbek RJ Jr, Golish SR, Rubino LJ, Oliviero JA, Hart JM, Miller MD. The graft/femoral tunnel angles in posterior cruciate ligament reconstruction: a comparison of three techniques for femoral tunnel placement. *J Knee Surg.* 2009;22(2):106-110.
32. Salzler MJ, Miller CD, Lin A, Herold S, Irrgang JJ, Harner CD. Arthroscopic PCL reconstruction leads in complications. *AAOS Now.* August 2013.

Please see videos on the accompanying website at www.routledge.com/9781617119996

32

Anatomic Reconstruction of the Posterolateral Corner of the Knee

Adam M. Johannsen, MD; Evan W. James, BS; and
Robert F. LaPrade, MD, PhD

Introduction

The complex anatomy of static and dynamic stabilizers in the posterolateral corner (PLC) of the knee creates a diagnostic and treatment challenge. These structures are injured in 5% to 9% of all knee injuries and up to 16% of all ligamentous knee injuries.[1-3] Injuries to the PLC are often caused by a direct or indirect blow to the anteromedial aspect of the knee, a contact or noncontact hyperextension injury, or a varus noncontact injury.[4,5] Concomitant injuries to the anterior cruciate ligament (ACL) and posterior cruciate ligament (PCL) are frequent, with isolated PLC injuries accounting for only 16% to 28% of all PLC injuries.[3-5] Despite an increased awareness, up to 70% of PLC injuries are missed acutely, leading to a critical delay in treatment.[3] Due to the inherent bony instability of the lateral compartment, which contributes to a lack of healing, surgical intervention is often required.[6-8] Primary repair of injured ligaments and tendons is only possible in the acute setting, whereas chronic PLC injuries and acute grade III (complete) injuries generally require surgical reconstruction.[9-11] In repair and reconstruction, the goal of surgery is anatomic restoration of these structures in order to best reproduce the native anatomy and biomechanics of the knee.

The primary stabilizers of the PLC include the fibular collateral ligament (FCL), popliteus tendon, and popliteofibular ligament.[1,12,13] Anatomic-based surgical reconstruction of these structures has been developed and validated through biomechanical and clinical outcome studies (Figure 32-1).[9,12,14-17] This chapter provides an overview of the diagnosis and indications for surgery following a PLC knee injury and presents a detailed description of an anatomic-based PLC surgical reconstruction technique.

Sgaglione NA, Lubowitz JH, Provencher MT, eds. *The Knee: AANA Advanced Arthroscopic Surgical Techniques* (pp 449-460).

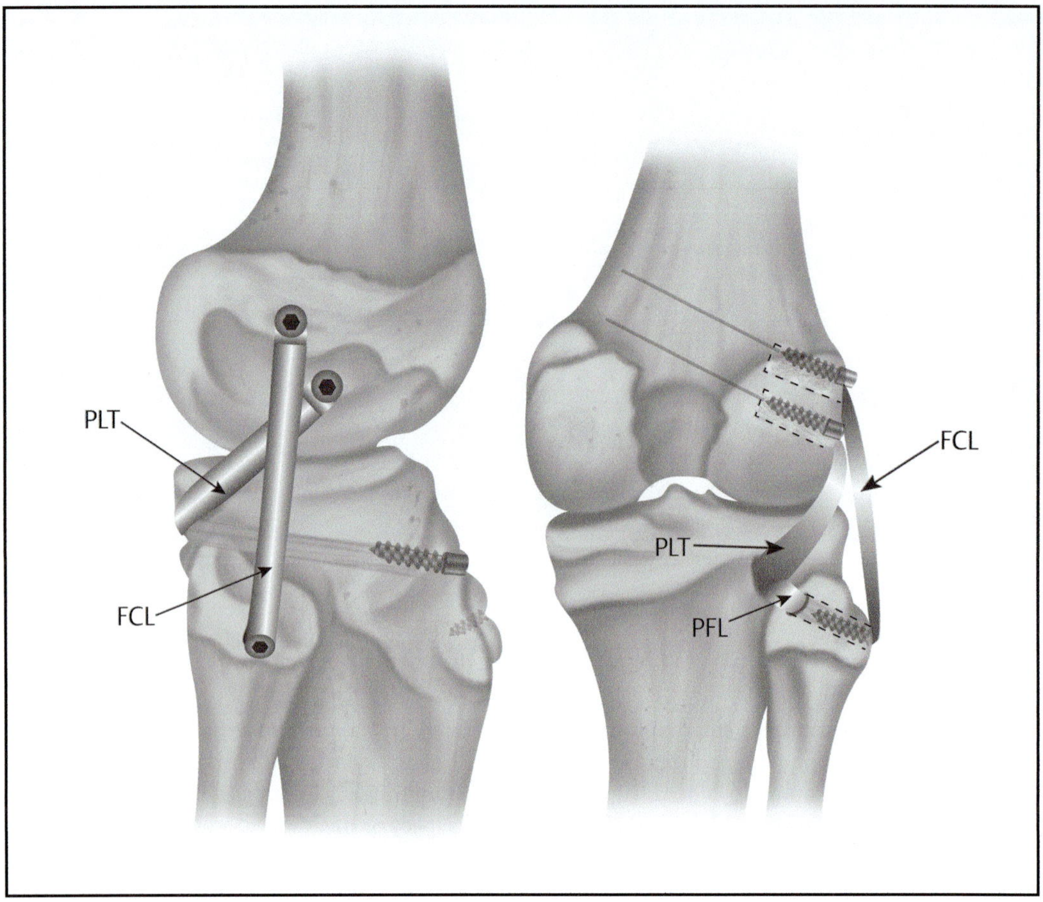

Figure 32-1. An anatomic-based PLC reconstruction of the popliteofibular ligament, popliteus tendon, and FCL.

Indications

There are several indications for surgical reconstruction of the PLC. The recommended treatment for grade I or II PLC knee injuries is generally nonoperative.[3,8,18] Operative indications include the following:

- Acute grade III PLC injuries that display significant varus and posterolateral rotary instability in the setting of functional instability and/or knee pain necessitate surgical intervention.[14] If these injuries are diagnosed acutely, the ligaments are of acceptable quality, and surgery is planned within the first 1 to 2 weeks after injury, primary repair of injured ligaments may occasionally be feasible. However, at about 3 weeks after injury, significant scar tissue develops, making repairs difficult, and reconstruction should be considered. In addition, injury to the popliteus muscle at the musculotendinous junction precludes repair.[10,11] Stannard et al[11] compared acute PLC repair vs surgical reconstruction and found a 28% higher failure rate with repair. Levy et al[10] reported similar results favoring anatomic reconstruction. The authors recommend anatomic surgical reconstruction for acute grade III PLC injuries in most instances, especially where tissue and injury pattern are not optimal for a repair.[19]

- Chronic grade III PLC injuries are unlikely to heal with primary repair or nonoperative measures and require surgical reconstruction.[10,11] Therefore, the authors recommend anatomic surgical reconstruction for chronic grade III PLC injuries.[19]
- Although total PLC reconstruction is indicated in cases of severe injury, isolated injuries to posterolateral structures, including the FCL, popliteus tendon, and popliteofibular ligament, are relatively common and must be ruled out before performing a total reconstruction. Isolated anatomic-based repair or reconstruction procedures may be used in cases of less-extensive injury.[20-22]

Controversial Indications

Genu varus in the setting of PLC injury is a difficult problem that creates a treatment challenge. Due to the stress of PLC structures in genu varus alignment, correction of malalignment is often necessitated prior to reconstruction. Without correction, there is a high risk of graft failure.[5,19,23,24] In addition, it has been shown that a proximal tibial osteotomy alone will resolve chronic PLC laxity in patients with genu varus 38% of the time.[25] Therefore, in the setting of genu varus, the authors recommend a 2-staged approach to correct the mechanical axis using a proximal tibial osteotomy and then to reassess for residual PLC laxity before proceeding with a PLC reconstruction.

Pertinent Physical Findings

The diagnosis of PLC injury is best made by a combination of history, physical examination, and imaging studies. Several physical examination maneuvers are important when assessing for PLC injury because no single test provides sufficient specificity or sensitivity to reliably predict PLC injury.

- External rotation recurvatum test: This test is performed by lifting the patient's big toe off the examination table and assesses for knee hyperextension as compared to the contralateral leg. A positive test may indicate severe ligament injury, most commonly combined ACL injury.[26]
- Varus stress test: This test should be performed at 0 and 30 degrees to assess for FCL and PLC injury (Figure 32-2). A positive varus stress test at 0 degrees usually indicates severe posterolateral ligament laxity. Greater than 1 cm of subjective varus gapping with the knee at 30 degrees indicates a grade III PLC injury.[18,19]
- Dial test: This test, also known as the posterolateral rotation test, should be performed at 30 and 90 degrees (Figure 32-3). In this test, the foot and ankle are externally rotated, and the rotation of the tibial tubercle is compared to the contralateral side. Some authors have advocated for a surgical intervention when there is a 15-degree discrepancy between legs.[17] Medial ligamentous knee injury may also cause a false-positive test and must be ruled out prior to intervention.[26]
- Reverse pivot shift test: In this test, the knee is flexed to 45 degrees, the foot is externally rotated, and a valgus force is applied to the knee. In this position, patients with PLC injury may sublux the knee. The knee is then slowly extended, and the test is considered positive if there is a palpable clunk of the knee relocating with extension. However, this test has been shown to have wide variability among healthy knees and must always be compared to the contralateral side.

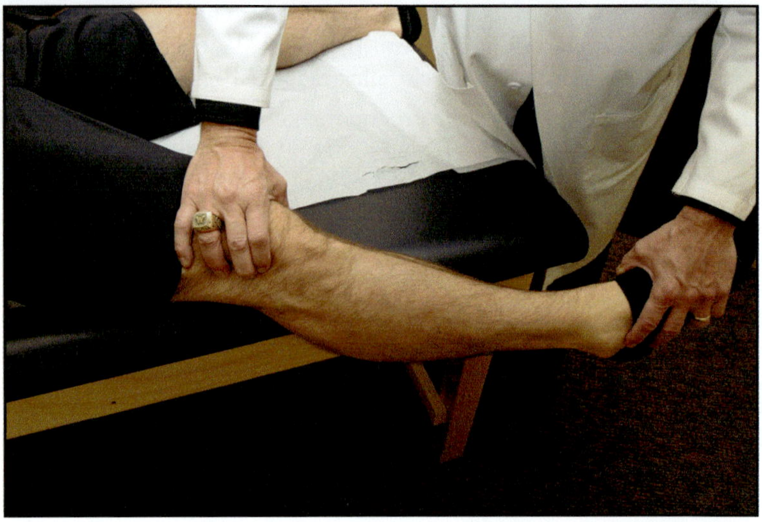

Figure 32-2. Image of a right leg demonstrating a varus stress test performed at 0 degrees of knee flexion. The test should be repeated at 30 degrees of flexion.

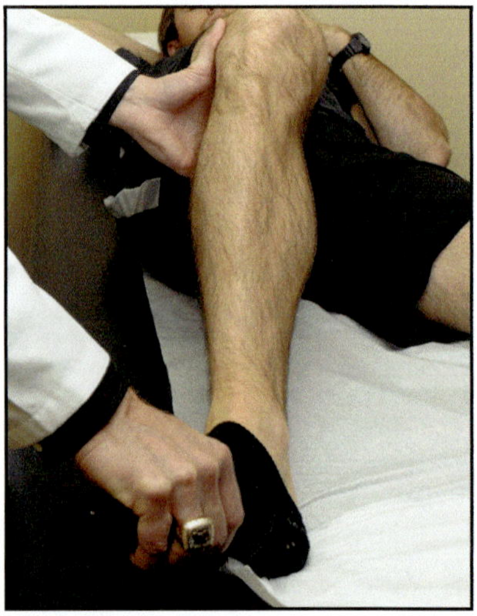

Figure 32-3. Image of a right knee dial test at 30 degrees of knee flexion. A positive test is defined as increased external rotation on the injured side compared to the contralateral side. The test should be repeated at 90 degrees of knee flexion.

- Posterolateral drawer test: This test is best used in assessing the integrity of the popliteus muscle complex. The knee is flexed to 90 degrees, and the foot is externally rotated 15 degrees. A posterior force is applied to the knee, and translation is compared to the contralateral side.
- Anterior and posterior stress examinations: The constellation of examination findings should be confirmed with increased anterior tibial translation on the Lachman maneuver and increased posterior tibial translation on the posterior drawer test. These findings can be present with isolated injury but may also indicate concomitant ACL or PCL injury.

The synergistic results of these tests provide the best clinical utility in diagnosing PLC injury. All of these tests should be used in the clinic and during the examination under anesthesia to confirm the findings.

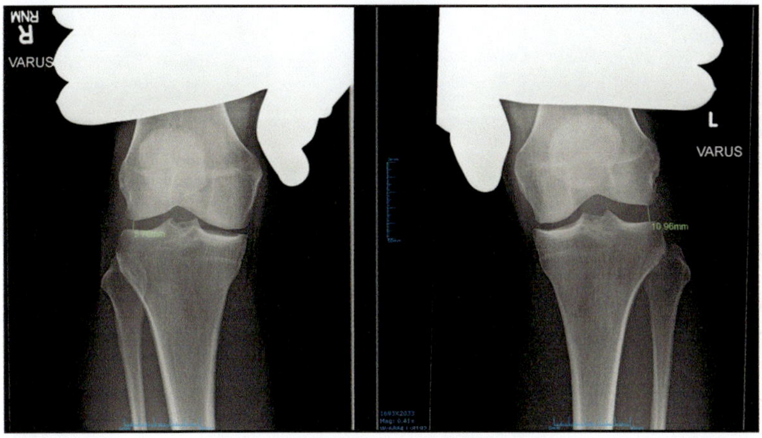

Figure 32-4. Preoperative varus stress x-rays of an injured (left) and noninjured (right) knee demonstrating a 5.2-mm side-to-side difference in varus gapping, indicative of a grade III PLC injury.

Pertinent Imaging

A combination of basic and advanced imaging modalities is necessary in the diagnosis of PLC knee injury.

X-Rays

Plain anteroposterior (AP) and varus stress x-rays can be helpful in assessing static and dynamic varus gapping. On varus stress x-rays at 20 degrees of knee flexion, the mean varus gapping in isolated FCL injured knees is 2.7 mm, as compared to a 4.0-mm gap in complete PLC-injured knees (Figure 32-4).[27] AP, lateral, sunrise, and tunnel x-rays are also necessary to rule out associated fracture, fibular head avulsion fractures, and osteoarthritis. Bilateral AP long-leg imaging is necessary to assess the alignment of the extremities. If genu varus is detected, a proximal tibial osteotomy is necessary to correct malalignment and to protect the PLC reconstruction.[25]

Magnetic Resonance Imaging

Magnetic resonance imaging (MRI) is warranted to assess ligamentous integrity and concomitant injuries to the ACL, PCL, menisci, and other knee structures. MRI has been shown to diagnose PLC injuries in 93% of cases when performed within 12 weeks of injury but has significantly lower predictive value in chronically injured knees.[3]

Equipment

In preparing for a PLC reconstruction, instruments for an open and arthroscopic procedure must be readily available. An operating table with removable ends or the ability to flex the end of the bed is required for proper patient positioning. An arthroscopy tower and arthroscopy equipment are needed to address cruciate and meniscal intra-articular pathology. Tool kits for cruciate reconstructions, meniscal repair, and microfracture should be readily available. An Adson pointed hemostat is useful to perform a common peroneal neurolysis. For the PLC reconstruction, a cruciate-aiming device is needed for placement and reaming of tunnels. A split Achilles allograft is the authors' preferred graft material. In addition to standard operating materials, reamers, bioabsorbable screws, and cannulated screws are needed for graft fixation. It is helpful if the operating room staff are well versed with these required materials and the flow and pace of the procedure.

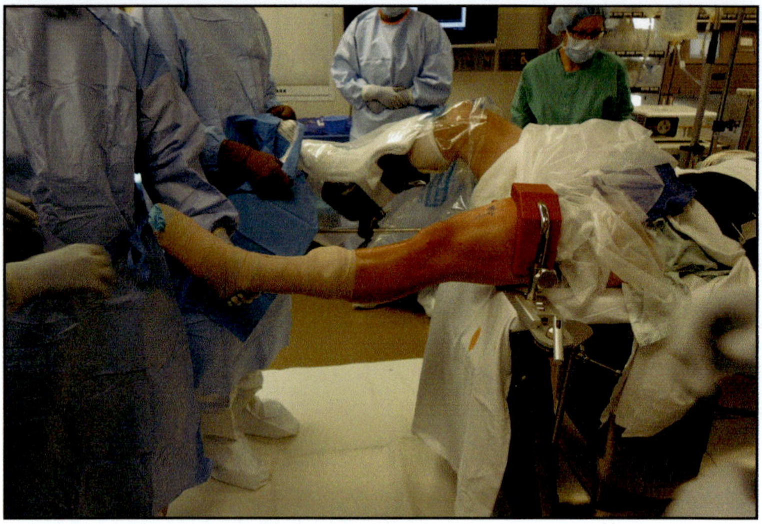

Figure 32-5. Operating room image of a preoperative, prepped left leg. The patient is positioned on the operating table with the nonsurgical leg abducted and held in a leg holder while the surgical leg hangs freely from the flexed end of the operating table. A tourniquet is placed on the proximal thigh.

Positioning and Portals

The patient should be in the supine position on the operating table. A leg holder is used to secure the nonoperative leg away and to the side of the surgical field. With the foot of the operating table flexed down, a tourniquet is placed around the proximal thigh while the distal thigh is secured using a leg holder (Figure 32-5). The surgical leg is allowed to hang freely from the edge of the operating table at approximately a 70-degree angle. The bed is raised to an appropriate height for the surgical team to allow for easy access to the lateral aspect of the knee. Once proper positioning is achieved, the surgical site is prepared and the procedure is ready to begin.

Step-by-Step Description of the Procedure

After the patient is brought into the operating room, general, epidural, or spinal anesthesia may be used in accordance with surgeon and patient preference. Prior to beginning the surgery, a thorough examination under anesthesia should be conducted, including the posterolateral drawer test, varus stress test at 0 and 30 degrees, external rotation recurvatum test, reverse pivot shift test, dial test, Lachman test, posterior drawer test, and assessment for other ligamentous injuries (Video). Upon confirmation of injury by physical examination, the patient may be prepped for surgery. The patient should be positioned supine with the surgical leg hanging from the lowered foot of the operating table. A tourniquet is placed on the proximal thigh. At this point, a time-out is performed to confirm patient identity, injury, and sidedness, and prophylactic antibiotics are given.

The fibular head, Gerdy's tubercle, tibial tubercle, lateral epicondyle, and predicted path of the common peroneal nerve should be marked with a marking pen prior to the incision. The superficial incision is a standard hockey stick incision beginning along the posterior midportion of the distal iliotibial band and extending distally across the knee to the anterior compartment (Video).[28] The incision should cross the knee at the level of Gerdy's tubercle. The incision is carried down through the subcutaneous tissue to the level of the iliotibial band. Next, meticulous dissection should occur posteriorly to identify the short and long heads of the biceps femoris. A common peroneal nerve neurolysis is critical to preserving neurologic function of the extremity, and neurolysis is necessary to gain access to the posteromedial fibular head and to prevent a postoperative foot drop due to postoperative swelling causing nerve compression (Figure 32-6). The common

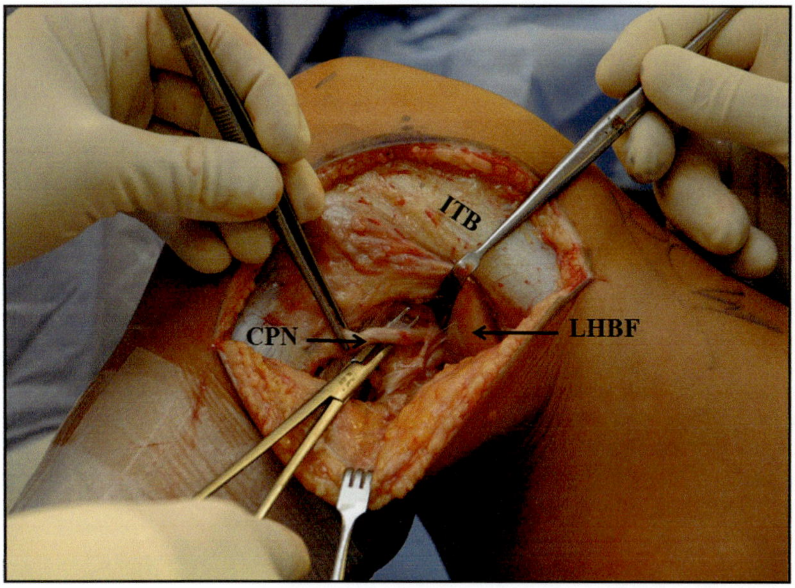

Figure 32-6. Intraoperative image of the surgical approach on a left knee. A standard lateral hockey stick incision is made, and peroneal neurolysis is performed to minimize the risk of iatrogenic injury (common peroneal nerve, forceps). The interval for the peroneal dissection is carried out between the long head of the biceps femoris and the peroneal muscle bellies. CPN, common peroneal nerve; ITB, iliotibial band; LHBF, long head of the biceps femoris muscle.

peroneal nerve is identified 2 to 3 cm distal to the long head of biceps femoris. When the nerve is not readily identifiable, it can be palpated 2 cm distal to the fibular head. The peroneal nerve is decompressed for up to 8 cm to minimize the risk of postoperative palsy secondary to swelling and to ensure that gentle traction to retract it from the surgical site will not injure the nerve.

Blunt dissection between the planes of the long head of the gastrocnemius and soleus is conducted to better expose the fibular head (Video). Through this interval, the posteromedial aspect of the fibular head (where the popliteofibular ligament inserts) and the musculotendinous junction of popliteus muscle can be readily identified. Next, an incision through the anterior arm of the long head of the biceps femoris proximal to the fibular head is created and extended through the biceps bursa. Through this incision, the midsubstance of the FCL is identified, as well as its attachment to the fibular head. A traction stitch is placed in the distal midsubstance of the FCL to assist with identification of the proximal femoral attachment later in the surgery. The fibular attachment of the FCL is now subperiosteally dissected off of the fibular head. A saddle should be identified on the posteromedial aspect of the fibular head, which denotes the insertion of the popliteofibular ligament on the posteromedial aspect of the fibular head.

With necessary identification and exposure conducted, the fibular head tunnel may now be drilled. The proper path of the tunnel should begin directly at the attachment of the FCL and continue through to the posteromedial downslope of the fibular styloid. Using a cruciate-aiming device, a guide pin is carefully directed along this path. A retractor should be inserted posterior and medial to the fibular head to prevent intrusion of the guide pin into the posterior neurovascular structures while drilling. After confirmation of proper guide pin placement, a 7-mm reamer is used to ream the fibular head tunnel. Finally, a passing suture is placed through the fibular tunnel to facilitate future graft passage.

The next portion of the procedure is aimed at reaming the tibial tunnel. Meticulous dissection of the distal attachment of the superficial layer of the iliotibial band is conducted to identify Gerdy's tubercle. Immediately distal and medial to Gerdy's tubercle is a small flat area. This area is also adjacent to the lateral aspect of the tibial tubercle. Sharp dissection is carried to bone in this area, and a rongeur is used to free the area of soft tissue. The anterior aperture of the tibial tunnel will emerge through this site. After the anterior site is prepared, attention is again directed toward the posterior aspect of the tibia. Through the interval between the gastroc-soleus complex, the

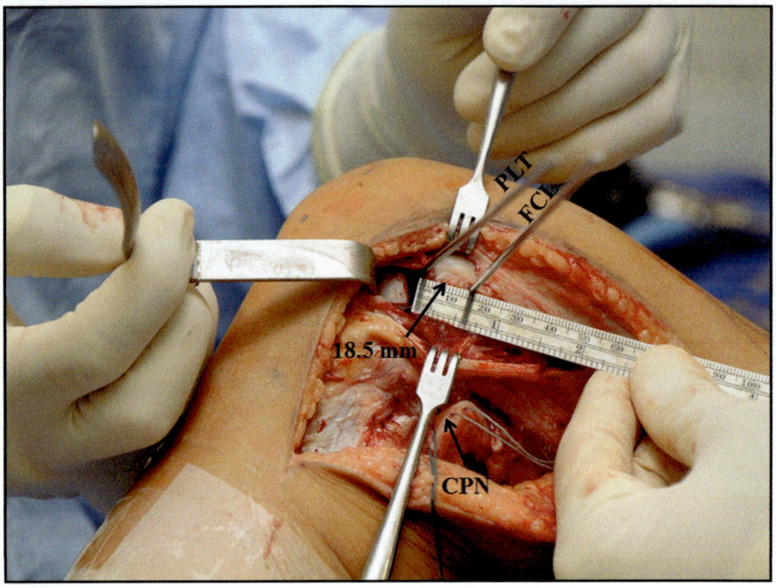

Figure 32-7. Intraoperative image of a left knee demonstrating the relationship between guide pins placed at the femoral attachments of the popliteus tendon and FCL. It is essential to confirm the correct positioning of the popliteus tendon and FCL guide pins at 18.5 mm apart. CPN, common peroneal nerve; FCL, fibular collateral ligament; PLT, popliteus tendon.

musculotendinous junction of the popliteus tendon is identified. At this level, approximately 1 cm medial and 1 cm proximal to the fibular tunnel, the tibial tunnel should exit. An obturator from the arthroscopy set may be placed through the fibular tunnel to assist in identifying the posterior tibial site. An ACL-aiming device is used to direct a guide pin from the flat area on the anterior tibia to the site at the musculotendinous junction of the popliteus on the posterior tibia. A retractor should be used to protect the neurovascular structures of the posterior knee from overpenetration of the guide pin. After confirmation of proper placement, the tibial tunnel may be reamed using a 9-mm diameter reamer.

Attention is now directed toward the femoral attachments of the PLC. Using traction on the suture placed in the FCL, the femoral attachment of the FCL may be palpated and identified. The superficial fibers of the iliotibial band are split in line with their fibers just anterior to the attachment of the FCL so that posterior traction on the fibers provides optimal exposure. The popliteus tendon inserts 18.5 mm anterior to the femoral FCL attachment.[13] Direct palpation of the anterior aspect of the popliteus tendon attachment in the anterior fifth and proximal half of the popliteal sulcus is performed, and a vertical incision through the lateral capsule of the knee is conducted to visually confirm the femoral popliteus tendon attachment. If this attachment is not readily identifiable, one can follow the direction of the fibular shaft across the knee when the knee is in 70 degrees of flexion. At this angle, the FCL courses parallel to the popliteus tendon. By traveling approximately 2 cm anterior to the FCL attachment, the popliteus tendon insertion is located. The proper location of the popliteus tendon is on the anterior fifth of the popliteal hiatus, which is 18.5 mm anterior to the FCL attachment (Figure 32-7).[13]

After both femoral attachment sites are identified, these tunnels may be reamed. First, a guide pin is passed through the FCL attachment anteromedially across the knee through the medial thigh. Care should be taken to direct the pin anteriorly so that the intercondylar notch, saphenous nerve, and any potential cruciate ligament femoral tunnels are avoided. A second guide pin is placed parallel to the FCL guide pin beginning at the anterior insertion of the popliteal tendon attachment.

After both guide pins have been passed, a critical step occurs in the procedure. The distance between guide pins is measured and should be 18.5 mm apart. Any significant variation from this distance may indicate nonanatomic positioning or misidentification of femoral attachments. Once this is confirmed, the femoral tunnels may be reamed. A 9-mm reamer should be used to

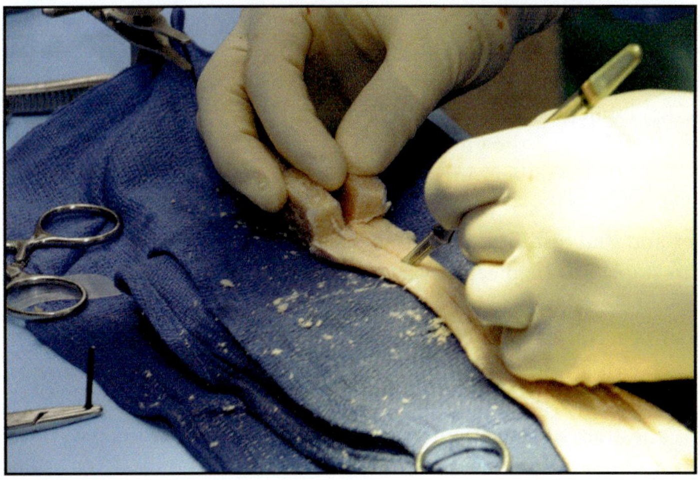

Figure 32-8. Split Achilles tendon allograft is preferred for an anatomic PLC reconstruction. The graft may be prepared on the back table by an assistant while any intra-articular pathology is addressed.

drill to a depth of 25 mm for both the popliteus and FCL tunnel. Passing sutures are then passed into both tunnels. After the femoral tunnels are completed, any intra-articular pathology, such as ACL reconstruction, PCL reconstruction, meniscectomy, meniscal repair, or articular cartilage repair, is conducted. In cruciate ligament reconstructions, the femoral attachments of the grafts should be fixed, but the tibial attachments should remain free due to risk of a fixed external rotation deformity.[29]

Although the surgeon is performing the intra-articular portion of the surgery, an assistant should prepare the PLC reconstruction grafts. The authors prefer to use a split Achilles tendon graft. The calcaneal portion is split down the middle, and 2 additional 9-by-25-mm bone plugs are harvested from the calcaneal bone graft for use in the femoral tunnels (Figure 32-8). The distal aspects of the Achilles tendon are tubularized for graft passing. Although the graft should be easily passable through a 7-mm tunnel, the initial 70-mm length of the FCL graft and 60 mm of the popliteus graft should remain thicker to best restore the strength of these ligaments and tendons, with only the portions passing through bone being slightly trimmed at the time of passing. Passing sutures are placed in the soft tissue end and bone plugs of the graft.

Once the graft is prepared, it may be passed in a femoral-to-tibial direction. Similar to an endoscopic ACL passage, the femoral ends of the graft are placed into the femoral tunnels, and passing sutures from the bone plugs are placed in the looped passing sutures. The bone plug sutures are pulled through, and tension is placed on the graft. A tight fit of the graft and bone plugs is confirmed, and the bone plugs are secured with screw fixation. In this technique, a 7-by-20-mm cannulated titanium screw is fitted to a handheld drill chuck, with approximately 3 cm of guide pin protruding past the screw. The guide pin is positioned at the margin between the bone plug and tunnel edge so that the screw is placed optimally between the bone plug and tunnel wall. After the screw is tightly fixed, secure purchase of the graft is verified with a firm lateral tug.

After femoral fixation, the popliteus tendon graft is passed distally along the popliteal hiatus and exits the knee in the interval between the lateral gastrocnemius and the soleus. The FCL graft is passed distally, medial (deep) to the superficial iliotibial band and lateral aponeurosis of the long head of the biceps femoris. The FCL graft is then passed through the fibular head tunnel and may be assisted with a suture or suture passer. If any further graft trimming is necessary to facilitate passage, this should occur now. If a PCL reconstruction is needed, the tibial graft fixation should occur prior to fibular or tibial fixation of the PLC grafts and should occur now.

To secure the FCL graft in the fibular tunnel, tension is applied to the graft end by pulling proximally, and a valgus force is applied to the knee in 20 degrees of knee flexion, with the knee in neutral rotation. The graft is fixed with a 7-mm bioabsorbable screw. Following fixation, a physical examination should be performed to ensure correction of varus instability. The remaining graft ends, which reconstruct the popliteus tendon and the popliteofibular ligament, are passed from posterior to anterior through the tibia. Each graft must be cycled to ensure no residual laxity is present and proper tension is being applied. In addition, the posterior entry site of the grafts is palpated to confirm that there is no bunching of the grafts. With the knee flexed to 60 degrees in neutral rotation and sufficient tension being applied to the grafts individually, the grafts are fixed in the tibial tunnel with a 9-mm bioabsorbable screw. A thorough examination under anesthesia, including the posterolateral drawer and dial test, occurs to make certain that posterolateral instability has been corrected. A backup staple can be placed over the tibial graft for maximal fixation in patients with osteopenic bone. Now that the PLC has been corrected, fixation of an ACL graft to the tibia can occur, and any other procedures can be finished.

Subcutaneous tissues are repaired with absorbable sutures, and a running absorbable suture is used to close the skin. Loose skin taping is a secondary measure to ensure adequate strength of closure. Prior to the termination of anesthesia, the patient's incisions are sterilely dressed, and the knee is placed in a knee immobilizer. This minimizes the chance of stress on the reconstruction while the patient awakens.

Postoperative Protocol

Following the procedure, patients should remain nonweightbearing for 6 weeks. For the first 2 weeks, quadriceps contraction sets and straight leg raises may be performed while the knee is in an immobilizer, and early passive range of motion (ROM) from 0 to 90 degrees is allowed up to 4 times per day. The goal is to achieve ROM to 90 degrees of knee flexion by 2 weeks. If the patient is able to perform straight leg raises with no extensor lag at 2 weeks, he or she may perform his or her quadriceps sets and straight leg raises out of the knee immobilizer for the rest of rehabilitation. After 2 weeks, ROM is gradually increased, and active ROM is allowed, with the goal of attaining maximum knee flexion and extension by 6 weeks. Activities or exercises that may lead to graft stress, including external rotation or varus gapping, should be avoided for 6 weeks. After 6 weeks, patients are allowed to progressively wean off crutches and begin weightbearing as tolerated if limping is absent. Stationary bicycle and low-resistance exercises may be initiated following successful knee flexion of 105 to 110 degrees. At 12 weeks, low-impact exercises, such as swimming, cycling, walking, and using an elliptical, are permissible, and the goal is full strength and ROM by 6 months. After 6 months, varus stress x-rays are obtained to assess for attenuation of the reconstruction grafts. At 7 months for an isolated PLC surgery, or 9 months for a combined PLC surgery, a full physical examination and assessment by the surgeon occurs, and full return to contact and pivot activities is allowed if cleared.

Potential Complications

As with all open procedures, infection and wound dehiscence are potential risks. However, with sterile technique and prophylactic antibiotics, this risk is minimized, and a recent report showed only 1 surgical site infection among 64 surgeries.[9] Common peroneal nerve laceration and neuropraxia is also a rare, but significant complication. Graft failure or residual posterolateral knee instability is a concern in any ligamentous reconstruction and has been shown to occur in approximately 5% of surgeries.[9] This is best assessed using varus stress x-rays.

Top Technical Pearls for the Procedure

1. Preoperative varus alignment: During the preoperative workup, it is essential to obtain standing long-leg x-rays. In patients with chronic PLC injury and varus alignment deformity, it is important to first correct the deformity with a proximal tibial osteotomy. If uncorrected, the reconstruction is at risk of stretching and failure.
2. Peroneal nerve neurolysis: Ensuring adequate exposure and neurolysis is critical when performing the procedure. Without adequate release, the nerve is at risk of neurologic damage from postoperative swelling and possible limb functional limitations.
3. Popliteus tendon attachment identification: This is a difficult and technically demanding portion of the procedure. However, one must properly identify the popliteus tendon attachment. Understanding the lateral condyle anatomy and relationships to the FCL will assist in proper identification and anatomic reconstruction.
4. Cruciate graft fixation: The order of cruciate graft fixation in a PLC reconstruction is important in restoring native knee kinematics. A PCL graft should be fixed to the tibia after the PLC grafts have been anchored at their femoral position but prior to the PLC grafts being fixed on the tibia or fibula. The ACL graft should not be fixed until after the PLC graft reconstruction has been completed. This prevents excess laxity in the ACL graft once the PLC has been stabilized and minimizes the risk of a fixed external rotation deformity.
5. Postoperative protocol: Early ROM exercises remain controversial following ligamentous reconstructions. Although immobilization minimizes the risk of graft failure in the acute healing phase, it also leads to excess scar tissue development and risks postoperative arthrofibrosis. Therefore, the authors recommend early passive ROM exercises to prevent these complications, with a gradual transition to active ROM at 2 weeks.

References

1. LaPrade RF. Introduction and incidence of posterolateral knee injuries. In: *Posterolateral Knee Injuries: Anatomy, Evaluation, and Treatment.* New York, NY: Thieme; 2006:1-8.
2. LaPrade RF, Wentorf FA, Fritts H, Gundry C, Hightower CD. A prospective magnetic resonance imaging study of the incidence of posterolateral and multiple ligament injuries in acute knee injuries presenting with a hemarthrosis. *Arthroscopy.* 2007;23(12):1341-1347.
3. Pacheco RJ, Ayre CA, Bollen SR. Posterolateral corner injuries of the knee: a serious injury commonly missed. *J Bone Joint Surg Br.* 2011;93(2):194-197.
4. Geeslin AG, LaPrade RF. Location of bone bruises and other osseous injuries associated with acute grade III isolated and combined posterolateral knee injuries. *Am J Sports Med.* 2010;38(12):2502-2508.
5. LaPrade RF, Terry GC. Injuries to the posterolateral aspect of the knee. Association of anatomic injury patterns with clinical instability. *Am J Sports Med.* 1997;25(4):433-438.
6. Baker CL Jr, Norwood LA, Hughston JC. Acute combined posterior cruciate and posterolateral instability of the knee. *Am J Sports Med.* 1984;12(3):204-208.
7. Fleming RE Jr, Blatz DJ, McCarroll JR. Posterior problems in the knee. Posterior cruciate insufficiency and posterolateral rotatory insufficiency. *Am J Sports Med.* 1981;9(2):107-113.
8. Hughston JC, Andrews JR, Cross MJ, Moschi A. Classification of knee ligament instabilities. Part II. The lateral compartment. *J Bone Joint Surg Am.* 1976;58(2):173-179.
9. LaPrade RF, Johansen S, Agel J, Risberg MA, Moksnes H, Engebretsen L. Outcomes of an anatomic posterolateral knee reconstruction. *J Bone Joint Surg Am.* 2010;92(1):16-22.

10. Levy BA, Dajani KA, Morgan JA, Shah JP, Dahm DL, Stuart MJ. Repair versus reconstruction of the fibular collateral ligament and posterolateral corner in the multiligament-injured knee. *Am J Sports Med.* 2010;38(4):804-809.
11. Stannard JP, Brown SL, Farris RC, McGwin G Jr, Volgas DA. The posterolateral corner of the knee: repair versus reconstruction. *Am J Sports Med.* 2005;33(6):881-888.
12. LaPrade RF, Bollom TS, Wentorf FA, Wills NJ, Meister K. Mechanical properties of the posterolateral structures of the knee. *Am J Sports Med.* 2005;33(9):1386-1391.
13. LaPrade RF, Ly TV, Wentorf FA, Engebretsen L. The posterolateral attachments of the knee: a qualitative and quantitative morphologic analysis of the fibular collateral ligament, popliteus tendon, popliteofibular ligament, and lateral gastrocnemius tendon. *Am J Sports Med.* 2003;31(6):854-860.
14. Geeslin AG, LaPrade RF. Outcomes of treatment of acute grade-III isolated and combined posterolateral knee injuries: a prospective case series and surgical technique. *J Bone Joint Surg Am.* 2011;93(18):1672-1683.
15. LaPrade RF, Johansen S, Engebretsen L. Outcomes of an anatomic posterolateral knee reconstruction: surgical technique. *J Bone Joint Surg Am.* 2011;93(1):10-20.
16. LaPrade RF, Johansen S, Wentorf FA, Engebretsen L, Esterberg JL, Tso A. An analysis of an anatomical posterolateral knee reconstruction: an in vitro biomechanical study and development of a surgical technique. *Am J Sports Med.* 2004;32(6):1405-1414.
17. Yoon KH, Bae DK, Ha JH, Park SW. Anatomic reconstructive surgery for posterolateral instability of the knee. *Arthroscopy.* 2006;22(2):159-165.
18. American Medical Association. *Standard Nomenclature of Athlete Injuries.* Chicago, IL: American Medical Association; 1966.
19. LaPrade RF, Wentorf F. Diagnosis and treatment of posterolateral knee injuries. *Clin Orthop Relat Res.* 2002;(402):110-121.
20. Horst PK, LaPrade RF. Anatomic reconstruction of chronic symptomatic anterolateral proximal tibiofibular joint instability. *Knee Surg Sports Traumatol Arthrosc.* 2010;18(11):1452-1455.
21. LaPrade RF, Spiridonov SI, Coobs PR, Ruckert PR, Griffith CJ. Fibular collateral ligament anatomical reconstructions: a prospective outcomes study. *Am J Sports Med.* 2010;38(10):2005-2011.
22. LaPrade RF, Wozniczka JK, Stellmaker MP, Wijdicks CA. Analysis of the static function of the popliteus tendon and evaluation of an anatomic reconstruction: the "fifth ligament" of the knee. *Am J Sports Med.* 2010;38(3):543-549.
23. Harner CD, Vogrin TM, Höher J, Ma CB, Woo SL. Biomechanical analysis of a posterior cruciate ligament reconstruction. Deficiency of the posterolateral structures as a cause of graft failure. *Am J Sports Med.* 2000;28(1):32-39.
24. Neuschwander DC, Drez D Jr, Paine RM. Simultaneous high tibial osteotomy and ACL reconstruction for combined genu varus and symptomatic ACL tear. *Orthopedics.* 1993;16(6):679-684.
25. Arthur A, LaPrade RF, Agel J. Proximal tibial opening wedge osteotomy as the initial treatment for chronic posterolateral corner deficiency in the varus knee: a prospective clinical study. *Am J Sports Med.* 2007;35(11):1844-1850.
26. LaPrade RF, Ly TV, Griffith C. The external rotation recurvatum test revisited: reevaluation of the sagittal plane tibiofemoral relationship. *Am J Sports Med.* 2008;36(4):709-712.
27. LaPrade RF, Engebretsen L, Johansen S, Wentorf FA, Kurtenbach C. The effect of a proximal tibial medial opening wedge osteotomy on posterolateral knee instability; a biomechanical study. *Am J Sports Med.* 2008;36(5):956-960.
28. Terry GC, LaPrade RF. The posterolateral aspect of the knee. Anatomy and surgical approach. *Am J Sports Med.* 1996;24(6):732-739.
29. Wentorf FA, LaPrade RF, Lewis JL, Resig S. The influence of the integrity of posterolateral structures on tibiofemoral orientation when an anterior cruciate ligament graft is tensioned. *Am J Sports Med.* 2002;30(6):796-799.

Please see videos on the accompanying website at www.routledge.com/9781617119996

33

Anatomic Reconstruction of the Posteromedial Corner and Medial Collateral Ligament

Andrew J. Blackman, MD; Paul L. Sousa, MD, MBA; and Bruce A. Levy, MD

Introduction

Although the majority of medial-sided ligamentous knee injuries are isolated and can be successfully managed nonoperatively, reconstruction of the medial collateral ligament (MCL) and other posteromedial structures of the knee (posterior oblique ligament [POL], posteromedial capsule [PMC], semimembranosus, medial head of gastrocnemius) is indicated for the management of multiligamentous injured knees. In addition, cases of chronic valgus instability and/or cases of anteromedial rotatory instability that have failed conservative management may require operative intervention. The authors' preferred technique for treatment of medial and posteromedial knee injuries includes anatomic reconstruction of the MCL[1] and anatomic repair of any additional ligamentous injuries. This chapter describes the technique in detail, along with the preoperative evaluation and postoperative course.

Indications

- Isolated medial-sided insufficiency
  - Persistent symptomatic instability despite nonoperative treatment
  - Intra-articular entrapment of the MCL
  - Stener lesion of the knee: Pes anserine tendons trapped deep to the MCL
- Multiligamentous injury
  - Asymmetric medial joint space opening with valgus stress

In the authors' practice, the majority of medial-sided reconstructions are performed in the setting of multiligamentous knee injuries; however, chronic isolated valgus and/or anteromedial rotatory instability are also potential indications. In the case of isolated, medial-sided insufficiency, patients are indicated for reconstruction if they have symptomatic instability that persists despite comprehensive nonsurgical treatment, including bracing. In addition, MCL entrapment

Sgaglione NA, Lubowitz JH, Provencher MT, eds. *The Knee: AANA Advanced Arthroscopic Surgical Techniques* (pp 461-469).

within the joint as well as distal MCL disruption with pes anserine tendons trapped deep to the MCL fiber—the so-called Stener lesion of the knee—are indications for operative management. In the multiligamentous injury setting, medial-sided reconstruction is indicated in patients with asymmetric medial joint space opening with valgus stress. If the knee demonstrates greater than 10 degrees of valgus opening in full extension, not only are the MCL and PMC injured, but both cruciate ligaments are likely disrupted. The decision to reconstruct the medial side may be made from preoperative stress radiographs; however, equivocal results present a unique circumstance. In this context, final determination of the need for medial-sided reconstruction is made after the cruciate ligaments have been reconstructed because the anterior cruciate ligament (ACL) and posterior cruciate ligament serve as secondary valgus stabilizers.

Controversial Indications

- Acute midsubstance MCL injury
- Asymmetric valgus laxity less than 3 mm

Many cases do not provide an absolute indication for medial-sided reconstruction. Acute medial-sided injuries in the multiligamentous setting can be treated with bracing, surgical repair, or reconstruction. The indication for reconstruction in this setting is based on the perceived irreparability of the medial-sided injury and/or its inability to heal with bracing. An acute, midsubstance, irreparable tear of the superficial MCL and POL has been suggested as an indication for medial-sided reconstruction,[2] although the authors' practice treats these injuries in a brace, saving reconstruction for patients for whom bracing fails.

In addition, the amount of asymmetric valgus laxity above which medial-sided reconstruction should be performed has not been well-delineated. In the setting of a multiligamentous reconstruction, valgus stability is checked after reconstruction of the cruciates by obtaining stress x-rays. A decision must be made about whether to proceed with medial-sided reconstruction based on the result of these stress views. Sectioning studies have shown that an isolated MCL injury will result in 3.1 mm of asymmetric laxity at 20 degrees of knee flexion, whereas a combined MCL-POL injury will result in 9.8 mm of asymmetric laxity.[3] As a result, the authors typically use asymmetric laxity greater than 3 mm as a cutoff to proceed with medial-sided reconstruction,[2] especially in the setting of valgus malalignment because valgus loads are associated with ACL injury and ACL graft failure.[4] Having said that, it is important to recognize that this treatment algorithm has not been validated clinically.

Pertinent Physical Findings

- MCL injury shows asymmetric joint space opening at 30 degrees of flexion.
- Asymmetric opening at 0 and 30 degrees suggests POL and MCL injury.
- Anteromedial rotatory instability indicates PMC involvement.

Physical examination may reveal swelling, tenderness, and/or ecchymosis over the MCL femoral or tibial insertions. Valgus stress applied at 0 and 30 degrees of knee flexion assesses the competency of the medial-sided structures. Examination of the contralateral knee is imperative for side-to-side comparison. Asymmetric medial joint space widening at 30 degrees of flexion is indicative of an MCL injury, which can be graded according to the amount of widening (3 to 5 mm = 1+; 6 to 10 mm = 2+; > 10 mm = 3+).[5] Increased joint space widening at 0 and 30 degrees is indicative of injury to the MCL and POL.[5]

It is also important to assess for anteromedial rotatory instability on physical examination because this will help distinguish an isolated MCL injury from a PMC injury. This can be accomplished with the anteromedial drawer test,[6] which is performed with the knee in 90 degrees of

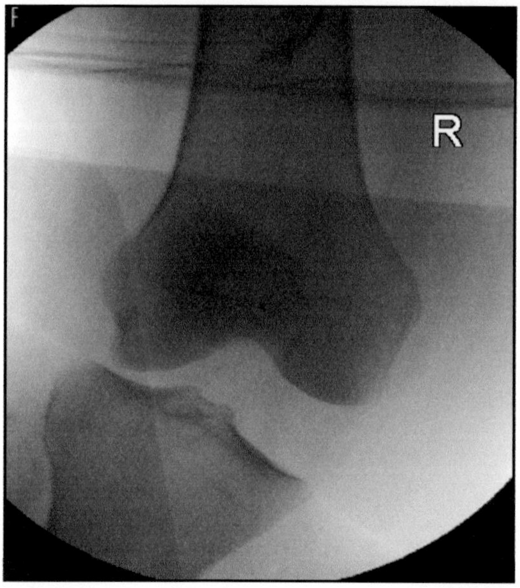

Figure 33-1. Fluoroscopic image of right knee under valgus stress showing substantial widening of the medial joint space, which is consistent with a combined MCL and PMC injury.

flexion with the foot fixed and externally rotated 10 to 15 degrees. In this position, an anteromedial rotatory force is applied to the proximal tibia, and any anterior subluxation of the medial tibial plateau relative to the medial femoral condyle is consistent with a PMC injury. It is important to discern how the tibia plateaus are moving relative to the femoral condyles during this test because increased tibial external rotation can be caused by increased anteromedial translation of the medial tibial plateau (anteromedial rotatory instability) or increased posterolateral translation of the lateral tibial plateau (posterolateral rotatory instability).

Pertinent Imaging

- Magnetic resonance imaging (MRI) is the modality of choice for evaluating medial-sided injuries.
- Valgus stress x-rays at 30 degrees help assess the extent of the injury.

Plain x-rays are often unremarkable in patients with medial-sided knee injuries. Full-length standing x-rays should be obtained when feasible to assess coronal plane alignment because patients with significant genu valgum may benefit from a varus-producing osteotomy. MRI is the modality of choice for imaging the medial-sided knee structures,[7,8] although MRI evaluation in the chronic setting can be difficult. For this reason, imaging results must be corroborated with clinical findings to arrive at an accurate diagnosis.

The authors routinely use valgus stress x-rays at 30 degrees of flexion, especially in the multiligamentous injury setting, to evaluate the competency of the MCL prior to surgery. Both knees must be imaged to provide a side-to-side comparison. LaPrade et al reported that an isolated superficial MCL injury will result in a side-to-side difference in joint space widening of 3.1 mm, whereas a complete medial-sided injury (superficial and deep MCL and POL) will result in 9.8 mm of asymmetric widening (Figure 33-1).[3]

Equipment

- Achilles tendon allograft with calcaneal bone block
- Fluoroscopy entering from the ipsilateral side of the table
- 9-mm reamer and guide pins
- Interference screw, metal or biocomposite, 7 by 20 mm
- Large straight hemostat
- Several threaded suture anchors, single or double loaded
- 4.5-mm cortical screws with 3.2-mm drill bit
- 18-mm spiked washer
- #2 nonabsorbable sutures
- 0 braided absorbable sutures
- Mersilene tape (Ethicon)

Positioning and Portals

For isolated medial-sided reconstruction, the patient is positioned supine on a radiolucent table with a foam ramp under the operative extremity. For a patient undergoing multiligamentous reconstruction, the patient is positioned supine with the foot of the table dropped to facilitate cruciate ligament reconstruction. Once the cruciate portion of the procedure is completed, the foot of the table is raised for the medial-sided reconstruction.

Step-by-Step Description of the Procedure

The authors' technique for medial-sided reconstruction includes allograft reconstruction of the MCL[1] using 3 anatomic insertion points: femoral, proximal tibial (12 mm from the joint line), and distal tibial (60 mm from the joint line) points.[9] This is combined with repair or imbrication of any other injured structures, including the POL/PMC, semimembranosus, medial head of the gastrocnemius, and meniscotibial ligaments. An Achilles tendon allograft with a 9-by-20-mm calcaneal bone plug is used for the MCL reconstruction.

Exposure to the medial side of the knee is dependent upon the pathology needing treatment and the presence of other concomitant procedures. Isolated MCL reconstruction can be accomplished through 2 small incisions over the femoral and tibial MCL insertions, tunneling the graft between the two, deep to the sartorial expansion (Figure 33-2).[1] Cases with concomitant medial-sided pathology may require a full open approach to the medial knee with full-thickness skin flaps so that all pathology can be identified and treated (Figure 33-3). This incision can be combined with those needed to treat other concomitant knee pathology, such as cruciate ligament insufficiency, chondral/meniscal injuries, and malalignment.

Distal exposure is obtained first. Dissection is carried down to the sartorial expansion, which is incised in line with and at the proximal border of the pes tendons. The expansion and the tendons are reflected distally to expose the underlying distal MCL tibial insertion, which is approximately 6 cm distal to the joint line.[9] This insertion is marked for later identification.

Proximal exposure is obtained next. Dissection is carried down to the crural fascia, at which point the femoral insertion of the superficial MCL is identified using fluoroscopic guidance (Figure 33-4).[10,11] This insertion is, on average, 3.2 mm proximal and 4.8 mm posterior to the

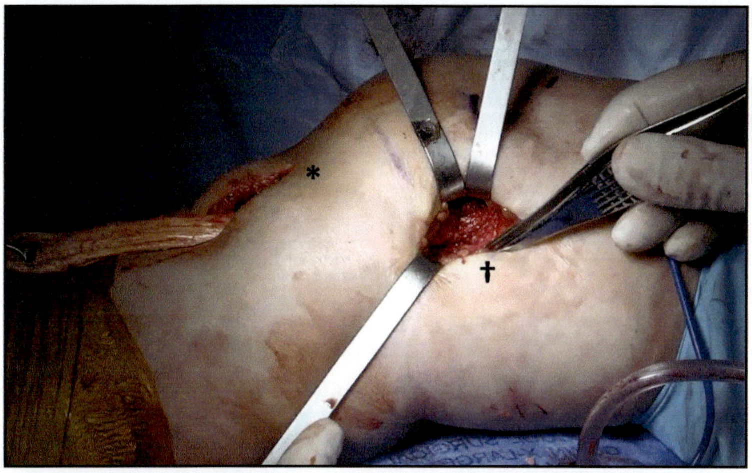

Figure 33-2. Intraoperative image of medial side of the right knee (anterior = up; distal = left) showing MCL reconstruction using a 2-incision technique, with the graft tunneled between the femoral (†) and tibial (*) incisions deep to the sartorial expansion.

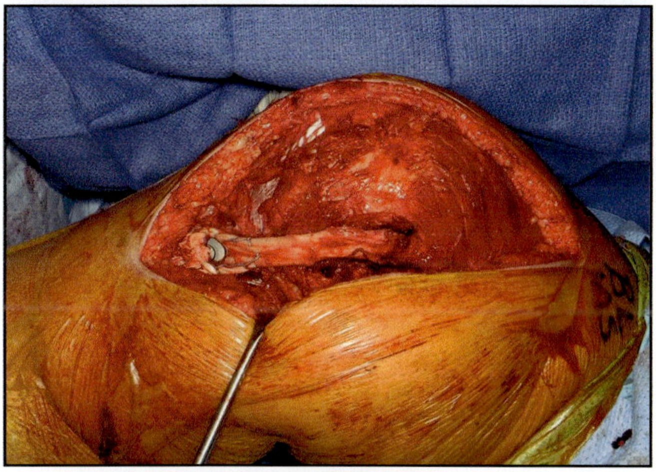

Figure 33-3. Intraoperative image of the medial side of the right knee (anterior = up; distal = left) showing MCL reconstruction using a 1-incision technique that can be used to treat concomitant knee pathology.

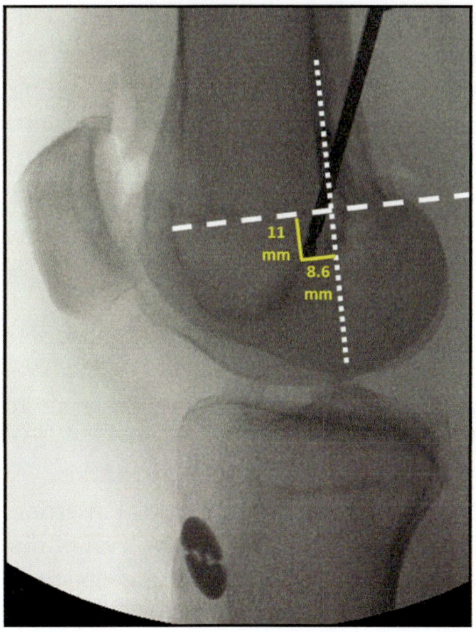

Figure 33-4. Fluoroscopic image of a right knee with a drill bit at the anatomic MCL femoral insertion, which is 8.6 mm anterior to the posterior femoral cortex extended (dotted line) and 11.0 mm distal to a line that is perpendicular to the posterior femoral cortex and intersected the most proximal extent of Blumensaat's line (dashed line).[10]

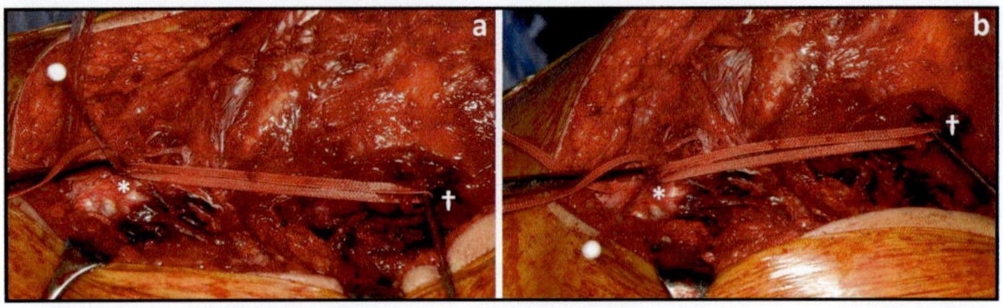

Figure 33-5. Intraoperative images of the medial side of a right knee (anterior = up; distal = left). During MCL reconstruction, isometry between the femoral (†) and distal tibial (*) attachments is confirmed in (A) extension and (B) flexion using Mersilene tape.

medial epicondyle,[9] which can be palpated and used as a reference point. It has been shown that the fluoroscopic and anatomic methods of determining the MCL femoral insertion have similar accuracy.[11] Identification of the femoral MCL insertion will help guide further dissection, which includes identification of the adductor magnus tendon, adductor tubercle, medial head of the gastrocnemius, semimembranosus insertion, POL, and PMC. Occasionally, higher-energy injury mechanisms can cause disruption of the meniscotibial ligaments with resultant meniscal extrusion on preoperative MRI. In these cases, these ligaments should be exposed as well to facilitate repair.

Disrupted or attenuated tissues are then repaired or imbricated, with the exception of the posteromedial capsule, which is imbricated after MCL reconstruction is complete. Single- or double-loaded threaded suture anchors are used for repair/imbrication. Meniscotibial ligament anchors are placed in the proximal tibia, just distal to the articular margin, and sutures are placed in a mattress configuration to repair the ligament and reduce the meniscus. Medial head of the gastrocnemius anchors are placed on the posteromedial distal femur, and semimembranosus anchors are placed on the posteromedial aspect of the tibial plateau.

Once any injured posteromedial knee structures have been repaired or imbricated, attention is turned to MCL reconstruction. A longitudinal split is made in the crural fascia at the posterior border of the native MCL. This is taken down to the bone, dividing the crural fascia and joint capsule. The posterior flap created by this split contains the PMC and the POL. This tissue is commonly attenuated or redundant due to valgus instability and will later be imbricated and repaired.

Next, 2.4-mm guide pins are inserted at the femoral and distal tibial MCL insertions. Isometry between the 2 points is examined by looping Mersilene tape between the 2 guide pins and cycling the knee in flexion and extension (Figure 33-5). The femoral insertion can be adjusted to achieve optimal isometry.

Next, a 9-by-25-mm socket is reamed over the femoral guide pin, and a bicortical 3.2-mm drill hole is made at the site of the distal tibial insertion. Then, 2 suture anchors are placed on the proximal medial tibia 12 mm distal to the joint line along the proposed course of the reconstructed MCL. These sutures are set aside to later restore the proximal MCL tibial attachment.

At this point, femoral fixation is obtained by inserting the calcaneal bone plug into the femoral socket and fixing with a 7-by-20-mm interference screw. Two suture anchors are placed on the posterior margin of the medial femoral condyle, just distal and anterior to the gastrocnemius tubercle at the femoral insertion of the POL/PMC.[9] Mattress sutures are passed into the attenuated capsular tissue in preparation for capsular imbrication, which will be performed after final graft fixation.

The graft is then tunneled distally beneath the sartorial expansion to the distal tibial insertion using a large straight hemostat. A 2-cm longitudinal split is made in the graft at the level of the distal MCL tibial insertion, and a #2 nonabsorbable suture is used to place a locking whip stitch up and down the graft, 2 to 3 cm proximal to this point. The graft is tensioned by pulling on the whip stitches with the knee held in varus at 20 degrees of flexion and is fixed at the distal tibial attachment site with a bicortical 4.5-mm screw and 18-mm spiked ligament washer (Figure 33-6).

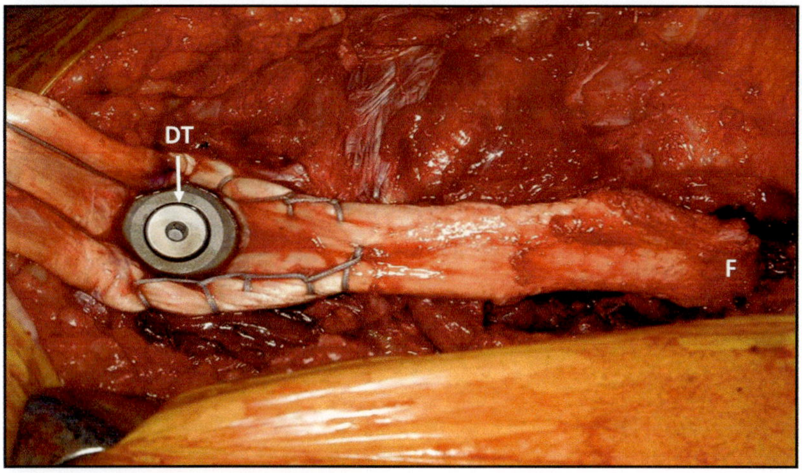

Figure 33-6. Intraoperative image of the medial side of a right knee after femoral (F) and distal tibial (DT) fixation of the MCL graft. Proximal tibial suture anchor fixation has not yet been performed.

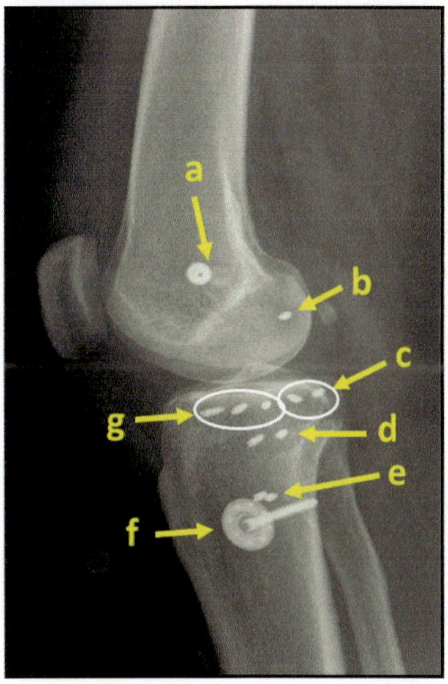

Figure 33-7. Lateral x-ray of a right knee. This case involved reconstruction of the MCL; imbrication of the PMC; and repair of semimembranosus, meniscotibial ligament, and distal MCL avulsions. (A) Bone block and interference screw for femoral insertion of MCL reconstruction. (B) PMC imbrication suture anchor. (C) Semimembranosus repair suture anchors. (D) Suture anchors for proximal tibial insertion of MCL reconstruction. (E) Distal MCL avulsion suture anchors. (F) Screw and washer for distal tibial insertion of MCL reconstruction. (G) Meniscotibial ligament suture anchors.

Fluoroscopy is used to confirm that the screw is bicortical. Excess graft is then trimmed, and the whip stitch suture ends are tied around the screw to achieve double fixation at the distal attachment. The sutures from the proximal tibial suture anchors are then passed through the graft in a mattress configuration and tied to recreate the proximal MCL tibial attachment. The previously placed posteromedial capsule sutures are tied to obtain capsular imbrication, and the longitudinal capsular split is closed with braided 0 absorbable suture. Fluoroscopy is used to confirm appropriate anchor and screw placement (Figure 33-7).

Postoperative Protocol

Postoperative restrictions may vary depending on concomitant injuries and procedures performed. Typically, the patient is placed into a hinged knee brace with a slight varus mold, which will be worn for 6 weeks after surgery until a custom, varus-molded knee orthosis is prescribed. The brace is recommended for the first year after surgery. Toe-touch weightbearing with the brace locked in extension is prescribed for the first 6 weeks. Range of motion and quadriceps activation exercises

Table 33-1. Potential Complications After Medial Collateral Ligament/Posteromedial Corner Reconstruction

- Injury to distal femoral physis: This technique contraindicated in the skeletally immature
- Injury to saphenous nerve and branches
- Persistent valgus or anteromedial rotatory instability
  - Graft failure
  - Fixation failure
  - Graft anisometry
  - Unidentified concomitant injury
- Range of motion loss
  - Arthrofibrosis
  - Graft anisometry

are begun 1 week postoperatively. At 6 weeks, weightbearing and strengthening programs are initiated, with the goal of full motion and normal gait by 12 weeks. Return to sports and other activities is individualized but is allowed no sooner than 1 year postoperatively after multiligamentous reconstruction. Chemical venous thromboembolism prophylaxis is indicated in all multiligamentous reconstruction patients and in isolated MCL reconstruction patients with risk factors.

Potential Complications

Recent reports suggest satisfactory results and a low complication rate after MCL/PMC reconstruction.[1,2,12] In addition to general postoperative complications after lower-extremity surgery (eg, superficial and deep infection, deep venous thrombosis, etc), there are several specific potential complications related to MCL/PMC reconstruction (Table 33-1).

Top Technical Pearls for the Procedure

1. Identify the femoral isometric point on lateral fluoroscopic view prior to proximal exposure.[10]
2. Localize the distal tibial insertion point (60 mm distal to the joint line) by identifying MCL fibers inserting on the proximal medial tibia.[9]
3. Ensure isometry between the proposed femoral and distal tibial insertion points prior to drilling tunnels.
4. Recreate proximal tibial MCL insertion (12 mm distal to joint line) with suture anchors.[9]
5. Repair/imbricate all concomitantly injured structures, including the POL, PMC, semimembranosus tendon, medial head of the gastrocnemius tendon, and meniscotibial ligament.

References

1. Marx RG, Hetsroni I. Surgical technique: medial collateral ligament reconstruction using Achilles allograft for combined knee ligament injury. *Clin Orthop Relat Res.* 2012;470(3):798-805.
2. Laprade RF, Wijdicks CA. Surgical technique: development of an anatomic medial knee reconstruction. *Clin Orthop Relat Res.* 2012;470(3):806-814.
3. Laprade RF, Bernhardson AS, Griffith CJ, Macalena JA, Wijdicks CA. Correlation of valgus stress radiographs with medial knee ligament injuries: an in vitro biomechanical study. *Am J Sports Med.* 2010;38(2):330-338.
4. Hetsroni I, Lyman S, Pearle AD, Marx RG. The effect of lateral opening wedge distal femoral osteotomy on medial knee opening: clinical and biomechanical factors. *Knee Surg Sports Traumatol Arthrosc.* 2014;22(7):1659-1665.
5. Wijdicks CA, Griffith CJ, Johansen S, Engebretsen L, LaPrade RF. Injuries to the medial collateral ligament and associated medial structures of the knee. *J Bone Joint Surg Am.* 2010;92(5):1266-1280.
6. Sims WF, Jacobson KE. The posteromedial corner of the knee: medial-sided injury patterns revisited. *Am J Sports Med.* 2004;32(2):337-345.
7. Stannard JP. Medial and posteromedial instability of the knee: evaluation, treatment, and results. *Sports Med Arthrosc.* 2010;18(4):263-268.
8. Tibor LM, Marchant MH Jr, Taylor DC, Hardaker WT Jr, Garrett WE Jr, Sekiya JK. Management of medial-sided knee injuries, part 2: posteromedial corner. *Am J Sports Med.* 2011;39(6):1332-1340.
9. LaPrade RF, Engebretsen AH, Ly TV, Johansen S, Wentorf FA, Engebretsen L. The anatomy of the medial part of the knee. *J Bone Joint Surg Am.* 2007;89(9):2000-2010.
10. Wijdicks CA, Griffith CJ, LaPrade RF, et al. Radiographic identification of the primary medial knee structures. *J Bone Joint Surg Am.* 2009;91(3):521-529.
11. Leiter JR, Levy BA, Stannard JP, et al. Accuracy and reliability of determining the isometric point of the knee for multiligament knee reconstruction. *Knee Surg Sports Traumatol Arthrosc.* 2014;22(9):2187-2193.
12. Kovachevich R, Shah JP, Arens AM, Stuart MJ, Dahm DL, Levy BA. Operative management of the medial collateral ligament in the multi-ligament injured knee: an evidence-based systematic review. *Knee Surg Sports Traumatol Arthrosc.* 2009;17(7):823-829.

Please see videos on the accompanying website at www.routledge.com/9781617119996

34

Treatment of Multiligament Knee Injuries

James P. Stannard, MD and Clayton W. Nuelle, MD

Introduction

The multiligament-injured knee is a complicated orthopedic injury that is typically the result of a high-energy force and often results in a knee dislocation. The mechanism may be from an athletic injury or from high-energy blunt trauma, such as a motor vehicle collision. The knee may dislocate or sublux at the time of injury as a result of the impact but frequently reduces prior to presentation to the treating physician. Even if the knee spontaneously reduces, the damage to the ligaments and other structures in and around the knee can be significant.[1,2]

Indications

- Any patient with a multiligament- (2 or more of the 4 major ligament complexes) injured knee who requires knee stability for ambulation or activities of daily living and who may tolerate potentially prolonged surgery
- Patients with 3 or more ligament complexes injured may require staged procedures or placement of a Compass Knee Hinge (Smith & Nephew).

Controversial Indications

- Patients with partial ligament complex injuries in conjunction with 1 or 2 complete ligament ruptures

Sgaglione NA, Lubowitz JH, Provencher MT, eds. *The Knee: AANA Advanced Arthroscopic Surgical Techniques* (pp 471-481).

Pertinent Physical Findings

The initial management of a patient with a multiligament-injured knee requires a thorough evaluation of associated injuries and comorbidities. In particular, a complete neurovascular examination should always be completed upon initial presentation. Vascular injury can lead to severe limb dysfunction, and tibial and/or peroneal nerve injury can be seen in up to 25% of dislocated knees.[3] The initial examination includes a bilateral pulse examination, with ankle-brachial indices obtained if pulses are asymmetric or there is asymmetric limb color or warmth. An ankle-brachial index less than 0.9 warrants further investigation, including arterial ultrasound or computed tomography angiography. Any subsequent necessary vascular repair or intervention should preclude any orthopedic procedure.[4] After other associated injuries have been identified and stabilized, indications for surgical management of multiligament injuries include any patient who requires knee stability for ambulation or activities of daily living. Contraindications include any patient medically unable to tolerate prolonged or multiple procedures or any patient with an active infection.

When formulating a treatment plan for a patient with a knee dislocation, it is necessary to consider multiple patient factors. Neurovascular status should always be assessed, as well as the degree of injury to the surrounding skin, other significant intra- and extra-articular injuries about the knee, and the overall spectrum of ligament injury. Patients with an abnormal vascular examination or severe soft tissue injury should be delayed from ligament repair or reconstruction until these injuries have stabilized. Associated fractures, such as tibial plateau or femoral condyle fractures, should also be stabilized prior to any soft tissue procedures.

Physical examination findings can be critical to the initial diagnosis of multiligament knee injuries, and include the following:

- Positive Lachman test to identify an anterior cruciate ligament (ACL) injury
- Positive posterior drawer sign and posterior tibial sag for a posterior cruciate ligament (PCL) injury[5,6]
- Varus and valgus stressing at 20 to 30 degrees should be performed to assess the lateral and medial collateral ligaments, respectively.
- Dial test for the posterolateral corner (PLC). This is performed with the patient prone and the knees flexed to 30 and 90 degrees. A side-to-side difference of 10 to 15 degrees with the knees at 30 degrees represents an isolated PLC tear, whereas a difference at 90 degrees represents a combined PLC and PCL injury.[7]
- For the posteromedial corner (PMC), anterior medial rotatory instability can be differentiated with an anterior drawer test with the foot in neutral rotation and an anterior drawer test with the foot in external rotation. An increase in the amount of anteromedial tibial rotation in external rotation represents a PMC injury.[8]

Pertinent Imaging

- Quality magnetic resonance imaging (MRI) of the knee to assess the extent of ligament injury and to identify other associated injuries, such as meniscal tears or chondral defects
- Stress x-rays (varus, valgus, and posterior), with comparison to the contralateral knee, can frequently be helpful to identify the degree of instability present in the medial and lateral corners and the PCL.
- Intraoperative fluoroscopic stress examinations can help confirm clinical and/or MRI findings.

After adequate imaging has been completed, a plan may be formulated regarding surgical timing, ligament repair vs reconstruction, the order of ligament reconstruction, and an assessment of any further surgeries potentially required.[9] Appropriate surgical timing and planning are necessary to prevent the poor outcomes that can result from multiligament injuries. Hospital readmission within 90 days and unplanned repeat surgeries can be as high as 4.8% and 28%, respectively.[10] Recurrent instability, arthrofibrosis, and persistent pain are the most frequent complications.[11-13]

Multiple techniques exist when planning operative treatment of knee dislocations, with studies demonstrating advantages and disadvantages to repair vs reconstruction and acute vs delayed management of these injuries. Repair vs reconstruction may be dictated by surgeon preference or by the degree of injury, but for highly unstable injuries with 3 or 4 ligaments involved, studies have shown benefit to reconstruction rather than repair, in particular reconstruction of the PMC and the PLC.[9,14-18] There are also times when the native ligaments and soft tissue are extremely hemorrhagic and difficult to define and, thus, cannot be repaired. When the native ligaments are identifiable or present, however, the authors prefer to repair the native tissue. Then they perform the planned reconstructions in addition to the repairs to give the best stability possible using a belt and suspenders approach.

When performing reconstructions, autograft or allograft may be used. Allograft is most frequently chosen in the multiligament knee to protect as much of the uninjured native anatomy surrounding the knee joint as possible. Many allograft options exist, including anterior and posterior tibialis tendons, hamstring tendon, quadriceps tendon, Achilles tendon, and patellar tendon. The specific grafts used may be dictated by the availability of the grafts, the number of ligaments being reconstructed, and the planned reconstruction techniques. Some techniques require different size grafts than others. For example, a 2-tailed PLC reconstruction requires a graft that will have plenty of length to complete the entire reconstruction. In contrast, a tibial inlay technique for a PCL reconstruction requires an appropriately sized bone block on one end of the tendon.

Timing and staging of operative intervention is the topic of some debate and may be influenced by other injuries or comorbidities, but, when possible, many authors prefer early (< 4 weeks) operative treatment to achieve good ligamentous stability and promote mobilization.[9,16,19] Early stabilization may result in decreased risk of arthrofibrosis, improved range of motion (ROM), and earlier rehabilitation. Ensuring the patient's swelling and skin will tolerate multiple incisions is important to define prior to any operation, because a poor tissue bed could lead to postoperative wound breakdown or infection.

For patients with a multiligament injury, the authors prefer an initial repair and/or reconstruction within 2 to 4 weeks of initial injury. Surgeons may choose to repair or reconstruct every ligament in one procedure or may delay one or more of the reconstructions in a staged fashion. In a 3- or 4-ligament injured knee, the authors recommend considering staging 2 separate procedures for the following reasons:

- Performing all reconstructions in a single procedure involves an extensive operation with a prolonged anesthesia time and a potential increased risk for infection.
- Some degree of stiffness may result after reconstructing multiple ligaments, and a planned return to the operating room allows for a manipulation under anesthesia and/or lysis of any adhesions that have developed, which aids the patient in his or her postoperative rehabilitation.
- By staging the procedures, different rehabilitation techniques can be used at different time points to maximize the patient's final ROM and return to function.

The preferred technique of the senior author is an early reconstruction of the PMC, PLC, and PCL, with a delayed reconstruction of the ACL 6 weeks after the index procedure. In addition, in the setting of the highly unstable knee, consideration is given to placing a Compass Knee Hinge. The Compass Knee Hinge consists of 2 carbon fiber rings bolted to multi-hole Rancho Cubes (Smith & Nephew) that are connected to the Schanz pins placed in the femur and tibia. The rings are connected by 2 calibrated hinges that align along either side of the knee joint. The rings are available in numerous sizes based on the size of the patient. The Compass Knee Hinge allows ROM in the sagittal plane while restricting motion in the coronal and axial planes. This allows early weightbearing and knee ROM while protecting the newly reconstructed ligaments. Studies have shown multiple benefits to using the Compass Knee Hinge after multiligament reconstructions, particularly in decreasing the potential for reconstruction failures vs knee bracing alone.[20-23] The Compass Knee Hinge is particularly helpful for 4-ligament knee injuries, multiligament injuries with associated fractures or fracture dislocations, preoperative flexion deformities greater than 15 degrees, or for chronic knee dislocations. When any of these situations are encountered or when planning multiple simultaneous reconstructions or staged procedures, the authors recommend considering the Compass Knee Hinge during the preoperative planning process.

Numerous techniques for the timing and specific types of reconstructions for multiligament knee injuries are available to surgeons. Regardless of the techniques used, with proper planning and preparation, a successful outcome can frequently be achieved in 1 or 2 operations.

Equipment

The equipment necessary depends on the number of ligaments being reconstructed and the techniques used by the surgeon. In general, standard arthroscopy equipment with a 30-degree arthroscope is sufficient for visualization during the arthroscopic portions of the procedure.

For allograft reconstruction, adequately sized grafts and a graft prep station with a tensioning device are necessary. For a PCL using a tibial inlay technique, the authors prefer an Achilles tendon with a bone block at a minimum length of 15 mm, width of 10 mm, and thickness of 10 mm. The thickness is crucial to avoid cracking the bone block when the screw is tightened. For a PLC reconstruction using a modified 2-tailed technique, the authors prefer an anterior or posterior tibialis tendon at least 27 cm in length. For a PMC reconstruction using a modified loop technique, the authors prefer a semitendinosus tendon. Finally, for an ACL reconstruction using a soft tissue, all-inside technique, the authors prefer a semitendinosus, anterior tibialis, or posterior tibialis graft with the goal of obtaining a final graft diameter 8.5 mm or greater.[24]

For the techniques used by the senior surgeon, cannulated drills, reamers, and taps in multiple sizes are necessary to create bone tunnels or sockets. Guide wires are necessary for screw placement. A nitinol wire is used for tap and screw placement, and a suture passer is necessary for suture and graft passage. A #2 nonabsorbable suture is used for the ends of the grafts. Cortical screws with washers, bioabsorbable screws, or suspensory button fixation may all be used for graft fixation depending on surgeon preference. For the PCL inlay technique, a 4.5-mm cannulated screw and washer is used to fix the bone block in the tibia, and absorbable interference screws are used to fix the soft tissue fixation in the femur (Figure 34-1). For the PMC, an absorbable biotenodesis screw is used to fix the graft in the femur, and a 4.5-mm screw and washer are used to fix the graft in the tibia. For the PLC, a 7-mm bioabsorbable screw secures the soft tissue graft in the tibia while a fully threaded 4.5- or 6.5-mm screw and washer secure the graft in the femur.

In addition to the mentioned screw fixation techniques, consideration may be given to reconstructions using suspensory fixation. This technique incorporates bone sockets instead of full bone tunnels, meaning more preserved bone stock and less chance of crossing or crowding bone tunnels during simultaneous reconstructions. It also eliminates the risk of screw cutout or screws or washers cutting soft tissue grafts. The senior author prefers suspensory fixation for the ACL reconstruction in the setting of multiligament knee reconstruction and has also begun incorporating the technique in PMC and PLC reconstructions.

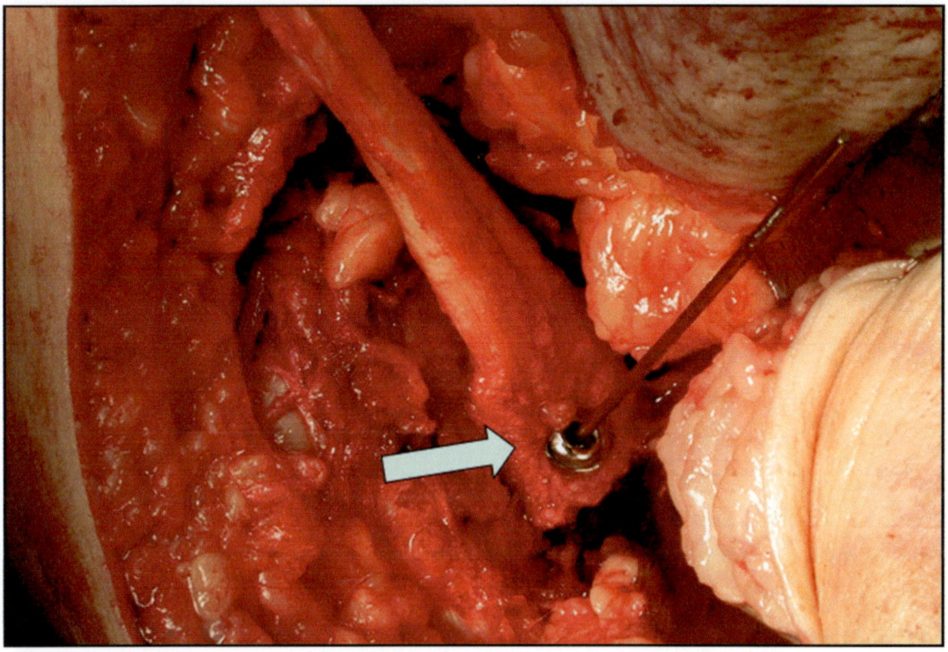

Figure 34-1. Intraoperative photograph from a posteromedial view of the posterior aspect of a right knee depicting screw fixation of a tibial inlay PCL bone block (arrow) with the thigh to the top and the lower leg to the bottom of the photograph.

Positioning and Portals

Patient positioning and portal placement is dictated by the number and specific ligaments being reconstructed. In the multiligament setting of 3 or 4 ligaments when the PCL is involved and either or both of the corners are to be reconstructed, it may be necessary to gain access to both sides of the knee via open approaches. Manipulation of the leg and knee into flexion or a figure-4 position may also be required at various points in the procedure. For these reasons, the authors do not recommend using any type of leg holder. They use a single post at the mid-thigh level for resistance during arthroscopy to gain access to the medial compartment but no other posts or metal clamps on or below the bed because these could interfere with any necessary fluoroscopy. The patient should be placed supine on a radiolucent bed. The authors initially use standard anterolateral and anteromedial arthroscopy portals. An outflow portal at the superomedial or superolateral border of the patella and accessory posteromedial or posterolateral portals may be incorporated as needed based on the planned reconstructions. When performing an open approach for a PCL or PMC reconstruction, the knee should be placed in the figure-4 position at approximately 70 degrees to help with retraction and prevent injury to the posterior neurovascular structures. Similarly, for a PLC reconstruction, the knee should be flexed to relax and protect the peroneal nerve.

Step-by-Step Description of the Procedure

For a multiligament knee reconstruction, the senior author prefers a modified loop technique for the PMC; a modified 2-tailed technique for the PLC; a double-bundle tibial inlay technique for the PCL; and a single-bundle, quadrupled tendon, suspensory fixation technique for the ACL.[25-28] The step-by-step details of each procedure have been described elsewhere and are not

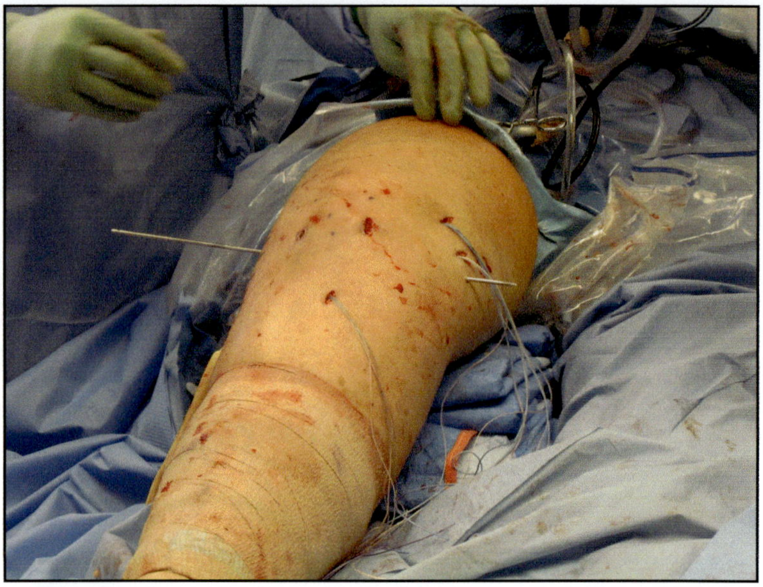

Figure 34-2. Intraoperative photograph demonstrating proper placement of a threaded centering wire from lateral to medial across a right knee for placement of a Compass Knee Hinge.

described here. Regardless of the techniques used, it is vital for the surgeon to attempt to achieve anatomic restoration of the ligament complexes being reconstructed. For the PMC, restoration of the superficial medial collateral ligament, posterior oblique ligament, and direct head of the semimembranosus attachment are necessary to restore function. For the PLC, the vital components are the lateral collateral ligament, popliteus, and popliteofibular ligament. When reconstructing multiple ligaments simultaneously, it is important to plan each step preoperatively to proceed as efficiently as possible intraoperatively. The authors recommend performing diagnostic arthroscopy first to identify and address any intra-articular pathology, such as chondral defects or meniscal tears, and then proceed with the open reconstructions. Femoral tunnels for the double-bundle PCL are created arthroscopically. The authors typically perform the posteromedial approach first and reconstruct the PCL, followed by the PMC reconstruction, then the posterolateral approach, and finally the PLC reconstruction. All of the reconstructions should be tensioned at the end of the overall procedure so the exact order can be adjusted based on the number of ligaments being reconstructed or by surgeon preference. A precise preoperative plan ensures optimal efficiency.

Application of the Compass Knee Hinge is relatively straightforward, but there are some critical steps required to ensure the Compass Knee Hinge functions appropriately. First, in the setting of a multiligament knee reconstruction including the PMC and/or the PLC that will also be combined with Compass Knee Hinge placement, it is necessary to place a centering wire for positioning of the Compass Knee Hinge and the femoral Schanz pins first prior to PMC or PLC reconstruction. The centering wire for the Compass Knee Hinge is placed through the isometric point in the femur where the reconstructions of the corners would also be placed (Figure 34-2). Positioning the wire frequently takes a number of passes to obtain the perfect position, so placing the wire after performing the PLC or PMC reconstructions is impossible and would damage the reconstructions. For this reason, application of the hinge must be completed in 2 phases.

The first step in the application requires finding the isometric point on the femur using fluoroscopy. To accomplish this, a perfect lateral view of the knee is obtained, with the isometric point at the intersection of a line drawn along the anterior aspect of the posterior femoral cortex with Blumensaat's line.[29] A long, threaded 2.5-mm wire is then drilled through the cortex at this point, with the wire appearing as a single dot on the lateral fluoroscopic view (Figure 34-3). Fluoroscopy should be used throughout to ensure exact placement of the wire. When the wire is well seated and in line, it is then drilled across the femur, parallel to the joint line. This

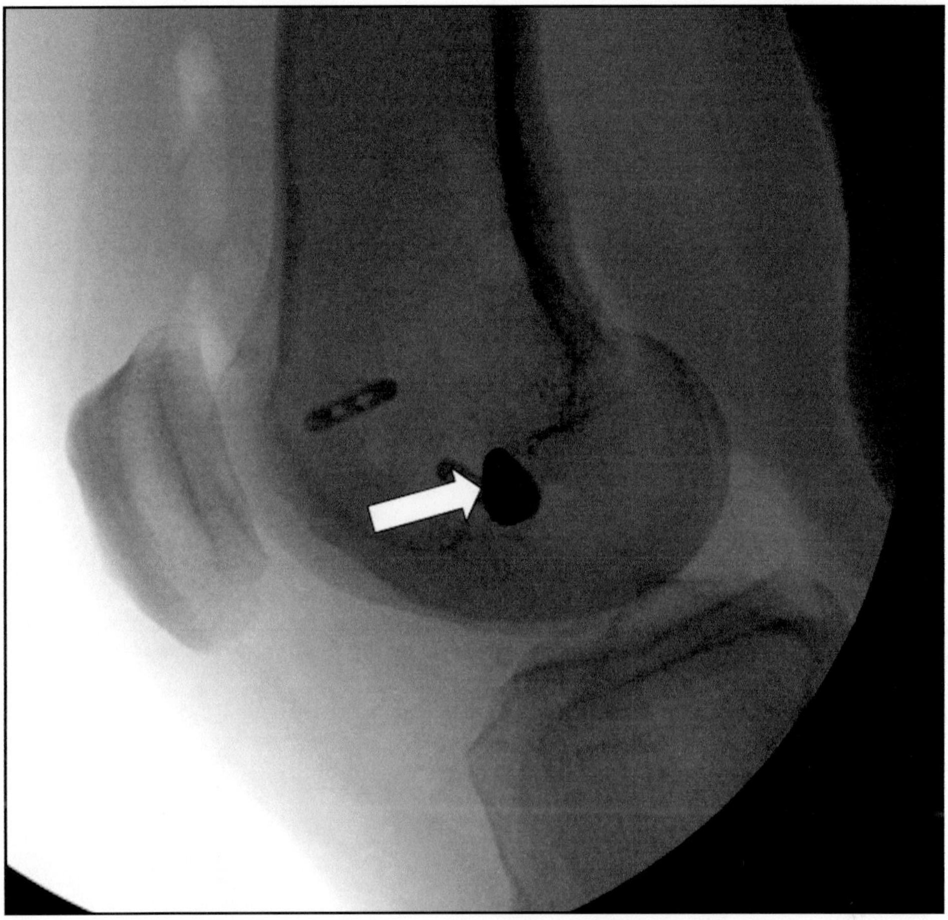

Figure 34-3. Lateral intraoperative fluoroscopic x-ray depicting centering wire placement across the femur for placement of a Compass Knee Hinge. The centering wire should appear as a single dot (arrow) at the isometric point of the knee.

placement is confirmed with an anteroposterior view of the knee. If it is not parallel to the joint line, it should be removed and revised. Precise placement of this centering wire is a critical step to appropriate placement and subsequent final functioning of the Compass Knee Hinge; it is critical to take the time to get adequate fluoroscopic views to ensure proper placement. After the wire is appropriately placed, the 2 femoral pins may then be placed. Construction of the hinge begins by placing the apparatus on the centering wire with the wire placed through the holes in the middle of the medial and lateral calibrated hinges (Figure 34-4). Rancho Cubes are then placed in the most posterior hole on the medial and lateral sides of the proximal side of the femoral carbon fiber ring, with a 1-hole cube used medially and a 3-hole cube laterally to avoid crossing of the pins in the femur. Triple trocar guides are then placed through the Rancho Cubes to allow drilling for the femoral pins. An adequate skin incision is made at the entry point of the trocar, and blunt dissection is carried out down to bone. A 4-mm drill is used to drill completely across the femur medially and laterally, and a 6-mm pin is then placed through each guide. A centering sleeve that is provided in the system is then placed over the pins to lock the Rancho Cube into place. At this point, the Compass Knee Hinge may be detached from the pins. Leaving the femoral pins and Rancho Cubes in place, the centering wire is removed, and the Compass Knee Hinge is placed on a sterile table to allow completion of the corner reconstructions.

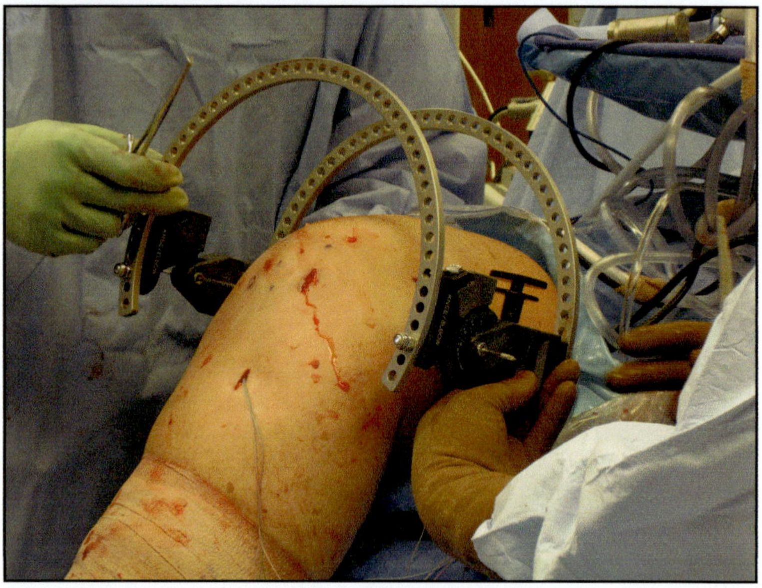

Figure 34-4. Intraoperative photograph demonstrating placement of a fully assembled Compass Knee Hinge on a centering wire previously placed across the femur in a right knee.

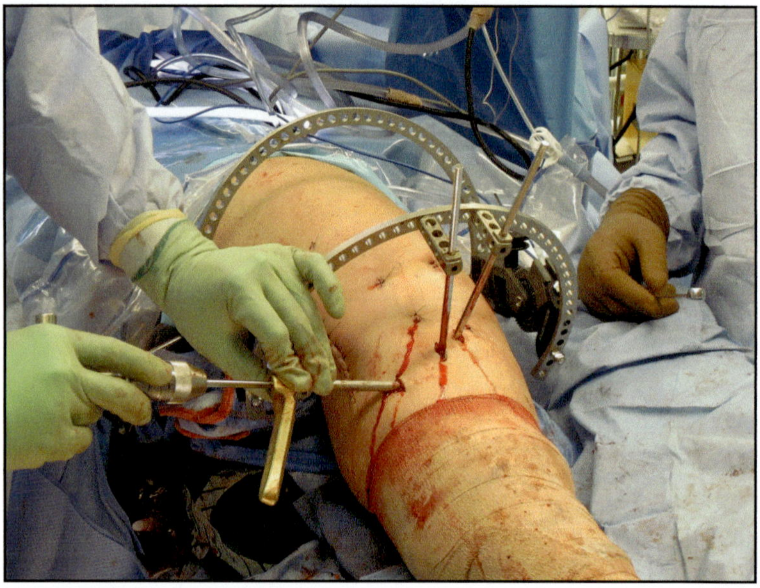

Figure 34-5. Intraoperative photograph demonstrating placement of tibial Schanz pins through guide sleeves in a right knee during placement of a Compass Knee Hinge, with the foot to the right in the image.

After the appropriate reconstructions have been completed, the Compass Knee Hinge is then remounted on the femoral pins through the same holes as before. Three-, 4-, or 5-hole Rancho Cubes are then placed on the distal aspect of the tibial ring in lateral, anterior, and anteromedial locations on the tibia, and the tibial pins are placed in a similar fashion as the femoral pins (Figure 34-5). Centering sleeves are placed over all the pins, and the femoral and tibial sleeves are all tightened to complete the application. The knee is then flexed to 90 degrees to ensure that there is no skin tension at the pin entry sites. If tension is present, the incisions may be extended to release the tension. The knee is then taken through a final ROM to ensure all pins and bolts are properly positioned and tightened and the ROM is adequate (Figure 34-6).

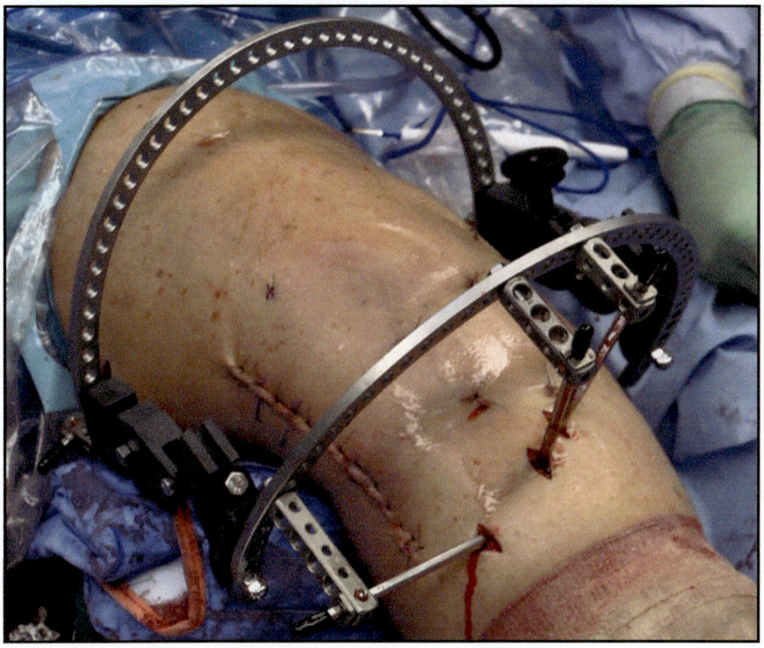

Figure 34-6. Intraoperative photograph demonstrating completion of placement of a Compass Knee Hinge around a right knee, with the thigh to the left and the foot to the right in the image.

Postoperative Protocol

The authors' postoperative protocol incorporates an early, progressive attempt to regain motion. Continuous passive motion machines set from 0 to 60 degrees are begun on postoperative day 1, and patients are allowed to bear weight immediately with a knee brace or the Compass Knee Hinge locked in extension. A combination of anesthetic epidurals, spinal or femoral blocks, and patient-controlled analgesia may be used for inpatient postoperative pain control. ROM is progressed as tolerated as quadriceps strength and function improve. When a Compass Knee Hinge is used, patients are asked to lock the hinge in full extension and in the maximum tolerable flexion for a least 1 hour every day. At 6 weeks, the Compass Knee Hinge is removed, and the ACL reconstruction is completed. After this point, the rehabilitation may then be primarily dictated by the surgeon's preferred ACL rehabilitation protocol.

Potential Complications

Appropriate preoperative physical examination, imaging, diagnosis, and planning are critical to avoid the many complications that may arise in the treatment of multiligament knee injuries. Adequate diagnosis of PMC and PLC injuries preoperatively is imperative because failure to reconstruct the corners in the setting of a multiligament knee injury can lead to persistent instability and early failure of ACL and/or PCL reconstruction. Surgical timing must be balanced with associated injuries and comorbidities because wound breakdown or infection can occur when the skin envelope and soft tissue swelling around the knee are inappropriate for surgery. Neurovascular injury to the saphenous nerve and vein, tibial nerve, and popliteal artery and vein can occur with the posteromedial approach to the knee during a PMC or a PCL reconstruction. Peroneal nerve injury can occur with the posterolateral approach to the knee during PLC reconstruction. Awareness of the pertinent anatomy and proper patient positioning are necessary to avoid these major neurovascular complications. Recurrent instability, arthrofibrosis, and persistent pain are all complications that may be encountered postoperatively but may be avoided with proper surgical planning, timing, and technique.

Top Technical Pearls for the Procedure

1. Appropriate preoperative imaging and stepwise planning is vital to success, and staged procedures (ie, PMC/PLC/PCL first, ACL 6 weeks later) may be required.
2. Consider using suspensory fixation techniques and bone sockets to minimize bone loss, graft damage, or screw loosening, and plan bone sockets/bone tunnels based on the type and number of reconstructions being performed (aim sockets/tunnels away from each other to avoid crossing).
3. For a posterolateral or PMC reconstruction, flex the knee during reconstruction to avoid injury to neurovascular structures.
4. Reconstructions of all ligaments should be anatomically based and seek to replicate the critical ligaments, and all grafts should be tensioned together at the end of the procedure, always beginning with the PCL.
5. If placing a Compass Knee Hinge, place the centering wire for reference prior to reconstructing the posteromedial or PLC.

References

1. Peskun CJ, Levy BA, Fanelli GC, et al. Diagnosis and management of knee dislocations. *Phys Sports Med.* 2010;4(38):101-111.
2. Wascher DC, Dvirnak PC, DeCoster TA. Knee dislocation: initial assessment and implications for treatment. *J Orthop Trauma.* 1997;11(7):525-529.
3. Niall DM, Nutton RW, Keating JF. Palsy of the common peroneal nerve after traumatic dislocation of the knee. *J Bone Joint Surg Br.* 2005;87(5):664-667.
4. Fanelli GC, Stannard JP, Stuart MJ, et al. Management of complex knee ligament injuries. *J Bone Joint Surg Am.* 2010;92(12):2235-2246.
5. Makhmalbaf H, Moradi A, Ganji S, Omidi-Kashani F. Accuracy of Lachman and anterior drawer tests for anterior cruciate ligament injuries. *Arch Bone Jt Surg.* 2013;1(2):94-97.
6. Feltham GT, Albright JP. The diagnosis of PCL injury: literature review and the introduction of two novel tests. *Iowa Orthop J.* 2001;21:36-42.
7. Jung YB, Lee YS, Jung HJ, Nam CH. Evaluation of posterolateral rotatory knee instability using the dial test according to tibial positioning. *Arthroscopy.* 2009;25(3):257-261.
8. LaPrade RF, Wijdicks CA. The management of injuries to the medial side of the knee. *J Orthop Sports Phys Ther.* 2010;42(3):221-233.
9. Levy BA, Dajani KA, Whelan DB, et al. Decision making in the multiligament-injured knee: an evidence based systemic review. *Arthroscopy.* 2009;25(4):430-438.
10. Wilson SM, Mehta N, Do HT, Ghomrawi H, Lyman S, Marx RG. Epidemiology of the multiligament knee reconstruction. *Clin Orthop Relat Res.* 2014;472(9):2603-2608.
11. Cole BJ, Harner CD. The multiple ligament injured knee. *Clin Sports Med.* 1999;18(1):241-262.
12. Yeh WL, Tu YK, Su JY, Hsu RW. Knee dislocation: treatment of high-velocity knee dislocation. *J Trauma.* 1999;46(4):693-701.
13. Noyes FR, Barber-Westin SD. Reconstruction of the anterior and posterior cruciate ligaments after knee dislocation. Use of early protected postoperative motion to decrease arthrofibrosis. *Am J Sports Med.* 1999;25(6):769-778.
14. Fanelli GC, Edson CJ. Arthroscopically assisted combined anterior and posterior cruciate ligament reconstruction in the multiple ligament injured knee: 2- to 10-year follow-up. *Arthroscopy.* 2002;18(7):703-714.
15. Bin SI, Nam TS. Surgical outcome of 2-stage management of multiple knee ligament injuries after knee dislocation. *Arthroscopy.* 2007;23(10):1066-1072.

16. Dwyer T, Marx RG, Whelan D. Outcomes of treatment of multiple ligament knee injuries. *J Knee Surg.* 2012;25(4):317-326.
17. Stannard JP, Brown SL, Farris RC, McGwin G Jr, Volgas DA. The posterolateral corner of the knee: repair versus reconstruction. *Am J Sports Med.* 2005;33(6):881-888.
18. Stannard JP, Black BS, Azbell C, Volgas DA. Posteromedial corner injury in knee dislocations. *J Knee Surg.* 2012;25(5):429-434.
19. Howells NR, Brunton LR, Robinson J, Porteus AJ, Eldridge JD, Murray JR. Acute knee dislocation: an evidenced based approach to the management of the multiligament injured knee. *Injury.* 2011;42(11):1198-1204.
20. Richter M, Lobenhoffer P. Chronic posterior knee dislocation: treatment with arthrolysis, posterior cruciate ligament reconstruction and hinged external fixation device. *Injury.* 1998;29(7):546-549.
21. Fitzpatrick DC, Sommers MB, Kam BC, Marsh JL, Bottlang M. Knee stability after articulated external fixation. *Am J Sports Med.* 2005;33(11):1735-1741.
22. Stannard JP, Sheils TM, McGwin G, Volgas DA, Alonso JE. Use of a hinged external knee fixator after surgery for knee dislocation. *Arthroscopy.* 2003;19(6):626-631.
23. Stannard JP, Nuelle CW, McGwin G, Volgas DA. Hinged external fixation in the treatment of knee dislocations: a prospective randomized study. *J Bone Joint Surg Am.* 2014;96(3):184-191.
24. Magnussen RA, Lawrence JT, West RL, Toth AP, Taylor DC, Garrett WE. Graft size and patient age are predictors of early revision after anterior cruciate ligament reconstruction with hamstring autograft. *Arthroscopy.* 2012;28(4):526-531.
25. Bonasia DE, Bruzzone M, Dettoni F, et al. Treatment of medial and posteromedial knee instability: indications, techniques, and review of the results. *Iowa Orth J.* 2012;32:173-183.
26. Stannard JP, Brown SL, Robinson JT, McGwin G Jr, Volgas DA. Reconstruction of the posterolateral corner of the knee. *Arthroscopy.* 2005;21(9):1051-1059.
27. Miller MD, Gordon WT. Posterior cruciate ligament reconstruction: tibial inlay technique—principles and procedure. *Oper Tech Sports Med.* 1999;7:127-133.
28. Lubowitz JH, Ahmad CS, Anderson K. All-inside anterior cruciate ligament graft-link technique: second-generation, no-incision anterior cruciate ligament reconstruction. *Arthroscopy.* 2011;27(5):717-727.
29. Stannard JP, Hammond A, Tunmire D, Clayton M, Johnson C, Moura C. Determining the isometric point of the knee. *J Knee Surg.* 2012;25(1):71-74.

Please see videos on the accompanying website at www.routledge.com/9781617119996

Financial Disclosures

Dr. David A. Abrutyn has no financial or proprietary interest in the materials presented herein.

Dr. Annunziato Amendola is a consultant for Arthrex, owns stock in Arthrosurface, and receives royalties from Arthrex, Arthrosurface, and Smith & Nephew.

Dr. Jack Anavian has no financial or proprietary interest in the materials presented herein.

Dr. Jack M. Bert has no financial or proprietary interest in the materials presented herein.

Dr. Timothy M. Bert is a consultant for Blue Belt Technologies.

Dr. Andrew J. Blackman has no financial or proprietary interest in the materials presented herein.

Dr. Trevor Born has no financial or proprietary interest in the materials presented herein.

Dr. Joel Boyd lists Arthrex as a financial disclosure.

Dr. Joseph Brunkhorst has no financial or proprietary interest in the materials presented herein.

Dr. William Bugbee is a consultant for and has received research support from Joint Restoration Foundation.

Dr. James M. Bullock has no financial or proprietary interest in the materials presented herein.

Dr. Joseph Carney has no financial or proprietary interest in the materials presented herein.

Dr. Thomas Carter's financial disclosures are Arthrex (royalties, consultant, fellowship support), Arthroscopy Association of North America (Board of Directors), Cayenne Medical (fellowship support), Osiris (stock, consultant, research support), Ossur (fellowship support), and RTI Biologics (consultant, research support).

Dr. Brian J. Cole is a board member/owner/officer/committee member (unpaid) for Carticept, Regentis, International Committee AANA, Educational Committee AANA, and the AAOS Board. His medical/orthopedic affiliations include *Journal of Shoulder and Elbow Surgery, Journal of Bone and Joint Surgery, Cartilage, American Journal of Sports Medicine, American Journal of Orthopedics*, and Elsevier. He receives royalties from Arthrex and DJ Ortho. He is a paid consultant to Zimmer, Arthrex, and DePuy. Dr. Cole receives research or institutional support from Arthrex, Zimmer, DePuy, Regentis, Smith & Nephew, and DJ Ortho. He receives financial/material support from Elsevier and WB Saunders, and receives fellowship support from Smith & Nephew.

Dr. Austin Crow has no financial or proprietary interest in the materials presented herein.

Dr. Umer R. Dasti has no financial or proprietary interest in the materials presented herein.

Dr. Julie A. Dodds is an Arthroscopy Association of North America board and committee member.

Dr. Ryan Dunlay has no financial or proprietary interest in the materials presented herein.

Dr. Neil C. Dunleavy has no financial or proprietary interest in the materials presented herein.

Dr. Paul Fadale has no financial or proprietary interest in the materials presented herein.

Dr. Gregory C. Fanelli has no financial or proprietary interest in the materials presented herein.

Dr. Jack Farr is a consultant for Genzyme, Zimmer, Osiris Therapeutics, Regeneration Technologies Inc, DePuy Mitek, and Arthrex. Royalties include Arthrex and DePuy Synthes. All other disclosures are up to date on AAOS.org.

Dr. Donald C. Fithian has no financial or proprietary interest in the materials presented herein.

Dr. Freddie H. Fu's Department of Orthopaedic Surgery receives research funding from Smith & Nephew for anatomic ACL reconstruction.

Dr. John P. Fulkerson has no financial or proprietary interest in the materials presented herein.

Dr. Theodore J. Ganley has no financial or proprietary interest in the materials presented herein.

Dr. Brian B. Gilmer has no financial or proprietary interest in the materials presented herein.

Dr. Andrew D. Goodwillie has no financial or proprietary interest in the materials presented herein.

Dr. Vipool K. Goradia has no financial or proprietary interest in the materials presented herein.

Dr. Nathan L. Grimm has no financial or proprietary interest in the materials presented herein.

Dr. Jeffrey Halbrecht has no financial or proprietary interest in the materials presented herein.

Dr. Christopher D. Harner receives education and research support from Smith & Nephew.

Dr. Nathan Jacobson has no financial or proprietary interest in the materials presented herein.

Evan W. James has no financial or proprietary interest in the materials presented herein.

Dr. Adam M. Johannsen has no financial or proprietary interest in the materials presented herein.

Dr. Darren L. Johnson is a consultant for Smith & Nephew.

Dr. Lanny L. Johnson has no financial or proprietary interest in the materials presented herein.

Dr. Ethan Kellum has no financial or proprietary interest in the materials presented herein.

Dr. Jason L. Koh has no financial or proprietary interest in the materials presented herein.

Dr. Peter R. Kurzweil is a consultant for Ceterix, Cayenne Medical, Orteq, Parcus, and Pierce Surgical.

Dr. Robert F. LaPrade is a consultant for Arthrex, Ossur, and Smith & Nephew and has received a grant from Health East Norway.

Dr. Bruce A. Levy has the following financial or proprietary interests in the materials presented herein: consultant for Arthrex; royalties from Arthrex and VOT Solutions; research support—Arthrex, Biomet, and Stryker; editorial board memberships: *Clinical Orthopaedics and Related Research*—deputy editor, *Arthroscopy*—Board of Trustees, *Knee Surgery, Sports, Trauma and Arthroscopy*—member.

Dr. Darius Lin has no financial or proprietary interest in the materials presented herein.

Dr. Robert Litchfield receives royalties from Arthrosurface, is on the speaker's bureau of Zimmer, and receives research and fellowship support from Smith & Nephew and Arthrex (fellowship).

Dr. James H. Lubowitz has no current consulting or royalty disclosures. (Past consulting or royalties include Arthrex and Smith & Nephew.) Taos Orthopaedic Institute Research Foundation receives educational grant support from Arthrex, Breg, DonJoy, Smith & Nephew, Stryker, and Tournier.

Dr. Jonathan R. Maher has no financial or proprietary interest in the materials presented herein.

Dr. Randy Mascarenhas has no financial or proprietary interest in the materials presented herein.

Dr. Taylor Mathis has no financial or proprietary interest in the materials presented herein.

Dr. Owen P. McGonigle has no financial or proprietary interest in the materials presented herein.

Dr. Sanjay Menon has no financial or proprietary interest in the materials presented herein.

David B. Merkow has no financial or proprietary interest in the materials presented herein.

Dr. Adam V. Metzler is a consultant for Smith & Nephew.

Dr. Ryan Michels has no financial or proprietary interest in the materials presented herein.

Dr. Mark Miller has no financial or proprietary interest in the materials presented herein.

Dr. Kai Mithoefer is a consultant for Osiris, Vericel, and Regentis.

Dr. Kevin R. Myers has no financial or proprietary interest in the materials presented herein.

Dr. Shane J. Nho is a consultant for Stryker, Pivot Medical, and Ossur. Stocks include Pivot, and he receives research support from Stryker and Allosource.

Dr. Clayton W. Nuelle has no financial or proprietary interest in the materials presented herein.

Dr. Benjamin R. Parker has no financial or proprietary interest in the materials presented herein.

Dr. Leon (Lonnie) Paulos has no financial or proprietary interest in the materials presented herein.

Dr. Matthew A. Pifer has no financial or proprietary interest in the materials presented herein.

Dr. John D. Polousky is a consultant for Allosource.

Dr. Matthew T. Provencher is a consultant for Arthrex and Joint Restoration Foundation.

Dr. John C. Richmond is a consultant for Histogenics Corp and DePuy Synthes.

Dr. V. Franklin Sechriest II has no financial or proprietary interest in the materials presented herein.

Dr. Nicholas A. Sgaglione receives royalties from Biomet Sports Medicine.

Dr. Kevin G. Shea has no financial or proprietary interest in the materials presented herein.

Dr. Walter Shelton has no financial or proprietary interest in the materials presented herein.

Dr. Robby Sikka has no financial or proprietary interest in the materials presented herein.

Dr. Patrick A. Smith is a consultant for Arthrex Inc.

Dr. Paul L. Sousa has no financial or proprietary interest in the materials presented herein.

Dr. Jeffrey T. Spang has no financial or proprietary interest in the materials presented herein.

Dr. James P. Stannard receives institutional research support from Smith & Nephew and Arthrex Inc and receives royalties from Thieme Publishing. Dr. Stannard is the Editor-in-Chief of *Journal of Knee Surgery*. He is also a consultant to Smith & Nephew, Regeneration Technologies Inc, Ellipse Technologies Inc, and DePuy Synthes. Dr. Stannard is also a board member of the AO Board of Trustees, the AO Research Review Commission, and the Orthopaedic Trauma Association. He is receiving support from a US Department of Defense research grant.

Dr. James Starman has no financial or proprietary interest in the materials presented herein.

Alexandra Styhl has no financial or proprietary interest in the materials presented herein.

Dr. Kentaro P. Suzuki has no financial or proprietary interest in the materials presented herein.

Annemarie K. Tilton has no financial or proprietary interest in the materials presented herein.

Dr. Garth N. Walker has no financial or proprietary interest in the materials presented herein.

Dr. Amanda L. Weller has no financial or proprietary interest in the materials presented herein.

Dr. Adam Wilson has no financial or proprietary interest in the materials presented herein.

Dr. Adam B. Yanke receives research funding from NuTech and Arthrex.

Dr. Kenneth R. Zaslav is a consultant for Vericel Inc, Cartiheal Inc, Lifenet Inc, and Aesculap Inc.

Index